ACID RELATED DISEASES

BIOLOGY AND TREATMENT

Second Edition

ACID RELATED DISEASES

BIOLOGY AND TREATMENT

Second Edition

Irvin M. Modlin, M.D., Ph.D., F.R.C.S.(Ed), F.R.C.S.(Eng), F.C.S.(SA), F.A.C.S.

Professor of Surgery
Director, Gastric Surgical Pathobiology Research Group
Department of Surgery
Yale University School of Medicine
New Haven, Connecticut

George Sachs, M.B., Ch.B., D.Sc.

Professor of Physiology and Medicine
Wilshire Chair in Medicine
University of California, Los Angeles, David Geffen School
    of Medicine at UCLA
Veterans Administration Medical Center
Los Angeles, California

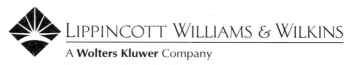

LIPPINCOTT WILLIAMS & WILKINS

A **Wolters Kluwer** Company

Philadelphia · Baltimore · New York · London
Buenos Aires · Hong Kong · Sydney · Tokyo

Managing Editors: Jennifer Kullgren, Mary Moore, and Jennifer Jett
Marketing Manager: Kate Rubin
Production Editor: Alyson Langlois, Silverchair Science + Communications, Inc.
Purchasing Manager, Clinical and Healthcare: Jennifer Jett
Compositor: Silverchair Science + Communications, Inc.
Printer: Walsworth Publishing Company

© 2004 by LIPPINCOTT WILLIAMS & WILKINS
530 Walnut Street,
Philadelphia, PA 19106 USA
LWW.com

Printed in the USA

Library of Congress Cataloging-in-Publication Data

Modlin, Irvin M.
    Acid related diseases : biology and treatment / Irvin M. Modlin, George Sachs.--2nd ed.
      p. ; cm.
    Includes bibliographical references and index.
    ISBN 0-7817-4123-8
     1. Peptic ulcer. 2. Gastroesophageal reflux. 3. Gastric acid. I. Sachs, George, 1935- II. Title.
    [DNLM: 1. Gastric Acid--secretion. 2. Peptic Ulcer--physiopathology. 3. Gastroesophageal Reflux--physiopathology. 4. Helicobacter pylori--pathogenicity. 5. Peptic Ulcer--drug therapy. WI 350 M692a 2003]
    RC821.M63 2003
    616.3'43--dc21

2003054341

03 04 05
1 2 3 4 5 6 7 8 9 10

In the uncertain hour before the morning
Near the ending of interminable night
At the recurrent end of the unending
After the dark dove with the flickering tongue
Had passed below the horizon of his homing . . .

We shall not cease from exploration
And the end of all our exploring
Will be to arrive where we started
And know the place for the first time.

T. S. Eliot
Four Quartets
Little Gidding

To Joyce, Steve, Andy, Paula, Lara, Oscar, Nicholas, Lucas, Natalie, Olivia, Teala, and Winston, whose occasional tolerances and continued support enabled us to perform this task.

—G.S.

To Maria, Alex, Jonny, and Mouton, without whose input this would not have been possible.

—I.M.M.

Contents

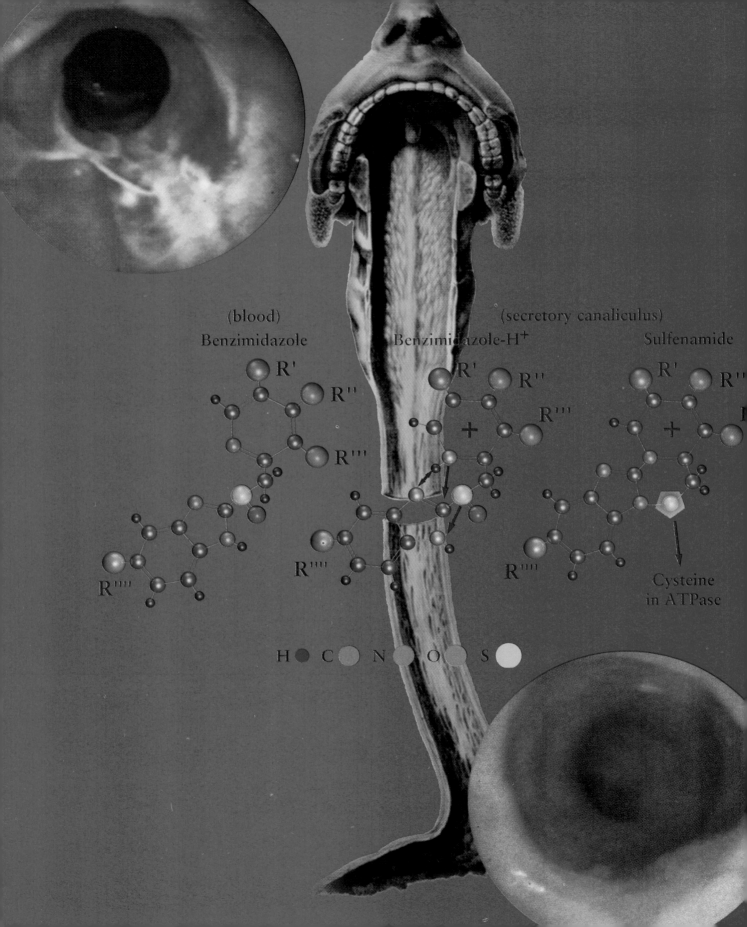

(blood)
Benzimidazole

R'
R''
R'''
R''''

(secretory canaliculus)
Benzimidazole-H+

R'   R''
R'''
+
R''''

Sulfenamide

R'   R''
+

Cysteine
in ATPase

H ● C ● N ● O ● S ●

PREFACE

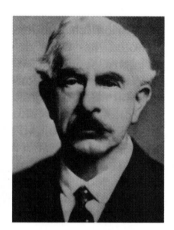

William Prout (1785–1850), in 1823, identified muriatic (hydrochloric) acid in the gastric juice of animals and humans.

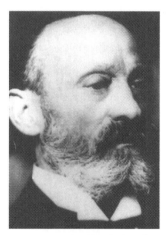

John Sydney Edkins (1863–1910), described in 1905 a chemical agent in the antrum that stimulated gastric acid secretion. He proposed that it be known as *gastrin*.

Ismar Boas (1858–1938), the founder of gastroenterology as a specialty and the editor of the first medical journal for digestive diseases.

The acid related diseases, duodenal and gastric ulcer and reflux esophagitis, have plagued man and animal throughout recorded history. It is a tribute to the scientific advances of the twentieth century that, whereas gastrectomy was introduced at the end of the nineteenth century and at the commencement of the twentieth, the statement "no acid, no ulcer" had just been enunciated. Now, at the beginning of the third millennium, we are able to control acid secretion at will and to cure duodenal and gastric ulcers of noniatrogenic origin by treating a gastric infection. It is likely that treatment of this infection may also reduce the incidence of gastric cancer and adequate acid suppression reduce the frequency of esophageal cancer.

Sustenance of life on this planet requires food, be it molecules or organisms. With the development of multicellular creatures came specialized organs for digestion and absorption. Acid was used very early as a means of preparing food for absorption, and the development of tubes entering and leaving the acid-producing organ was also an early evolutionary happening.

The modern esophagus, stomach, and duodenum have specialized epithelial and neuroendocrine cells, specialized musculature and specialized innervation, each to enable effective and trouble-free digestion and passage of food for further processing and absorption by the small intestine. Although we have progressed far in our understanding of the mechanistic function of these organs in day-to-day existence, there is certain to be as much that is yet to be learned as that which we already know.

It is surprising that it took civilized man so long to learn the fundamentals of mammalian biology, exemplified by events such as William Harvey's description of the route of circulation or William Prout's proof that the stomach produces hydrochloric acid. Replacement of superstition with scientific method had to wait in the Western world until the passing of the Middle Ages with the fall of Constantinople in 1453.

The digestive tract before Leonardo and Vesalius remained simply an object of ill-understood function as suggested by the terminology employed by Shakespeare and other dramatists of his time. Thus, in keeping with Greek and Roman usage, the stomach (*ventriculus*) was equated with the belly (*venter*) as noted in the parable about "the belly and the members" in Coriolanus or the episodes of Falstaff and Justice Greedy (Massinger). Indeed, the stomach was most often characterized as involved with gluttony or drinking by the Elizabethans, whereas the Persian poets such as Saadi noted that an empty belly supported mental and spiritual activity. Later thoughts on the stomach suggested that the entire gastrointestinal tract was associated with pluck and courage ("guts"). It is of interest to note that an old Latin adage declared the stomach to be the mother of all invention!

The identification of gastric acidity as an internally generated event and its relationship to digestion was a phenomenon of the early nineteenth century. Studies of gastric function in those days are epitomized by the studies of Beaumont on a gastric fistula patient. The subsequent squabbles as to whether the acid was lactic or whether the gastric juice actually contained acid were settled

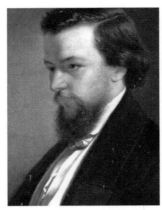

Theodor Billroth (1829–1894), an accomplished violinist, music critic, poet, scholar, and surgical teacher. His consummate surgical skills enabled the first successful gastrectomy in 1881.

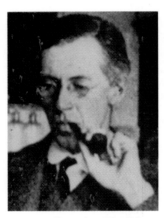

Sir Henry Hallett Dale (1875–1968), a pioneer in the isolation of histamine and the determination of its function. Awarded the Nobel Prize for his work on acetylcholine.

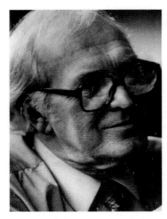

Sir James Black (c. 1990), awarded the Nobel Prize in 1988 for developing the concept of H₂ receptor antagonists and their therapeutic utility.

by the contributions of William Prout in 1823. The understanding of the central regulation of gastric digestive activity began with the work of Ivan Pavlov, who utilized gastric fistula dogs to study the nervous mechanisms that governed gastrointestinal secretion. The discovery by W. Bayliss and his brother-in-law, E. Starling, in 1902, of the hormone secretin and its stimulatory effect on pancreatic secretion established the basis for hormonal regulation of gastric secretion. Edkins was a man before his time in his discovery of gastrin, and his descriptions of a spiral bacteria in the feline stomach remain virtually unacknowledged to this time.

The recognition in this first part of the century that mucosal damage was caused by acid and that this acid could be decreased by luminal neutralization resulted in a wave of enthusiasm for antacid preparations, bland diets, and milk infusion as therapeutic options. Surgery was probably the most effective means of treating recurrent peptic ulcer until the development of specific pharmacological agents. By 1881, Billroth (successfully), Péan, and Rydiger (unsuccessfully) had resected the stomach, and Wölfler had in principle developed the procedure of gastroenterostomy. By the turn of this century, Moynihan of Leeds had transformed the treatment of peptic ulcer disease into a unique surgical discipline and refuted the notion of Naunyn that such intervention was little more than an autopsy *in vivo*. With expanding understanding of the regulation of acid secretion, gastrectomy was successively replaced by vagotomy (pioneered by Latarjet and extended by Dragstedt), then selective vagotomy by Griffith and Harkins in 1957 and, finally, in 1967, Holle and Hart and Amdrup introduced highly selective vagotomy.

One decade later, the introduction of drugs capable of blocking acid secretion by H_2 receptor antagonism revolutionized the management of the disease process and almost obliterated surgery as a therapeutic option for peptic ulcer except in cases of emergency. Gastroesophageal reflux disease, however, may still be treated even today by mechanical (laparoscopic or endoscopic) forms of fundoplication, given that pharmaceutical normalization of the lower esophageal sphincter pressure has not been achieved.

The identification of the molecular basis of acid secretion—the proton pump—resulted in development of a new class of therapeutic agents—the proton pump inhibitors. By identifying the pump as a target, an effective inhibition of acid secretion with predictable therapeutic efficacy has been achieved.

Most recently, the description of *Helicobacter pylori* in the gastric mucosa and its correlation with ulcer disease has suddenly and unexpectedly led to dramatic advances in the curing of peptic ulcer disease. It has also become clear that an infection predisposes to a form of gastric neoplasia. We still await a simple therapeutic regimen for eradication of this organism, but this will undoubtedly happen.

Even though acid related diseases are now being effectively treated, problems that derive from abnormalities of esophageal and gastric biology, such as cancer of these organs, are still virtually untreatable, although now more preventable. The current advances that have been made in genomic biology and those ongoing in the area of proteonomics hold much promise in these areas in the twenty-first century.

This book is focused on gastric biology. It takes a historical path to introduce present-day discoveries and concepts and uses these concepts to explain modern-day treatment of acid related disease. Indeed, without an understanding of the direction from which we have come, it will not be easy to perceive where our future direction lies.

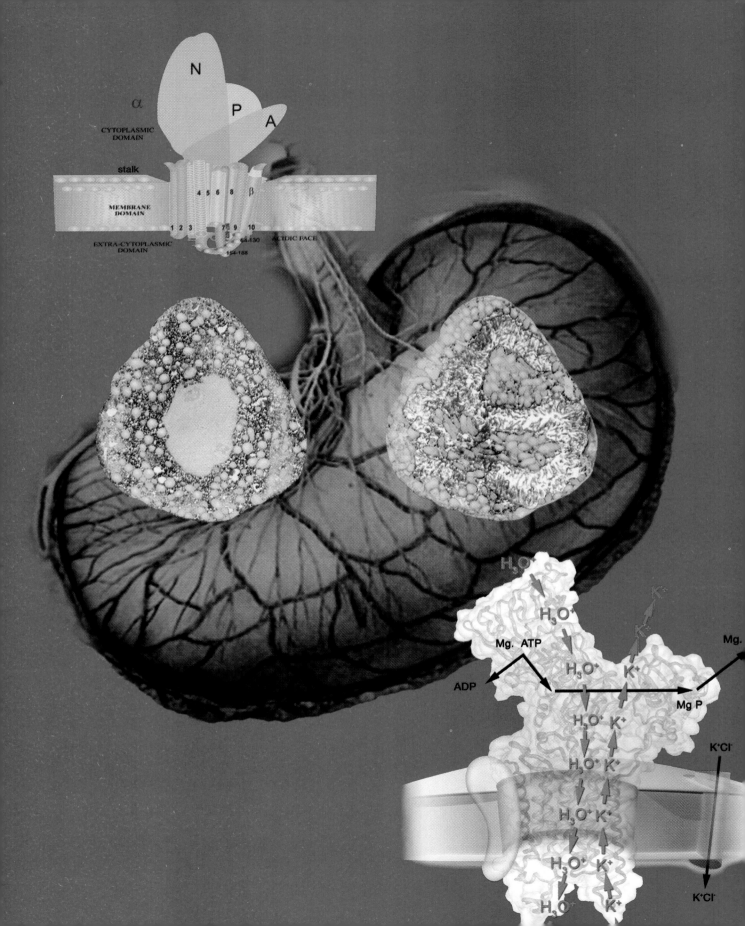

Acknowledgments

Numerous institutions and individuals have generously provided us with access to material and allowed its usage. These include the Yale University School of Medicine Library, the *Yale Journal of Biology and Medicine*, the Huntarian Museum and Library of the Royal College of Surgeons of England, the Royal Society of Medicine, the Royal College of Physicians of England, and the Welcome Institute for the History of Medicine.

A number of individuals, including Herbert Helander, Nils Lambrecht, David Scott, Nicholas Wright, Robert Genta, Neal Seymour, Nat Soper, Laura Tang, Mark Kidd, Jeff Kraut, Jai Moo Shin, Keith Munson, Olga Vagin, David Weeks, and Joe Pisegna, contributed either personal material, scientific information, or their valuable time. Innumerable colleagues, scientific collaborators, and friends have generously provided us with the benefit of their years of experience in the discussion of information emanating from their research efforts—*ars gratia artis*. Special thanks to Dennis Ninneman, without whose support this project would not have been possible.

We are both entirely responsible for any errors, oversights, and misinterpretations of either the history or scientific data expressed in this text, although Dr. Sachs believes any such possibility to be so remote as to hardly warrant consideration. At a personal level, I wish to acknowledge William Prout, whose original work in Edinburgh engendered in me so monstrous a curiosity regarding the subject of acidophiles. His initial extraordinary observation that the atomic weights of all elements would be exact multiples of hydrogen stimulated more investigation than almost any other generalization that has ever been made in the field of chemistry; his subsequent identification of the presence of free hydrochloric acid in the stomach in 1823 remains one of the classics of physiology. The subsequent extraordinary contributions by Peter Mitchell on the subject of chemiosmotic proton circuits in biologic membranes provided the intellectual impetus not only to resolve the membrane biology of the proton pump, but to develop therapeutic applications of considerable relevance to clinical medicine.

The credo of the application of the scientific method to the resolution of clinically relevant problems embraces the progress made in the resolution of acid peptic disease—a worldwide disease entity of major proportions. Thus, the conceptual expansion of the initial early nineteenth-century experiments of Prout have culminated in the elucidation of the proton pump not only as a biochemical entity, but also as a therapeutic target of considerable relevance. Such events are best summarized in the words of Peter Mitchell: "When seen retrospectively, the evolution of ideas and knowledge, like organic evolution, tends to take on a deceptively logical and inevitable appearance. But, as it actually happens, the quest for truth through the test of imaginary concepts against reality is bound to be an uncertain and hazardous adventure entailing disappointments as well as pleasant surprises." We hope that the contents of this book afford the reader not only pleasure and information, but also the opportunity to reflect on the application of science to the resolution of acid peptic disease.

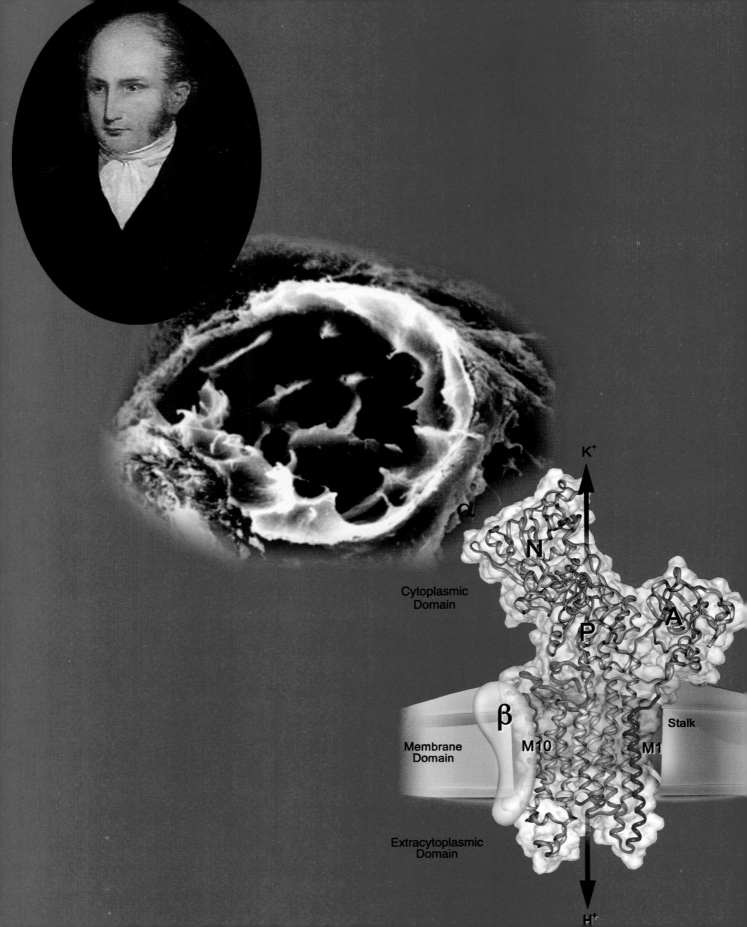

THE PRODUCTION OF ACID IN THE STOMACH

CHAPTER 1
THE DISCOVERY OF ACID

In the earliest times, physicians believed that the individual organs were the seats of separate spiritual agencies that in a divine manner controlled bodily function. Given the clearly perceived importance of food, the stomach was thus highly placed in the pantheon of lay regard. The ancient Greeks proposed that digestion was a process of concoction or heating, and, in this evolution, food was converted initially to chyle and then to the four humors (blood, phlegm, and yellow and black bile) before use by the mortal body. Hippocrates had, in fact, called the process of digestion *pepsis* and proposed that it was not dissimilar to the preparation of food by cooking. Galenic physiology proposed that successive cooking processes occurred sequentially in the stomach, intestine, and liver until food was finally converted into blood, and, indeed, such notions were commonly held until the eighteenth century.

The question of acid in the stomach

The early Greeks were not aware of acids in the modern sense of chemistry but identified them only as bitter-sour liquids. Diocles of Carystos (circa 350 BC) specified sour eruptions, watery spitting, gas, heartburn, and epigastric hunger pains radiating to the back (with occasional splashing noises and vomiting) as symptoms of illness originating in the stomach. Three hundred years later, Celsus (30 BC–25 AD), although more an encyclopedist than a physician, recognized that certain foods were acidic and recommended that *"if the stomach is infested with an ulcer . . . , light and gelatinous food must be used . . . and everything acrid and acid is to be avoided."*

There appears to have been little further development in understanding the function of the stomach and the real nature of digestive processes until the sixteenth century. Philippus Aureolus Theophrastus Bombastus von Hohenheim (also known as Paracelsus) was born in Ensiedeln near Zürich in 1493. He was an alchemist-physician and a proponent of chemical pharmacology and therapeutics who had enormous influence on the medical thinking of his day. Indeed, the origin of modern rational therapeutic strategy may be regarded as having been initiated by Paracelsus.

Hippocrates (460–370 BC) provided Greek medicine with its scientific spirit and ethical ideals. He practiced on the island of Kos, where he developed a school of medicine that crystallized the loose knowledge of the Coan and Cinidian schools into systematic science. His philosophies permeated society and formed the basis of rational medical thought for centuries thereafter. In early Greek pathology, the efforts of the body to bring the humors from a raw, fermented status (apepsia) to a normal status (pepsis) were associated with the idea of cookery or coction, a view of the digestive process that survived until the seventeenth century.

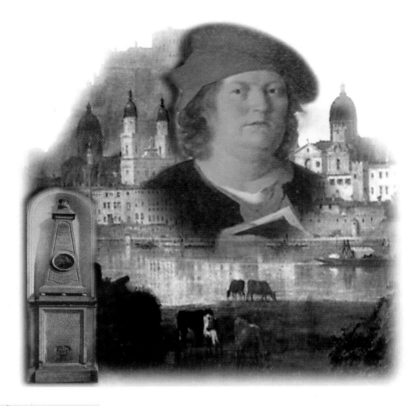

Paracelsus (1493–1541) underwent medical training in Ferrara (1515) and subsequently taught at Freiburg and Strasbourg (1525). He was appointed Professor of Medicine in Basel in 1527 and publicly burned the books of Galen and Avicenna. He rejected the old notion of the four elements—earth, air, fire, and water. Instead, he proposed that the forces of energy that governed the universe were the archei and maintained that physiologic processes, diseases, and drugs were chemical changes governed by the chief archeus.

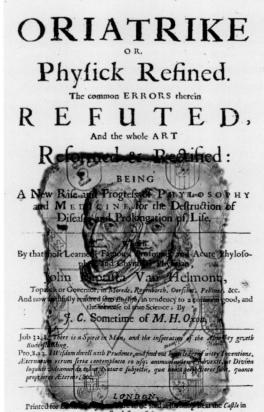

Paracelsus believed that there was acid in the stomach and that its presence was necessary for digestion, although he asserted that it was ingested. This conviction that gastric acid was of extracorporeal origin would, of course, subsequently be proven to be wrong. Nevertheless, he recognized the importance of chemistry and its relation to disease, rejecting Galenism and the mysticism of humors and health and insisting on the development of rational rather than alchemic strategies for symptom or disease management.

Jean Baptiste van Helmont (1577–1644) of Belgium founded the Iatrochemical School. This maintained that the principal archeus, Blas, was controlled by the sensitive and motive soul, *anima sensitiva motivaque*, in the "pit of the stomach" (solar plexus). From this site, all chemical physiologic processes were regulated. He believed that digestion began in the stomach by the intermittent fermentation of acid and that, thereafter, a number of other fermentation processes took place, including that of bile in the duodenum. In further observations, he recognized that

Jean Baptiste van Helmont (1577–1644), founder of the Iatrochemical School, proposed that acid might be a mineral acid, such as nitric or hydrochloric acid. He produced *spiritus salis marini*—spirits of sea salt (hydrochloric acid)—by distillation of salt and clay and noted that it could dissolve human kidney stones (*duelech*) in much the same manner as juice from the stomach of a bird.

Iatromechanical representation of the *"hand* that feeds." This representation of mechanical devices as the components of the human organism was applied in the most extreme fashion by the Neapolitan mathematician Giovanni Alfonso Borelli (1608–1679) (bottom left). In his view, locomotion, respiration, and digestion (the grinding and crushing action of the stomach) were purely mechanical processes. This mechanical allegory was expanded to an extreme form by G. Baglivi (top right) (1668–1706), who proposed that the body was a machine that could be regarded as being composed of numerous smaller machines. Thus, the teeth were scissors, the chest a bellows, the stomach a flask, the viscera and glands sieves, and the heart and vessels a system of waterworks.

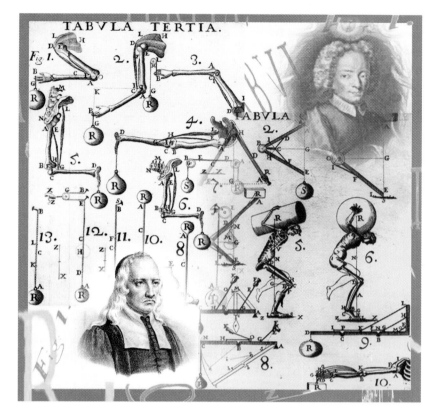

acid alone did not decompose food *in vitro*, and he postulated the existence of another agent typified as a ferment. In this respect, his prescience was noteworthy in first considering the concept of an enzyme adjunct to the digestive process.

The Iatromathematical School

The chemical views propounded by Paracelsus, van Helmont, and others were strongly opposed by the Iatromathematical School, which maintained that all physiologic happenings should be treated as fixed consequences of the laws of physics. This group included such individuals as Descartes, Borelli, Sanctorius, Pitcairn, and Boerhaave, all noteworthy for their intellectual and philosophical contributions to medicine and science.

Thus, Borelli (1608–1679) and his disciples favored the view that the stomach was but a mechanical mill, grinding up its contents into chyme. Mobius denied the existence of gastric acid, and Archibald Pitcairn interpreted all function in terms of mechanical activity, believing the teeth to be scissors, the stomach a fermenting vat, and the lungs and heart to be bellows and a pump, respectively.

The members of the Iatromathematical School cared little for the new science of chemistry, and their postulates faded into such sterile eccentricities as the proposal by Pitcairn to base the whole of medical practice on mechanical principles. Thus, in 1727, Pitcairn questioned the Iatrochemical group: "... *Why upon the digestion of food upon the stomach, which is easily [as] digestible as the food, yet the stomach itself should not be dissolved?*" This prescient question was, of course, irresolvable, and almost 250 years would pass before an explanation based on the "gastric barrier" would even approach resolution of this issue.

The nature of digestive agents

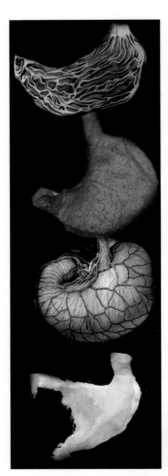

A series of depictions of the stomach demonstrating the rugula of the gastric mucosa (top), blood vessels (center two icons), and a partially digested stomach (bottom).

Attempts to define the nature of digestive agents were aided first by the ingenuity of investigators in developing methods of obtaining gastric juice and second by the development and recognition of indicator dyes capable of crudely defining acids and alkalis. These vegetable-derived substances changed color when exposed to appropriate acids or alkalis and allowed identification of the nature of the material being tested. In particular, controversy centered on the chemical nature of the acid in the stomach and the debate as to whether it was primarily secreted by the stomach or derived in some way from ingested food. Thus, one school of thought proposed acid as a vital product of the stomach and the other maintained it was either ingested or represented a product of the "corruption" of food.

Methods of obtaining gastric secretion

Necropsy of animals

In 1692, Viridet experimented with dogs, cats, squirrels, hares, pigs, and eagles. The animals were killed either after a meal or fasting, and the gastric contents were collected by opening the abdomen. Viridet noted that *solutio heliotropii* (tincture of heliotrope) could, by turning red, indicate the presence of acid. In a classic study, he killed a specially fattened pig and poured tincture of heliotrope down its throat.

The blue color was noted to be preserved "even to the entrance of the stomach"; in the stomach, however, an intense red solution was evident. Viridet reported that the stomach smelled of acid and that this resembled the odor of fermentation. He also noted that, in humans, acid could be recognized in the esophagus, but this was because of regurgitation of the contents of the stom-

Various anatomical depictions of the stomach by Bougery (center) and Cruveilhier (circled). Depictions by Bougery of the muscles of the outer and inner walls, the gastric folds, and nerve supply to the lesser curvature are placed in the corners of the picture. Cruveilhier's drawings depict gastric pathology and include cancer (top), perforated stomach (right), ulcer (bottom), and blood supply (left).

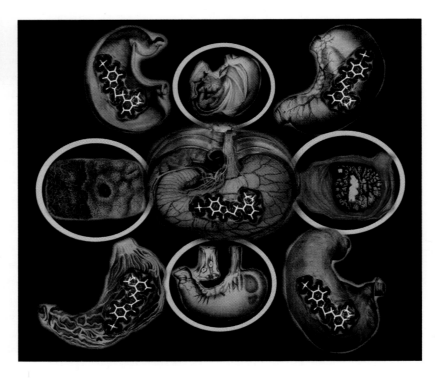

The French were considerably interested in digestion, both at scientific and epicurean levels. R. A. F. Réaumur (1683–1757) (top left) studied the digestion of birds, particularly his own pet buzzard (bottom left), in detail and concluded that their stomachs secreted acid that was necessary for digestion. The premature demise of his experimental model resulted in Réaumur's loss of interest in the subject of digestion, and he thereafter turned his skills to the development of a novel technique for strengthening steel. Anthelme Brillat-Savarin (1755–1826) (bottom right) studied digestion and its effect on the higher senses by compiling an exotic compendium of culinary information and dining etiquette. His reflections on the physiology of taste background and the relationship of food to human behavior are still regarded as definitive among those who believe that the gut-brain axis is modulated and amplified by a malolactic acid transduction system.

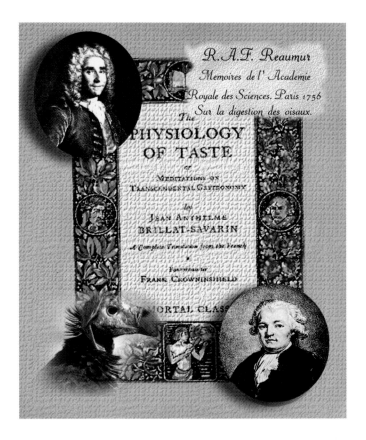

ach. "*We experience it by an acid in the mouth,*" he wrote. Of particular interest was his further comment, "*The condition was not a natural one.*"

The use of sponges

In 1752, Réaumur, the French naturalist, noted that birds of prey vomited indigestible objects, such as feathers and bones. Seizing on this observation, he experimented with a tame buzzard by feeding it small, hollow metal tubes containing a variety of foods. When the tubes were recovered, it was apparent that the food had dissolved without putrefaction, leaving a bitter yellow fluid. To further study the nature of this fluid, Réaumur placed sponges in the small metal tubes and, on recovery, squeezed these to obtain the gastric juice. The latter was a sour fluid that turned blue (litmus) paper red. Having identified an acidic reaction, Réaumur attempted to study *in vitro* digestion by incubating the gastric juice with meat. The meat, however, failed to digest completely, although he noted that the gastric juice had prevented the onset of "corruption." He interpreted the failure of this study to indicate that either digestion required a high temperature or that the gastric juice required constant renewal. Alternatively, it was possible that, in the *in vitro* situation, the evaporation of a volatile acid had taken place. At this stage, the pet buzzard died, and Réaumur ceased his studies with birds.

Self-induced emesis

In 1760, Reuss found that, even with preliminary alkalization of the stomach, the ingestion of a meal of meat and vegetables resulted in secretion of

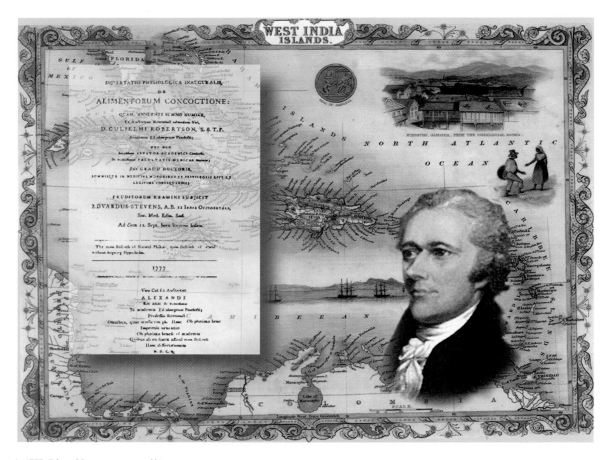

In 1777, Edward Stevens presented his inaugural thesis *De Alimentorum Concoctione* to the University of Edinburgh. He may have been the illegitimate half-brother of Alexander Hamilton (1755–1804) and was born on the island of St. Croix in the Leeward Islands. After graduating from Kings College in New York (now Columbia University) in 1774, he pursued his further medical studies in Scotland from 1775. His thesis was dedicated to Alexander *tertius* Monro. During the time he studied at Edinburgh, he became the president of the medical student society. He subsequently returned to become a professor of medicine at Columbia in New York and thereafter Consul General in Santo Domingo. He failed to further pursue investigative studies of the stomach.

acid. The vomit had an acid taste and turned an infusion of "*campanules à feuilles rondes*" red. Gosse, in 1783, repeated the studies more elegantly. He had, as a child, developed the faculty of aerophagy and self-induced emesis, whereas Reuss required the ingestion of an emetic. By inducing emesis at specific times after eating, Gosse was able to demonstrate that digestion began within 30 minutes of eating and was concluded by approximately 2 hours. Although Gosse was not able to find acid or alkaline gastric juice, he was, however, able to report that some food was partially digestible, whereas other food was completely digestible. He suggested that secretion occurred by a mechanical process whereby food stretched the internal lining of the stomach.

An experiment with *in vitro* digestion

Edward Stevens was the first to undertake an experiment of *in vitro* digestion successfully. He thus proved that the gastric juice itself contained the active principle necessary for the assimilation of food. Stevens obtained the services of a Hungarian Hussar who was visiting Edinburgh and whose means of livelihood was to entertain the populace by swallowing stones and then regurgitating them. Using perforated silver spheres so constructed as to hold meats, vegetables, worms, and leeches, Stevens observed that all were digested by the time the tubes passed through the rectum. He did not use a sponge and, thus, did not attempt to extract gastric juice and evaluate the presence of acid.

The Jesuit abbot Lazzaro Spallanzani (1729–1799) (bottom left) was Professor of Physics and Mathematics at the College of San Carlo in Modena. Over the course of his life, he undertook important studies on the gastric secretion of a wide variety of animals and concluded that digestion was a chemical process dependent on both the digestive power of saliva and the solvent properties of gastric juice. His recognition that the process of gastric digestion was not due to putrefaction but represented an active process was an important contribution. In collaboration with Professor Carminati of Pavia and the chemist Scopoli, Spallanzani was able to conclude that gastric juice from crows contained *"pure water, some soapy and gelatinous animal substances . . . and that the gastric juice distinctly turned tincture of heliotrope red."* John Hunter (right), whose comments on digestion in *Observations on Certain Parts of the Animal Oeconomy* (London, 1786) were translated into Italian by Antonio Scarpa, evoked a sharp response from the abbot, who assumed divine support for his digestive position. Their disagreement as to the presence or absence of acid in the gastric juice and whether the process of digestion required heat was finally resolved amicably in the form of a polemic letter addressed to Leopoldo Caldani (background), published in Milan in 1788. Presumably, the limited nature of the chemical techniques available to both resulted in a misunderstanding that was subsequently resolved by mutual agreement.

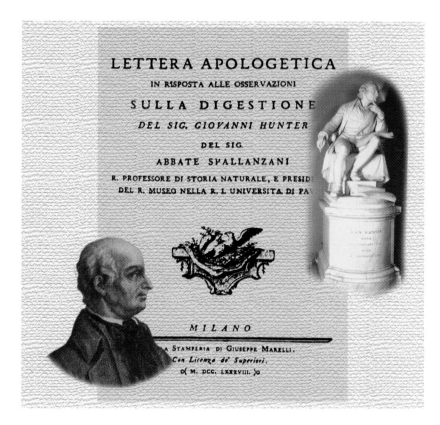

Digestion is a chemical process

In 1780, Lazzaro Spallanzani, who was the professor of Natural History in Pavia, published his extensive observations in the field of digestion. He had used the methods of Réaumur on fish, frogs, snakes, cattle, horses, cats, dogs, and himself. In 1783, he finally proved that digestion *in vitro* as well as *in vivo* was a chemical process, but he asserted that gastric juice was neutral.

The results of Spallanzani bear comment, because the studies were performed in great detail and with considerable care. He initially swallowed linen bags containing food and bread and collected them for examination after they had been passed *per rectum*. Later, he substituted small metal tubes to avoid any possibility of trituration. In both instances, he could find no trace of remaining food. At this time, it was believed that three types of fermentation existed: vinous, acid, and putrid. Because he could find no evidence of fermentation, Spallanzani postulated that digestion was by an acid or a putrefactive principle. The latter he disregarded, because gastric juice prevented putrefaction and, according to the results of his experiments, there had been no evidence of putrefaction.

Spallanzani, however, was uncertain about his findings regarding the acidity of gastric juice and collaborated with a number of colleagues to resolve this question. In 1785, Spallanzani undertook studies with Carminati, the professor of medicine at Pavia, which yielded novel information. Carminati was probably the first to detect the acidity of the contents of a meal. He said:

Albert von Haller (1708–1777) was a pupil of Boerhaave and the professor of anatomy, medicine, and botany in Gottingen from 1736 to 1753. In his 17 years in Gottingen, he wrote approximately 13,000 scientific papers and ultimately produced his masterpiece, *Elementa Physiologicae Corporis Humanae* (1759–1766), which confirmed his reputation as the physiologist of his age. von Haller recognized the use of bile in the digestion of fat but declared that gastric juice was not acid, alkaline, or a ferment and believed that any acid found in the gastric juice was from the degeneration of food.

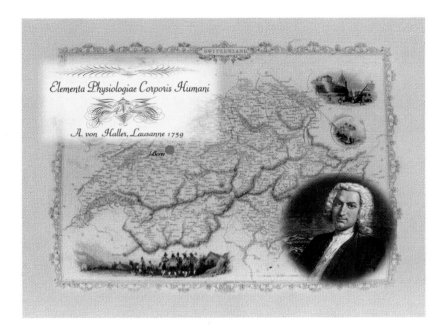

It is clear that the human gastric juice is neutral as the physiologists, such as von Haller and Spallanzani, have taught; that this is true in crows, in dogs, and in cats which eat and digest with equal facility both animal and vegetable substances; and that in fact this humor consists of a water, a small amount of marine salt, and an animal substance. I had already recognized in 20 crows that the gastric juice was neutral when I obtained in July two crows whose gastric juice distinctly turned tincture of heliotrope red, produced immediate and complete curdling of milk, and, in every way, proved similar to that of carnivorous animals. The novelty of this led me to inquire into its cause and I found that the birds for many days past had been fed exclusively on meat. . . . The same happened in dogs and cats fed entirely on meat for ten or more days as in the crows. Their gastric juice had all the properties of that of crows on a meat diet.

As a result of these findings, Carminati advised Spallanzani to test birds on a meat-free diet, and in this study he identified marine acid in the juice squeezed from sponges fed to five ravens that were fed on vegetables for 15 days. Later, Brugnatelli, in 1786, and Werner, in 1800, found the contents of the stomachs of sheep, cats, fish, and birds to be acid. Despite the relatively clear evidence produced by Spallanzani and his colleagues that there was acid in the stomach and that it was hydrochloric acid, considerable controversy persisted. Indeed, many of the investigators of this era not only reversed their positions on the subject a number of times during their investigations but also differed vehemently on their interpretation of the data. Thus, even among the minds of the most eminent physicians of the day, confusion reigned, not only as to the presence of acid, but also as to the exact nature of the substance.

Prout and the proton

The final resolution to the question of the exact nature of acid produced by the stomach was provided in 1823 by William Prout, a brilliant physician with diverse interests outside of medicine. Prout was productive in the fields of chemistry, meteorology, physiology, and clinical medicine. In addition, he was one of the first scientists to apply chemical analysis to biologic materials. He was, thus, able to demonstrate circadian rhythms in his own expired carbon dioxide as well as to propose that the destruction of tissues produced excretory materials, such as uric acid, urea, and carbonic acid. In 1827, he developed a classification of foods into subgroups: saccharinous (carbohydrates), oleaginous (fats), and albuminous (proteins).

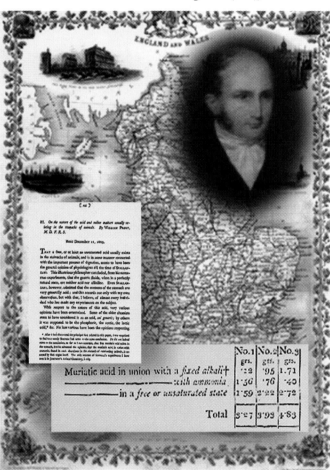

Frontispiece of Prout's original manuscript presented at the Royal Society (London, 1823). This piece of work irrefutably demonstrated that acid in humans and other animals was hydrochloric. The gastric juice was provided by the surgeon, Sir Astley Cooper of Guy's Hospital.

William Prout (1785–1850) was born in Horton, a remote village of Gloucestershire, England. Having studied at Guy's Hospital in London, he became a member of the Royal College of Physicians as well as a fellow of the Royal Medical Chirurgical Society. On December 11, 1823, at the Royal Society of Medicine, he presented his landmark paper, *On the Nature of Acid and Saline Matters Usually Existing in the Stomachs of Animals*. This presentation was unique in two ways. First, Prout had specifically identified hydrochloric acid in the gastric juice of many species (man, dog, rabbit, horse, calf, and hare), and second, he was able to quantify the free and total hydrochloric acid and chloride present. The acid was measured by neutralization with a potash solution of known strength and the chloride by titration with silver nitrate.

So advanced were his ideas that in addition he proposed that chloride may be secreted from blood to lumen by electrical means and that, when gastric acid was secreted, the blood would become alkaline (now recognized as the postprandial alkaline tide). More than 100 years were to elapse before his latter proposal was confirmed.

Apart from his definitive resolution of the nature of gastric acid, Prout was the first to propose that the atomic weights of all elements would be multiples of that of hydrogen (Prout's Hypothesis).

CHAPTER 2
THE DISCOVERY OF ION PUMPS

Mammalian plasma and organelle membranes are composed of phospholipids arranged in a bilayer such that the charged head groups face outward toward the water phase and the fatty acids are internal, making a hydrophobic core. For charged or hydrophilic molecules to cross the bilayer, pathways must be established to allow these molecules to move across the membrane without encountering the hydrophobic barrier. Transport proteins allow such molecules to move across the part of the protein that is placed across the hydrophobic core of the membrane, the membrane domain of the protein. In this way, these hydrophilic molecules pass across the membrane without contacting the hydrocarbon phase of the cell membranes. The ion or hydrophilic substance must be enclosed by the membrane domain of the protein; therefore, there are several chains of amino acids that surround the transported species. Transport proteins, therefore, are often rather large proteins with several amphipathic sequences of approximately twenty-one amino acids that are threaded in and out through the membrane, forming a polytopic integral membrane protein. Some of these membrane sequences are structural scaffolds, and some are responsible for the movement of molecules across the membrane. Several channel and pump proteins have been crystallized and their structure obtained by X-ray diffraction at high resolution. In this way, a description of structure-function can be generated at the atomic level.

Some transporters allow molecules to diffuse down their concentration gradient, resulting in passive transport; some couple diffusion in one direction to another molecule (usually an ion) diffusing in the opposite direction, resulting in countertransport; some couple diffusion in one direction to another molecule moving downhill in the same direction to give cotransport. There is group translocation, conversion of a diffusing substance to a different chemical on the other side of the membrane. Some, like the gastric acid pump or the sodium pump, couple energy-yielding reactions, such as the breakdown of adenosine triphosphate (ATP), directly to ion transport to produce primary active transport.

Acid secretion by the stomach was long recognized as an active transport process, because the concentration of hydrogen ions in the gastric juice is approximately 10^6 times higher than that in the blood. In the 1920s, the colored cytochrome oxidoreductases were discovered by Keilin and Hartree. They postulated the presence of a cytochrome chain such that electrons were transferred from a substrate, such as succinic acid, stepwise down the respiratory chain consisting of cytochrome b, then c, and then a_3, eventually reaching oxygen. This chain of oxidoreductases accounted for mitochondrial oxidation of substrates. Plant physiologists then suggested that similarly oriented oxidoreductases across a membrane could separate H^+ and electrons.

This concept was then applied to acid secretion by the stomach and was known as the redox hypothesis of acid secretion. Inherent in the redox hypothesis is development of a current across the membrane, providing an

Na⁺ or H⁺,K⁺ ATPase in E₁ Conformation

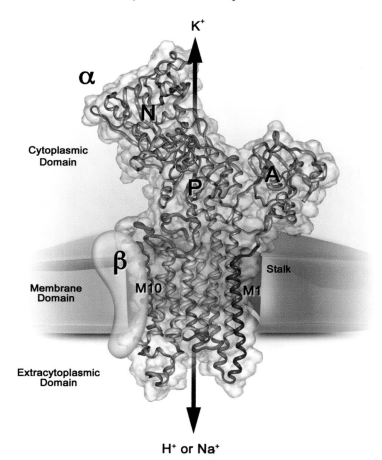

A schematic representation of a transport ATPase composed of two subunits, a catalytic or α subunit and a structural or β subunit, exchanging either intracellular Na⁺ or H⁺ for K⁺ outside the cell. The alpha subunit is shown as having a large cytoplasmic domain consisting of N, the nucleotide binding domain; P, the phosphorylation domain; and A, the activation domain. MgATP binds to the N domain and phosphorylates the P domain, and then there is a conformational change in the A and P domains that is transmitted to the membrane domain with ten membrane-spanning helices. The extracytoplasmic domain contains five loops connecting the membrane segments. The figure illustrates the general similarity between the Na⁺ and H⁺ pumps, as well as that they both have a β subunit, in contrast to other P-type ATPases.

electrogenic mechanism (i.e., voltage and current generating) for acid secretion across the membrane containing the pump. This electrogenic mechanism for acid secretion dominated thinking in the 1950s and early 1960s, largely due to the contributions of electrophysiologists such as Warren Rehm, first in Louisville and then in Birmingham, and Robert Davies in Sheffield. The experimental basis for this belief depended on measurements of transepithelial potential and resistance during changes in acid secretion in the *in vitro* frog mucosa.

Another strong proponent of this idea was E. J. Conway in Dublin, who had participated in a classic series of experiments just before World War II in Cambridge proving active transport of Na⁺ and K⁺ across cell membranes. Coincidentally, he was later responsible for developing an assay for urease and showed the presence of urease in the stomach. This urease was not recognized as the property of an infective organism, *Helicobacter pylori*, for another 40 years!

Bioenergetics and chemi-osmosis

A gastric ulcer contracted by a scientist working in transport before effective therapy facilitated one of the major conceptual revolutions in biology. ATP had been discovered by Engelhardt in the Soviet Union in 1939 as the major chemical energy store in biology. It was soon recognized that there were two major sources of ATP: glycolysis (substrate-level phosphorylation, described by Ephraim Racker in 1949) and oxidative phosphorylation in mitochondria. An enormous amount of effort was spent trying to specify the mitochondrial "substrate" that transferred high-energy phosphate to adenosine diphosphate (ADP) to account for oxidative phosphorylation. However, in 1961, Ephraim Racker isolated the mitochondrial ATPase and showed that it was composed of two sectors: a membrane sector, F_0, and a mitochondrial matrix sector, F_1. This ATPase is involved in bioenergetic conservation.

In 1957, Peter Mitchell, whose work had focused on transport in bacteria, acquired a severe gastric ulcer (due to the excessive consumption of haggis?) while Reader in Zoology at Edinburgh University. He postulated to his students that acid secretion by the stomach was due to the splitting of water by a vectorial ATPase, so that H^+ was extruded and OH^- was retained in the cell. In reading about the redox hypothesis of acid secretion, he realized that if redox pumps of mitochondria were oriented across the membrane, they would generate a gradient of H^+ or an electrical potential able to move H^+ inward across the mitochondrial membrane across a variety of proteins. With his vectorial ATPase running in reverse, an inward flow of H^+ would result in the synthesis of ATP. This simple idea changed the concept of substrate-level oxidative phosphorylation into a proton–electrochemical gradient mechanism for ATP synthesis by mitochondria, chloroplasts, and aerobic bacteria using the F_1F_0 ATPase running as an ATP synthase driven by the inwardly directed (outward in the case of chloroplasts) electrochemical gradient of H^+ (proton motive force).

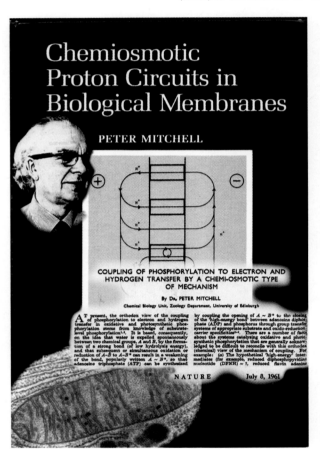

Peter Mitchell: His chemiosmotic hypothesis, wherein ATP was synthesized by an electrochemical gradient of hydrogen ions across bacterial, mitochondrial, and chloroplast membranes, revolutionized bioenergetics.

This chemiosmotic hypothesis was elegantly proven 12 years later by reconstituting a light-driven proton pump, bacterial rhodopsin, with the mitochondrial F_1F_0 ATPase in liposome membranes. Shining light on these vesicles in the presence of ADP and inorganic phosphate resulted in the synthesis of ATP. ATP synthesis in this reconstituted system had to be due to the gradient of H^+ generated by the rhodopsin oriented inside out in these vesicles moving across the inside-out ATPase. This experiment was also performed in Ephraim Racker's laboratory.

A representation of the key experiment proving the chemiosmotic hypothesis. At the bottom is the light-activated electrogenic proton pump, bacterial rhodopsin, and on the top the F_1F_0 ATP synthase. When light is shone on the vesicles coreconstituted with these two pumps in the presence of ADP and inorganic phosphate (Pi), ATP synthesis was observed. The only linkage between the two sets of structures is the electrochemical gradient of protons induced by illumination.

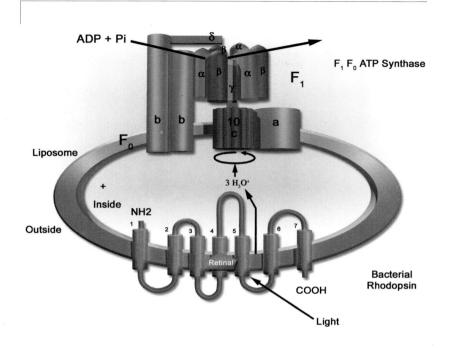

It is interesting that Peter Mitchell also conceived of the correct model for bacterial flagellar motion as being driven by a rotating proton motor, a concept later applied to the mechanism of the F_1F_0 ATPase.

P ATPases

The sodium pump, the Na,K ATPase, was discovered by Jens Skou in 1957. It was recognized as the mechanism for maintaining Na and K gradients across cell membranes because of stimulation of ATP hydrolysis by the simultaneous presence of Na^+ and K^+ and by its inhibition by a cardiac glycoside, strophanthidin, a specific inhibitor of the formation of Na^+ and K^+ gradients. These cardiac glycosides have been in use since the eighteenth century for treatment of congestive heart failure with dropsy (fluid accumulating in the limbs) as a presenting sign. Seminal work by Robin Post established the mechanism of the sodium pump as being driven by phosphorylation (energization)–dephosphorylation (deenergization) of the enzyme and the exchange of $3Na^+$ for $2K^+$. This pump is, therefore, electrogenic.

The positive inotropic effect of digitalis on the heart is now recognized to be somewhat indirect. When the Na^+ pump in the heart is inhibited, cell Na^+ increases, and K^+ decreases. The cell potential is maintained by the $[K]_i/[K]_o$ ratio and, therefore, starts to fall. The $3Na^+/Ca^{2+}$ exchanger, which moves Ca^{2+} out of heart cells, slows both because of the fall of the inward Na gradient and the decrease in membrane potential. The increase in $[Ca^{2+}]_i$ increases the force of contraction of the myocyte. In the normal heart, there is always risk of induction of arrhythmia due to the depolarization and inappropriate activation of voltage-dependent membrane channels. In the failing heart, there is danger

Pantoprazole, one of the PPIs, is used for treatment of acid related disease. It is also available in intravenous formation.

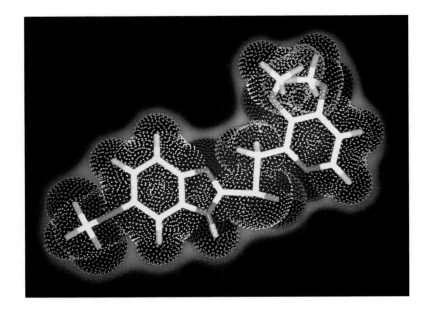

of Ca^{2+} overload. Nevertheless, digoxin is still in wide use today to treat left-sided heart failure as a specific inhibitor of the Na,K ATPase.

This discovery was followed by the description of the Ca^{2+} ATPases, found both in intracellular membranes, such as the sarcoplasmic reticulum (SERCA ATPases), and on the plasma membrane (PM Ca^{2+} ATPases). These are also considered to be electrogenic, exchanging $2Ca^{2+}$ for $2H^+$. The PM Ca^{2+} ATPases are uniquely regulated by the binding of calmodulin to the C-terminal region of this single-subunit enzyme.

Studies on acid secretion by isolated frog mucosae in the 1960s had started to point toward an ATP- rather than a redox-based mechanism. In the early 1970s, a K^+-stimulated ATPase was found in a frog stomach. A K^+-dependent acid transport was found in isolated gastric vesicles. Then it was shown that the mechanism of this ATPase was similar to that of the Na^+ pump but was an electroneutral ATP-driven H^+ for K^+ exchange. Previous data that were interpreted as demonstrating electrogenic acid secretion were explained as due to enhancement of a KCl conductive pathway with stimulation of acid secretion, thus providing the electrical response that was thought to demonstrate electrogenicity of gastric acid secretion. Permeabilized gastric parietal cells in rabbit gastric glands were able to secrete acid when ATP was added to the bathing solution in the presence of high concentrations of K^+. The ATP dependence and involvement of the H,K ATPase in acid secretion by the parietal cell was finally established and confirmed by the inhibition of acid secretion by proton pump inhibitors targeted to the H,K ATPase.

Recognition of the mechanism of acid secretion then led to the development of a new class of antiulcer drugs, the substituted pyridyl methylsulfinyl benzimidazoles, one of which is shown in the figure above. These are now the mainstay for treatment of most acid related diseases. Both the sodium pump and the acid pump remain specific drug targets, digoxin for the former, proton pump inhibitors for the latter.

CHAPTER 3
ION-MOTIVE ADENOSINE TRIPHOSPHATASES

Various ATPases that drive the transport of cations across biologic membranes have been described. The classes of ion-motive ATPases thus far described are listed in the following table and can be classified into multi-subunit and single- or two-subunit types, the F_1F_0 and V-ATPases representing the former and the P type the latter. The class of ATPases represented by the P glycoproteins or ABC transporters will not be discussed here.

The different types of ATPases that pump ions across membranes. The F_1F_0 ATPases pump protons or synthesize ATP from proton gradients; the V-type ATPases pump protons into acidic intracellular organelles; the P-type ATPases pump small ions like Na^+, K^+, H^+, Mg^{2+}, and Ca^{2+} as P_2-type ATPases; and the P_1 ATPases pump divalent cations such as Cu, Co, Zn, or Ni out of the cell.

Classes of Ion-Motive ATPases			
F_1F_0	V type	P type	
Mitochondria	Brain	Small cation	Transition metals
Chloroplasts	Renal	Na^+, K^+, H^+	Cu, Co, Zn
Bacteria		Ca^{2+}, Mg^{2+}	Ni

They have cytoplasmic domains that bind ATP and that transduce the energy from ATP hydrolysis into conformational changes, enabling binding of the ion from the cytoplasmic face of the membrane, movement of the ion into the membrane domain, and release of the ion from the exoplasmic face of the membrane. The cytoplasmic domain of the P-type ATPases or the cytoplasmic or intramitochondrial subunits of the V or F_1F_0 ATPases contain the energy-transduction sequences that transmit the ATP-induced conformational changes via a stalk region to the membrane domain. Their sequence, or that of one or more of their subunits, contains several relatively hydrophobic amino acid clusters of approximately twenty-one amino acids that are membrane inserted. These membrane segments form the transmembrane domain of these pumps and contain the ion-binding site and the ion pathway across the membrane. These segments are arranged as a compact cluster of membrane-inserted segments with varying degrees of tilt. Although the details of the ion transport mechanism of these pumps are still being explored, it is now apparent that alterations in tilt, and perhaps also rotation, of one or more of the membrane segments underlie the ion transport mechanism across the membrane domains.

Multimeric pumps

F_1F_0 type of ATPases/ATP synthases

The F_1F_0 type of ATPases/ATP synthases is found in the inner bacterial, chloroplast, and mitochondrial membranes and catalyzes the synthesis of ATP from ADP and inorganic phosphate (P_i) by dissipation of the electrochemical gradient of H^+ generated across these membranes by oriented redox pumps. Working in reverse, they are able to pump H^+.

These are multi-subunit pumps with a cytoplasmic domain consisting of a trimer of two subunits (α and β) as well as three other peptides (γ, δ, and ϵ) connected to a three-subunit membrane domain (a, b_2, c_{9-12}), as shown in the following figure. The γ subunit connects the F_0 to the center of the α-β trimer. The remarkable rotary mechanism of this ATP synthase has been deduced by kinetic analysis, cross-linking studies, and high-resolution crystals of the α-β trimer. It is thought that H_3O^+ traverses part of the membrane domain of the a subunit of F_0 driven by the electrochemical gradient for H^+. Three or four H^+ are then donated to the c subunit (assembled as a nonamer or decamer), initiating a single-step ratchet-like rotation of the c complex. This forces a rotation of the γ subunit, altering the conformation successively of each dimer of the F_1 α-β trimeric complex. After this step rotation, the H_3O^+ is dispersed into the inner mitochondrial space. The two b subunits are attached to the δ subunit that sits on top of the α-β trimer. Hence, the α-β trimer is fixed. The c and the ε subunits are attached to the γ subunit. The c complex (c, γ, ε) is mobile.

F_1 F_0 ATPase/Synthase

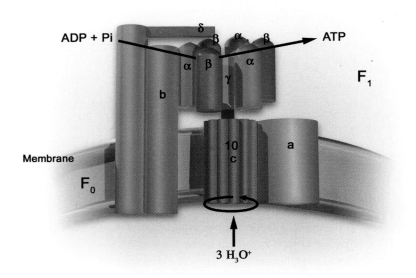

A model of the ATP synthase, the effector of the chemiosmotic mechanism. A potential and a hydrogen ion gradient is created across the inner membrane of mitochondria, bacteria, and chloroplasts by redox reactions. The energy of this proton motive force is translated into ATP synthesis by rotation of the cluster of c subunits of the F_0, and this rotation is transmitted via the γ stalk to the α-β trimers of the F_1 complex. The catalytic complex contains three α-β trimers that rotate with transmission of hydronium ions inward through the c subunit complex of the F_0 sector. The two b subunits tether the α-β trimers via the δ subunit, and the a subunit is fixed, allowing rotation of the c complex, thus rotating the γ stalk.

The γ-subunit rotation results in a relative change in affinity for the binding of ADP and P_i relative to ATP by decreasing the binding affinity of the latter, allowing release of ATP from the α-β monomer. Hence, the driving force for ATP synthesis is cyclic changes in the relative affinities of the various substrates, ATP, ADP, and P_i. Operating in reverse, the synthase acts as an electrogenic proton pump. This is the only cation pump that appears to function physiologically in a reversible manner.

V-type ATPases

This rotational paradigm probably extends to the V-type ATPases, which are also multi-subunit pumps. These are electrogenic proton-transport multi-subunit ATPases present in a variety of membranes and are responsible for acid secretion into various intracellular compartments (lysosomes, Golgi, neurosecretory granules), into the lumen of the proximal tubule and the renal collecting duct, or across the ruffled border of the osteoclast. In contrast to the F_1F_0 ATPases, they are unable to synthesize ATP and, hence, operate only in the proton pumping direction.

The minimal pH of the compartment that these pumps are able to generate is approximately 4.0. There are two major subtypes in mammals—the renal and the brain isoforms—but more subtypes may be discovered. The V ATPase contains seven to ten subunits organized into two distinct domains. The cytoplasmic domain contains five different subunits with molecular weights between 72 and 26 kDa, and the membrane domain contains two different subunits with molecular masses of approximately 20 and 16 kDa. The A cytoplasmic subunit (molecular mass of 72 kDa), in cooperation with the B cytoplasmic subunit (molecular mass of 57 kDa), contains the catalytic site, and the membrane subunits a and c conduct protons across the membrane. Recently, three variants of a 116-kDa subunit have been cloned, suggesting a larger family of V-type ATPases.

Oligomeric pumps

P-type ATPases

The enzyme class to which the gastric H,K ATPase belongs is called the *P-type ATPase family*. These enzymes are phosphorylated and dephosphorylated during their enzyme cycles. Enzymes of this family with similar functions, namely transport or countertransport of small cations or transition metals across membranes, often have similar amino acid sequences in regions that perform the same function, such as the binding of ATP or the sequence that is phosphorylated during the transport cycle. These are signature sequences.

Often, the arrangement of their transmembrane segments is retained to give a similar placement of relatively hydrophobic regions, producing recognizable transmembrane footprints. There are three subfamilies within the family of P-type ATPases: The Kdp ATPase of *Escherichia coli*, responsible for K^+ uptake by the microbe, is composed of three subunits, one of which is phosphorylated. Another type, the P_2 ATPases, transport small cations such as Na^+, K^+, H^+, Ca^{2+}, and Mg^{2+}. The third type, the P_1 ATPases, transport transition metals such as Cu^{2+}, Cd^{2+}, Zn^{2+}, or Co^{2+}. The P_1 ATPases have eight transmembrane segments, compared to the ten transmembrane segments in the P_2 ATPases. They do, however, share the phosphorylation and ATP-binding signature sequences, which has enabled their identification by library screening. They have a similar mechanism of transport. They bind the extruded ion at high affinity along with Mg^{2+} ATP. Phosphorylation of the enzyme by ATP follows. A conformational change results, with the outwardly transported ion moving into the membrane domain, becoming "occluded," and then appearing at the outside face, but now bound with low affinity. The outwardly transported ion is then released. In the countertransport pumps, there is binding of the inwardly transported cation with high affinity, and this cation then moves into the cell across the membrane domain, as the pump dephosphorylates and the inward-bound cation is released from a lower-affinity state on rebinding of ATP. Binding and transport of the counterion are essential for the cycling of these pumps.

Transition metal P-type ATPases

There are many transition metals that are toxic to bacteria; thus, various P-type ATPases have evolved to aid in export of toxic cations, such as Cd^{2+}. Also, some transition metals are essential to life, and pumps have appeared that import Cu^{2+}. At high concentrations, Cu^{2+} is also toxic, and Cu^{2+} export pumps are present in bacteria and even in humans, such as ATP7A and ATP7B, mutations of which are responsible for disorders of copper hemostasis, such as those found in Menkes' or Wilson's diseases, respectively. These enzymes have eight transmembrane segments. Three of these transition metal pumps are present in the *H. pylori* genome, and they have all been cloned. One appears to be able to function as a Cu^{2+}-export ATPase; the function of the others is not known. The phosphorylation consensus sequence and ATP-binding domains are present in the cytoplasmic loop between the fifth and sixth transmembrane domains in these pumps, compared to the site between the fourth and fifth membrane segments of the P_2-type ATPases. It is pumps such as these in *H. pylori* that might become targets of drugs designed to eradicate this organism by monotherapy.

Alkali cation ATPases

There are several mammalian members of alkali cation ATPases: the Na,K ATPases, the H,K ATPases, the SERCA (sarcoplasmic and endoplasmic reticulum), Ca^{2+}-transport ATPases, and the PM (plasma membrane) Ca^{2+} ATPase. The fungal H^+ ATPases also belong to this family. Characteristically, the mammalian enzymes all perform countertransport—exchange of a cellular cation with an extracellular cation. The fungal enzymes transport only H^+ outward. The parietal cell possesses a variety of these small alkali cation ATPases, each subserving a different function, but the pump of clinical interest is the pump responsible for acid secretion, the H,K ATPase.

SERCA ATPases

The SERCA ATPases are thought to be Ca^{2+}/H^+ exchange pumps that are found in sarcoplasmic and endoplasmic reticula and are responsible in part for calcium homeostasis in cell cytoplasm by sequestration of Ca^{2+} in the intracellular stores of the endoplasmic reticulum and for removal of Ca^{2+} into the sarcoplasmic reticulum after a contraction. As with the other P-type ATPases, there are various isoforms of the sarcoplasmic reticulum ATPase, differing in their expression in fast- and slow-twitch skeletal muscle (SERCA-1 and SERCA-2). The endoplasmic reticulum Ca^{2+} ATPase has the usual ten transmembrane segments plus an additional transmembrane segment at the C-terminal end. This latter segment is probably used as a retention signal, keeping the pump in the endoplasmic reticulum. It does not seem that they require association with any other protein for stable expression in intracellular membranes. Their homology with the Na,K or H,K ATPases is approximately 25%, although their topographic profile is very similar.

The crystal structure of the SERCA ATPase is available at 2.6 Å resolution and has formed the basis of modeling of the other P_2-type ATPases. Justification for the use of this E_1 crystal to model the three-dimensional structure of the other pumps is based on several observations. The SERCA ATPase was crystallized in the presence of high Ca^{2+} ion, and the binding sites for Ca^{2+} were seen directly. Similar conserved sites in the other ATPases have been mutated and shown also to be involved in cation binding. Further, cleavage sites in the presence of Fe^{3+}, peroxide, and ascorbate have been identified for the Na,K and H,K ATPase, and these sites conform almost exactly to the sites predicted by the crystal structure of the SERCA ATPase in the E_1 conformation and by models of the Ca^{2+}-pump cytoplasmic domain in the E_2 conformation.

Plasma membrane Ca^{2+} ATPases

There are four genes encoding isoforms of the PM Ca^{2+} ATPase, and alternative splicing generates other isoforms of this single-subunit plasma-membrane transport ATPase. These Ca^{2+}-transport ATPases are regulated by calmodulin and a variety of kinases and afford cells the ability to regulate cytoplasmic calcium by

The SERCA Ca ATPase

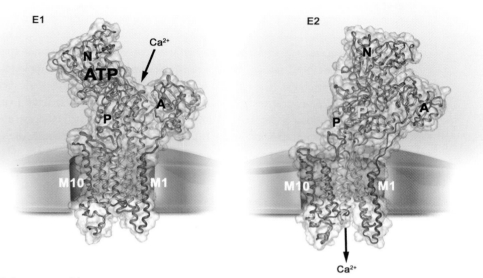

The high-resolution structure of the SERCA Ca^{2+} ATPase in two conformations. On the left is the E$_1$ conformation, where there is access of Ca^{2+} from the cytoplasmic side binding to sites in the membrane domain. On the right is the enzyme in the E$_2$ conformation, where Ca^{2+} is released to the outside of the pump. There are large changes in the three cytoplasmic domains, N (nucleotide binding) and P (phosphorylation), which are formed from the large cytoplasmic loop between M$_4$ and M$_5$, and the A domain (N terminus and M$_{2-3}$ cytoplasmic loop), where these move relative to each other in different states of the enzyme and will be discussed in detail for the gastric H,K ATPase. These conformational changes in the cytoplasmic domain are transmitted to the membrane domain, allowing changes in sidedness and affinity of the ion-binding region. The membrane and cytoplasmic conformation of the E$_1$ form is open towards the inside of the cell and the outside surface is closed. In the E$_2$ conformation, the cytoplasmic surface is closed and the membrane domain is open towards the outside of the cell. These changes result in outward transport of the ion.

extrusion of the cation across the plasma membrane. They have approximately 20% homology with the Na,K and H,K ATPase α subunits.

Na,K ATPases

There are four isoforms of the Na,K ATPases that all extrude Na$^+$ and reabsorb K$^+$, with a three-for-two stoichiometry. This unequal stoichiometry generates a potential across the cell membrane, inside negative. They consist of two tightly but noncovalently associated subunits—the α subunit, composed of approximately 1,000 amino acids, and the β subunit, composed of approximately 300 amino acids—that is N glycosylated at three or more sites in the extracytoplasmic region. The β1 isoform has 3 N-linked glycosylation sites; the β2 isoform has six or seven such sites on the outside surface. All of these sodium pumps generate a transmembrane current and membrane potential. Although pump current generates a potential difference across the plasma membrane, inside negative, a major component of the plasma membrane potential is due to the outward K$^+$ gradient generated by the pump. A variety of K$^+$ channels determine the K$^+$ conductance across the membrane.

Because many cell processes depend on inward electrogenic cotransport of Na$^+$ with nutrients such as amino acids or glucose, the generation of a transmembrane potential, inside negative, is of physiologic importance not only for maintenance of a transmembrane potential due to the outward K$^+$ gradient, but also for nutrition of the cell and, in the case of the heart, regulation of [Ca^{2+}]$_i$ by calcium channels or Ca^{2+}/H$^+$ exchange.

There are four isoforms of the α subunit: α1, α2, α3, and α4. The α subunit contains ten transmembrane segments. The N-terminal and C-terminal segments are cytoplasmic, and the loop between the fourth and fifth segments contains approximately 400 amino acids, with the phosphorylation consensus site and

ATP-binding domain present in this region. The α subunit is, therefore, the catalytic domain of the sodium pump, similar to the gastric H,K ATPase.

There are also three isoforms of the β subunit: β1, β2, and β3. Presumably, each isoform is expressed along with its α partner and assembled in the endoplasmic reticulum as an α-β heterodimer. The β subunit has a single transmembrane segment and is a type II membrane protein, with the N-terminal cytoplasmic and the C-terminal sequence extracytoplasmic. There are three N-linked glycosylation consensus sequences (NXT or NXS) and three disulfide bonds in the extracytoplasmic domain of the β subunit. The function of the β subunit of this ATPase is not very clear. Alteration of its structure by disulfide reduction inhibits ATPase activity. In its absence, the α subunit is unstable and does not reach the plasma membrane, so it is required for structural stability. Why the α subunit is unstable in the absence of the β subunit is not obvious, because the plasma membrane Ca^{2+} ATPase has similar topology but does not require a β subunit for stable plasma membrane expression. It seems that membrane insertion of the M5 and subsequent domains depends on expression of the β subunit. Only the K^+ countertransport pumps require a β subunit, and modification of this protein modifies pump kinetics.

The three isoforms of the Na^+ pump are differentially expressed in various tissues, with, therefore, specialized functions. The α1-β1 isoform is the most common form and is regarded as the housekeeper for maintenance of Na^+ gradients. The other isoforms vary in their affinity for ions and cardiac glycosides. The α2-β2 isoform may be the target for cardiac glycosides in the heart. The expression of the other isoforms may relate to their coupling to other transporters. For example, the α4 isoform is expressed in spermatozoa membranes and may be closely coupled to an Na^+/H^+ exchanger, allowing rapid regulation of internal pH in the face of external acidity.

The H,K ATPases

There are three or four isoforms of the H,K ATPases that are known. They are also α-β heterodimers. The H,K α1-β1 is the gastric H,K ATPase. The α subunit contains the phosphorylation consensus sequence and ATP-binding domain. The β subunit has six or seven N-linked glycosylation consensus sequences that are glycosylated, and expression of this subunit is required for stabilizing the α subunit and appropriate trafficking and sorting to the tubulovesicles of the parietal cell. The α subunit is approximately 75% homologous to the α subunit of the Na^+ pump, and the β subunit is approximately 40% homologous to the β2 subunit of the Na^+ pump.

The H,K colonic α2 ATPase has a similar (75%) homology to the gastric and Na^+ pumps and, although called an H,K ATPase, may transport Na^+ rather than H^+, but does absorb K^+. The H,K α2-β2 is found in colon, brain, and kidney. This enzyme may be misnamed, because although it has been shown that it is upregulated in the kidney with K^+ depletion, there is no evidence that proton transport is catalyzed by this pump in the kidney. The β subunit used by this isoform was initially considered unique but when cloned from the colon is identical to the β3 subunit.

The toad bladder H,K ATPase is the third isoform and is closely allied to the gastric H,K ATPase α3, but has a unique β subunit. Another homolog is an ATPase cloned from human skin, ATPAL1. It is 86% homologous to the colonic isoform and is also found in the kidney and the brain and lesser amounts in the colon. There does not appear to be a unique β sequence associated with this ATPase. Recently it has been shown that this ATPAL1 isoform is associated with the β1 isoform of the Na^+/K^+ ATPase.

CHAPTER 4
THE GASTRIC ACID PUMP

The gastric H,K ATPase exchanges H$^+$ for K$^+$ at equal stoichiometry. Even though the outward and inward parts of the transport cycle are electrogenic, pump transport is electroneutral and does not generate a transmembrane potential. The general transport process that the α subunit of this pump catalyzes is shown in the following figure. More detail has been gleaned from homology analysis with the structure of the Ca^{2+} ATPase and by site-directed mutagenesis to elucidate the binding region of the K$^+$-competitive inhibitor—the 1,2α imidazo-pyridine SCH28080—and from binding of the proton pump inhibitors (PPIs) to different cysteines accessible from the luminal surface of the catalytic subunit.

The transport reactions of the gastric H,K ATPase. As a function of binding MgATP and H$^+$ or hydronium (H$_3$O$^+$) ion, the export of protons or hydronium ions occurs after phosphorylation. In the presence of K$^+$ extracellularly enabled by the presence of a KCl channel in the canalicular membrane, K$^+$ binds to the outward conformation of the phosphorylated pump. The K$^+$ is then transported inwardly during the dephosphorylation step. In the absence of K$^+$, the pump stops in the E$_2$P conformation.

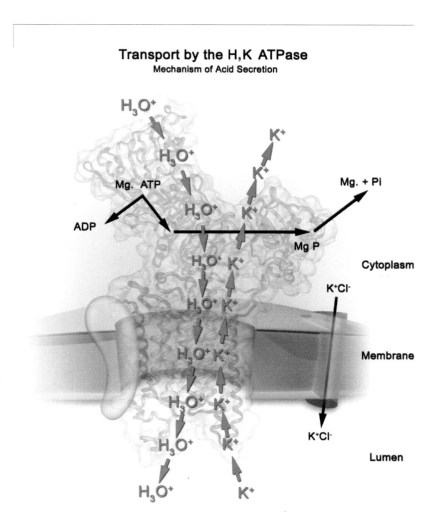

Transport by the H,K ATPase
Mechanism of Acid Secretion

Reaction pathway of the H,K ATPase

The Na,K ATPase exchanges intracellular sodium ions for extracellular potassium ions, the gastric ATPase H_3O^+ for extracellular potassium, and the sarcoplasmic or endoplasmic reticular Ca^{2+} pump two cytoplasmic Ca^{2+} for $2H^+$ in the sarcoplasmic reticulum. In the outward reaction transporting Na^+, H^+, or Ca^{2+}, the catalytic subunit is phosphorylated by ATP, and in the inward reaction, the phosphoenzyme is dephosphorylated by K^+ or H^+ (in the case of the sarcoplasmic reticulum Ca^{2+} ATPase). To achieve uphill transport at a significant rate, there has to be a decrease in binding-site affinity on the side of the membrane from which the ion is transported and reorientation of this site toward the side to which the ion is transported.

A conceptual model for this H^+ outward and K^+ inward transport that is supported experimentally is that the transported ion enters the membrane domain from one side and binds to a site with relatively high affinity with phosphorylation to provide the transporting conformation. Then the membrane domain closes to occlude the ion to provide the occluded conformation. Another conformational change then opens the membrane domain to allow the ion to be removed from the cytoplasm to escape from the other side of the membrane from

Transport-Catalysis Coupling

Transport-catalysis coupling in the gastric H,K ATPase, in which hydronium ions and MgATP bind to the cytoplasmic face of the enzyme; then the enzyme phosphorylates, moving the hydronium ion into the membrane domain and then out to the exoplasmic face. The hydronium ion is released, and then K^+ binds and, with dephosphorylation, moves into the membrane domain and thence to the cytoplasmic face of the enzyme.

a lower-affinity state of the ion-binding site. Binding of the counter-transported ion induces the converse changes in affinity and conformation, the ion binding with relatively high affinity to the outside face, occluding, and releasing from the low-affinity state to the cytoplasm.

The experiment on the Na^+ pump that established occlusion took advantage of the fact that this enzyme forms a phosphorylated intermediate. In the presence of 100 mM of Na^+ and ATP, phosphoenzyme is formed at a constant rate. Various other cations can substitute for K^+ in the dephosphorylation reaction, such as Rb^+, Cs^+, or NH_4^+. These are K^+ surrogates. If the concentration of these cations is set to give equal rates of dephosphorylation, but the enzyme turns over at a different rate, the rate-limiting step must be subsequent to dephosphorylation and before rephosphorylation. It was postulated that this step was the unbinding of the occluded cation present in the membrane domain of the dephosphorylated enzyme.

This hypothesis was then shown to be correct by demonstrating the binding of $^{86}Rb^+$ to the pump in the presence of ouabain and showing that the addition of ATP resulted in deocclusion. Similar binding of cation has also been demonstrated for the sarcoplasmic reticulum Ca^{2+} ATPase and the gastric H,K ATPase, establishing the mechanistic similarity of these enzymes.

The scheme of their reaction is shown in the figure illustrating the kinetic steps for the H,K ATPase. This shows that the enzyme exists in three major conformations, with ion-binding sites facing inward [the "in" conformation (E_1)], ion-binding sites facing outward [the "out" conformation (E_2)], and ion sites occluded (the "occ" conformation). The transition between these conformations is driven by ATP binding, transphosphorylation, and dephosphorylation.

Kinetics of the H,K ATPase

Kinetic studies on the H,K ATPase have defined the reaction steps shown in the figure illustrating the H^+ and K^+ transport steps. Understanding of the overall catalytic cycle of this ion pump has facilitated a mechanistic description of the process of acid secretion by the stomach. From this derives our understanding of stimulation of acid secretion and the processes inhibited by the PPIs.

The key structural change in the ion-binding site, apart from sidedness, is the size of the ion it can accommodate. In the "in" conformation, the smaller hydronium ion, H_3O^+, is accommodated. In the "out" conformation, the smaller ion is weakly bound compared to the larger, partially hydrated K^+. Experimental evidence for the reaction cycle described above has been obtained using rapid kinetic analysis of the rate of formation and destruction of phosphoenzyme generated from ^{32}P-ATP at different pH and potassium concentrations.

The rate of formation of the phosphoenzyme and the K^+-dependent rate of breakdown are sufficiently fast to allow the phosphoenzyme to be an intermediate in the overall ATPase reaction. The initial step is the reversible binding of ATP to the enzyme in the absence of added K^+ ion, followed by a Mg^{2+}- (and proton-) dependent transfer of the terminal phosphate of ATP to the catalytic subunit (E_1–P•H^+). The Mg^{2+} remains occluded until dephosphorylation. Increasing the hydrogen ion concentration on the ATP-binding face of the vesicles accelerates phosphorylation, whereas increasing the potassium ion concentration inhibits phosphorylation. Increasing the hydrogen ion concentration reduced K^+ inhibition of the phosphorylation rate. Decreasing the hydrogen ion concentration accelerated dephosphorylation in the absence of K^+, and K^+ on the luminal surface accelerated dephosphorylation. Increasing K^+ concentrations at constant ATP decreased the rate of phosphorylation, and increasing ATP concentrations at constant K^+ concentration accelerated ATPase activity and increased the steady-state phosphoenzyme level. Therefore, inhibition by the alkali cations is due to cation stabilization of a dephosphorylated E_1 form at a cytosolically accessible cation-binding site. Occlusion was demonstrated directly by showing ^{86}Rb binding to the enzyme at a low temperature that was released by the addition of ATP.

The addition of K^+ to the enzyme-bound acylphosphate results in a two-step dephosphorylation. The faster initial step is dependent on the concentration of K^+. The second phase of EP breakdown is accelerated in the presence of K^+, but at K^+ concentrations exceeding 500 µM, the rate becomes independent of K^+ concentration. This shows that two forms of EP exist. The first form, E_1P, is K^+ insensitive and converts spontaneously to E_2P, the K^+-sensitive form. ATP binding to the H,K ATPase occurs in both the E_1 and the E_2 states, but with a lower affinity in the E_2 state. As for the Na^+ pump, various cations, such as Rb^+, Cs^+, NH_4^+, and Tl^+, can act as K^+ substitutes or surrogates. As will be seen later, the design of K^+-competitive inhibitors of the H,K ATPase takes advantage of the surrogate properties of NH_4^+. At higher concentrations of K^+, the rate of hydrolysis slows as the removal of K^+ from the E_1 conformation of the pump becomes rate limiting.

Membrane potential and the H,K ATPase

The gastric H,K ATPase is electroneutral, in contrast to the Na,K ATPase, because the number of H^+ ions exported is the same as the number of K^+ ions imported. However, each half of the reaction cycle generates an equal but opposite membrane potential as the ion traverses the membrane domain.

The H^+ for K^+ stoichiometry of the H,K ATPase was reported to be one or two per ATP hydrolyzed. The H^+:ATP ratio was independent of external KCl and ATP concentrations. If care is taken to measure initial rates in tight vesicles, the ratio is 1ATP:2H:2K, at pH 6.1. Because at full pH gradient the stoichiometry must fall to 1ATP:1H:1K, this pump displays a variable stoichiometry. This can be explained if at least two carboxylic amino acids are involved in ion binding and one of them stays protonated as the pH of the acid space falls to below the negative logarithm of the acid ionization constant (pK_a) of one of the carboxylic acid residues. Since the ion binding sites face into the center of the ion transport pathway that is hydrophilic, the pK_a is likely to be between 3.0 and 4.0. Hence, the stoichiometry will fall to 1:1 at a pH of approximately 3.0.

2D structure of the gastric H,K ATPase

Eventually, a complete description of the mechanism of the H,K ATPase will include a detailed three-dimensional structure of this enzyme with the changes seen on binding ATP, phosphorylation, and ion binding and transport, as have been obtained for the SERCA ATPase.

The catalytic subunit is similar in general structure to that of other mammalian small cation P-type ATPases. Composed of 1,034 or 1,035 amino acids, it has a large cytoplasmic domain, a connecting stalk or energy transduction domain, a transmembrane domain, and a small extracytoplasmic domain. The β subunit has an N-terminal cytoplasmic sequence of approximately 60 amino acids, a transmembrane domain of approximately 30 amino acids, and a C-terminal domain containing approximately 200 amino acids with seven N-linked glycosylation sites. Although the function of the pumps that have been sequenced is usually known, it is not possible by inspection of the sequence to predict which ion is transported by which sequence. In the 1980s, when complementary deoxyribonucleic acid (cDNA) and, hence, amino acid sequences became available, there was hope that linear sequence would provide mechanistic clues as to protein function. Amino acid sequencing has enabled enormous advances in the fields of phenotyping cells, analyzing families of proteins, and defining interacting proteins and signature sequences but has not fully enabled functional or mechanistic analysis. Biochemical, molecular, and structural features are necessary in addition to be able to call the function of a protein sequence.

The catalytic α and β subunit amino acid sequence

The primary sequences of the α subunits deduced from cDNA have been reported for several species such as pig, rat, rabbit, and human. The hog gastric H,K ATPase, a subunit sequence deduced from its cDNA, consists of 1,034 amino acids and has a molecular weight (MWt) of 114,285 Da. The sequence, based on the known N-terminal amino acid sequence, is one less than the cDNA-derived sequence and begins with glycine. The degree of conservation among the α subunits is extremely high (over 97% identity). The human gastric H,K ATPase gene has 22 exons and encodes a protein of 1,035 residues, including the initiator methionine residue (MWt = 114,047). These H,K ATPase α subunits show high homology (~60% identity) with the Na,K ATPase catalytic α subunit. The distal colon K^+ ATPase α subunit, H,K α2, has also been sequenced and shares 75% homology with both the H,K and Na,K ATPases.

The amino acid sequence derived from the cDNA for the hog enzyme is shown in the figure. The sequences for this enzyme and of the sodium pump are 75% homologous. Regions of identity are the phosphorylation consensus sequence and the ATP-binding domain; many of the cytoplasmic regions have high homology compared to the transmembrane regions. It is remarkable that, even with the detailed knowledge of the amino acid sequence, the function of the protein must be measured experimentally and cannot be predicted.

The β subunit

The primary sequences of the β subunits have been reported for rabbit, hog, rat, mouse, and human enzymes and contain approximately 290 amino acids. The hydropathy profile of the β subunit is less ambiguous than that of the α subunit. There is one membrane-spanning region predicted by the hydropathy analysis,

Gastric H,K ATPase

Catalytic subunit

Beta subunit

The amino acid sequence of the α (right) and β (left) subunits of the gastric H,K ATPase, illustrating the transmembrane segments (ten in the α subunit, one in the β subunit) and regions of identity or homology with the Na,K ATPase. The region of interaction of the two subunits is with the beginning of the eighth transmembrane segment and two regions of the β subunit, as illustrated. The amino acids are colored red for carboxylic acids, blue for positively charged amino acids, pink for hydrophilic residues, and yellow for cysteine. These 1,034 amino acids provide the information for the ion selectivity of this pump as compared to the sodium pump. Many mutations have been made that have no measurable effect, but this sequence has been approximately 97% conserved throughout evolution.

The amino acid sequence of the H,K ATPase placed on a model of the enzyme. The single-letter code is used for the amino acids. This is the three-dimensional representation of the figures above showing linear sequence. The picture on the top shows the three cytoplasmic domains (green, N nucleotide binding; white, P phosphorylation domain; blue, activation domain). The picture on the bottom shows the membrane domain (dark blue, M1; yellow, M5; red, M10).

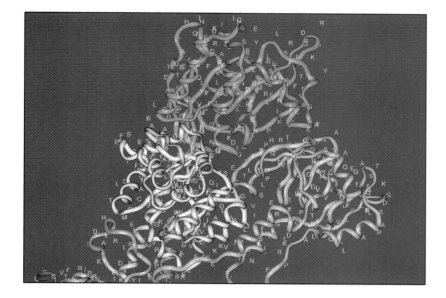

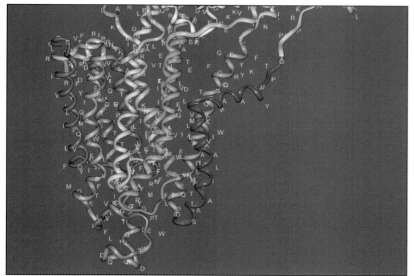

which is located at the region between positions 38 and 63 near the N terminus. Tryptic digestion of the intact gastric H,K ATPase produces only one small cleavage of the N-terminal segment of the β subunit on sodium dodecyl sulfate (SDS) gels. Wheat germ agglutinin (WGA) binding of the β subunit is retained due to the N-linked sugar residues. These data indicate that most of the β subunit is extracytoplasmic and glycosylated. When lyophilized hog vesicles are cleaved by trypsin followed by reduction, a small, nonglycosylated peptide fragment is seen on SDS gels with the N-terminal sequence AQPHYS, which represents the C-terminal region beginning at position 236 in the pig sequence. This small fragment is found neither after trypsinolysis of intact vesicles nor in the absence of reducing agents. A disulfide bridge must therefore connect this cleaved fragment to the β subunit containing the carbohydrates. The C-terminal end of the disulfide is at position 262. This leaves little room for an additional membrane-spanning α helix. Hence, the β subunit has only one membrane-spanning segment.

Region of association of the α and β subunits

The β subunit of both the Na,K and H,K ATPases is necessary for targeting the complex from the endoplasmic reticulum to the plasma membrane. It also stabilizes a functional form of both the gastric H,K and Na,K ATPases. The region of association of the two subunits helps explain this functional association, and this association is apparently vital for stable membrane folding of the α subunit. The β subunit, however, can traffic to the plasma membrane in the absence of the α subunit.

In the case of the Na,K ATPase, the last 161 amino acids of the α subunit are essential for effective association with the β subunit. Further, the last four or five C-terminal hydrophobic amino acids of the Na⁺-pump β subunit are essential for interaction with the α subunit, whereas the last few hydrophilic amino acids are not. Expression of the Na⁺-pump α subunit, along with the β subunit of either the sodium or proton pump in *Xenopus* oocytes, has shown that the β subunit of the gastric proton pump can act as a surrogate for the β subunit of the sodium pump for membrane targeting and ^{86}Rb⁺ uptake. This implies homology in the associative domains of the β subunits of the two pumps. The H,K ATPase α subunit requires its β subunit for efficient cell-surface expression. Expression of chimers of the α subunits of the Na,K and Ca²⁺ ATPases showed that the C-terminal half of the α subunit assembled with the β subunit.

A model of the arrangement of the α and β subunits of the H,K ATPase showing the region of the β subunit associated with the outside face of M_8, and vice versa. The ion transport domain is between transmembrane helices 4, 5, and 6. On the figure are the two specific regions of association of the β subunit with the outside surface of TM8. These are the peptide chains between amino acid 907 and 922 in the α subunit and between amino acid 64 and 130 and amino acid 154 and 188 in the β subunit.

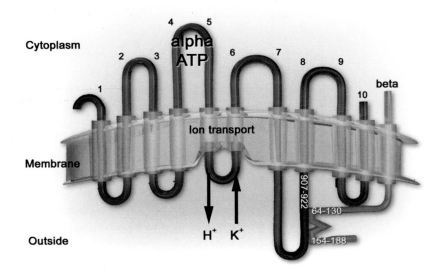

Arrangement of Alpha and Beta Subunits of the H,K ATPase

Cytoplasm

alpha
ATP

beta

Membrane

Ion transport

Outside

H⁺ K⁺

907-922

64-130

154-188

To specify the region of the α subunit associated with the β subunit, the tryptic digest was solubilized using nonionic detergents such as NP-40 or $C_{12}E_8$. These detergents allow the holoenzyme to retain ATPase activity. The tryptic fragments were then adsorbed to a WGA-affinity column. After elution of the peptides not associated with the β subunit binding to the WGA column, elution of the β subunit with 0.1 N acetic acid eluted almost quantitatively the M7/loop/M8 sector of the α subunit. These data show that this region of the α subunit is tightly associated with the β subunit such that nonionic detergents are unable to dissociate it from the β subunit.

If tryptic digestion is carried out in the presence of K$^+$, a fragment of 19 to 21 kDa is produced that contains the M7 segment and continues to the C-terminal region of the enzyme. When this digest is solubilized and passed over the WGA column, as outlined above, in addition to the 19- to 21-kDa fragment, a fragment representing the M5/loop/M6 sector is now also retained by the β subunit. Hence, provided there is no hydrolysis between M8 and M9, an additional interaction is present between the α and β subunits comprising regions of the M5, 6 and M9, 10 regions of the α subunit. The antibody mAb 146-14 also recognizes the region of the α subunit at the extracytoplasmic face of the M7 segment as well as a region of the β subunit enclosed by the second disulfide bridge. These data suggest interaction between these regions such that this assembled region is presented during generation of antibody, a finding consistent with the association found by WGA-column chromatography.

If the tryptic digestion is carried out on solubilized enzyme, WGA fractionation of FMI-labeled tryptic fragments of detergent-solubilized H,K ATPase showed that a fragment Leu 854 to Arg 922 of the α subunit was a major fragment bound to the β subunit.

Yeast two-hybrid analysis for protein association is a method that uses a split nuclear-transcription factor (β-galactosidase) to determine interactions between different proteins or different fragments. The binding domain and activating domain of the factor are expressed on separate vectors, and different fragments of the cDNA sequence are ligated onto one or another vector. When there is interaction, the β-galactosidase gene is expressed and can be assayed either by the development of a blue color or by a direct luminescent enzyme assay. Yeast two-hybrid system showed that only the region containing a part of TM7, the loop, and part of TM8 was capable of giving positive interaction signals with the ectodomain of the β subunit in agreement with the data from digestion.

The sequence in the extracytoplasmic loop close to TM8, namely Arg 897 to Thr 928, was identified as being the site of interaction using this method. Hence, we deduced that there is strong interaction within the sequence Arg 897 to Arg 922 in the α subunit and the extracytoplasmic domain of the β subunit. Using yeast two-hybrid analysis, two different sequences in the β subunit, Gln 64 to Val 126 and Ala 156 to Arg 188, were identified as containing association domains in the extracytoplasmic sequence of the β subunit.

The reactive sites of the catalytic subunit

The gastric α subunit has conserved sequences along with the other P-type ATPases for the ATP-binding site, the phosphorylation site, the pyridoxal 5'-phosphate–binding site, and the fluorescein isothiocyanate (FITC)-binding site. These sites are in the ATP-binding domain in the large cytoplasmic loop between membrane-spanning segments 4 and 5.

In the case of the hog gastric H,K ATPase, pyridoxal 5'-phosphate bound at Lys 497 of the a subunit in the absence but not the presence of ATP, suggesting that Lys 497 is present in the ATP-binding site or in its vicinity. The phosphorylation site was observed to be at Asp 386. FITC covalently labels the Na,K and the gastric H,K ATPases in the absence of ATP. The binding site of FITC was at Lys 518. However, several additional lysines, such as those at positions 497 and 783, were shown to react with FITC during the inactivation of the Na,K ATPase and to be protected from reaction with FITC when ATP was present in the incubation. Based on these data, similar lysines of the H,K ATPase could be near or in the ATP-binding site, which is, therefore, formed by several nonadjacent stretches of the cytoplasmic amino acid sequence.

The crystal structure of the SERCA ATPase and modeling based on two-dimensional crystals have also revealed the changes in the cytoplasmic conformation that occur on binding ATP and phosphorylation. The cytoplasmic domain consists of three distinct regions: the N or nucleotide binding domain, the P or phosphorylation domain, and the A domain, consisting of the N terminus and the cytoplasmic loop between M2 and M3. In the E_1 configuration, these domains are well separated. On binding ATP and the transported cation, there is transient closer association between the N and P domains to allow phosphorylation. Then, as the N domain moves away, the A domain moves toward the P domain and in so doing generates the E_2 form of these pumps. In this transition, the ion-binding site transits from inward to outward facing, and the exported ion is released. With binding of the counter-ion, the pump dephosphorylates, and the ion-binding site and cytoplasmic domains return to the E_1 state, allowing release of the counter-ion into the cytoplasm of the cell.

The membrane domain of the catalytic subunit

The hydropathy plot of the H,K ATPase is shown in the following figure and is similar in all the P-type ATPases that transport the small cations, H^+, Na^+, K^+, Ca^{2+}, and Mg^{2+}. This plot defines the potential transmembrane or membrane-inserted segments; the methods that have been used to define these segments of the acid pump are also illustrated in this figure.

The membrane domain of the enzyme contains the ion-transport pathways. There must be a hydrophilic pathway in the membrane domain that the ions can traverse as the cytoplasmic domain changes conformation as a function of phosphorylation and dephosphorylation.

It can be seen that there are five regions of hydrophobicity, suggesting the possible presence of ten membrane segments. These have been established experimentally by determining the residual membrane domains after removal of the cytoplasmic sectors by tryptic digestion of cytoplasmic side

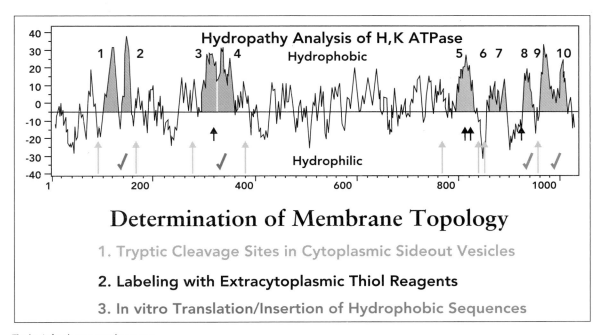

Determination of Membrane Topology

1. Tryptic Cleavage Sites in Cytoplasmic Sideout Vesicles

2. Labeling with Extracytoplasmic Thiol Reagents

3. In vitro Translation/Insertion of Hydrophobic Sequences

The basis for the ten-membrane segment model of the gastric H,K ATPase is shown. The hydropathy plot provides evidence for 8, 9, or 10 predicted membrane sequences. Experimental evidence for membrane segments 1 to 8 was provided by labeling of the enzyme with either omeprazole or a photoaffinity derivative of SCH28080 followed by tryptic digestion and sequencing of the labeled tryptic fragments. Evidence for membrane segments 9 and 10 was obtained by showing membrane insertion of these segments after *in vitro* translation in the presence of microsomal membranes.

out vesicles, by *in vitro* translation scanning, and by sites of labeling with extracytoplasmic inhibitors of the enzyme, such as the PPIs or the acid-pump antagonists. The two-dimensional model that results from such analyses shows the presence of a large cytoplasmic domain, a membrane domain with ten transmembrane segments for the α subunit, and one transmembrane segment for the β subunit.

This is shown in the next figure, and reflects the information that was obtained before high-resolution images of the SERCA ATPase. These are shown in the third figure, where the details of the different domains in two different conformations can be distinguished. The cytoplasmic domain has three subdomains, the N (nucleotide binding), the P (phosphorylation), and A (activation) domains. There are ten transmembrane segments. In the ion-binding site accessible from the inside of the cell (E_1 conformation), the N, P, and A domains are separated, and the ion site is open toward the inside. In the state where ions are released to the outside, the P and A domains are close together, and the ion site is exposed to the outside, allowing outward transport of the proton.

Transport region of the membrane domain

To establish the regions of the membrane domain transporting H_3O^+ outward and K^+ inward, a variety of sites have been mutated in this pump. Measurements have been made of enzyme activity, cation binding (occlusion), and transport in these mutants. In the membrane domain, mutations, especially of carboxylic and hydrophilic amino acids in the region of M4, 5, 6, and 8, affect ion binding and transport. It is, therefore, considered that these transmembrane sequences enclose the ion pathway across the membrane.

Gastric H,K ATPase

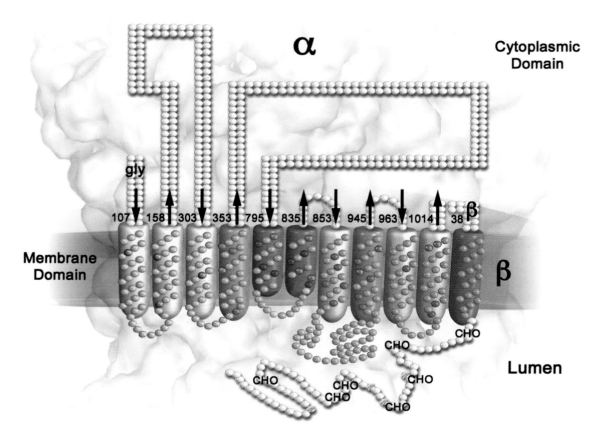

A two-dimensional diagram of the H,K ATPase showing the arrangement of charged (acid, colored red) groups in the membrane domain clustered in M4, 5, 6, and 8 (the putative ion-binding sites) and the association of the α and β subunits. The cytoplasmic domain is composed of the N terminus and the loop between M2 and M3 (the A domain) and the large segment between M4 and M5 [containing the N (nucleotide-binding) domain and the P (phosphorylation) domain].

The carboxylic and other hydrophilic side chains of the amino acids in M4, 5, 6, and perhaps M8 provide binding sites for the cations. When the amino acid sequences of the Na,K, H,K, and sarcoplasmic reticulum Ca ATPases are compared, there is conservation of several of these carboxylic or hydrophilic amino acids in certain transmembrane segments. The carboxylic acids in TM4, 5, 6, and 8 are conserved, as well as the motifs surrounding these amino acids, suggesting a commonality of functions such as ion binding.

M5/M6 domain, a part of the transport region of the catalytic subunit

As discussed above, this region of the membrane domain of the enzyme is thought to be intimately involved with the ion-transport pathway. This inference is based on studies of site-directed mutagenesis, extractability from digested membranes, and conformationally sensitive cutting sites at the N-terminal end of this region. There is also the binding site for the covalent inhibi-

The Ion Binding Domain of the Gastric H,K ATPase

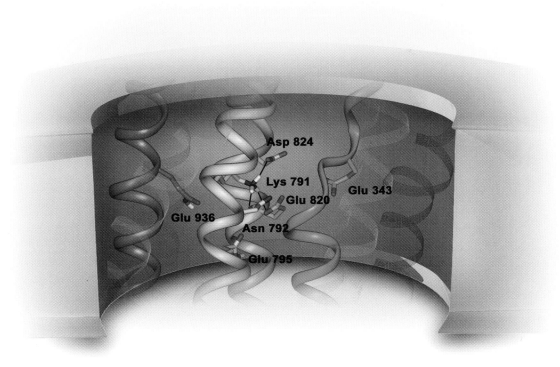

A representation of the ion-binding domain of the gastric H,K ATPase, with the carboxylic acids present in M4 (solid green), 5 (light yellow), 6 (dark yellow), and 8 (brown) illustrated as well as the lysine in M5, unique to the gastric H,K ATPase. The segments not involved in ion binding are shown as strands, whereas the helices involved in transport are shown as opaque colored ribbons and are TM4, 5, and 8.

tors—the substituted pyridyl methylsulfinyl benzimidazoles, the PPI class of drugs. These are thiophilic reagents and can, therefore, bind covalently to the –SH group of cysteines. There are two cysteines in the M5/M6 domain, at positions 813 and 822. The use of radioactive omeprazole has established that the cysteine involved in inhibition by this antiulcer drug is found at position 813. Although omeprazole also binds to cysteine at position 892, this is outside the transport domain and not related to inhibition.

Site-directed mutagenesis and structural modeling of the H,K ATPase membrane domain based on the Ca^{2+} ATPase structure has allowed definition of the amino acids involved in the binding of K^+ or NH_4^+ as the counterion. Carboxylic acids in the fourth, fifth, and sixth membrane domains, and perhaps one in the eighth transmembrane domain, form part of the ion-binding region, as illustrated in the figure. It should be noted that the cytoplasmic end of TM6 contains an expanded α helix, whereas the TM5 helix extends deep into the cytoplasmic P domain. Presumably, motion of TM6 relative to TM5 alters the "sidedness" and size of the ion-binding region, providing directional transport with appropriate changes in affinity for the primary and countertransported ion.

Transport by H,K ATPase

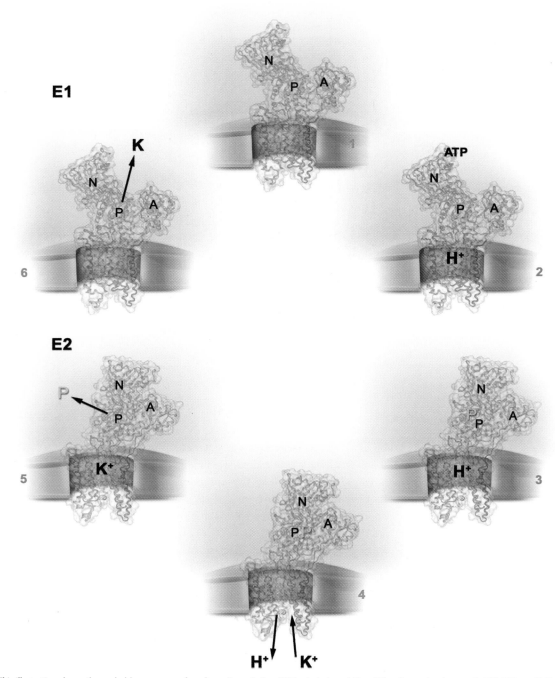

This illustration shows the probable sequence of conformations during ATP hydrolysis and H and K exchange by the gastric H,K ATPase. (1) The conformation of the pump prior to binding of MgATP and H+, with the cytoplasmic N, P, and A subdomains separated the E_1 form of the pump (2). Binding of ATP to the N cytoplasmic subdomain and H+ to the ion binding sites between M4, 5, and 6. (3) The occluded state E-P with H bound in the membrane and the P domain phosphorylated (the phosphate is colored yellow). (4) The E_2-P form with the ion site facing outward able to release H+ and bind K+. (5) K binding to the outside-facing conformation with release of phosphate back to the cytoplasm. (6) Regeneration of the E_1 form of the pump along with transport of K+ back into the cell.

Structural changes of the gastric acid pump and transport

The relationship between the cytoplasmic domain and the transmembrane domain changes as a function of the transport conformation. This statement is based on the findings with fluorescent probes that change their quantum yield as a function of the hydrophobicity of their environment. When the H,K ATPase is in the ion-binding site "in" conformation, the distance between the inner boundary of the cytoplasmic domain and the inner boundary of the membrane domain is small. With the ion-binding site in the "out" conformation, this distance increases as measured by the K^+-dependent quenching of fluorescence of FITC bound to Lys 516 of the amino acid sequence. Conversely, the distance between the outer edge of the membrane domain and the inner surface is larger with the ion site "in" conformation and smaller with the ion site "out" conformation. The enzyme, therefore, contracts its cytoplasmic domain as the ion is transported outward, and associated with this is a degree of extrusion of the membrane domain. As the countertransported ion binds to the outside surface, the outside binding site moves towards the cytoplasm.

There is evidence that the more mobile part of the membrane domain is the fifth and sixth transmembrane segment pair and its connecting loop. For example, tryptic cleavage of cytoplasmic side out vesicles cuts the cytoplasmic chain before M5 at different places depending on either the length of digestion or the absence or presence of K^+. The first N-terminal cutting site is at position 776, and then at 784, and finally at 792 after longer digestion or in the presence of K^+, whereas the C-terminal cutting site does not change. After digestion in the presence of K^+ when the residual membrane domain is treated at pH 10.0, of the five transmembrane segment pairs, first the M5/M6 is removed and then TM7/loop/TM8. *In vitro* translation of TM5/TM6 also shows that these relatively hydrophilic membrane segments probably do not interact fully with the hydrophobic lipid phase but more with the protein surface of other transmembrane segments. TM7 also does not act as a membrane-insertion sequence in *in vitro* translation. The cluster of M5/M6 and TM7/TM8 may provide the flexibility within the membrane domain that is necessary for transport competence.

Model of conformation and transport

The SERCA crystal structure available in the E_1 and E_2 conformations has allowed modeling of the different conformations of the H,K ATPase, perhaps explaining the mechanism of transport. In the figure on the left, with the binding of ATP and H^+, the P domain phosphorylates and a large conformational change occurs in the cytoplasmic domain, visualized as approach of the A and P domains. Associated with this change, there is a change of sidedness of the ion-binding site, with an ion-transport pathway now facing the lumen in the E_2 conformation. After the proton leaves, K binds, and then the pump dephosphorylates, allowing the E_1 conformation to reappear.

This P-type ATPase is the enzyme that is inhibited by the PPIs. Their target is found in the outside-facing surface of the transport segment of the pump, and their mechanism will be discussed in a subsequent section of this book.

SUGGESTED READING

Ahn KY, Kone BC. Expression and cellular localization of mRNA encoding the "gastric" isoform of H,K-ATPase alpha-subunit in rat kidney. *Am J Physiol* 1995;268:F99–F109.

Andersen J, Vilsen B. Structure-function relationships of cation translocation by Ca^{2+} and Na,K-ATPases studied by site directed mutagenesis. *FEBS Lett* 1995;359:101–106.

Asano S, Matsuda S, Hoshina S, et al. A chimeric gastric H^+,K^+-ATPase inhibitable with both ouabain and SCH 28080. *J Biol Chem* 1999;274:6848–6854.

Asano S, Tega Y, Konishi K, et al. Functional expression of gastric $H^+,K^{(+)}$-ATPase and site-directed mutagenesis of the putative cation binding site and catalytic center. *J Biol Chem* 1996;171:2740–2745.

Auer M, Scarbrough GA, Kuhlbrandt W. Three-dimensional map of the plasma membrane H^+-ATPase in the open conformation. *Nature* 1998;392:840–843.

Bamberg K, Mercier F, Reuben MA, et al. cDNA cloning and membrane topology of the rabbit gastric $H^+,K^{(+)}$-ATPase alpha-subunit. *Biochim Biophys Acta* 1992;1131:69–77.

Bamberg K, Sachs G. Topological analysis of the H,K ATPase using in vitro translation. *J Biol Chem* 1994;269:16909–16919.

Bayle D, Weeks D, Sachs G. The membrane topology of the rat sarcoplasmic and endoplasmic reticulum calcium ATPases by in vitro translation scanning. *J Biol Chem* 1995;270:25678–25684.

Berglindh T, Helander HF, Obrink KJ. Effects of secretagogues on oxygen consumption, aminopyrine accumulation and morphology in isolated gastric glands. *Acta Physiol Scand* 1976;97:401.

Besancon M, Shin JM, Mercier F, et al. Membrane topology and omeprazole labeling of the gastric H,K-adenosinetri–phosphatase. *Biochemistry* 1993;32:2345–2355.

Besancon M, Simon A, Sachs G, et al. Sites of reaction of the gastric H,K-ATPase with extracytoplasmic thiol reagents. *J Biol Chem* 1997;272:22438–22446.

Clarke DM, Loo TW, Maclennan DM. Functional consequences of alterations to polar amino acids located in the transmembrane domain of the Ca-ATPase of the Sarcoplasmic reticulum. *J Biol Chem* 1990;265:6262–6267.

Claros MG, von Heijne G. TopPred II, an improved software for membrane protein structure predictions. *Comput Appl Biosci* 1994;10:685–686.

Celsus AC. Of the disorders of the stomach and their cures. In: *De Medicina*, book IV. London: Wilson and Durham, 1756:196–201. Griene J, translator.

Cyrklaff M, Auer M, Kuhlbrandt W, et al. 2-D structure of the *Neurospora crassa* plasma membrane ATPase as determined by electron cryomicroscopy. *EMBO J* 1995;14:1854–1857.

Davies RE. The mechanism of hydrochloric acid production by the stomach. *Biol Revs* 1951;26:87.

Dibona DR, Ito S, Berglindh T, et al. Cellular site of gastric acid secretion. *Proc Natl Acad Sci U S A* 1979;76:6689.

Feng J, Lingrel JB. Analysis of amino acid residues in the H5-H6 transmembrane and extracellular domains of Na,K-ATPase alpha subunit identifies threonine 797 as a determinant of ouabain sensitivity. *Biochemistry* 1994;33:4218–4224.

Forte JG, Ganser A, Beesley R, et al. Unique enzymes of purified microsomes from pig fundic mucosa. *Gastroenterology* 1975;69:175–189.

Forte JG, Soll A. Cell biology of hydrochloric acid secretion. In: Forte JG, Schultz SG, eds. *Handbook of physiology. The gastrointestinal system III*. Bethesda, MD: American Physiological Society, 1989:207–228.

Forte TM, Machen TE, Forte JG. Ultrastructural changes in oxyntic cells associated with secretory function. A membrane recycling hypothesis. *Gastroenterology* 1977;73:941.

Foster M. Van Helmont and the rise of the chemical physiology. In: *Lectures on the history of physiology*. Boston: Cambridge University Press, 1924:120–143.

Fulton JF. René Antoine Ferchault de Réaumur. In: *Selected readings in the history of physiology*. Springfield, IL: Charles C. Thomas, 1966:68–170.

Garrison FH. The seventeenth century. In: *The history of medicine*. Philadelphia: WB Saunders, 1963:257–258.

Gibert AJ, Hersey SJ. Morphometric analysis of parietal cell membrane transformations in isolated gastric glands. *J Membr Biol* 1982;67:113–124.

Glynn IM, Karlish SJ. Occluded ions in active transport. *Annu Rev Biochem* 1990;59:171.

Golgi C. Sur la fine organisation des glandes peptiques des mammiferes. *Arch Ital Biol* 1893;19:448.

Helander HF. The cells of the gastric mucosa. *Int Rev Cytol* 1981;70:217–289.

Helander HF, Hirschowitz BI. Quantitative ultrastructural studies on gastric parietal cells. *Gastroenterology* 1972;63:951.

Henderson R, Baldwin JM, Ceska TA, et al. Model for the structure of bacteriorhodopsin based on high-resolution electron-cryo-microscopy. *J Mol Biol* 1990;213:899–929.

Hermsen HP, Swarts HG, Koenderink JB, et al. The negative charge of glutamic acid-820 in the gastric H^+,K^+-ATPase alpha-subunit is essential for K^+ activiation of the enzyme activitiy. *Biochem J* 1998;331:465–472.

Hersey SJ, Perez A, Matheravidathu S, et al. Gastric H^+K^+-ATPase in situ, evidence for compartmentalization. *Am J Physiol* 1989;257:G539.

Hippocrates. *The genuine works of Hippocrates*. London: Sydenham Soc., 1899:155–161. Adams F, translator.

Ife RJ, Brown TH, Blurton P, et al. Reversible inhibitors of the gastric H,K-ATPase. 5. Substituted 2,4-diaminoquinazolines and thienopyrimidines. *J Med Chem* 1995;38:2763–2773.

Ito S. Functional gastric morphology. In: Johnson LR, ed. *Physiology of the gastrointestinal tract*, 2nd ed, vol 1. New York: Raven Press, 1987:817.

Ito S, Schofield GC. Studies on the depletion and accumulation of microvilli and changes in the tubulovesicular compartment of mouse parietal cells in relation to gastric acid secretion. *J Cell Biol* 1974;63:364.

Jewell EA, Lingrel JB. Site directed mutagenesis of the Na,K ATPase. Consequences of the substitutions of negatively charged amino acids localized in the transmembrane domains. *Biochemistry* 1993;32:13523–13530.

Jewell-Motz EA, LIngrel JB. Site-directed mutagenesis of the Na,K-ATPase: consequences of substitutions of negatively-charged amino acids localized in the transmembrane domains. *Biochemistry* 1993;32:13523–13530.

Kuntzweiler TA, Wallick ET, Johnson CL, et al. Glutamic acid 327 in the sheep alpha 1 isoform of $H^+,K^{(+)}$-ATPase stabilizes a $K^{(+)}$-induced conformational change. *J Biol Chem* 1995;270:2993–3000.

Lambrecht N, Corbett Z, Bayle D, et al. Identification of the site of inhibition by omeprazole of a alpha-beta fusion protein of the H,K-ATPase using site-directed mutagenesis. *J Biol Chem* 1998;273:13719–13728.

Lee J, Simpson G, Scholes P. An ATPase from dog gastric mucosa: changes of outer pH in suspensions of dog membrane vesicles accompanying ATP hydrolysis. *Biochem Biophys Res Commun* 1974;60:825–832.

Lundegardh H. Investigations as to the absorption and accumulation of inorganic ions. *Ann Agric Coll Sweden* 1940;8:233.

MacLennan DH, Brandl CJ, Koreczak B, et al. Amino acid sequence of the Ca^{2+} Mg^{2+} dependent ATPase from rabbit muscle sarcoplasmic reticulum, deduced from its complementary DNA sequence. *Nature* 1985;316:696–700.

Maeda M, Ishizaki J, Futai M. cDNA cloning and sequence determination of pig gastric ($H^+ + K^+$)-ATPase. *Biochem Biophys Res Commun* 1988;157:203–209.

Melchers K, Weitzenegger T, Buhmann A, et al. Cloning and membrane topology of a P type ATPase from *Helicobacter pylori*. *J Biol Chem* 1996;271:446–457.

Mercier F, Bayle D, Besancon M, et al. Antibody epitope mapping of the gastric H,K-ATPase. *Biochim Biophys Acta* 1993;1149:151–165.

Mitchell P. Chemiosmotic coupling in oxidative and photosynthetic phosphorylation. *Biol Rev Camb Philos Soc* 1966;41:445–502.

Modlin IM. From Prout to the proton pump—a history of the science of gastric acid secretion and the surgery of peptic ulcer. *Surg Gynecol Obstet* 1990;170:81–96.

Munson KB, Lambrecht N, Sachs G. Effects of mutations in M4 of the gastric H^+,K^+-ATPase on inhibition kinetics of SCH28080. Biochemistry 2000;39:2997–3004.

Munson K, Vagin O, Sachs G, et al. Molecular modeling of SCH28080 binding to the gastric H,K-ATPase and MgATP interactions with SERCA- and Na,K-ATPases. *Ann N Y Acad Sci* 2003;986:106–110.

Patchornik G, Goldshleger R, Karlish SJ. The complex ATP-$Fe^{(2+)}$ serves as a specific affinity cleavage reagent in ATP-$Mg^{(2+)}$ sites of Na,K-ATPase: altered ligation of $Fe^{(2+)}$ ($Mg^{(2+)}$) ions accompanies the $E(1) \rightarrow E(2)$ conformational change. *Proc Natl Acad Sci U S A* 2000;97:11954–11959.

Pitcairn A. A dissertation upon the motion which reduces the aliment in the stomach to a form proper for the supply of blood. In: *The whole works*. London: J. Pemberton, 1727:106–138. Sewell G, Desaguliers JT, translators.

Post RL. A reminiscence about sodium, potassium-ATPase. *Ann N Y Acad Sci* 1974;242:6–11.

Prout W. On the nature of the acid and saline matters usually existing in the stomach of animals. *Philos Trans* 1824;114:45.

Rabon EC, Reuben MA. The mechanism and structure of the gastric H,K-ATPase. *Annu Rev Physiol* 1990;52:321–344.

Rabon EC, Smillie K, Seru V, et al. Rubidium occlusion within tryptic peptides of the H,K-ATPase. *J Biol Chem* 1993;268:8012–8018.

Racker E. Resolution and reconstitution of biological pathways from 1919 to 1984. *Fed Proc* 1983;42:2899–2909.

de Reaumur RAF. Sur la digestion des oiseaux. *Mem Acad Roy d Sc Paris* 1752:266.

Rehm WS, Sanders SS. Electrical events during activation and inhibition of gastric HCl secretion. *Gastroenterology* 1977;73:959–969.

Reti L. How old is hydrochloric acid? *Chymia* 1965;10:11–23.

Reuben MA, Lasater LS, Sachs G. Characterization of a beta subunit of the gastric $H^+/K^{(+)}$-transporting ATPase. *Proc Natl Acad Sci U S A* 1990;87:6767–6771.

Sachs G, Chang HH, Rabon E, et al. A nonelectrogenic H^+ pump in plasma membranes of hog stomach. *J Biol Chem* 1976;251:7690–7698.

Schertler GFX, Villa C, Henderson R. Projection structure of rhodopsin. *Nature* 1993;362:770–772.

Scott DR, Helander HF, Hersey SJ, et al. The site of acid secretion in the mammalian parietal cell. *Biochim Biophys Acta* 1993;1146:73.

Shin JM, Kajimura M, Arguello JM, et al. Biochemical identification of transmembrane segments of the Ca^{2+}-ATPase of sarcoplasmic reticulum. *J Biol Chem* 1993;269:22533–22537.

Shull GE. cDNA cloning of the beta-subunit of the rat gastric H,K-ATPase. *J Biol Chem* 1990;265:12123–12126.

Shull GE, Lingrel JB. Molecular cloning of the rat stomach ($H^+ + K^+$)-ATPase. *J Biol Chem* 1986;261:16788–16791.

Skou JC. The influence of some cations on an adenosine triphosphatase from peripheral nerves. *Biochim Biophys Acta* 1957;23:394–401.

Smith DL, Tao T, Maguire ME. Membrane topology of a P-type ATPase. The MgtB magnesium transport protein of *Salmonella typhimurium. J Biol Chem* 1993;268:22469–22479.

Smolka A, Helander HF, Sachs G. Monoclonal antibodies against gastric H+,K+ ATPase. *Am J Physiol* 1983;245:G589.

Spallanzani AL. Della digestione degli animali. In: *Fisica Animale*. Venice, 1782.

Spallanzani AL. *Dissertazioni de fisica animale e vegetabile.* Modena: Società Tipografica, 1780.

Stewart B, Wallmark B, Sachs G. The interaction of H+ and K+ with the partial reactions of gastric H,K-ATPase. *J Biol Chem* 1981;256:2682–2690.

Swarts HG, Klaassen CH, de Boer M, et al. Role of negatively charged residues in the fifth and sixth transmembrane domains of the catalytic subunit of gastric H+,K+-ATPase. *J Biol Chem* 1996;271:29764–29772.

Toh BH, Gleeson PA, Simpson RJ, et al. The 60- to 90-kDa parietal cell autoantigen associated with autoimmune gastritis is a beta subunit of the gastric H+/K+-ATPase (proton pump). *Proc Natl Acad Sci U S A* 1990;87:6418–6422.

Toyoshima C, Nakasako M, Nomura H, et al. Crystal structure of the calcium pump of sarcoplasmic reticulum at 2.6 A resolution. *Nature* 2000;405:647–655.

Toyoshima C, Nomura H. Structural changes in the calcium pump accompanying the dissociation of calcium. *Nature* 2002;418:605–611.

Toyoshima C, Sasabe H, Stokes DL. Three-dimensional cryo-electron microscopy of the calcium ion pump in the sarcoplasmic reticulum membrane [published erratum appears in *Nature* 1993;363(6426):286] *Nature* 1993;362:467–471.

Vagin O, Munson K, Lambrecht N, et al. Mutational analysis of the K+-competitive inhibitor site of gastric H,K-ATPase. *Biochemistry* 2001;40:7480–7490.

Walderhaug MO, Post RL, Saccomani G, et al. Structural relatedness of three ion-transport adenosine triphosphatases around their active sites of phosphorylation. *J Biol Chem* 1985;260:3852–3859.

Wang SG, Eakle KA, Levenson R, et al. Na+-K+-ATPase alpha-subunit containing Q905-V930 of gastric H+-K+-ATPase alpha preferentially assembles with H+-K+-ATPase beta. *Am J Physiol* 1997;272:C923–930.

Wolosin JM, Forte JG. Stimulation of oxyntic cell triggers K+ and Cl− conductances in apical H+-K+-ATPase membrane. *Am J Physiol* 1984;246:C537–C545.

Xu C, Rice WJ, He W, et al. A structural model for the catalytic cycle of Ca(2+) ATPase. *J Mol Biol* 2002;316:201–211.

Yao X, Thibodeau A, Forte JG. Ezrin-calpain I interactions in gastric parietal cells. *Am J Physiol* 1993; 265:C36.

Zhang P, Toyoshima C, Yonekra K, et al. Structure of the calcium pump from sarcoplasmic reticulum at 8A resolution. *Nature* 1998;992:835–839.

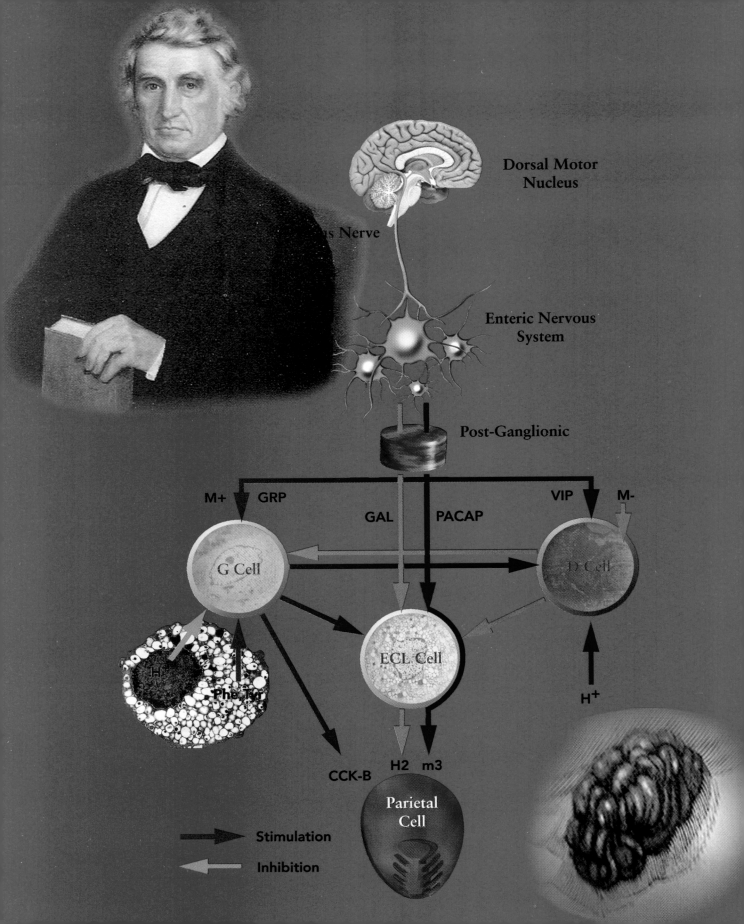

THE REGULATION OF GASTRIC ACID SECRETION

CHAPTER 1
TOWARDS AN UNDERSTANDING OF THE PHYSIOLOGY OF THE STOMACH

Gastric fistulae: a unique opportunity

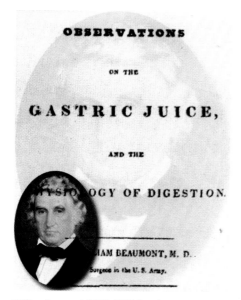

William Beaumont (1785–1853) (inset) and the frontispiece of his book. His contributions are best summarized by William Osler in the preface of Jesse Meyer's book *Life and Letters of Dr. William Beaumont*: "The man was greater than his work . . . The pioneer physiologist of the United States and the first to make a contribution of enduring value, his work remains a model of patient, persevering research. The highest praise that we can give is to say that his life fulfilled the ideal with which he set out, and which he so well expressed in the sentence: 'Truth, like beauty, is when unadorned adorned the most, and in prosecuting these experiments and enquiries I believe I have been guided by its light.'"

William Beaumont and the case of Alexis St. Martin

William Beaumont was born on November 25, 1785, in Lebanon, Connecticut, and began his study of medicine at the age of 22 years. In the War of 1812, he accepted a position in the Army as an acting surgeon's mate and saw active service. In 1819, after a brief spell in practice, his former colleague, Joseph Lovell, who had now become Surgeon General, offered Beaumont a commission, and he was assigned to Fort Mackinac.

Fort Mackinac was located on the island of Michel Mackinac at the junction of lakes Huron and Michigan. Beaumont was the only physician within 300 miles and was often busy because of frequent brawls among Native Americans and fur traders. On the morning of June 6, 1822, a 19-year-old voyageur, Alexis St. Martin, was accidentally shot in the left upper abdomen and chest. Beaumont was called to see the victim and noted a disastrous wound. He thought the chances of survival were slim and remarked, *"The man cannot live 36 hours; I will come and see him by and by."*

Surprisingly, St. Martin survived, and after approximately 10 months, his wound was largely healed, but a gastric fistula remained. During this time, Beaumont had been actively involved in the care of St. Martin. By this stage, St. Martin had become penniless; the county authorities, refusing further support, proposed transporting him 1,500 miles back to his birthplace in Canada. Beaumont opposed the proposal, fearing for the safety of his patient and wishing to study his condition further. In April of 1823, Beaumont moved his patient into his own home, where he remained for almost 2 years under constant care and attention. In 1824, Beaumont had sent his commanding officer (Surgeon General Lovell) a manuscript concerning this patient. It was published in the Medical Recorder as *A Case of Wounded Stomach* by Joseph Lovell, Surgeon General, U.S.A. The oversight resulting in Beaumont's omission as an author was soon remedied, and he was instated as a coauthor.

At this stage, Beaumont recognized the unique opportunity that St. Martin's gastric fistula presented and began his epic investigation into gastric function and digestion. In 1826, his first paper was published, but, unfortunately, further studies were curtailed by his military transfer to Fort Niagara and the disappearance of St. Martin into Canada. It took Beaumont until 1829 to locate St. Martin and arrange a job for him with the American Fur Company. Under the auspices of the company, St. Martin was sent to Fort Crawford on the Upper Mississippi River, where Beaumont was then stationed. During the next 2 years, many experiments were performed, but not long afterward, St. Martin and his family became so homesick and discontented that they returned to Canada.

William Beaumont (right) was born on November 25, 1785, in Lebanon, Connecticut, and began his study of medicine at the age of 22 years. During the War of 1812, he accepted a position in the army as an acting surgeon's mate and thereafter returned to civilian life. His investigation of the gastric fistula (inset) of Alexis St. Martin (left) at Fort Mackinac (background) led to the elucidation of the basics of gastric physiology and the process of digestion. Martin was an unwilling experimental subject, and Beaumont secured his services by signing him up as an employee of the military (inserted document).

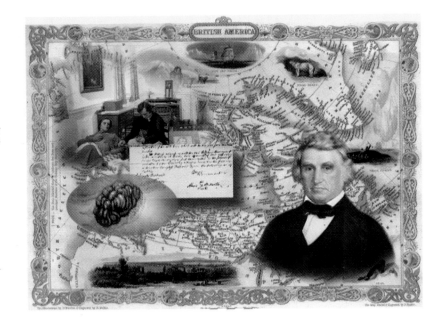

Studying St. Martin had by now become an obsession for Beaumont, and he attempted to travel to Europe with him for further scientific investigation. Although this proposed trip failed, he was, with the help of Lovell, able to enlist St. Martin in the United States Army to forestall any further episodes of abscondment, which would hence be regarded as desertion. Thereafter, Beaumont entered into a formal written agreement with St. Martin as his "human guinea pig." In return for allowing the study of his stomach and digestion, St. Martin was to receive board, lodging, and a certain sum of money for the year.

Despite being an unpleasant and dissolute person to work with, St. Martin was studied by Beaumont without further interruption until November 1, 1833. At this stage, he again disappeared into Canada, and Beaumont was

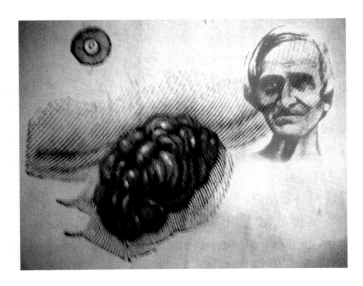

The gastric fistula of Alexis St. Martin. Through this "window in the stomach," Beaumont was able to peer into the chamber of acid secretion and elucidate the principles of gastric digestion. Despite his reprobate behavior and the serious medical problem constituted by the fistula, St. Martin (inset) actually outlived Beaumont.

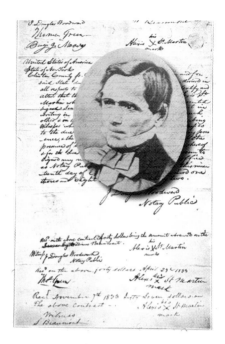

Alexis St. Martin at the age of 67 years (inset). In a novel and creative attempt to permanently secure the services of his patient, Beaumont arranged a contract (background) whereby St. Martin was used by the U.S. Army and paid as an experimental subject.

never able again to work with him. St. Martin died at the age of 83 and, in fact, outlived his physician, Beaumont, by several years.

Beaumont studied the physiologic manifestation of digestion and produced a classic text on the subject in 1833. Despite his lack of training as a physiologist and his relatively unsophisticated medical background, Beaumont's work remained a model on the subject. In essence, by 1833, Beaumont had been able to outline the basic principles of digestion in a human and establish the presence of hydrochloric acid in gastric juice.

Although the studies of a patient with gastric fistula were unique for North America in the nineteenth century, in Europe, similar observations had been made previously. In 1797, Jacob Anton Helm of Vienna studied a 58-year-old woman, Therese Petz of Breitenwaida, who had a spontaneous gastric fistula. Using a hired person, Zyriak Sieddeler, and himself, with his own brother as a control, Helm performed meticulous studies of digestion, intragastric temperature, and salivary function. Helm had no skills in chemistry, and he did not measure acid, nor was he able to demonstrate a change in the color of dye to indicate the presence of acid.

Similarly, in 1801, Rouilly transferred to the care of Dupuytren and Bichat in Paris a patient, Madeline Gore, with a gastric fistula. Gore's gastric juice was analyzed by Clarion, a professor of chemistry, who performed the first quantitative assessment of gastric juice. Clarion found neither acid nor alkali and concluded that gastric juice was identical to saliva. This conclusion remained dogma in the French medical profession so that, even in 1812, when Montegre reported acid in fasting and meal-stimulated gastric juice, he attributed this acid to the digestion of food and saliva.

The gastric fistula of Madeline Gore (right). At the age of 20 years, she fell down stone stairs and thereafter always walked bent over to the left. Eighteen years later, she developed a lump over her stomach that broke down and became a fistula through which food passed. The gastric fistula of Therese Petz (left), with the frontispiece of the *Gesundheits–Taschenbuch* of 1803, documenting Jacob Helm of Vienna's experience with this patient. She died in 1802 after having been studied for 5 years. Helm's report documented digestion and to a large extent repeated observations that had previously been detailed by Spallanzani and Gosse.

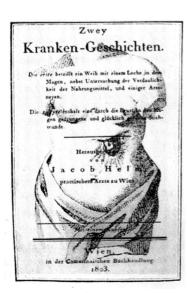

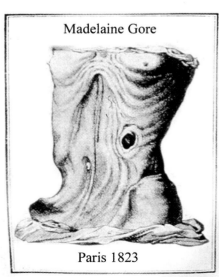

By the sixteenth century, there still existed considerable controversy as to the events that occurred in the lumen of the stomach. A number of reactionary and thoughtful individuals, including Paracelsus, Van Helmont, and Spallanzani, had written effectively about their individual concepts of gastric function. Their ideas ranged from chemical principles of an undefined nature, to *archei* (spirits), to the presence of acid, as proposed by Spallanzani. Many investigators in numerous countries considered the fundamental problem of digestion at many different levels. Of particular interest was the philosophic approach used by individuals who, although learned, had no formal training in science. Most interesting among these was the gourmand Brillat-Savarin.

Jean Anthelme Brillat-Savarin (1755–1826)

The preoccupation of the French with food was never better exemplified than in the life and writings of the gourmet Brillat-Savarin. Indeed, his philosophic observation antedated by many years the concept of the central modulation of gastric secretion.

He worked in Paris for years on a book called *The Physiology of Taste*, which was finally published in 1825. It consisted of a series of thoughtful essays that detailed his ideas regarding the preparation of food, its role in philosophy and life, and the role of digestion and different foods in behavior. Chapters include discussions of osmazomes, the erotic power of truffles, the nature of digestion, and the dangers of acids. Much of the content of this work reflects Savarin's interactions with philosophers and physicians of his time. Indeed, guests at his table included Napoleon's physician Corvisart, the surgeon Dupuytren, the pathologist Cruveilhier, and other great literary and scientific minds of his time. Conversations among these individuals would no doubt have provided Brillat-Savarin with considerable information regarding the chemistry of food and its relationship to the physiology of digestion.

Jean Anthelme Brillat-Savarin (1755–1826) (bottom) and the frontispiece of his monumental contribution to the art of gastronomy. Savarin spent 2 years in America (as a refugee from the French revolution), initially in New York, where he taught language and played violin in an orchestra at the John Street theatre. Because New York failed to satisfy his intellectual and culinary tastes, he subsequently moved to Hartford, Connecticut, where he spent 2 years becoming familiar with American culture (sic) and food before returning to France. He believed that the chemical nature of food profoundly influenced human physiology and emotional behavior.

The question of acid in the stomach had been a vexatious one for many years. Opinions had ranged from there being no acid in the stomach at all to its originating from the pancreas. Physicians of the fifteenth and sixteenth centuries felt that any acid present in the stomach was the result of putrefaction or fermentation and did not in any way reflect an active secretory process of the body or the stomach itself. It was, however, the general opinion of physiologists up to the time of Spallanzani that a free, or at least unsaturated, acid usually existed in the stomach and was necessary for digestion. Indeed, the studies of Edward Stevens in Edinburgh and Lazzaro Spallanzani in Pavia had concluded that the antiseptic powers of gastric juices invalidated the possibility of fermentation as a means of gastric digestion.

A second controversial issue surrounded what the exact nature of the acid might be. Johann Tholde had first described the acid known as *hydrochloric acid*, although it had also been called *muriatic acid* for many years. The detection of this substance in the stomach was first reported by William Prout in 1823. At a meeting of the Royal Society in London on December 11, 1823, in a lucid and elegant

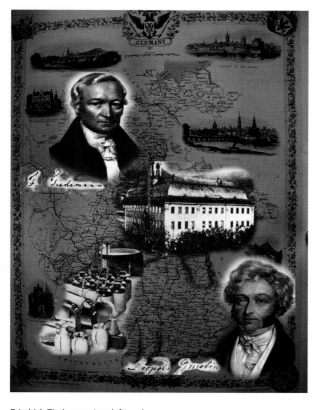

Friedrich Tiedemann (top left) and Leopold Gmelin (bottom right) of Heidelberg (center), Germany, collaborated on a series of remarkable discoveries in the field of human digestion. Together they identified that the intestines and other organs participate in the process, and not only the stomach, as previously believed. In addition, they demonstrated that digestion involved chemical transformation (the conversion of starch into glucose) and not merely dissolution, and that hydrochloric acid (bottom left) acted as a powerful agent of digestion in the stomach. They thus confirmed the earlier observations of Prout in regard to the presence of hydrochloric (muriatic) acid in the stomach.

discourse, he provided incontrovertible evidence that gastric juice of many different animals (hares, dogs, horses, cats) contained hydrochloric (muriatic) acid. In addition, Prout demonstrated that the same acid was present in dyspeptic patients, and that the amount of this acid appeared to be related to the degree of dyspepsia. Thus, the subject of the exact nature of the acid in gastric juice appeared to be resolved. Unfortunately, however, this was not to be the case, because physiologists as eminent as Claude Bernard were of the opinion that lactic acid (a product of fermentation) was present in gastric contents. Indeed, as late as 1885, Ewald and Boas reported that all acid present in the stomach at the beginning of a meal was lactic. It was their theory that hydrochloric acid gradually replaced the lactic acid during eating, with the result that, by the end of a meal, only hydrochloric acid was evident.

The French Académie des Sciences was interested in the exact nature of acid in the stomach and established an essay contest for which it offered a prize of 3,000 Francs for the answer to this question. A panel of distinguished judges was selected to evaluate the essays. One year later, the prize was awarded jointly to Leuret and Lassaigne of Paris and Tiedemann and Gmelin of Heidelberg. Leuret and Lassaigne declared that the acid in gastric juice was lactic, whereas Tiedemann and Gmelin confirmed Prout's earlier observations that it was hydrochloric acid. When asked to share the prize, the Germans declined and withdrew, having been offended by the contradiction provided by the judges. At this time, Berzelius was regarded as the ranking authority on chemistry in Europe. As a result, his comments on the literature were anxiously scanned by authors in an attempt to gauge the level of acceptance of their thoughts. Thus, Wöhler, in a letter of May 17, 1828, told Berzelius how pleased Tiedemann and Leopold Gmelin were to have noted in the *Årsberättelser* 7, 297 the deprecatory comments of Berzelius about the "*unbedeutende Arbeit*" of Leuret and Lassaigne.

The publication in Paris of the studies of Leuret and Lassaigne in 1825 defined their contribution to gastrointestinal physiology. Although they presciently noted that duodenal acid stimulated pancreatic secretion, they erroneously concluded that the stomach secreted lactic acid. Nevertheless, the French Academy of Science judged their work to be of adequate merit to share the prize with Tiedemann and Gmelin of Heidelberg, who had correctly concluded that Prout of London was correct and that gastric juice contained hydrochloric acid.

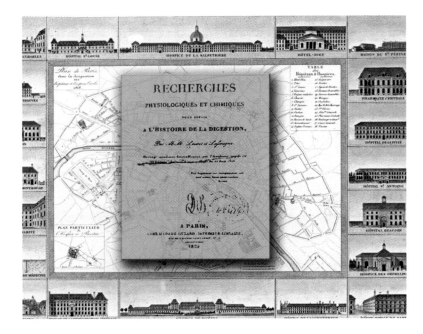

The work of Leuret and Lassaigne was not inconsequential. Their experimental studies on dogs demonstrated for the first time that acid introduced into the duodenum elicited the secretion of pancreatic juice and bile.

Seventy years later, in 1894, a student of Pavlov, Ivan Leukich Dolinsky, rediscovered this effect and noted that acid in the duodenum of the dog stimulated pancreatic secretion. It was on the basis of the earlier French observations that William Bayliss and his brother-in-law, Ernest Starling, on the afternoon of January 16, 1901, tested Dolinsky's thesis and proved the existence of chemical messengers (hormones) that regulated secretion.

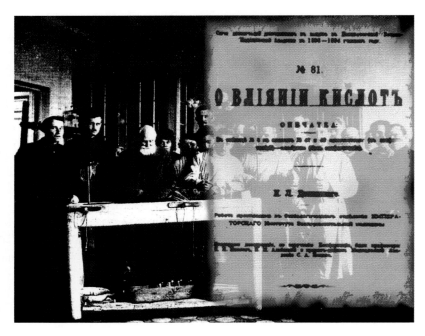

In 1894, Dolinsky, a member of Pavlov's laboratory group (background) published his thesis (right) accurately detailing the ability of acid in the duodenum to stimulate pancreatic secretion. Unfortunately, his fervent adherence to the Pavlovian concept of "nervism" led him to the erroneous conclusion that the mechanism of the phenomenon was neural in origin.

Concepts of digestion

Claude Bernard (1813–1878) was born of a modest family in the town of Saint Julien on the Rhône; he attended a Jesuit college at Villefranche and then became a pharmacist's assistant in Lyon. Bernard is best known for his book on experimental physiology, in which he outlined a number of the major concepts that he felt were critical to the pursuit of physiologic science. In particular, his delineation of the "milieu intérieur" has remained one of the critical physiologic observations ever made.

Apart from his numerous contributions, which included the identification of the glycogenic function of the liver and the delineation of the vasomotor mechanism, Bernard was noted for his contributions to the study of digestion. Before his work, it had been held that gastric digestion itself encompassed all digestive physiology. Bernard, however, demonstrated that "*gastric digestion is only a preparatory act*" and in particular delineated the enzymatic role of the pancreas. He demonstrated that pancreatic juice emulsified fat, converted starch into sugar, and was a solvent for proteins undigested by the stomach. Bernard was a creative investigator and had adopted Nicholas Blondlot's canine model of the gastric fistula for the study of gastric secretion. In 1840, Blondlot of Nancy, a surgeon, had used Bernard's innovative experimental model to determine that there was no acid or chloride in the stomach and concluded that the active principle was 1% calcium phosphate. Blondlot had been inspired to devise his canine model after reading of Beaumont's studies of Alexis St. Martin. His innovative work in this area was later taken up by Pavlov, who constructed a series of vagally innervated and denervated pouches to evaluate the effects of neural regulation on gastric secretion. This was the so-called Pavlov pouch, which formed the basis of many of the subsequent experimental models used by the great physiologist and his pupils.

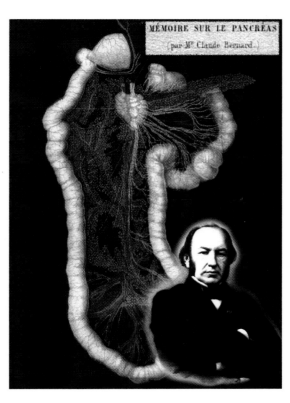

Before Bernard's work on the pancreas, it had been held that gastric digestion itself encompassed all digestive physiology. Bernard, however, identified that "*gastric digestion is only a preparatory act*" and in particular delineated the enzymatic role of the pancreas. This work was published in 1856 as the *Mémoire sur le Pancreas* (top) (*Memoir on the Pancreas: And the Role of Pancreatic Juice in Digestive Processes Particularly in the Digestion of Neutral Fat*). The seminal observations of Bernard on the digestive actions of the pancreas have been eponymously credited by naming the inner layer of cells lining the acinar complex the *glandular layer of Bernard*.

Vagal function and gastric function

Investigations on the vagus nerve began 2,000 years ago. Marinus, in the first century AD, studied the anatomy of the vagi and was the first to assign to the cranial nerves a numeric sequence. Although none of the original work by Mari-

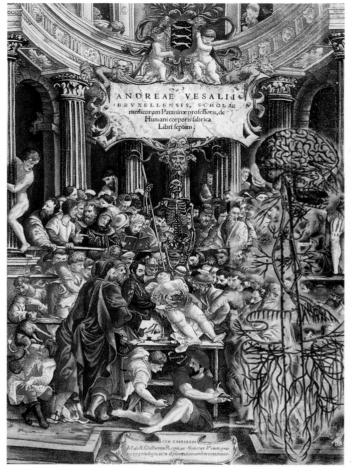

The Vesalian (1543) concept of the distribution of the vagus nerve (right) to the viscera was contained in *De Humani Corporis Fabrica Libri* (1543). The book was dedicated to the Holy Roman Emperor, Charles V, and was printed by Johannes Oporinus of Basel, the printing blocks having been carried by mule over the Alps from Padua. They survived intact in the library of Munich until July 16, 1944, when the building was destroyed by an Allied air raid. The unique treatise of Vesalius provided the basis for a completely novel understanding of human anatomy. Its illustrations were undertaken by Jan Stephan van Calcar, a fellow Belgian and one-time pupil of Titian. Vesalius was a unique individual who combined intellectual vigor with clinical acumen. He epitomized the early traditional role of the surgeon as a clinician whose knowledge of anatomy facilitated surgical intervention. In the colored frontispiece, Vesalius is depicted as the demonstrator, while Calcar included himself as the artist in the front row. (Copyright J. Norman & Co., Inc.)

nus survives today, Galen cited his studies in the second-century anatomy text *On the Usefulness of the Parts of the Body.*

Galen, who was born in Pergamon Mysia, which is now part of Turkey, in 130 AD, expanded on the work of Marinus by speculating on the possible function of the nerves to the stomach:

The stomach must have very accurate perception of the need for food and drink. Hence, most of these nerves seem to be distributed to its so-called [cardiac] orifice and afterwards to all the other portions of it as far as its lower end.

The anatomy of the vagus undoubtedly contributed to the name applied to it. The term *vagus*, or *per vagum*, means "wandering part." A more anatomically correct name was given to the nerve in the early nineteenth century, when the term *pneumogastric* appeared in the French and Italian literature. It then became a frequent term in the English and American literature. In Germany, however, the nerve was always referred to as the vagus. Thus, by the end of the nineteenth century, when German scientific research attained prominence, the term *pneumogastric* fell from common usage in the surgical community.

Once its anatomy became better defined, studies into vagal function were initiated. In 1814, Brodie published some of the first known experiments on vagal physiology and gastric function. In the report of his findings to the Royal Society of London, he noted that his work was inspired by Edward Home's report of "*some facts which render it probable that the various animal secretions are dependent on the influence of the nervous system.*" Home, in fact, studied secretion in the electric eel:

Since in these fish the abundance of nerves connected with the electrical organs proves that this power resides in them, and since the arrangement of many nerves in animal bodies has evidently no connexion with sensation, it seems not improbable that these may answer the purpose of supplying and regulating the organs of secretion.

Thus, the observation by Home of the electric eel inspired Brodie to be the first to perform the surgical procedure that is now accepted as a vagotomy. The pioneering work of Brodie, however, was not on humans but on a total of four dogs. His first experiment was a bilateral cervical vagotomy.

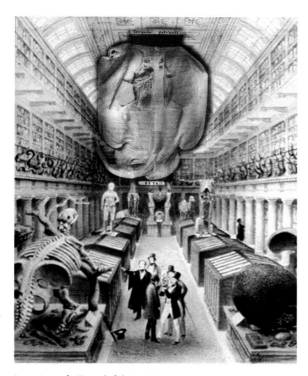

A specimen of a Torpedo fish (c. 1810) (top) from the original collection of John Hunter at the Royal College of Surgeons of England (background). It was used to study the concept of the "electrical activity" that resided in nerves.

He noted that this operation prevented arsenic-stimulated gastric secretion but was complicated by the development of severe respiratory compromise. To remedy the subsequent respiratory embarrassment, he modified his procedure to that of a subdiaphragmatic vagotomy. With the latter operation, the animals no longer experienced the "laborious breathing" and circulatory arrest observed during cervical vagotomy.

The earlier findings of "no watery or mucous fluid in the stomach or small intestines" seen with the cervical vagotomy were confirmed in the animals that underwent abdominal vagotomy. Brodie concluded *"that the suppression of secretion in all of them was to be attributed solely to the division of the nerves: and all of the facts which have been stated sufficiently demonstrate, that the secretions of the stomach are very much under the control of the nervous system."* This observation was a watershed in the history of gastrointestinal physiology, as the concept of nervous control of gastrointestinal secretion had not been previously demonstrated.

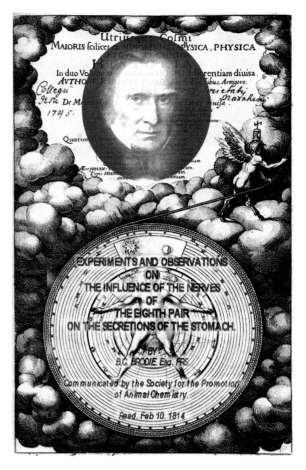

The frontispiece of the original description by Brodie of the effects of the VIII nerve. Because not all the cranial nerves had been recognized and different authors used their own individual schemata, the vagus was referred to as the VIII nerve until the reclassification by Thomas Sommering of the nomenclature in 1791.

Ivan Pavlov as a youth (inset). Born in 1849, the first son of an impoverished priest in Ryazan, Russia, he was awarded a Nobel Prize in 1904 for research on the activity of the digestive glands. Pavlov regarded his initial studies with the physiologist Elie Tsyon as his inspiration and his subsequent work with Heidenhain of Breslau and Ludwig of Leipzig as having been critical to his success. The scientific rigor of his thought was dramatically amplified by his unusual ambidextrous surgical skills as well as his ability to devise unique experimental models (background). It was often stated that surgery in the experimental laboratory of Pavlov was safer than that in most Russian medical facilities of the time.

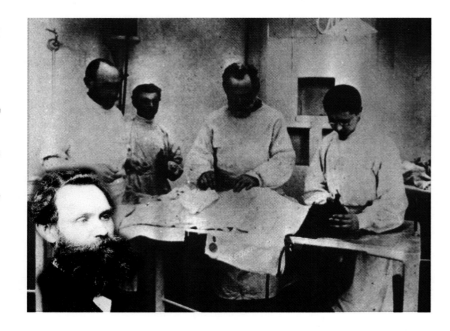

Pavlov's delineation of vagal function

Later in the nineteenth century, Rokitansky and Bernard confirmed the findings of Brodie when they observed decreased gastric secretion and motility after vagotomy. Despite the contributions of these eminent physiologists, the modern era of the study of vagal physiology was initiated and dominated by Ivan P. Pavlov. Although he achieved principal recognition for his investigation of conditioned reflexes, his methods and the results of his observations on vagal function laid the foundation for the subsequent study of the nervous control of gastrointestinal function.

Pavlov was a graduate of the Medico-Chirurgical Academy in St. Petersburg, Russia, in the late nineteenth century. His scientific philosophy was greatly influenced by the work of Lister and Pasteur. Pavlov's theory of "nervism" was a momentous postulate for the times in which he lived. He explained it as "*a physiological theory which tries to prove that the nervous system controls the greatest possible number of bodily activities.*" It was from the hypothesis of nervism that Pavlov investigated the effects of vagal stimuli on gastric secretion.

A vagally innervated Pavlov pouch (top right, bottom left). These studies were undertaken by P. P. Khigine in collaboration with Pavlov. Confusion arose as to the authorship, because the work was performed by P. P. Khizhin, but, when it was published, Pavlov's name was omitted, and the student's name translated into the French form, Khigine. In keeping with the creative nature of Pavlov was the strategy whereby the dogs used for studies provided gastric juice that served as a source of research income for the laboratory. Thus, large volumes of the juice were sold to Germany, where it was used as a rejuvenant medication for elderly men seeking to restore their vital fluids and potency.

Initially, he examined the work of his predecessors and recognized that most of their experiments used cervical separation of the vagi. With this protocol,

Pavlov observed that most of the body functions of the animals "came to a standstill." The first studies performed in his newly created modern operating rooms generated canine surgical models with diverted cervical esophagi.

Thus, Pavlov devised a simple method for studying the cephalic phase of gastric function. The dogs were then fed and their gastric outputs measured. It was evident that up to 700 mL of the "purest gastric juice" was secreted by the stomachs of the dogs after the sham feeding. After cervical esophageal diversion, subdiaphragmatic vagotomy was undertaken, and it was evident that secretion of gastric juice was dramatically reduced after sham feeding. "*It is obvious,*" Pavlov concluded, "*that the effect of feeding was transmitted by nervous channels to the gastric glands.*" Final confirmation of this finding was obtained by excitation of the vagi of the dogs with electrical impulses and the observation of increased gastric secretion.

Ulcer models and EGF

In 1940, the genesis of the ulcer disease was still unknown. Controversy continued regarding the role of the vagus or of chemical regulators in generating increased acid secretion. Without a defined regulatory system for acid secretion, no rational understanding of ulcer biology could be derived. Experimental models of ulcers had been produced under a number of circumstances. Anton Wölfer, who had performed the first gastrojejunostomy as treatment for peptic ulcer in Theodor Billroth's Vienna clinic in 1881, noted that an ulcer at the stoma followed in up to 34% of his patients.

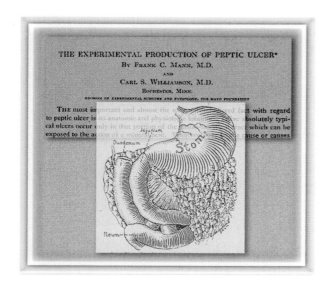

Subsequently, Frank Mann of the Mayo Clinic noted that the neostomal ulcers resulting from gastrojejunostomy reflected a critical relevance of the anatomic and physiologic location of the lesion. He devised the Mann-Williamson experimental operation, which was used for the next 30 years as the basic test for a new procedure to prevent or cure a peptic ulcer.

The procedure was constructed to enable the duodenum to drain its secretions and those of the pancreas and liver at a distance from the pylorus. Ten of the first 14 of Mann's and Williamson's dogs had chronic ulcers at the point where the gastric contents impinged on the jejunal mucosa. At this stage, the beneficial effects of urogastrone, which had been identified by David J. Sandweiss, a gastroenterologist at the Harper Hospital in Detroit, were studied. He had noted that out of 70,310 gravid women admitted to the hospital, only one exhibited a peptic ulcer and proposed that a substance secreted in the urine of pregnant women might be used in the treatment of peptic ulcer disease. Sandweiss and his colleagues were able to demonstrate some signs of fibroblastic proliferation and healing of ulcers in dogs and some amelioration of symptoms in humans.

The initial report of Williamson and Mann detailing the technique of the experimental preparation they had devised to generate peptic ulcer disease (top). The subsequent widespread usage of the Mann-Williamson model provided the experimental surgical basis for the evaluation of the role of acid in the genesis of ulcer disease (bottom).

By 1940, Gray had prepared a pyrogen-free inhibitor from the urine and named it *urogastrone*. In 1967, Harry Gregory of Imperial Chemical Industries, in a preliminary report, stated that he had prepared a pure urogastrone that consisted of 28 amino acids. In 1975, however, he published a composition of urogastrone that had a sequence of 53 amino acids and was similar to epidermal growth factor. In this paper, Gregory commented that, more than 30 years previously, Sandweiss had observed that urogastrone *"produced a beneficial effect on experimental ulcers by promoting fibroblastic proliferation and epithelialization of the mucosa."*

The role of histamine

The first experiments with histamine

The regulation of acid secretion, however, was to require a completely different route to establish a therapeutic basis for management. The unwitting initiator of the research that would lead finally to the development of the H_2 receptor antagonists was Henry Dale.

Working with the chemist George Barger, Dale applied Kutscher's silver method to a specimen of ergot dialysatum and *"isolated a few centigrams of the picrate of an intensively active base, which produced a characteristic action on the cat's non-pregnant uterus in a minute dose."* Barger and Dale identified the base as beta-imidazolylethylamine and compared it with an authentic sample that had been obtained by the putrefaction of histidine.

The supplement of the *Oxford English Dictionary* attributes the first use of the term *histamine* to the *Journal of Chemistry*, civ.,

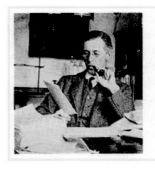

"Beta-1, as we called it, is, of course, the now almost too familiar histamine; and this was always the obvious name for it. Somebody, however, had objected to its use, as infringing his trademark rights in a name to which its resemblance was, in fact, only distant. Later somebody called it histamine and then the road was clear."

Henry Hallett Dale (c. 1915). At the age of 29 years, Dale accepted a research position at the Welcome Physiological Laboratory to obtain finances to marry. His employer, Henry Williams, in a letter to him requested *"that when Dale could find the opportunity for it without interfering with plans of his own, it would give him special satisfaction if he (Dale) would make an attempt to clear up the problem of ergot . . . ."* In 1936, Dale was awarded the Nobel Prize for his contribution with Otto Loewi to the chemical transmission of nerve impulses (acetylcholine). The Nazi government subsequently demanded that Loewi surrender the prize to the Third Reich to secure safe passage from Vienna!

1913. Dale worked extensively in the area of the pharmacologic and physiologic actions of histamine between 1910 and 1927 but failed to detect his role in promoting acid secretion by the glands of the stomach.

It remained for Leon Popielski, a student of Pavlov, to identify the acid-secretory effects of histamine. After leaving Pavlov's laboratory in 1901, Popielski had been placed in charge of the military bacteriologic laboratory in Moscow. His initial work was on the mechanism of the intravenous injection of Witte's peptone (a peptic digest of fibrin) in causing a fall in blood pressure. This research continued after he had become the Professor of Pharmacology at the University of Lemberg, and Popielski believed that he had identified a substance, *"vaso dilantine,"* as a component of Witte's peptone distinct from histamine or choline. On October 28, 1916, in the course of experiments on the effect of the injection of an extract of the pituitary gland on gastric secretion, Popielski injected 32 mg of beta-imidazolylethylamine hydrochloride subcutaneously into a dog with a gastric fistula. Over the next 5.75 hours, the dog secreted 937.5 mL of gastric juice having a maximum acidity of 0.166 N. Because similarly stimulated secretion was unaffected by section of the vagus

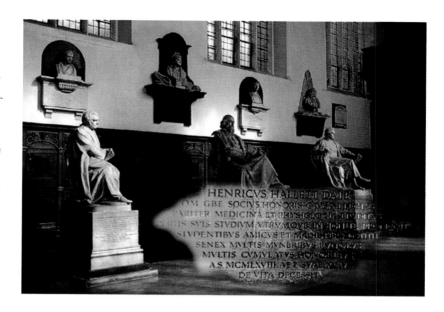

The antechamber of Trinity Chapel, Cambridge (background), with the memorial epitaph of Dale (inset). It reads, "*Sir Henry Hallett Dale O.M., G.B.E., Honorary Fellow. Equally learned in medicine and in physiology, he signally advanced both disciplines by his discoveries. He stood by his students as friend and teacher. After a long life with many responsibilities he died in 1968 at the age of ninety-three.*" The inscription on the base of the statue of Isaac Newton (left), "*Qui genus humanum ingenio superavit*" ("*He surpassed the race of men in understanding*"), is applicable in terms of the contributions of Dale to biochemistry. Despite his elucidation of the subject of histamine in 1936, he and Otto Loewi were jointly awarded the Nobel Prize for their discoveries relating to the chemical transmission (acetylcholine) of nerve impulses.

or by atropine, Popielski concluded that beta-imidazolylethylamine acts directly on the gastric glands.

Due to World War I, Popielski's paper describing these results was unfortunately not published until 1920.

Clinical relevance of histamine in gastric secretion

The key protagonist in the elucidation of the role of histamine and its clinical relevance in gastric secretion was Charlie Code. Code had grown up in Winnipeg and received an M.D. degree from the University of Manitoba in 1933. He worked at the Mayo Clinic with Frank Mann, then obtained support to study in London, where he first worked with Charles Lovatt Evans at the University College of London. In his further studies with Sir Henry Dale at the National Institutes for Medical Research, Code demonstrated that 70% to 100% of histamine in unclotted blood is in the white-cell layer, and that clotting liberates 60% to 90% of this into the serum.

Code continued to be fascinated by the effect of histamine and its bioactivity. Because its rapid disappearance from the blood made it difficult to study, he developed the technique of suspending histamine in beeswax that was then injected subcutaneously. The biologic test for the effectiveness of histamine liberation was to measure the acid secretion of the animal. In these studies of histamine-stimulated acid secretion from the Heidenhain pouches of dogs, Code was assisted by the surgeons Owen Wangensteen and Richard Varco. It became apparent that, with increasing doses of histamine and increasing acid secretion, duodenal ulcers could be initiated not only in dogs, but also in a number of other animal species, including chickens, woodchucks, calves, monkeys, and rabbits. Code concluded that the experiments incriminated gastric juice as the factor in the production of peptic ulcer and noted the relationship of histamine to this event.

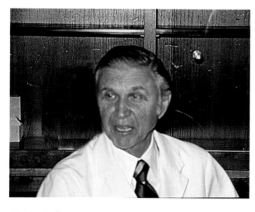

Charles Code (c. 1978). Using a unique blend of perceptive inquiry, rigorous investigative methodology, and shrewd common sense, Code carefully defined the role of histamine as a principal physiologic regulator of parietal cell secretion. In addition to his delineation of histamine as a secretory agonist, he postulated the presence of a gastric "histaminocyte" and explored the mechanisms of mucosal injury, thus providing the basis for defining the pathogenesis of the ulcer lesion.

The establishment of the role of acid in the genesis of peptic ulceration was supported by studies undertaken jointly by I. N. Marks (left) and W. Card (right) of Cape Town and Edinburgh, respectively, who concluded that acid secretion was a function of parietal cell mass. They established that histamine stimulation could be used to assess the function of the parietal cell mass. This work facilitated the recognition that acid output, parietal cell mass, and peptic ulceration were inextricably linked. As a result of these physio-pathologic observations, a rational basis was provided for the consideration of acid reduction—initially surgically and subsequently by pharmacotherapeutic means—as a definitive intervention in the management of acid peptic disease.

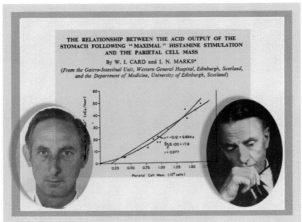

Parietal cell mass, acid secretion, and histamine

The precise relationship of histamine to acid secretion was firmly established by Andrew Kay of Glasgow, who had developed the augmented histamine test. Mepyramine maleate was used to block the systemic effects of histamine. The ability of histamine to stimulate acid secretion was measured at a dose of 0.1 mg per 10.0 kg of body weight and maximal acid secretion determined in different groups of patients. The dose-response curves for acid secretion in human subjects in response to intravenous infusion of histamine were subsequently determined by Wilfred Card of the Western General Hospital in Edinburgh in conjunction with I. N. Marks.

Marks and Card then applied their method of estimating parietal cell mass to 17 patients with duodenal ulceration, chronic gastric ulceration, or carcinoma of the stomach whose stomachs had been removed at surgery. They were able to establish that the maximal acid output correlated with the parietal cell mass using quadratic-equation analysis. Thereafter, Marks, working with Simon Komarov and Harry Shay at the Fels Research Institute of the Temple University of Philadelphia, was able to correlate the maximal secretory response of dogs to the estimated total parietal cell mass of each stomach.

The identification of effective antihistaminic agents

Parallel to the evaluation of the pathogenesis of peptic ulcer disease and the pharmacology of histamine, a strong interest developed in identifying agents that might prevent the action of histamine. By 1957, a long list of antihistaminic agents had been proposed and studied by Keir and his colleagues, without identification of an agent effective in the inhibition of acid secretion. In 1966, A. S. F. Ash and H. O. Schild of University College London stated

The structure of histamine and the various modifications undertaken to produce cimetidine, a clinically effective H$_2$ receptor blocking agent without the serious side effects of the earlier compounds.

At present, no specific antagonist is known for the secretory stimulant action of histamine in the stomach.

Ash and Schild suggested the symbol H_1 for receptors that are specifically antagonized by low concentrations of antihistaminic drugs, implying that there is another class of histamine receptors that mediates the acid secretory action of histamine.

At this stage, James Black, a pharmacologist working for Smith Kline and French in Welwyn Garden City, England, provided an observation of considerable significance. After synthesizing and testing "about 700 compounds," his group in 1972 announced that a compound (burimamide), which possessed an imidazole ring but with a side chain much bulkier than that of histamine, antagonized the responses to histamine that were not antagonized by drugs acting on the H_1 receptor. Included in these responses was the inhibition of the secretion of acid. Black, therefore, proposed that there existed a homogeneous population of non-H_1 receptors, which he chose to term *H_2 receptors*.

It was evident that burimamide inhibited pentagastrin-stimulated, as well as histamine-stimulated, acid secretion, and Black suggested that H_2 blockade might resolve the long-debated question of whether histamine was the final common mediator of acid secretion.

The presence of histamine in the gastric mucosa

Thus, the wheel had turned the full circle from Pavlovian nervism to the moment of the chemical mediator. It was now clear that there was a chemical phase of the stimulation of gastric secretion in addition to the nervous phase that Pavlov had done so much to establish.

At a Ciba Foundation symposium held in honor of Sir Henry Dale in London on April 6 and 7, 1955, Charlie Code began his contribution by saying:

An overwhelming mass of decisive evidence is now available showing that stimulation of gastric secretion is a physiological function of histamine.

The evidence for histamine being present in the gastric mucosa had initially been presented by John Jacob Abel on April 25, 1919. Abel was convinced that all the *"motilines, peristaltic hormones, vaso dilantins and histamine-like substances in tissues were one and the same substance—histamine."*

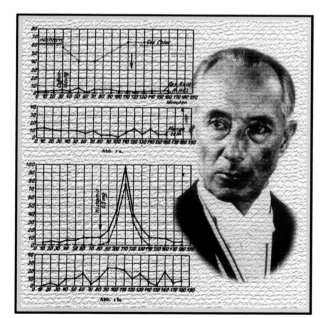

Gerhard Katsch of Greifswald (1887–1961). Katsch introduced quantitative gastric function tests (1925) with fractionated sampling using caffeine or histamine ("kinetic method") to evaluate gastric secretory capacity. In addition to his contributions to gastroenterology, he founded the first center in Germany for the education and care of diabetics.

He succeeded in isolating and identifying histamine as the pictrate in extracts of the pituitary gland and stated that *"histamine is the essential therapeutically active constituent of the hypophysis."* Subsequently, Code demonstrated significantly more histamine in the oxyntic mucosa than in the antrum. Wilhelm Feldberg and Jeffrey Harris then sought the cellular locus of histamine in the gastric mucosa. The highest concentration was identified as near the lumen, where the parietal cells are at their

Histamine staining of the enterochromaffin-like (ECL) cells (red arrows) in rat gastric mucosa. Their apparently random distribution in the gastric gland belies the fact that each ECL cell exhibits a dendritic arborization that forms a syncytium to envelop a number of parietal cells. Thus, when activated by gastrin, each ECL cell releases histamine from its processes and stimulates an aggregation of parietal cells.

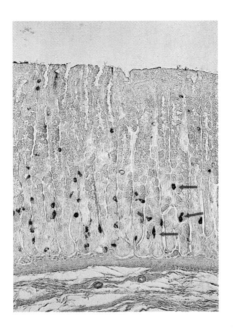

greatest density, and in the region of the muscularis mucosa. In 1959, A. N. Smith, a Glasgow surgeon, found a similar distribution of histamine in the human gastric mucosa and noted that histamine had no higher concentration in tissues from patients with duodenal ulcer and high rates of acid secretion than in those from patients with gastric cancer and low rates of acid secretion.

R. Thunberg of Lund used a fluorescent method for detecting histamine in the mucosa and noted a high concentration in the region of the parietal cells and a low concentration in the submucosa. He noted that the cells in the submucosa were definitely mast cells, but those lying close to the parietal cells did not stain like mast cells.

Charles Herbert Best (1899–1978) (c. 1928) was born in Maine, the son of a physician who had joined the Canadian artillery during World War I, and thus qualified for Canadian citizenship. Best was still a medical student at the University of Toronto when he joined Frederick Banting in his work to isolate the pancreatic hormone insulin and apply it to the treatment of diabetes. The work had personal significance for Best, as his favorite aunt had recently died of the disease. Best finished his medical degree in 1925, 2 years after Banting and the physiology professor J. J. Macleod received the Nobel Prize for the work. Banting, who felt that Best should have been recognized by the Nobel Prize committee as well, gave half of his monetary award to Best. Macleod then shared his with J. B. Collip, the chemist who had worked with them to purify insulin for clinical trials. After continuing his studies in Canada, the United States, and Europe, Best returned to the University of Toronto in 1929 and became the chairman of the physiology department. After the death of Banting in 1941, Best was appointed director of the Banting-Best Department of Medicine Research. During this period, he worked extensively in the area of histamine and described the enzyme histaminase.

J. PHYSIOL LXX, 1930

THE INACTIVATION OF HISTAMINE.

BY C. H. BEST AND E. W. McHENRY

(From the Department of Physiological Hygiene, University of Toronto.)

THE transient effects produced [...] travenous or subcutaneous injection of small or moderate [...] ine suggest that the body may possess an efficient [...] n or inactivation of this substance. When histami[...] intravenously, relatively large amounts can be adm[...] appearance of the characteristic signs which the [...] f small quantities to the same animal produce. It [...] t very little histamine is found in the urine even aft[...] njection of large doses of the substance [Oehme, 191[...]ty that the amine may be eliminated by passage from th[...] to the intestine has not been investigated.

Eugen Werle had demonstrated in 1936 that an enzyme present in guinea pig tissues converts histidine to histamine by decarboxylating the substrate. The activity of this enzyme was characterized as the histamine-forming capacity, and it was believed that histamine formation and histamine storage occurred in the same cells. In 1965, R. S. Levine of Yale demonstrated that when histidine decarboxylase (HDC) was blocked with a hydrazino analog of histidine, the histamine concentration within the gastric mucosa of the rat was reduced. Kahlson was convinced that histamine was essential for exciting gastric secretion and demonstrated that histamine-forming capacity is labile. He demonstrated that the histamine content of the mucosa falls slightly when the rat is fed and reaches its nadir when the histamine-forming capacity is at its maximum.

Charles Best, who was later to achieve fame for his work in the area of insulin, had noted that histamine in fresh ox or horse lung rapidly disappears when the tissues autolyze at 37°C. Best demonstrated that the disappearance of histamine is inhibited by cyanide and concluded that an oxidated process ruptures the imidazole ring. He called the enzyme *histaminase*, but it was subsequently renamed *diamine oxidase* after it was noted to inactivate histamine

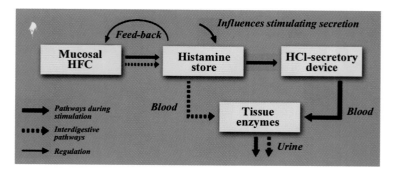

A model of histamine synthesis and mobilization in the gastric mucosa, as described by G. Kahlson in 1964. He postulated a feedback control of the histamine-forming capacity (HFC) of the mucosa by the histamine content of the mucosa itself. Some 30 years later, the validity of this prescient suggestion appears substantiated by the identification of different histamine receptor subtypes on the enterochromaffin-like cell and their ability to regulate histamine secretion.

by oxidative deamination. Code asserted that histaminase was absent from the gastric mucosa, and that histamine brought by the blood or released within the mucosa is in a preferred position, *"a most propitious and essential circumstance if minute amounts of histamine are to have their full effects on the secretory cells."*

Studying histamine in the gastric juice of dogs and cats, Nils Emmelin and Georg Kahlson noted that it was present in the juice whether spontaneously secreted or in response to stimulation of the vagus, injection of acetyl choline, or during the cephalic phase of digestion. They therefore concluded that the parietal cell activity, no matter how stimulated, involved liberation of histamine into gastric juice, and that histamine was the final common mediator.

The discovery of hormones

In 1902, Bayliss and Starling opened a new era in physiologic thought by demonstrating that there existed, besides the nervous system, a hormonal system for the integration of organ function. Before this proposal, it had been assumed that the physiologic regulation of function was entirely of neural origin. Three years later, Starling, in the delivery of his famous Croonian lectures to the Royal College of Physicians of London on "The Chemical Correlations of the Functions of the Body," was able to cite the discovery of gastrin as the second example, after secretin, of a hormone. In 1825, François Leuret and Jean Louis Lassaigne had demonstrated that, after applying vinegar to the first part of the small intestine, biliary and pancreatic juice secretion was rapidly initiated. They postulated, *"If an acid stimulates duodenal secretions and dilates the ducts of the liver and pancreas, chyme ought to do the same thing for it is always acid."*

Some 70 years later, the fact that acid in the duodenum stimulates pancreatic secretion was rediscovered in Pavlov's St. Petersburg laboratory by his student, Ivan Leukich Dolinsky.

Secretin and gastrin

On the afternoon of January 16, 1901, William Bayliss and his brother-in-law, Ernest Starling, repeated Dolinsky's original experiments. Bayliss' and Starling's conclusions were that acid liberated a chemical messenger from cells of the duodenal and jejunal mucosa, and that the messenger's traveling through the blood excited the pancreas to secrete. They named this substance *secretin* and, some years later, at the suggestion of William Hardy, used the word *hormone* to characterize a chemical messenger of this type.

In subsequent studies, they demonstrated that extracts from the mucosa of the small intestines of dogs, cats, rabbits, oxen, monkeys, frogs, and humans stimu-

Although the neural regulation of digestive activity was initially defined by Pavlov, the discovery of secretin by W. M. Bayliss (bottom left) and E. H. Starling (center right) and the elucidation of the concept of a chemical messenger system ushered in a new era of understanding of the regulation of gastrointestinal function. Bayliss was a modest and retiring individual not given to public appearances, preferring the solitude and intellectual solace of libraries and laboratories to the flurry of public debate and the power of the podium. His text, *Principles of General Physiology* (1914) (bottom), was regarded as a monumental classic of general physiology and earned him high regard. A measure of the man may be gained from the anecdote that, when offered a knighthood, he initially declined the invitation to the investiture because it clashed with a meeting of the Physiological Society! Ernest Starling was cut from a different cloth and, although as intellectually gifted as Bayliss, possessed none of his brother-in-law's reticence and understated demeanor. Rapier tongued, outspoken, and vivacious, his rhetoric and impressive public persona both inspired colleagues and awed opponents who dared to disagree. Creative, innovative, and disputatious he was, although a natural leader and a gifted administrator, hampered by sharp elbows. The presentation of the Croonian Lectures of 1905 (top) epitomized his genius and led directly to the development of an entirely novel discipline—endocrinology. Among the veritable cornucopia of scientific discoveries made by Bayliss and Starling, the masterful understatement of Charles Martin (top left) in describing the experiment that first demonstrated a chemical messenger best sums up the tenor of the time and the individuals. His meticulous experimental notes of January 16, 1901, close with the immortal line *"It was a great afternoon."* Thus was born endocrinology!

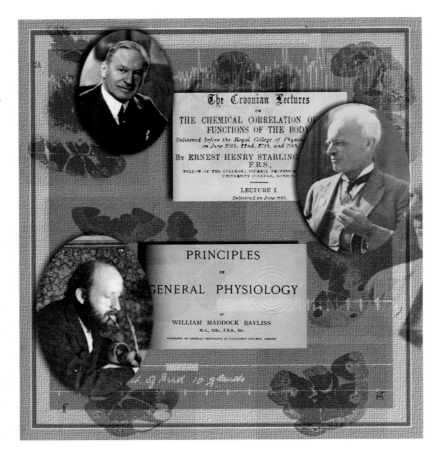

lated the secretion of normal pancreatic juice, whereas extracts of the ileum did not. In addition, they noted that secretin did not stimulate secretion of gastric juice or of succus entericus, but that it probably stimulated secretion of bile.

These observations stimulated John Sidney Edkins, a teacher of physiology at St. Bartholomew's Hospital Medical School in London, to evaluate the control of gastric secretion. Even before the studies of Bayliss and Starling and their description of secretin, Edkins had sensed that absorbed peptones might liberate a chemical messenger. His ruminations in this area led him to conclude that there might well be a "gastric secretin." On May 18, 1905, he obtained sufficient evidence to make a preliminary communication to the Royal Society on this matter. His recognition that there might be in the gastric mucosa a preformed substance that is absorbed into the portal stream and returned to the circulation to stimulate the fundic oxyntic glands was a critical hypothesis. In a modest paper entitled *On the Chemical Mechanisms of Gastric Secretion*, he described how various extracts of antral mucosa potently stimulated gastric secretion in anesthetized cats. It was unfortunate for Edkins that a large number of distinguished investigators provided substantial and "apparently incontrovertible" evidence in support of the theory that the active principal in his extract was histamine.

More than a quarter of a century was to elapse before Simon Komarov, in 1938, recognized the sad trick that nature had played on Edkins. In antral

William Bate Hardy (1864–1934). He was an avid sailor, brilliant histologist, and unorthodox thinker. Thus, F. Gowland Hopkins, in his obituary notice in the *Lancet* of 1934, noted that *"his mind was little trammeled by either tradition or the orthodox views of his day."* Hardy was the first to suggest the use of the word *hormone*, which he derived from the Greek term *hormaein* (to set in motion, excite, stimulate), to describe the agents of the chemical messenger system. Starling thereafter adopted it as a descriptive term for his proposal of a novel class of chemical messengers that would act via the blood stream.

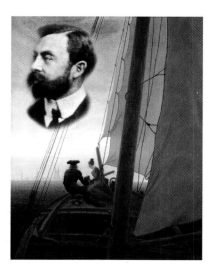

mucosa, there are both histamine and a protein-like substance with a bioactivity that mimics the action of histamine on gastric acid secretion. Komarov precipitated with trichloroacetic acid, a diluted acid extract of antral mucosa, and obtained a protein-free fraction that was histamine-free, yet strongly stimulated gastric-acid secretion. He thus rediscovered the antral hormone originally noted by Edkins.

Nevertheless, the concept of a hormonally mediated regulatory system in the gastrointestinal tract remained a considerable issue for Pavlov and the supporters of the nervism doctrine. In his biography of Pavlov, Babkin noted the turbulence generated by the observations of Bayliss and Starling as well as Edkins.

The frontispiece (center) of J. S. Edkins' (top left) epic communication, which documented the existence of a novel antral stimulant of acid secretion-gastrin (1905). Edkins entered Cambridge University as a scholar of Caius College in 1881. Such was his ability that he was awarded two scholarships: one in mathematics and the other in natural sciences. After Cambridge, he worked with C. S. Sherrington (who was later to attain a Nobel Prize in Neurophysiology) (top right) in Liverpool. Edkins taught with great distinction at St. Bartholomew's in London and subsequently became Chairman of Physiology at Bedford College for Women in 1914. In this capacity, he was responsible for training the majority of women physiologists in England between 1914 and 1930. Apart from his fundamental observations with regard to gastrin, he worked with Langley on pepsin and helped deduce the nature of pepsinogen exocytosis. It is of particular note that he was not only a great oarsman but also a superb croquet player and President of the British croquet association from 1935 to 1937. The last subject that Edkins investigated in 1923 was the presence of spiral bacteria (*Spirella regaudi*) in the gastric mucosa and their relevance to digestion.

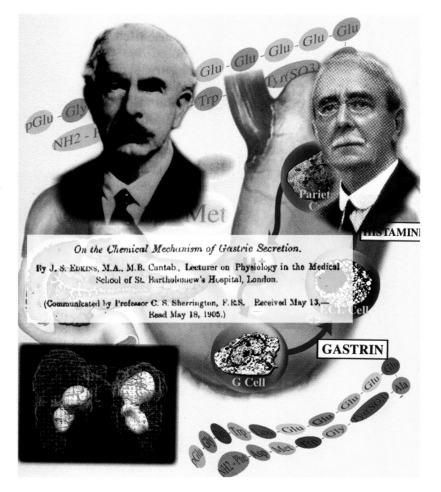

On the Chemical Mechanism of Gastric Secretion.

By J. S. EDKINS, M.A., M.B. Cantab., Lecturer on Physiology in the Medical School of St. Bartholomew's Hospital, London.

(Communicated by Professor C. S. Sherrington, F.R.S. Received May 13,— Read May 18, 1905.)

GASTRIN

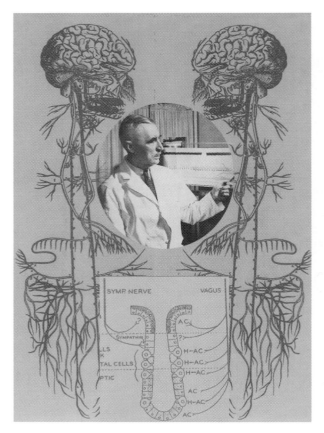

Boris Babkin (center), a pupil of Pavlov, translated the Russian scientist's views into English and was responsible for disseminating many of his ideas in North America. Babkin, himself, developed novel theories regarding the parasympathetic innervation (bottom) of the gastric glands.

I think it was in the fall of 1902 that Pavlov asked V. V. Savich to repeat the secretin experiments of Bayliss and Starling. The effect was self evident. Then, without a word, Pavlov disappeared into his study. He returned half an hour later and said: "Of course, they are right. It is clear that we did not take out an exclusive patent for the discovery of truth."

Subsequent to this admission, a series of experiments were undertaken using a unique dog model that Pavlov himself had constructed. In three successive operations, a Pavlov pouch, then a gastric fistula and a duodenal fistula were produced. In the third operation, Pavlov sectioned the pylorus between two clamps, closing both the pyloric and duodenal stumps. Because the stomach was now separated from the small intestine, continuity was established by connecting the gastric and duodenal fistulas with a glass and rubber cannula.

The experiments demonstrated that food substances (and in particular meat extracts) in the stomach stimulated acid secretion by the Pavlov pouch. This led to the conclusion that the stomach might not be a single organ but represents a body component with one function and a pyloric unit with a separate biologic responsibility. Thereafter, the pars pylorica was resected and confirmed histologically to have been completely removed. In a subsequent set of experiments, when meat extract was put into the antrectomized stomach, the Pavlov pouch failed to secrete. It was then concluded that chemical stimuli act on the mucosa of the pylorus and not on that of the body of the stomach.

In a subsequent series of experiments, Pavlov made a pouch of the pyloric antrum in a dog that also had a gastric fistula and a gastroenterostomy. He noted that introduction of chemical substances, such as meat extract, into an isolated and either innervated or denervated pyloric pouch resulted in a flow of gastric juice from the fundus. Sadly, neither Pavlov nor any of his immediate students sought to identify the nature of the chemical messenger that linked the pyloric mucosa and the oxyntic cells.

The chemical identification of gastrin: Komarov

Simon Komarov had spent 3 years (1910–1913) in Pavlov's St. Petersburg laboratory. During this time, he had met with Babkin, who had come from the United States to work with Pavlov. When Babkin became the Professor of Physiology at McGill University in 1930, he hired Komarov as his research assistant to work on the organic constituents of gastric secretion, particularly mucus. It was at Babkin's instigation and with his support that Komarov undertook the series of studies that allowed him to finally identify and isolate

Klemensiewicz pouch (left) (1875). Because it was difficult to study gastric juice without contamination by saliva, food, or duodenal content, Rudolf Klemensiewicz of Graz constructed an isolated antral pouch. He noted *succus pyloricus* to be alkaline and viscous and different from the secretion of the fundus. Rudolf Heidenhain, in 1879, was so impressed by this technique that he subsequently constructed a pouch from the acid-secreting segment of a canine stomach and noted the juice to be acid and contain pepsin. Pavlov's pouches (*B*) (right) (1906) were examples not only of his intellectual ingenuity but also his surgical dexterity, which was much aided by his ambidexterity. In three successive operations, a Pavlov pouch and gastric fistula were constructed, followed by a duodenal fistula and then separation of the pyloric area from the corpus. In *C*, a similar technique was used to produce an entirely separate pyloric pouch. Pavlov noted that placing meat extract in this "antral" pouch caused increased gastric secretion from the fundic pouch. This observation was consistent with Edkins' "gastrin" hypothesis, but Pavlov did not pursue the issue of the nature of a chemical link, being of the fixed persuasion that "nervism" was the only reasonable explanation.

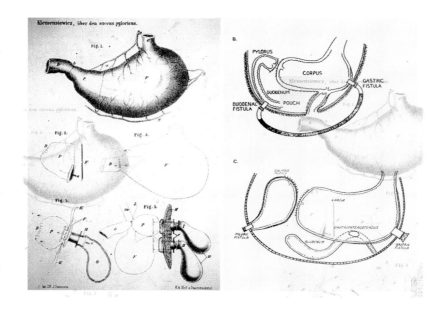

the active extract of the antrum as gastrin. Komarov was a meticulous chemist, and, at crucial stages in his extraction procedure, he assayed the product by injecting it intravenously into anesthetized cats. He used boiled, minced hog antral mucosa extracted in 0.15 N HCl and, after filtering the extract, precipitated the active component with trichloroacetic acid. The acid was removed with organic solvents, and the active components were redissolved in saline solution and once more precipitated by salting out with NaCl.

After numerous tedious repetitions of precipitation, extraction, salting out, and further extraction, a powder that was a protein in nature was obtained.

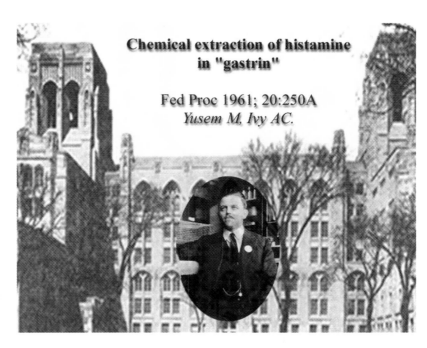

Andrew C. Ivy (center) had an illustrious physiologic career at the University of Chicago (background) and the Northwestern University Medical School before his dalliance with the discredited anticancer drug Krebiozen led to a considerable period of decline. One of the manifestations of this was Ivy's insistence that gastrin was in fact a heparin-histamine complex (top). It was only after Gregory sent Ivy a sample of synthetic gastrin (after 1965) that was tested and found to be highly active that Ivy repudiated his prior claim and acknowledged the existence of gastrin as an antral hormone.

Simon Komarov (1892–1964) was originally a student of Pavlov. In 1938, while at McGill University (bottom right) he worked with Babkin (also a former pupil of Pavlov). Babkin was born in Kursk, Russia, in 1877 and in 1901 began postgraduate study in the History of Medicine at the Military-Medical Academy in St. Petersburg. Babkin had decided that clinical medicine as such held no interest for him, although the science of medicine itself had great attraction. He thus hoped to combine his study of Medical History with actual experience in its clinical and experimental aspects. With this in mind, he initially entered the laboratory of Pavlov at the Institute of Experimental Medicine. Although Pavlov regarded Babkin's avowal of an interest in medical history, which he considered purely academic, with rather vehement contempt, he nevertheless agreed to let Babkin work in his laboratory. Babkin was thus initiated into the methods of physiologic research, and his interest subsequently grew to such an extent that its study soon superseded his progress not only in the clinical aspects of medicine, but also in medical history itself. By 1902, Babkin had decided to become a physiologist and in this capacity remained as an assistant in Pavlov's laboratory until 1912. The influence of this period was considerable and is clearly reflected in the research interests pursued by Babkin for the rest of his life. In 1912, he was appointed to the Chair of Animal Physiology at the Agricultural Institute of Novo Alexandria, and in 1915, he accepted a position at the University of Odessa as Professor of Physiology. However, in 1922, Babkin was forced to leave Russia for political reasons and went to London, where he worked for a time in the laboratory of Ernest Starling. After emigrating to America, Babkin received an appointment as Professor of Physiology at Dalhousie University,

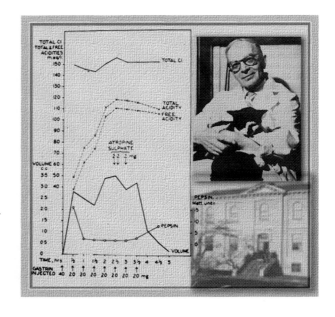

Halifax, a position that he held until 1928 when he moved to McGill, where he remained until 1946. Komarov (top right) successfully documented that gastrin existed as a chemical entity separate from histamine and thereby validated the work that Edkins had presented 3 decades previously. A graph (left) from Komarov's original publication of 1942 (*Revue Canadienne de Biologie*) demonstrates the acid response of an anesthetized cat to an intravenous injection of "gastrin" (histamine-free antral, mucosal extract) and the effect of atropine on the response. It is apocryphally reported that the widow of Edkins attended a subsequent presentation of this work and at the conclusion of the lecture expressed gratitude to Komarov for the vindication of her husband's original observations.

Komarov said it was free of choline and "organic crystalloids" but could say nothing further about its chemical nature. The product did not lower the blood pressure of anesthetized cats when injected intravenously and, therefore, did not contain histamine. Komarov believed that he was justified in calling it *gastrin* for this reason:

In all cases without exception the pyloric preparation, injected in quantities equal to 5 gm of mucosa, elicited a copious secretion of gastric juice, which was characterized by high acidity and low peptic power and which was not affected by atropine even in large doses.

Komarov, in addition, identified a small amount of gastrin in the duodenal mucosa but none in the jejunal mucosa. These facts were long used to explain the intestinal phase of gastric secretion. He also noted that there was no gastrin evident in the oxyntic mucosa but a small amount present in the mucosa of the cardia. Once his manuscript had been published in 1938, it was evident that all parties, except Ivy, accepted the reality of gastrin as a chemical and physiologic entity.

The isolation and characterization of gastrin

Thereafter, the further thrust of investigation in the area of gastrin related to attempts to isolate and purify the substance. Gregory and Tracy were the first

G. W. Kenner (center) of the Robert Robinson Laboratories at Liverpool (top) was instrumental in leading the group that first synthesized gastrin (top and center demonstrate the different moieties that were synthesized using a variety of chemical steps [elongation, curtius degradation, selective saponification, or azide coupling and ammonolysis]). This publication appeared in *Nature* on December 5, 1964 (bottom). In this work, the L-forms of amino acids were used.

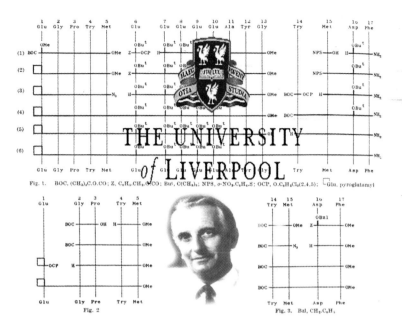

THE ANTRAL HORMONE GASTRIN

December 5, 1964   NATURE

J. C. ANDERSON
MOIRA A. BARTON
R. A. GREGORY
P. M. HARDY   Robert Robinson Laboratories   J. S. MORLEY
G. W. KENNER   and Physiological Laboratory,   Imperial Chemical Industries, Ltd.,
J. K. MACLEOD   University of Liverpool.   Pharmaceuticals Division,
J. PRESTON   Alderley Park.
R. C. SHEPPARD

to devise a method of extracting gastrin using trichloroacetic acid in acetone. This produced a histamine-free preparation and, by using adsorption on a column of calcium phosphate gel and displacement by a gradient of phosphate, they obtained a product sufficiently pure to be tested on human subjects. Unfortunately, although the substance was more potent than histamine on a weight basis, it was apparent on paper electrophoresis that it was inhomogeneous. Thereafter, they extracted a gastrin-like substance from a small pancreatic tumor of a patient with Zollinger-Ellison syndrome. Gregory demonstrated this work on April 26, 1962, at a meeting in New York at which Simon Komarov was the chairman.

The data on the amino acid composition and molecular weight indicated to Gregory that gastrin was a heptadecapeptide of approximately 2,114 daltons. On Christmas Day, 1962, Gregory and Tracy noted that they had identified two gastrins instead of one. These were called *gastrin I* and *gastrin II*. With the help of Kenner, they published the structure of the two gastrins in the December 5, 1964, issue of *Nature* and noted that the difference was that the tyrosine on gastrin II was sulfated.

Rod Gregory (c. 1975) (top left) of London obtained a Rockefeller Traveling Scholarship (1939–1940) to work with A. C. Ivy in Chicago in the hope that exposure to North American science would provide him with a broader scientific perspective. Because he had previously been working in the field of cardiac physiology, he decided to translate the 1928 edition of Babkin's text *Die Aussere Sekretion der Verdauungsdrusen* to broaden his knowledge of gastrointestinal physiology. Before his investigation of gastrin, he explored the subject of histamine with C. Code at the Mayo Clinic and had become intrigued by the nature of the regulation of acid secretion. On his return to the United Kingdom, Gregory pursued the idea of identifying the chemical nature of gastrin. Despite the fact that he was a British citizen working in Liverpool, he was on good terms with his American counterparts and thus received a substantial grant from the U.S. Public Health Service. This support enabled him to purchase numerous items of capital equipment necessary to fully undertake the isolation and characterization of gastrin. In addition, he and his coworker, Hilda Tracy (bottom left), signed a contract with a Liverpool firm that made pork pies and, as a result, were able to acquire for extraction purposes up to 600 hog antra weekly for 6 months. Despite this huge load of material, the system worked well enough that, by the end of 18 months, they had accumulated hundreds of milligrams of pure gastrin. On Christmas Day, 1962, Gregory and Tracy noted that they had identified not one but two gastrins, which they imaginatively proceeded to name *gastrin I* and *gastrin II*. Of interest was the observation that the tyrosine on gastrin II was sulfated. Gregory subsequently presented this work on April 26, 1962, at a meeting in New York at which Simon Komarov was chairman. The data on the amino acid composition and molecular weight indicated to Gregory that gastrin was a heptadecapeptide of approximately 2,114 daltons, and, with the help of Kenner, they published the structure of the two gastrins in the December 5 (1964) issue of *Nature*. The diagram on the right shows the structure and sequence of gastrin, which he determined with the help of Tracy. To facilitate communication, the peptide sequences are numbered from the N-terminal amino acid. Big gastrin, cholecystokinin, and cerulein share many physiologic properties because they possess the same C-terminal tetrapeptide.

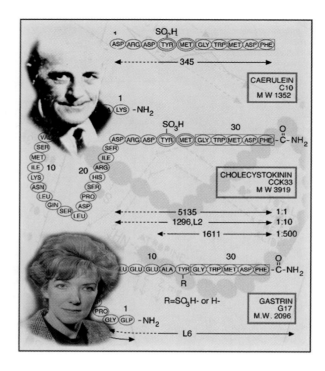

Clinical and biologic relevance of gastrin

It now remained to determine the clinical and biologic relevance of gastrin. In 1958, Solomon Berson and Rosalyn Yalow published their manuscript documenting the use of radioimmunoassay to measure plasma insulin. In 1967, James McGuigan used the principle of this methodology to devise a radioimmunoassay for gastrin. He refined the methodology further by developing a double-antibody technique and was able to measure gastrin in human serum. Similar studies were undertaken by Jack Hansky and Cain, and it was apparent that different gastrin levels were evident in fasting versus fed patients or individuals with the Zollinger-Ellison syndrome.

The technique of the gastrin radioimmunoassay was further modified by Yalow and Berson, and it became apparent that plasma levels could differentiate between patients with various disease states. In addition, it was evident that hypergastrinemia associated with achlorhydria could be inhibited by oral administration of 300 mL of 0.1 N HCl by straw or by stomach tube. This confirmed the role of luminal pH in the regulation of antral gastrin secretion and of a class of HCl to antral glands.

The cellular site of gastrin secretion

Little, however, was known of the precise cellular site of gastrin secretion until 1967, when Enrico Solcia of the University of Pavia described a cell (the G cell) in the antral mucosa that he proposed as the site of gastrin secretion.

The measurement of gastrin in the blood was a direct result of the development of radioimmunoassay (RIA) by Solomon Berson (center) and his assistant Rosalyn (Sussman) Yalow (top left). Yalow was born in New York on July 19, 1921, to unschooled parents who both believed that the key to the future was education. In 1950, Yalow began a 22-year partnership with Dr. Solomon A. Berson, and their first joint efforts were in the use of radioisotopes to analyze blood for evidence of thyroid and other diseases and to observe the distribution of globin and serum proteins. Over the years, Yalow and Berson developed a system by which they would tag a known sample of a hormone with a radioisotope and in this fashion developed the exciting investigational tool of RIA, primarily for the study of diabetes. Surprisingly, this revolutionary diagnostic process was largely ignored when Yalow and Berson published it in 1959. They later expanded their methods to include the observation of hormones, especially insulin and subsequently gastrin. In 1977, Yalow received the Nobel Prize for this work, because Berson had died tragically some years previously. As such, she became only the second woman, after Marie Curie, to receive the Nobel Prize for medicine. Of interest is the fact that neither Yalow nor Berson applied for a patent on RIA, preferring to make it available to the scientific community. Gastrin RIA enabled the physicians to identify hypergastrinemia and further developments, such as the use of an intravenous secretin bolus (graph), facilitated the identification of the neoplastic source of gastrin from gastrin-secreting lesions. Using this principle, James McGuigan (bottom right) in 1967 developed a similar strategy for a gastrin RIA by developing a double antibody technique and was able to measure gastrin in human serum. The classic standard plot indicating the percentage of total radioactivity precipitated with goat anti-gastrin antibodies in varying concentrations of ^{125}I-labeled human gastrin is shown (center). His manuscript in the *New England Journal of Medicine* in 1968 (bottom) described a greater than tenfold increase ($p < .0001$) level in fasting serum gastrin levels in three patients with Zollinger-Ellison syndrome. In addition, he was able to identify gastrin immunohistochemically in an extract derived from a pancreatic islet-cell tumor of one of the patients. Further refinements of the gastrin RIA technique by Yalow and Berson enabled a precise determination of plasma levels and, in addition, enabled an appreciation of the different molecular forms of gastrin present in the circulation.

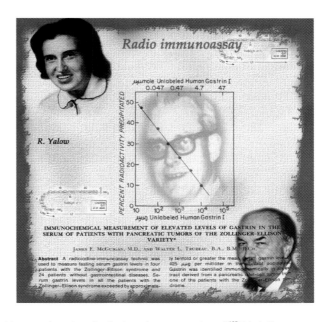

He noted that the G cell had a distribution corresponding to that of gastrin, being most numerous in the mid-part of the pyloric glands. It was bottle shaped, with a narrow neck extending to the lumen of the glands between mucous-secreting cells, and its luminal surface was covered with a fringe of microvilli. Specific secretory granules, protein in nature, were present in the basal part of the cells, which exhibited a well-developed Golgi complex.

Using direct-immunofluorescence methodology, McGuigan was able to demonstrate that these cells contained gastrin. He noted that the immunofluorescence in the granules of the cytoplasm of the cells in the pyloric glands exhibited a distribution that corresponded to that of the G cells.

Subsequently, both A. G. E. Pearse and W. Creutzfeldt conclusively demonstrated that the cells showing immunofluorescence when treated with a gastrin antibody were the argyrophil G cells.

After the morphologic and immunocytochemical localization of these G cells, numerous investigators attempted to relate alteration of the numbers of these cells to various disease processes. The condition of G-cell hyperplasia was initially thought to represent a cause of peptic ulcer disease, whereas in conditions of achlorhydria, significant hyperplasia of the G cells was felt to be related to the hypergastrinemia that accompanied pernicious anemia and atrophic gastritis.

Immunofluorescent identification of gastrin cells. The use of immunofluorescent-labeled antibodies to a specific peptide allowed a more precise identification of the secretory granules of a particular endocrine cell. This technique has become a critical adjunct in the histologic identification of the precise nature of cells comprising various neoplasms.

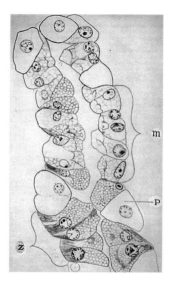

Neck of a gastric gland from a human stomach (R. R. Bensley, 1928). By the beginning of the second decade of the twentieth century, it had become apparent that intact organ physiology possessed scientific limitations, and as a consequence, histology became a major tool in the identification and assessment of the individual cell types that constituted whole organ function. (m, neck chief cells; p, parietal cells; z, body chief cells.)

Linkage between gastrin and histamine: the ECL cell as the source of histamine

Although the discovery of secretin by William Bayliss and Ernest Starling of London in 1902 provided the first scientific evidence that the gut was an endocrine organ, some of the histologic and pathologic aspects had been described before Starling's proposal. In 1867, Paul Langerhans of Berlin noted clumps of cells in the pancreas that were separate from the acini. These were later named the *islands* or *islets of Langerhans*. The next year, Rudolf Heidenhain of Breslau, Prussia found enterochromaffin (EC) cells in the gastric mucosa, and in 1897, Nikolai Kulchitsky in Russia noted similar cells in the crypts of Lieberkuhn in the intestinal mucosa. The early literature thus abounds with complex descriptions of Heidenhain cells, Nicolas cells, Kulchitsky cells, Nussbaum cells, Ciaccio cells, Schmidt cells, Feyrter cells, and Plenk cells. Broadly, these cells were codified according to their staining properties (enterochromaffin, argentaffin, argyrophil, pale or yellow cells) and recognized simply as being morphologically different from other intestinal mucosal epithelial cells. Later, in 1914, Pierre Masson of Montreal found them to be argentaffin and suggested that they formed "a diffuse endocrine gland" in the intestines. Unfortunately, 14 years later, he proposed that these cells were neurocrine, and that they originated in the intestinal mucosa and subsequently migrated into the nerves. In the 1930s, Friedrich Feyrter of Gdansk, Poland, also described a diffuse endocrine organ that included the gastroenteropancreatic (GEP) argentaffin cells and also many argyrophil cells. To these he attributed a paracrine function. Much later, Everson Pearse of London incorporated all of these different cell types into a group colliquation identified as the *amine precursor uptake decarboxylation (APUD) series.*

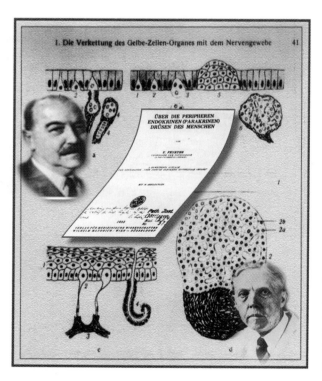

In 1930, F. Feyrter (top left) of Gdansk proposed the existence of a diffuse system of neuroendocrine cells in the gastrointestinal tract (center). Thereafter, P. Masson (1880–1959) (bottom right) described in detail the characteristics of the cells that formed the basis of the diffuse neuroendocrine system (background). In addition, Masson proposed that the enterochromaffin cells in the crypts of Lieberkuhn (which had been identified by N. Kulchitsky in 1897) were the progenitors of neuroendocrine tumors of the gut (carcinoids).

A careful perusal of the early writings and drawings of Heidenhain suggests that in 1870 he had first noticed the existence of the enterochromaffin-like (ECL) cell, although he was not able to define its role. Heidenhain's classic research on the structure of the gastric gland had noted that the "Labzellen" (rennin cells) were separate from a second type of cells that he termed *Hauptzellen*, which formed the complete lining to the gland. Because he felt the Labzellen were more peripheral, he therefore renamed them as *Belegzellen*. These two types of

Rudolf Peter Heidenhain (1834–1897) was the eldest of 22 children of the physician Heinrich Jacob Heidenhain (1808–1868). Born January 29, 1834, in Marienwerder, East Prussia, he died October 13, 1897, in Breslau, Germany, having revolutionized many spheres of physiology. After completion of his secondary education in his native town at the age of 16 years, he began the study of nature on an estate near his home but soon turned to medicine at the University of Königsberg. He subsequently studied at a number of institutions before undertaking, in 1867, a systematic investigation of the physiology of glands and of the secretory and absorption process, which remained his chief field of interest for the rest of his life. Heidenhain noted in the stomach two types of cells in the gastric glands and demonstrated that one produced pepsin and the other hydrochloric acid. Of particular interest was his identification of a third type of small, granulated, yellow-staining cell on the surface of the gastric glands—almost certainly the enterochromaffin-like cell of today. To facilitate investigation of the gastric secretory process, he devised a gastric pouch, later improved by Ivan Petrovich Pavlov (1849–1936), who worked for some time in Heidenhain's laboratory and always held Heidenhain in great esteem.

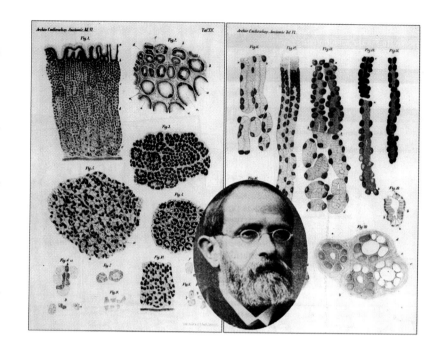

cells identified by R. Heidenhain, and independently by Rollett, are now known as the parietal cell (*Belegzelle*) and the chief cell (*Hauptzelle*). It is, however, of particular interest to note that, in addition to these cell types, Heidenhain identified a "*third type of cell in the form of minute oval elements found adhering to the external surface of the epithelial tube (gastric gland) and particularly conspicuous in preparations made with bichromate solutions in which they stained a deep yellow color.*" These cells were noted to occupy a parietal position on the surface of the glands in the rabbits and numerous other animals studied by Heidenhain and were particularly notable for the deep yellow stain that they took on with bichromate solutions. Similar observations were noted by Nicolas (1891), Kull (1924), and others in various portions of the alimentary tract and studied by Kull under the name of the cells of Nicolas. Harvey and Bentley found that, in fresh preparations, these cells were closely studded with minute granules that stained crimson in neutral red or blue in the various Nile blues used by them as indicators. They possessed a centrally located nucleus similar to that of other epithelial cells and were in all probability the same cells described by Twort (1924) under the title *The Demonstration of a Hitherto Undescribed Type of Cell in the Glands of the Stomach*. Similar cells, but in a somewhat different position in the gastric gland, were identified by Nussbaum and Stohr and presumably may have represented other endocrine cell types of the fundus of the stomach.

By 1969, Forssmann was able to recognize at least five different types of endocrine cells both by ultrastructures and immunohistology (serotonin-, glucagon-, catecholamine-, gastrin-, and secretin-containing cells). This observation contradicted the previous prevailing opinion that the enterochromaffin cell was the only endocrine cell type to be found in the gastric mucosa and that its sole product was serotonin. Indeed, within 2 years, Hakanson and Capella

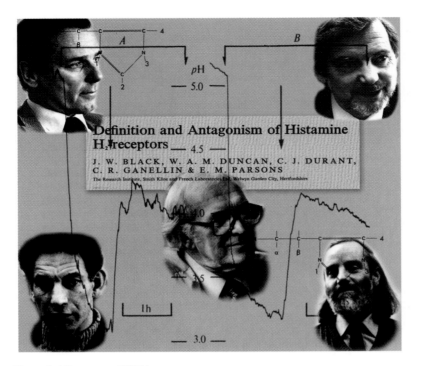

The seminal *Nature* paper (1972) from Black's group (center). In the background is a graphical depiction of rat gastric secretion and its response to burimamide. Injection of the antagonist reversed 90% of acid output and could be maintained over the experimental period. Black's coauthors included (from top left, clockwise) Duncan, Durant, Parsons, and Ganellin.

independently identified the existence of histamine-storing argyrophil cells in the murine stomach and noted their equivalents in other mammals and fish. The description in 1971 of the ECL histamine-containing cell of the fundus of the stomach constitutes the first precise recognition of the cell in this era.

The histamine-2 receptor

The synthesis of H_1 histamine antagonists had inaugurated the era of novel chemicals acting as agonists or antagonists of small molecule ligands that were useful clinically. The recognition that adrenergic receptors were divided into α and β subtypes led Black to the synthesis of the first β adrenergic antagonist, propranolol. It had been recognized that H_1 antagonists were relatively inactive against gastric acid secretion, and Keir postulated the presence of an H_2 receptor subtype in the gastric mucosa. Black and his colleagues after 8 years synthesized the first H_2 receptor antagonist, burimamide. The chemical difference between H_1 and H_2 antagonists is that the former contain major modifications of the imidazole ring, the latter modifications of the ethylamine side chain. The first successful H_2 antagonist, cimetidine, was launched in 1977.

A pure preparation of isolated enterochromaffin-like (ECL) cells (background), identified with fluorescent-labeled histamine antibody. The intact gastric gland (right) demonstrates the integrated relationship of the cell system, and the electron micrograph reveals the ultrastructural characteristics of the ECL cells and their secretory granules and vesicles (bottom left). The novel ability to produce a pure isolated ECL cell preparation from a gastric gland has facilitated the evolution of the investigation of the role of this cell in the regulation of parietal cell secretion. Because it contains substances other than histamine, it may have as-yet-unanticipated biologic functions in fundic mucosa.

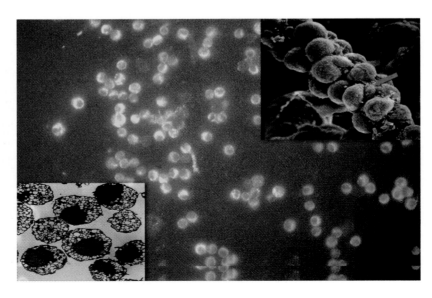

CHAPTER 2
GASTRIC ACID SECRETION

One of the unique properties of the mammalian stomach is its ability to secrete large quantities of 0.16 N hydrochloric acid. This secretory process represents one element in an elaborate system that allows higher organisms to regulate their food intake. Gastric acid secretion represents the outcome of several regulatory signals. Secretion can be initiated by a wide variety of factors related to the ingestion of food and the caloric status of the individual. In most current texts of physiology, the regulation of acid secretion is considered to occur in "phases," which were previously termed the *cephalic, gastric,* and *intestinal phases* and believed to function in an overlapping manner in the regulation of acid secretion.

The terms implied that individual regulatory mechanisms originated in the central nervous system (CNS) (cephalic phase) or in the periphery (gastric and intestinal phases). Because our current understanding of such mechanisms recognizes that both the central and peripheral components function as parts of an overlapping and integrated process, the use of the term *phase* has become inaccurate. The central regulation of acid secretion involves the cortical and spinal cord structures; *peripheral regulation* is defined as neural, endocrine, and paracrine pathways. In this section, we initially discuss the general principles of regulation of gastric acid secretion by the brain, nerves, and endocrine or paracrine cells. Thereafter, we detail the transmitters and their effects on individual cells. Finally, we outline regulation at the level of the parietal cell.

Neural and Endocrine Regulation

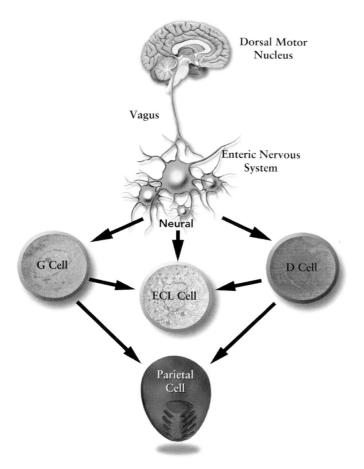

An illustration of the regions of regulation of gastric acid secretion, divided into central dorsal motor nucleus, enteric nervous system, neural, endocrine, and paracrine. Impulses flow down the vagus from the dorsal motor nucleus to the enteric nervous system in the wall of the stomach. From there, acetylcholine is released to the G cell, D cell, and parietal cell and PACAP to the ECL cell.

The complexity of neural, endocrine, and paracrine regulation is illustrated in the following table, which displays ligands that have been shown to affect gastric acid secretion by direct action on gastric mucosal cells as well as their probable cellular site of action.

There is, therefore, a remarkable number of ligands used to control acid secretion in the gastric mucosa, showing that the process of digestion of food has been refined over the course of evolution to a remarkably exact system.

The various ligands that have been shown to affect functions of isolated gastric cells. All of these also affect acid secretion *in vivo*, but understanding of their pathways has required studies on isolated cells, glands, and organs.

Receptors on Gastric Cells					
	Cell Type				
Receptor	**ECL**	**G**	**D**	**Parietal**	**Chief**
CCK$_1$	No	No	Yes	No	Yes
CCK$_2$	Yes	Yes	Yes	Yes	No
PACAP	Yes	?	VIP	?	Yes
M$_1$, M$_3$, M$_5$	No	Yes	No	Yes	Yes
M$_{2,4}$	No	No	Yes	No	No
GRP	No	Yes	Some	?	?
SST	Yes	Yes	Yes	Yes	Yes
Ca	?	Yes	?	?	?
Y$_1$	Yes	?	?	?	?
Gal	Yes	?	?	?	?
Histamine	H$_3$	No	H$_3$	H$_2$	Species
CGRP	No	No	Perhaps	No	No
Amino acids	No	Yes	No	No	No
pH	No	Perhaps	Perhaps	No	No

Central regulation

The CNS, particularly via the vagus, is responsible for the initiation of acid secretion. Although it is well recognized that the sight, smell, taste, or thought of food can stimulate acid secretion, it is less appreciated that hypoglycemia itself comprises virtually the strongest central stimulus for acid secretion. Thus, insulin is a powerful stimulant, and its effect is mimicked by 2-deoxy-glucose, which, by forming 2-deoxyglucose-6-phosphate, effectively acts to inhibit glucose metabolism in the regulatory centers of the CNS.

There are two crucial events necessary for stimulation of acid secretion: activation of the parietal cell and increased blood flow. The stimulation of blood flow depends on the release of nitric oxide (NO) from the endothelial cells in the gastric vasculature, and this may be due to stimulation by calcitonin gene–related peptide (CGRP) or by histamine acting at an H$_2$ receptor. Activation of the parietal cell depends on vagal stimulation of the enteric nervous system (ENS). All the interneuronal connections in the ENS are muscarinic, because adequate doses of atropine ablate acid secretion induced by sham feeding or even thyroid-releasing hormone (TRH) central injection. H$_2$ antagonists in the rat can block only 60% of acid secretion due to sham feeding; therefore, pathways other than those impinging on the ECL cell account for 40% of central stimulation of acid secretion.

There are several regions within the CNS responsible for detecting and transmitting central stimuli. The dorsomotor nucleus of the vagus (DMNV), the hypothalamus, and the nucleus tractus solitarius (NTS) have been identified as central structures that are key participants in the regulatory process. The final integration of central stimuli appears to occur in the DMNV, which supplies stimulatory efferent fibers to the stomach via the vagus nerve. Its destruction eliminates central stimulation of acid secretion, whereas electrical stimulation results in a strong secretory response. The DMNV appears to function as a central integrator of function and does not appear to initiate stimulation itself but rather integrates central sensory input that arises primarily from the hypothalamus or as visceral sensory input from the NTS. Vagal efferents to the stomach arise also from the nucleus ambiguus (NA), but these appear to be primarily involved in regulating motility rather than secretion.

In the hypothalamus, several sites have been identified as exerting stimulatory and inhibitory influences on acid secretion. The ventromedial hypothalamus (VMH) appears to exert a tonic inhibitory influence, because its ablation enhances secretion, whereas electrical stimulation suppresses secretion. The VMH appears to function by inhibiting the stimulatory signals arising from the lateral hypothalamus (LH) and adjacent medial forebrain bundle (MFB). The latter two structures mediate the response to the hypoglycemic stimulation of acid secretion. Both direct and indirect connections from the LH and MFB to the DMNV have been identified.

The NTS also responds directly to glucose deprivation and initiates stimulation of acid secretion mediated via the DMNV. In addition to the glucose deprivation response, the NTS also receives other major neural inputs that include taste fibers and visceral afferents, which presumably participate in the modulation of the secretory process. The former probably initiate acid secretion related to taste. Visceral afferent input to the NTS arises primarily from synapses in the inferior ganglion of the vagus. Greater than 95% of vagal neural fibers are afferent rather than efferent. This means that visceral sensory input to the CNS plays an important part in the continuous central modulation of gastric function and is necessary to assure integration of CNS and peripheral mechanisms.

Sensory information from the stomach is relayed to the CNS by both vagal afferent fibers and sympathetic afferent fibers. The sensory receptors of the stomach consist primarily of unmyelinated nerve endings that detect mechanical (distention and touch), chemical, and thermal stimuli. Receptive fields for the

In the early 1940s, Cornell University professors Harold Wolff and Stewart Wolf studied the response of the human stomach to a range of emotions precipitated by stressful situations in everyday life. These interests, which were focused on peptic ulceration, were facilitated by the availability of Tom (bottom), a patient with a large gastric fistula (center left). The investigations of Tom became a model for the study of human physiology with the voluntary cooperation of a patient and were later detailed in *Time* magazine.

sympathetic afferents appear to lie mainly within the smooth muscle layers and surrounding blood vessels. Despite this location, the sensory fibers are more sensitive to chemical (e.g., bradykinin) than to mechanical stimulation. The recognition that bradykinin is a mediator of inflammatory responses suggests that these sympathetic afferents encode painful sensations associated with gastritis and ulcers. This concept was initially recognized by Wolff and Wolff in their observations of Tom, a patient with a permanent gastric fistula. Except for major distention, the normal stomach is relatively insensitive to mechanical and chemical stimuli, at least in terms of pain. On the other hand, inflamed regions of the mucosa are quite sensitive to the application of chemicals and even light touch. It is thus likely that the pain associated with gastritis may arise from the release of inflammatory mediators or the sensitization of sympathetic sensory fibers. In this respect, the observation that the sympathetic receptors that respond to bradykinin also respond to capsaicin, the irritant component of cayenne pepper, may be of relevance. Capsaicin is a sensory neurotoxin that exerts its effects by opening calcium channels in the plasma membrane of sensory nerve endings. This first results in stimulation of the nerve, but prolonged application leads to degeneration of the nerve fiber and loss of sensation.

Vagal afferent fibers are found in the smooth muscle layers and the mucosa of the stomach. The receptors in the muscle layers are primarily tension or stretch receptors capable of detecting motility changes. Although these receptors detect and regulate motility of the muscle layers, they also are involved in the vagovagal reflexes (the so-called long reflexes) associated with distention-dependent secretory activity, an important element in the peripheral regulation of acid secretion.

Neural regulation of acid secretion

The primary function of the peripheral neural regulatory mechanisms is to modulate and integrate the stimuli (histamine and gastrin) that act directly on the parietal cell itself. This section, therefore, addresses the known neuronal factors involved in regulation of the parietal cell, directly or indirectly.

Cholinergic

The efferent fibers of the vagus nerve do not innervate the parietal cells directly but synapse with ganglion cells of the ENS. It is thus likely that the CNS serves to modulate the ENS regulatory mechanisms, because there exists a great numeric disparity between efferent vagal fibers and ganglia of the ENS. Approximately 2,000 vagal fibers synapse with an estimated 10 million ganglia, suggesting that, rather than exerting any direct control of parietal cell function, an intermediate class of modulators exists.

The majority of the cell bodies of enteric neurons are found in the two plexuses, the myenteric (Auerbach's plexus) and the submucosal (Meissner's plexus). Because the enteric plexuses of the stomach have not been studied in as much detail as those of the small and large intestines, a description of the organization and function of the gastric enteric neurons relies often on information gleaned from other segments of the gastrointestinal tract.

The myenteric plexus lies between the circular and longitudinal layers of smooth muscle and is primarily associated with coordination of motility. The

Regulation of Parietal Cell Function

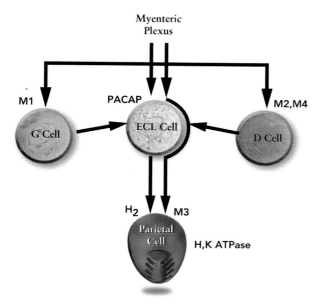

The actions of acetylcholine on the regulatory mechanisms of acid secretion. Atropine ablates acid secretion, emphasizing the importance of muscarinic receptors. Pirenzepine and telenzepine are M_1 antagonists also effective on acid secretion, suggesting that the transmission in the myenteric plexus is via an M_1 receptor. Vagal stimulation releases PACAP at the ECL cell and acetylcholine at the G and D cells. In the latter, vagal stimulation is inhibitory, suggesting the presence of either M_2 or M_4 receptors. Acetylcholine is also released at the parietal cell, stimulating acid secretion by binding to an M_3 receptor. As a consequence of PACAP or muscarinic stimulation, the ECL cell releases histamine, which stimulates the parietal cell at an H_2 receptor.

submucosal neurons supply nerve fibers directly to the mucosal cells, as well as to the loosely arranged smooth muscle cells contained within the submucosal layer. The submucosal ganglia receive a variety of synaptic inputs, which include projections from the myenteric plexus as well as extrinsic nerve fibers that consist primarily of postganglionic sympathetic fibers.

An important feature of the ENS, as with other components of the autonomic nervous system, is that the postganglionic nerve fibers are polymodal, releasing two or more neurotransmitters. Individual nerve fibers may thus contain both a conventional neurotransmitter [e.g., acetylcholine (ACh) or norepinephrine] and one or more neuropeptides, such as pituitary adenylate cyclase–activating peptide (PACAP), galanin, or calcitonin gene–releasing peptide (CGRP). Whether both types of transmitter are released simultaneously or differentially is unclear, but this configuration provides opportunity for a single nerve fiber to engender a number of diverse responses. Another feature of many postganglionic nerve fibers of the ENS is that transmitter release can occur along an extended length of the nerve axon. This reflects the existence of periodic swellings or varicosities along the axon that are assumed to be the sites for transmitter release. Postganglionic nerve fibers and epithelial cells of the stomach do not exhibit conventional synapses, usually evident at the neuromuscular junction, although some nerve fibers terminate near the mucosal cells. This spatial organization suggests that transmitters are released into the extracellular space and diffuse to nearby cells, where they may act if appropriate cellular receptors are present. The advantage of regional rather than conventional synapses is activation of several cells but possibly a number of divergent cell types, as well as obviation of the formation of new synapses as the epithelial or endocrine cells are replaced.

ACh exhibits a number of different actions when it is released from postganglionic nerve fibers in the fundic mucosa. Regional release of ACh activates parietal cells directly by binding to an M_3-subtype muscarinic receptor. In the gastric antrum, ACh is able to stimulate all the G cells to secrete gastrin. This hormone is conveyed via the systemic circulation to the fundus. At this site, gastrin activates the ECL cell via a gastrin/cholecystokinin (CCK_2) receptor to release histamine. In the antrum, ACh also inhibits the release of somatostatin from D cells, which removes a tonic inhibition of gastrin release and thus indirectly augments acid secretion by elevation of gastrin.

Adrenergic

There is some evidence that the sympathetic fibers in the gastric mucosa are involved in regulation of blood flow and perhaps also are able to stimulate ECL cell release of histamine. In general, sympathetic innervation appears to play a minor role in regulation of gastric function.

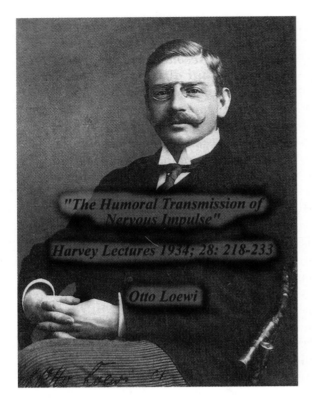

"The Humoral Transmission of Nervous Impulse"

Harvey Lectures 1934; 28: 218-233

Otto Loewi

Otto Loewi (1873–1961) was a German physiologist who used the isolated frog-heart preparation in his studies. Between 1920 and 1934, he was able to demonstrate that the transmission of impulses was caused by the release of a chemical substance, a transmitter. These publications were introduced by a short paper of only four pages, "Uber humorale Über-tragbarkeit der Herznervenwirkung" (On humoral transmission of the action of heart nerves), in 1921. This work was summarized 13 years later in the Harvey Lectures (center). Loewi was also able to clarify two mechanisms of eminent therapeutic importance: the blockade and the augmentation of nerve action by certain drugs. In 1936, Loewi (with Henry Dale) was awarded the Nobel Prize for his contribution to the chemical transmission of nerve impulses (acetylcholine).

Vittorio Erspamer (b. 1909) (top left) investigated biogenic amines and bioactive peptides both in invertebrates and lower vertebrates (especially frogs). He succeeded in identifying, defining the chemical structure, chemically synthesizing, and studying at pharmacologic level a great number of biogenic amines. The discovery of some of these peptides paved the way for the discovery of analogous peptides in mammals that act as neurotransmitters/neuromodulators, neurohormones, and hormones (bombesin in acid secretion).

Peptidergic pathways

A variety of neuropeptides have been shown to affect acid secretion, such as gastrin-releasing peptide (GRP), CGRP, galanin, and PACAP. Some of these are targeted to one or another of the gastric endocrine cells. A problem that has arisen in interpretation of *in vivo* data is that both activating and inhibitory peptides can be released at the same time, thus confounding analysis of possible physiologic consequences of their release.

Gastrin-releasing peptide

GRP is a member of the subfamily of peptides that terminate with Leu-Met-NH$_2$ and is 27 amino acids in length. Immunoreactivity is found in nerves but not in endocrine cells in the intestine, but it is also found in endocrine cells in the stomach. Vagal stimulation increases GRP in the venous outflow of the stomach, and GRP antibodies or antagonists reduce gastrin release, whether caused by vagal stimulation or peptone meals. There is, therefore, good evidence that GRP is an important noncholinergic neural mediator of gastrin secretion. The release of somatostatin that is observed after GRP administration may be indirect, perhaps due to the effect of the elevated gastrin on the fundic D cell. Hence, it is not surprising that the maximal effect of GRP on acid secretion is found in the lower regions of the dose-response curve, because at higher levels, somatostatin release probably predominates. GRP stimulates Ca^{2+} signaling in an isolated G cell preparation. It might be expected that GRP would stimulate fundic but not antral D cells.

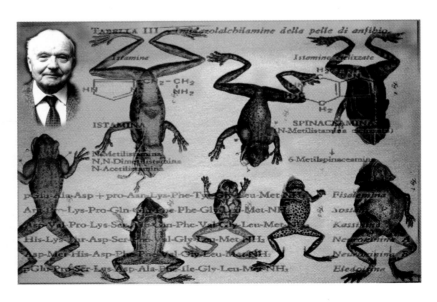

Calcitonin gene–related peptide

CGRP is a 37-residue peptide with a disulfide bridge and a C-terminal amide. CGRP immunoreactive afferent nerve fibers are found in the gastric myenteric plexus, muscle, submucosal blood vessels, and mucosa. The peptide inhibits gastric acid secretion, whether given centrally or peripherally. The latter is probably due to stimulation of somatostatin release; no effect has been found in isolated rat ECL cells. Inhibition of acid secretion by injected CGRP must be due to effects on either antral or fundic D cells, or both.

ECL Cell Stimulation/Inhibition

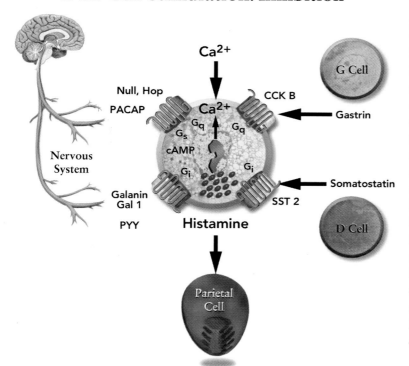

Major neural and endocrine regulation of ECL cell histamine release, showing PACAP and galanin/PYY as the neural and gastrin (G) and somatostatin (SST) as the endocrine mediators. The ECL cell is shown as the master cell of regulation of gastric acid secretion. It is stimulated by PACAP released by the postganglionic neurons of the enteric plexus and by gastrin released from the antral G cell. Galanin and PYY released from the ENS and somatostatin released by the D cell act as inhibitory influences on the ECL cell.

Galanin

Galanin is a 29–amino acid peptide found in nerve endings in the gastric mucosa that inhibits basal- and pentagastrin-stimulated acid secretion. There are three isoforms of the galanin receptor, one of which apparently stimulates and two of which inhibit calcium signaling. Galanin inhibits gastrin release but also inhibits gastrin-stimulated acid secretion. It does not inhibit bethanechol- or histamine-stimulated acid secretion. It therefore has an additional site of action distal to the G cell. Galanin interferes with stimulation of the ECL cell by a pertussis toxin (PTX)–sensitive pathway. This peptide has dual sites of inhibitory effect—both the G and ECL cells.

PACAP

PACAP is the newest member of the vasoactive intestinal peptide (VIP)/glucagon/secretin family. It is released from nerves, although their location in the gastrointestinal tract is not known. The PACAP receptor exists as several splice variants, and PACAP stimulates Ca^{2+} signaling in pancreatic acinar cells, showing that this receptor is coupled to both adenylate cyclase and phospholipase C. PACAP stimulates calcium signals and histamine release from the ECL cell. Several variants of this receptor have been shown to be present by reverse transcriptase–polymerase chain reaction (RT-PCR) of an ECL cell cDNA library.

Whereas injection of PACAP inhibits acid secretion, when this is done in the presence of antisomatostatin antibody, stimulation of acid secretion results. D cells have VIP receptors; hence, injection of PACAP will nonselectively release somatostatin. Local neural release will result in ECL cell stimulation and acid secretion. VIP nerves are presumably those that stimulate the D cell. PACAP also stimulates ECL cell growth as effectively as gastrin. Presumably, its release is acute, that of gastrin chronic.

The CCK_2 and the PACAP receptors appear to be functionally the most important in terms of stimulation of histamine release from the ECL cell—the former endocrine, the latter neural.

Vasopressin

This peptide also inhibits gastric acid secretion, but only in the intact animal. Its action is exerted on gastric mucosal blood flow. On stimulation, there is a large increase in mucosal perfusion, and this is essential for normal acid secretion. If blood flow is impeded, with consequent relative hypoxia of the parietal cell, acid secretion is also inhibited.

Paracrine regulation

Histamine

Initially, it was proposed that histamine is released from mucosal mast cells, but more recent studies indicate that gastric histamine is released from a specialized endocrine cell of the stomach, the ECL cell. The release of histamine from the ECL cell is regulated by various factors involving neural, endocrine, paracrine, and autocrine pathways, such as PACAP and galanin.

Somatostatin

The peptide is released from both fundic and antral D cells. The latter are more numerous. Somatostatin release is used almost universally as a downregulator of cellular function and, therefore, although a peptide, must have a short half-life to ensure organ specificity. This allows classification of this inhibitor as a paracrine mediator of acid secretion.

Endocrine regulation

Gastrin

Gastrin is the major stimulatory peptide for histamine release from the ECL cell. It is present in the G cells of the antral gland, in approximately the midregion in the human stomach. It is released from the G cell in response to aromatic amino acids or amines in the gastric lumen and in response to cholinergic stimulation or GRP released from postganglionic fibers of the vagus nerve. Acidification of the gastric lumen inhibits gastrin release. Although its effect on gastric acid secretion has been relegated to a secondary effect by stimulation of histamine release from the ECL cell, gastrin remains the major endocrine regulator of gastric acid secretion. Changes in circulating gastrin account for much of the gastric response to feeding.

Cholecystokinin

The peptide is present in both the pancreas and duodenum and has a broad spectrum of activities. Of particular interest in terms of gastric physiology is its ability to stimulate the D cell and the chief cell of the gastric mucosa at high

In 1943, Harper and Raper (bottom right) demonstrated that extracts of the mucosa of the upper intestine contained a substance that, on intravenous administration, stimulated the pancreas to secrete enzymes (amylase) as opposed to secretin, which stimulated water and bicarbonate secretion. In addition, no effect on volume output was noted. The British researchers proposed the name *pancreozymin* to describe the former (background). Thereafter, in 1966, the peptide chemists Jorpes and Mutt demonstrated that CCK and pancreozymin shared the same chemical structure and that the two biologic effects—of gall bladder contraction and pancreatic enzyme secretion—were induced by this agent.

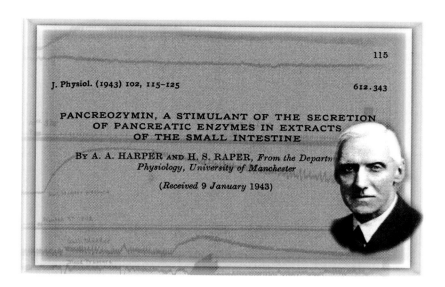

affinity on a CCK_1 receptor. It is approximately equally as effective as gastrin in stimulation of ECL cell Ca^{2+} signaling and histamine release, but the CCK_1 octapeptide (nonsulfated) does not result in growth stimulation of the ECL cell *in vitro*.

Peptide YY

Peptide YY (PYY) was first isolated from the intestine. PYY and neural peptide (NPY) interact with three receptor subtypes: Y_1, Y_2, and Y_3. PYY is released by meals, and relatively large doses have been shown to inhibit gastrin-stimulated acid secretion. This peptide may be a component of enterogastrone, a complex group of factors released during the intestinal phase of digestion, resulting in inhibition of gastric acid secretion. The ECL contains the Y_1-receptor subtype, and histamine release and calcium signaling are inhibited by PYY.

Enterogastrone

Gastric inhibitory peptide (GIP) and glucagon-like peptide (GLP) are thought to be components of the factors released during the intestinal phase of digestion that inhibit acid secretion. Relatively high doses of GIP and GLP inhibited gastrin-induced signaling and histamine release from ECL cells.

Secretin

A complex feedback mechanism exists communicating to the stomach from the intestine. Secretin inhibits gastric acid secretion, presumably in part by stimulation of the D cell. However, it also inhibits, at least in some species, histamine-stimulated acid secretion, indicating a direct action on the parietal cell.

Control of gastric acidity

The interaction of the triumvirate of the ECL cell, G cell, and D cell serves to regulate the release of histamine, as illustrated in the simplified model of the figure.

Because histamine, together with ACh and possibly gastrin, is responsible for the activation of the parietal cell, and somatostatin, epidermal growth factor (EGF), galanin, and secretin inhibit the parietal cell, the secretion of acid represents an example of neural, endocrine, and paracrine positive and negative interactions. The overall goal of these processes is to regulate the acidity of the gastric contents. The regulatory mechanisms must be able to detect the intragastric pH and respond with celerity and accuracy.

The only known mechanism that at this time corresponds to such a requirement is the suppression of gastrin release by pH less than 3.0. The low pH may, in fact, be detected by the antral D cell and then release of somatostatin that results in the suppression of gastrin secretion. This relatively simple feedback loop between acid secretion and gastrin release appears to function *in vivo*, as indicated by the observation that disruption of the loop by antisecretory agents, such as H_2 receptor antagonists or pump inhibitors, cul-

Gastric Acid Stimulation

A schematic model illustrating the regulation of acid secretion by interactions of the ECL, G, and D cells with each other and with the parietal cell. Blue arrows indicate stimulation of the cells, red arrows indicate inhibition of the cells toward which they are pointing. Smell, taste, and other influences increase vagal outflow from the dorsal motor nucleus of the hypothalamus. The vagal impulses are transmitted to the enteric neurons in the wall of the stomach. Secretory stimulation is then enabled by postganglionic fibers that release PACAP at the ECL cell and acetylcholine and gastrin-releasing peptide (GRP) at the G cells and the parietal cell. The G cell is also stimulated to release the hormone gastrin by the aromatic amino acids, phenylalanine and tyrosine, in the gastric lumen. Gastrin stimulates the ECL cell and the D cell. Release of histamine from the ECL cell stimulates the parietal cell at the H_2 receptor as does acetylcholine at an M_3 receptor. There is a gastrin (CCK_2) receptor on the parietal cell, but its role in stimulation of acid secretion is controversial. M+ indicates muscarinic stimulation, and M– indicates muscarinic inhibition.

minates in hypergastrinemia. Although the pH dependence of gastrin secretion represents the major known mechanism for control of gastric acidity, it is unlikely that so simple a feedback loop can account fully for the maintenance of gastric pH. Other mechanisms must be present, if only to regulate those types of acid secretion that are independent of gastrin (e.g., due to direct ACh stimulation of the parietal cell).

Cellular regulation

The interplay between the different regulatory cells of the stomach has been largely elucidated by studies of responses to injection of substances *in vivo* and by studies of responses of isolated cells either in terms of calcium signaling or release of ligand. The figure summarizes many of the observations to be discussed.

Some of the receptors defined on the gastric endocrine/paracrine system. The ECL and G cells upregulate acid secretion, and the D cell inhibits acid secretion. The ECL cell expresses the CCK_2 or gastrin receptor and the somatostatin type 2 receptor and PAC1, the PACAP receptor. The G cells express a stimulatory muscarinic receptor subtype not known and a stimulatory GRP receptor and an inhibitory somatostatin type 2 receptor. The D cell has stimulatory CCK_1 and CCK_2 receptors and inhibitory muscarinic (either M_2 or M_4) receptors.

Receptors of Gastric Endocrine Cells

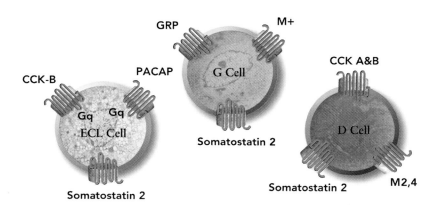

Endocrine cells

The gastric mucosa is endowed with a rich array of endocrine cell types. At least seven distinct endocrine cells have been identified based on ultrastructural features: the enterochromaffin (EC) cell, the ECL cell, the D cell, the A cell, the P cell, the G cell, and the X cell. As a group they represent approximately 2% of the cells in the fundic mucosa of the rat, whereas in humans, they are somewhat less numerous (0.5% to 1.0%). In total, they constitute an endocrine organ approximately equal in size to the endocrine pancreas.

In humans, EC cells are found in the antrum and oxyntic mucosa. Their main secretory product is 5-hydroxytryptamine (5-HT). It is this monoamine that reduces silver and chromium, constituting the argentaffin and chromaffin reactions, respectively. D cells secrete somatostatin and are distributed throughout the antral and oxyntic mucosa but are more numerous in the antrum. They display argyrophilic staining (i.e., they accumulate silver precipitates from a silver nitrate solution when treated with an exogenous

A cartoon of the principal endocrine cells of the antrum and fundus (background). Enrico Solcia (top right) of Pavia was an important contributor to the initial identification of the neuroendocrine cells of the stomach. Subsequently, Steven Bloom (center) and Julia Pollack (bottom left) of London were instrumental in elucidating the physiology and defining the histologic characteristics of the gastric neuroendocrine regulatory system. From this basis emerged the understanding of the critical biologic relationship between the antral G cell and the fundic ECL cell in the modulation of acid secretion.

Endocrine Cell Isolation and Evaluation

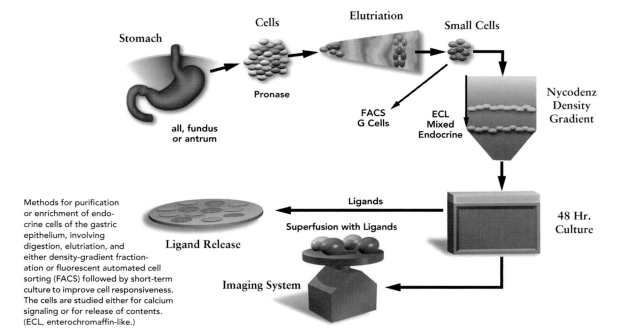

Methods for purification or enrichment of endocrine cells of the gastric epithelium, involving digestion, elutriation, and either density-gradient fractionation or fluorescent automated cell sorting (FACS) followed by short-term culture to improve cell responsiveness. The cells are studied either for calcium signaling or for release of contents. (ECL, enterochromaffin-like.)

reducing agent) and may be labeled immunohistochemically using antisomatostatin antibodies. Gastrin-producing G cells are located in the antrum. They are argyrophilic and may be labeled using antibodies against gastrin. The X cells, the function of which remains unknown, are found almost exclusively in the oxyntic gastric mucosa. They are stained with amylin antisera and the Grimelius silver stain. D1 cells are so named because on electron microscopy they display granules resembling those found in D cells. Similarly, P cells have granules that resemble those of pulmonary endocrine cells. Both of these cell types are found in the antral and oxyntic mucosa in humans, and their biologic functions remain to be delineated.

Definitive study of the regulation of these cells has been difficult due to the fact that each group comprises less than 1% of the total mucosal fraction, and they cross talk. It has been difficult to obtain pure preparations, except in the case of the ECL cell. A number of strategies have been used to produce enriched endocrine cell populations. Highly purified endocrine cells are necessary to prevent cross talk between cells when studying effects of ligands on release of transmitters. Single-cell video imaging under superfusion conditions allows measurement of signaling in the absence of cross talk, even in relatively impure preparations, provided that the cells being studied can be definitely identified. A means of purification or enrichment of different gastric endocrine cells is presented in the figure. This strategy has been applied most successfully to the ECL cell of rat mucosa, producing a preparation containing up to 90% ECL cells. Because this cell plays a central role in the stimulation of acid secretion, it forms the major focus of our analysis of gastric endocrine cells.

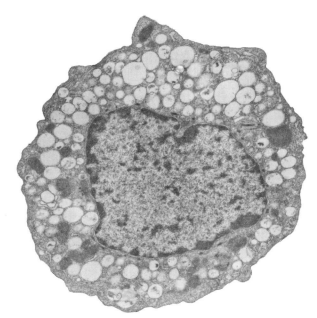

An electron micrograph of an isolated ECL cell showing the electron-translucent histamine-containing acidic vacuoles.

The ECL cell

General characteristics

The ECL cell is the critical interface between the peripheral and central regulation of acid secretion. Its pivotal role is achieved by the secretion of histamine, which appears to be predominantly activated by gastrin although influenced by PACAP and many other factors. There is evidence for at least four activating receptors in the ECL cell population isolated from rat gastric mucosa. The CCK_2 and PACAP receptors are likely to be dominant in positive regulation of ECL function and, therefore, histamine-dependent acid secretion, as shown in the figure below. Much of cholinergic mediation of acid secretion may be due to the direct effects of ACh on the parietal cell itself, as discussed later.

Somatostatin and galanin are major local inhibitors, with secretin and PYY playing a putative role.

The ECL cells comprise approximately one-third of the endocrine cells in the oxyntic (acid-secreting) mucosa of most vertebrates. They are small, 8- to 10-μm– diameter cells that contain numerous electron-translucent cytoplasmic vesicles, many of which have an electron-dense core. ECL cells store histamine and contain histidine decarboxylase (HDC), the enzyme required for histamine synthesis. The obvious role of the ECL cells is to release histamine, which acts as a paracrine agent to stimulate the parietal cells. It has been demonstrated that the vesicles contain other regulatory compounds, such as chromogranin and pancreastatin, but neither the specific compounds nor their functional significance has been defined.

The ECL cells are subepithelial and are not in direct contact with the lumen of the stomach. They are therefore not affected directly by gastric contents. The other cell type of the oxyntic mucosa that contains histamine is the mast cell that, in different forms, is found throughout the gastrointestinal tract. It was initially thought that a specialized type of mast cell was

Receptors for activation and inhibition of the ECL cell showing the refinement of regulation of one of the paracrine cells, the ECL cell, involved in regulation of acid secretion. It remains difficult to determine which of these regulators is functioning at any particular stage of gastric digestion.

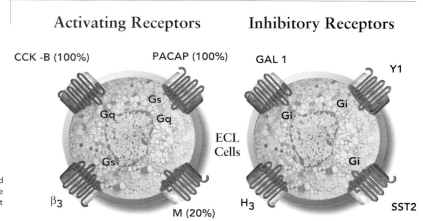

Activating Receptors

CCK -B (100%)
PACAP (100%)
Gs
Gq
Gq
Gs
β_3
M (20%)

ECL Cells

Inhibitory Receptors

GAL 1
Y1
Gi
Gi
Gi
Gi
H_3
SST2

responsible for releasing the histamine associated with acid secretion, because the mast cells were regarded as a traditional source of histamine released in response to inflammatory processes. This mistaken assumption was refuted by the recent development of preparations of isolated purified ECL cells, which allowed conclusive identification of the ECL cell as the source of the gastric histamine responsible for acid secretion. Although the role of the mast cell in acid secretion has been repudiated, it remains the cellular source of the histamine released during gastric inflammatory events.

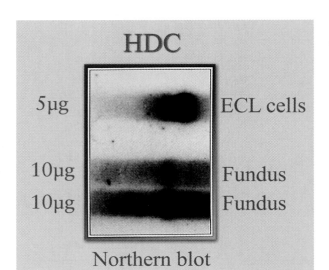

A Northern blot of gastric fundus and ECL cells demonstrating the large amount of HDC in the ECL cells.

ECL cells can be identified by silver staining techniques and more specifically by immunocytochemistry using antibodies against histamine or HDC. In mammals, the ECL cells are only found in the acid-secreting fundic mucosa, where they are most evident in the basal third of the mucosa. Their location is peripheral in the gastric gland and, although they are found in proximity to parietal cells, they appear to be particularly associated with chief cell–rich areas. They were initially defined in 1967 by Hakanson and Owman, who coined the term *enterochromaffin-like cell*. ECL cells constitute the major endocrine cell type in normal human gastric oxyntic mucosa, constituting 30% ± 9% of the endocrine cell mass of this region. ECL cells display immunoreactivity for antibodies against a wide array of markers, including chromogranin A, neuron-specific enolase, calbindin, and the α subunit of human chorionic gonadotropin.

ECL cells take up and decarboxylate a variety of aromatic amino acids [e.g., exogenous 5-HT, L-3,4-dihydroxyphenylalanine (L-DOPA)] and store the respective amines formed. This ability categorizes ECL cells as belonging to the APUD family of endocrine cells. The histamine-forming enzyme, HDC, can be detected together with histamine in ECL cells.

ECL cells exhibit a unique and characteristic structure. They are irregular in shape, with numerous and prominent cytoplasmic extensions. There is a large, eccentrically located nucleus surrounded by numerous electron-translucent vesicles with eccentric granules. Additionally, electron-dense granules are present. The distinction between these two cytoplasmic inclusions may reflect either stages in the processing of one product or the packaging of different products to different organelles. The transparent vesicle generates an internal acidity and accumulates histamine, driven by the acid gradient.

ECL cell function

The response of the ECL cell to a variety of agents can be divided into three phases—acute, intermediate, and chronic—relating to release of histamine, histamine homeostasis, and cellular response to histamine demand, as shown in the next figure.

The major receptors on the rat ECL cell and the different phases of ECL cell responses to gastrin and PACAP. Histamine release is virtually instantaneous, histidine decarboxylase is rapidly upregulated, and after some hours, ECL cell DNA synthesis is stimulated after gastrin administration.

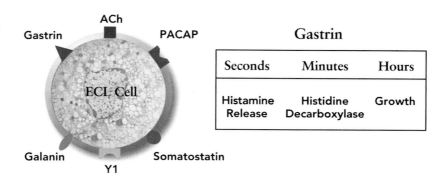

Major Receptors on ECL Cells

Gastrin		
Seconds	Minutes	Hours
Histamine Release	Histidine Decarboxylase	Growth

Not only is the ECL cell the central player on the stage of acid secretion, but it has also stolen much of the limelight from other regulatory cells due to now-outdated questions as to the safety of PPIs.

ECL Cell

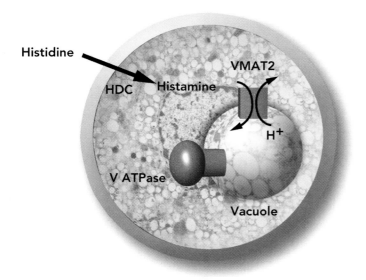

Histamine biosynthesis and accumulation in the secretory vacuoles of the ECL cell. Histidine is taken up and decarboxylated to histamine by HDC. The histamine is accumulated in the vacuole due to the H⁺ gradient formed by a V-type ATPase and the presence of a histamine countertransport protein in the vacuolar membrane.

Histamine

Of all the agents identified in or secreted by the ECL cell, histamine is the most physiologically relevant. The principal regulator of histamine secretion is gastrin. In the isolated ECL cell, preparation stimulation of histamine release by the addition of gastrin is detectable within 5 minutes. An initial peak at 5 minutes is evident and thereafter release is linear for at least 60 minutes. An overall three- to fivefold increase of histamine over baseline is detectable. The EC_{50} for gastrin stimulation of histamine release is 3×10^{-10} M, and CCK is equipotent in the stimulation of histamine release. Histamine release can be blocked by a variety of CCK_2 antagonists (L365,260, $IC_{50} = 5 \times 10^{-8}$ M), but very high concentrations of CCK_1 antagonists (L364,718) are required for blockade of histamine secretion, consistent with the presence of a CCK_2 receptor rather than a CCK_1 receptor on the ECL cell membrane. The general tyrosine kinase inhibitor, genistein (10^{-4} M), had no effect on gastrin-stimulated histamine secretion, although it blocked gastrin-induced proliferation.

The accumulation of histamine within the granules of the ECL cell depends on an acid gradient generated by a V-type ATPase driving histamine uptake across an amine transporter. The vesicular monoamine transporter (VMAT) $VMAT_2$ subtype, but not the $VMAT_1$ subtype, is expressed in the fundic epithelium, perhaps because of some preference for diamines, such as histamine. The expression of $VMAT_2$ is upregulated in low-acid states, probably by a mechanism secondary to hypergastrinemia. Current information is consistent with an ECL cell localization of this $VMAT_2$ subtype in the rat gastric corpus.

The ECL cell possesses the enzyme HDC, which is the only enzyme involved in histamine biosynthesis. The enzyme is stimulated *in vivo* by a gastrin-induced increase in gene transcription. It has been proposed that the rapid elevation induced by gastrin *in vitro* suggests that, besides an increase in gene transcription, there may also be activation of preexisting enzyme, as has been described in the regulation of other decarboxylases.

Stimulation of histamine release

Histamine is released by a direct action of gastrin at physiologic concentrations. The gastrin receptor associated with histamine release has been characterized pharmacologically as being of the CCK_2 subtype. The CCK_2 subtype receptor recently has been cloned from canine parietal cells and rat brain as well as rodent ECL cells and shows typical signature sequences for a guanine nucleotide binding protein (G protein)–coupled receptor, as does the CCK_1 subtype receptor. Typically, trimeric G protein–coupled receptors are linked to alterations of intracellular cyclic adenosine monophosphate (cAMP) or calcium. Gastrin stimulation of the ECL cells was shown to be associated with an elevation of intracellular calcium.

Histamine release from isolated ECL cells is also stimulated by PACAP as effectively as gastrin. This neuropeptide elevates intracellular Ca to a level similar to that of gastrin, with essentially the same time course as shown in the figure.

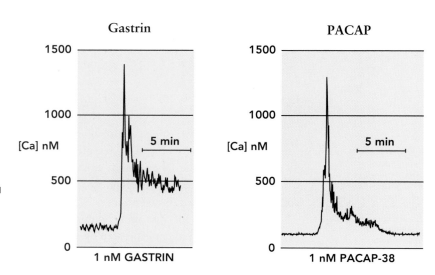

Ca2+ Signaling in ECL Cells

The regulation of $[Ca^{2+}]_i$ by PACAP and gastrin in the ECL cell, showing the characteristic biphasic response. The initial transient is due to release of Ca^{2+} from intracellular stores; the steady state is due to enhanced Ca^{2+} entry from the medium.

Given that, at best, ACh is a weak stimulant of a population of ECL cells, PACAP may be the significant neural mediator of histamine release by the ECL cell.

Forskolin, a stimulant of cAMP production, is also effective in releasing histamine; the action of PACAP may combine both cAMP and Ca^{2+} elevation. Although injection of PACAP appears to inhibit acid secretion, simultaneous administration of somatostatin-neutralizing antibody turns this inhibition into stimulation. Hence, injected PACAP may stimulate both the D cell and ECL cell, a finding also found in *in vitro* models. This D cell stimulation is presumably at a VIP receptor, whereas the stimulation of the ECL cell is at a PACAP receptor.

The physiologic significance of ECL cell stimulation by β-adrenergic agonists is unclear but may indicate multiple neural factors for regulation of the function of this cell. There is some evidence that the β-receptor on the ECL cell is of the β3 subtype.

The amount of histamine released from a single ECL cell is extremely small. The total histamine content of an ECL cell is estimated to be on the order of 30 fmol, and approximately 3% of the content, or 1 fmol, is released per hour under constant stimulation *in vitro*. It is not surprising, therefore, that it has been difficult to detect histamine in the blood during acid secretion, or that the histamine release from ECL cells does not result in any systemic effects. The local concentration of histamine required to maximally stimulate the parietal cells is on the order of 1 pM. After ECL cell stimulation, this concentration must be achieved within a few minutes, suggesting that the volume of extracellular fluid supplied by a single ECL cell must be exceedingly small (1 nL or less). Thus, the distance over which a single ECL cell regulates acid secretion may be very limited, perhaps only a few microns. Because the ECL cells are distributed primarily in the lower portion of oxyntic glands, it is possible that activation of more distant parietal cells may be achieved either by the cells having long dendritic processes or by transport of histamine in the microcirculation. At present, there is little evidence to support either postulate.

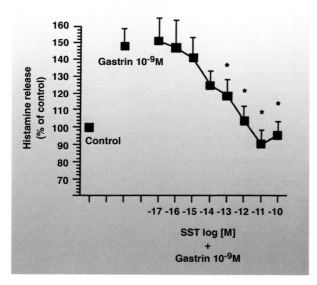

Effect of Somatostatin on Gastrin-Stimulated Histamine Release

The inhibition of gastrin-stimulated histamine release from ECL cells due to somatostatin (SST). Identification of SST led to the delineation of its role in inhibition of various secretory processes in the GI tract. The antral SST containing D cells communicate with the lumen of the antral gland and release SST in response to acidification of the lumen. The fundic D cells that do not communicate with the lumen of the fundic gland inhibit ECL cell release of histamine and are regulated by gastrin and are inhibited by acetylcholine released by postganglionic fibers of the enteric nervous system. The SST receptor is coupled to the trimeric G protein G_i that is able to inhibit both Ca^{2+} and cAMP signaling.

Interleukin 1-β, an inflammatory lymphokine involved in gastritis, induces histamine secretion from ECL cells. It is proposed that interleukin 1-β may be responsible for modulating peripheral acid secretion during *H. pylori* infection.

Inhibition of histamine release

Somatostatin at physiologic concentrations inhibits gastrin stimulation of histamine release from ECL cells. Natural somatostatin, somatostatin-14, and a synthetic agonist selective for the subtype-2 somatostatin receptor were effective in inhibiting histamine release and the steady-state rise of $[Ca^{2+}]_i$ due to stimulation by gastrin. This result indicates that somatostatin acts through a subtype-2 receptor to block gastrin-induced calcium entry into the ECL cell. Somatostatin is known to be a physiologic inhibitor of acid secretion, and its inhibition of histamine release would account for this inhibitory action. PTX, pertussin toxin, preincubation blocks the action of somatostatin, showing that the G7 receptor–binding somatostatin is G_i coupled.

Somatostatin inhibits acid secretion *in vivo* also by blocking gastrin release from antral G cells. Somatostatin inhibits histamine-stimulated acid secretion *in vitro* in isolated gastric glands and parietal cells where the release of gastrin is not involved. It has been suggested that somatostatin acts directly on the parietal cells, but part of the inhibitory action could result from somatostatin modulation of ECL cell activity.

The exact source of somatostatin acting on the oxyntic mucosa has been a matter of some debate, because cells containing somatostatin—D cells—are present both in the antrum and in the oxyntic mucosa. Additionally, postganglionic nerve fibers in the submucosa contain somatostatin, which may act as a neural transmitter. Because mucosal D cells, both in the antrum and in the fundus, possess elongated basal processes, somatostatin released locally may function as a paracrine regulator.

In addition to somatostatin, the release of histamine from ECL cells is inhibited by histamine itself. The histamine H_3 receptor agonist, α-methylhistamine, inhibited, whereas the H_3 receptor antagonist, thioperamide, potentiated gastrin-stimulated histamine release. This suggests an autocrine-feedback regulation of ECL function, but this has not been shown to occur physiologically.

The neuropeptide galanin is found in gastric neurons and gastric nerves. It potently inhibits histamine release from ECL cells and may be the important neural mediator for shutdown of ECL cell function at the end of gastric digestion. The figure illustrates the inhibition of histamine release found when galanin is added to a purified rat ECL cell preparation. Tolerance is also found in the galanin response of ECL cells.

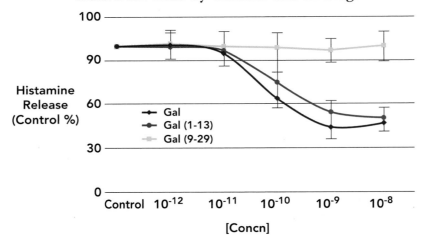

Inhibition of Gastrin-Stimulated Histamine Release from ECL Cells by Galanin and Analogs

The effect of galanin and galanin fragments on histamine release from ECL cells, showing that galanin is an effective neuropeptide inhibitor of ECL cell function and that the receptor is a galanin (Gal) 1 receptor subtype, based on a lack of response to Gal 9-29.

Human gastric mucosa expresses galanin-receptor messenger ribonucleic acid (mRNA), and this peptide may be important in neurally mediated inhibition of acid secretion. To determine whether galanin affects the ECL cell directly, the effect of the peptide was measured on calcium signaling and histamine release. Galanin dose dependently inhibited gastrin-stimulated histamine release with an IC_{50} of 10^{-10} M, as did the N-terminal (1-13) fragment of galanin with tenfold lower affinity. PTX partially blocked this inhibitory effect, as did one galanin inhibitor, galantide, but not other galanin inhibitors, such as galanin spantide I or galanin (1-13)-pro-pro-(ala-leu)$_2$-ala. Both Ca^{2+} release and elevation of Ca^{2+} entry due to gastrin stimulation of the CCK_2 receptor were blocked by equimolar concentrations of galanin. Inhibition of gastrin-stimulated histamine release from the ECL cell is the likely mechanism of acid-secretory inhibition by galanin *in vivo*. The pharmacology of this galanin receptor on the ECL cell distinguishes it from the brain receptor.

PYY is a peptide released from intestinal endocrine cells and has been found to be an effective inhibitor of calcium signaling and histamine release in isolated rat ECL cell preparations. Gastrin-stimulated histamine release was inhibited with an IC_{50} of 2×10^{-9} M. The finding of inhibition of histamine release and of calcium entry by PYY and [Pro34]-PYY and no effect of PYY (3-36) identified the presence of an inhibitory Y_1 receptor subtype. RT-PCR of ECL cell RNA showed that the receptor was the nontruncated Y_1 isoform. The inhibitory action of PYY and related peptides on gastrin-stimulated histamine release and calcium signaling was abolished by pretreatment with PTX at 200 ng per mL. Additive, but not synergistic, inhibitory effects of PYY and somatostatin on gastrin-stimulated histamine release were observed. Therefore, activation of a Y_1 inhibitory receptor subtype present on the gastric ECL cell that inhibits gastrin-induced ECL cell histamine release and Ca^{2+} entry by activation of a G_i or G_o class of protein may account for inhibition of gastric acid secretion by PYY released from the small intestine (enterogastrone).

The insulin receptor–related receptor (IRR) is a member of the insulin-receptor family and has a primary structure similar to the insulin receptor (IR) and the insulin-like growth factor-1 receptor (IGF-1R). In contrast to the widespread expression of IR and IGF-1R, the expression of IRR mRNA is highly restricted to the kidney (cortical collecting duct of the kidney) and stomach (oxyntic gland area). Using *in situ* hybridization, IRR mRNA has been localized to the basal third of oxyntic fundic glands, where it was colocalized with mRNA for HDC, a marker for ECL cells. Although the function of IRR is not known, the localization of the IRR to the ECL cell suggests that it may play an important role in these cells.

The following table summarizes some of the properties of the major inhibitors of ECL cell function that have been described.

The inhibitory ligands for the enterochromaffin-like cell, showing the subtype expressed and their effects on calcium and histamine, as well as their pertussis toxin sensitivity (G_i coupling). This table shows the inhibitory effects of the ligands on ECL cell responses.

Ligands	Inhibitors of ECL Cells			
	Gal	PYY	SS	His 3
Receptor Sub-type	Galanin 1	Y_1	$SSTR_2$	H_3
Ca^{2+}/Release	Yes	No	Yes	Yes
Ca^{2+}/Entry	Yes	Yes	Yes	Yes
Histamine/Basal	Yes	No	Yes	?
Histamine/ Stimulated	Partial	Partial	Complete	Complete
PTX Sensitive	Partial	Partial	Complete	?

Signal transduction

The cascade of the second messenger system for histamine release in the ECL cell has not been characterized. Isolated ECL cells studied in a perfusion chamber exhibit a biphasic increase in intracellular calcium when exposed to gastrin or PACAP. An early transient, presumably due to the release of calcium from intracellular stores, is followed by a steady-state increment due to calcium entry. Blockade of calcium entry by La^{3+} blocks histamine release. It is likely that the increase in cell calcium causes the activation of a variety of calcium-dependent signaling pathways, including protein kinase C. The C kinase activator, the phorbol ester tetradecanoyl-13-phorbol acetate (TPA) stimulates histamine release, supporting the proposal that this protein kinase is a component of the calcium-dependent histamine-stimulation pathway. Because forskolin (an intracellular stimulant of adenylate cyclase) is also a potent agonist of histamine release, a role for cAMP in histamine secretion is likely. This proposal is supported by increased cAMP levels in forskolin-stimulated ECL cells.

Stimulation of ECL cells by gastrin results in granule exocytosis. The granule membrane contains a V-type ATPase that generates an electrochemical gradient of protons at the expense of ATP. The identification of red fluorescent acridine orange-loaded granules dependent on this acid gradient may be used to assess ECL cell enrichment during the preparation of isolated ECL cells from the gastric fundic mucosa. This pump is electrogenic and therefore requires an ion conductance in parallel to generate an acid gradient. Because the histamine granule is acidic, it is likely that this is due to either a K^+ or Cl^- conductance in its membrane. It is probable that the chloride ion serves as the co-ion for the H^+ transported by the V-ATPase in the membrane of the secretory granule, because the cytoplasm of the cell has a high K^+ concentration, and a K^+ gradient would be in the incorrect direction for it to function as an effective co-ion. During exocytosis, the granule membrane fuses with the ECL cell plasma membrane and in doing so acquires a Cl^- conductance. Whole-cell current analysis of the ECL cell has shown a resting potential of approximately −50 mV, in contrast to the mast cell, which has a potential close to zero. This potential is due largely to the activity of a depolarization-activated K^+ current, which also maintains the potential difference after stimulation of exocytosis. Gastrin, CCK-8, and TPA, which all increase histamine secretion, presumably by stimulation of exocytosis, activate a Cl^- current that is thought to represent the fusion of the histamine vesicle with the plasma membrane. Increased medium $[K^+]$ has been noted to result in stimulation of histamine release.

The formation of histamine-containing vesicles involves accumulation of histamine via the H^+/histamine antiporter, which results in accumulation of active osmolytes. The vesicles grow in size during the process of fluid accumulation, consistent with their accumulation of histamine. When the ECL cells are activated by acute gastrin stimulation, both histamine and pancreastatin in the vesicles are released via exocytosis.

Histidine decarboxylase regulation

A role for histamine-regulated HDC activity in histamine secretion was initially postulated by Kahlson in 1964. Histamine secretion and synthesis are intimately coupled, and store depletion is often the signal for enzyme synthesis. HDC activation may be initiated by such an event. A second possibility is that the secretory signal cascade initiated by ligand binding results in enzyme activation. The initial histamine secretory response (exocytosis) is followed by a linear HDC activation, suggesting that HDC activity is responsive to histamine secretion. However, the synthesis of newly transcribed HDC mRNA may also occur in an *in vitro* setting and thus play a role in the synthesis of histamine.

Gastrin appears to play a significant role in the regulation of HDC. HDC is a homodimeric pyridoxal phosphate–dependent enzyme that produces the physiologic 1,4-diamine histamine. Mammalian HDCs exhibit extensive homology with the aromatic amino acid decarboxylase that produces serotonin and tryptamine. These enzymes share common catalytic properties. However, there is little sequence homology between these enzymes and the putrescine-producing ornithine decarboxylase (ODC). Both HDC and ODC have short half-lives, and there is a PGST (proline-glutamyl-serine-threonine) region that confers constitutive degradation and polyamine responsiveness in both proteins. Histamine, indeed, is known to behave like a polyamine analog and is able to regulate ODC, intracellular polyamine levels, and cell growth *in vivo* and *in vitro*.

In vivo studies indicate that ECL cell HDC activity and histamine concentration are directly dependent on circulating gastrin levels. Gastrin-induced activation of HDC is associated with a progressive increase in the level of HDC mRNA *in vivo*. This gastrin-evoked increase in HDC mRNA was slower and less marked than the increase in HDC activity. Fasting reduced HDC message by three- to fourfold after 48 hours, whereas refeeding induced a rapid increase in message that was detectable within 30 minutes by RT-PCR. HDC enzymatic activity and mRNA abundance varied in parallel, suggesting that HDC mRNA was important in the overall regulation of gastric mucosal HDC activity.

In an isolated culture of ECL cells, a linear increase in gastrin-stimulated HDC activity was noted over 60 minutes. HDC levels were elevated up to threefold during this time. In a similar system of acutely isolated ECL cells, it has been noted that gastrin stimulated HDC activity with an EC_{50} of 10^{-10} M and an EC_{max} of 10^{-8} M. Maximal stimulation resulted in a time-dependent increase of HDC activity, with linear kinetics up to 30 minutes, and no further increase between 30 and 60 minutes. In basophil leukemia cells, phorbol esters have been noted to increase HDC gene expression after 2 to 4 hours of incubation by 50% due to increased protein synthesis. The accelerated time course and amplified levels of HDC noted in ECL cells suggest that a second factor, such as posttranslational activation of HDC, might be involved, rather than only stimulation of HDC synthesis.

ECL cell ontogeny

Studies using an o-phthalaldehyde method (low sensitivity and specificity for histamine detection) failed to detect developing ECL cells in embryonic gastric mucosa. Detectable ECL cells only appeared at the end of the first postnatal week. After birth, an accelerated production of ECL cells was evident until postnatal day 21 (P21), by which time levels and distribution were similar to those noted in adult animals. During this period of expansion, ECL cells undergo a number of developmental and structural changes. By P3, mucosal ECL cells display long, thin processes traversing the length of gastric glands, making contact with glandular cells. By P7, an increase in the overall proportion of ECL cells possessing "paracrine-processes" was evident, and by P14, almost no histamine or HDC immunoreactive cells were detectable in the upper third of gastric glands. These now displayed a morphology similar to that of adult rats. By P14, the majority of ECL cells had formed aggregates in the basal parts of the glands.

Regulation of ECL cell proliferation

The biologic relevance of ECL cell hyperplasia or carcinoids had been recognized for many years in the context of the massive hypergastrinemia associated with pernicious anemia and atrophic gastritis. Growth of ECL cells assumed more significance when identified in the context of the elevated gastrin levels associated with the use of the PPI class of drugs in rats. Use of high doses of these drugs or high-dose histamine receptor antagonists resulted in ECL cell hyperplasia and even carcinoids after a 2-year treatment. This was not seen in mice or dogs and has not been seen in humans. The effect in rats was shown to be due to hypergastrinemia and not to any direct effect of the drugs. Nevertheless, the long-term consequences, if any, of the effects of sustained hypergastrinemia in the human species may not be apparent for many years. To date, however, despite careful surveillance, there does not appear to be any deleterious effect of administration of PPIs up to and beyond a decade.

The following section evaluates a series of ligands known to influence ECL cell proliferation.

1. Gastrin

It is apparent that, in addition to stimulating histamine release, gastrin acts as a trophic factor for the ECL cell. Indeed, the hypertrophic and hyperplastic responses of the ECL cell to gastrin became notorious due to the development of ECL cell carcinoids after life-long therapy with antisecretory drugs in rats. Although first thought to be a side effect of specific antisecretory agents, it is now apparent that ECL cell proliferation may occur in any condition resulting in a prolonged elevation of plasma gastrin levels.

The response of the ECL cell to gastrin may be regarded as exhibiting acute, intermediate, and chronic phases within which histamine secretion, HDC activation, and, lastly, DNA synthesis occur. Of particular relevance here is the ability of gastrin to stimulate ECL cell hypertrophy, hyperplasia, and ultimately neoplasia. The life-long administration (2 years) of high doses of acid-inhibitory agents in rats is associated with the development of ECL tumors (ECLoma, gastric carcinoids). The changes that the ECL cell undergoes during this time range from a diffuse hyperplasia through focal aggregation of cells to structures of a more solid appearance, culminating in gastric carcinoids. The rat ECL cell exhibits a four- to fivefold increase in numbers, compared with an approximately 30% increase in the oxyntic mucosal thickness in response to gastrin. No other oxyntic endocrine cell increases in number in response to gastrin.

In rats treated with the H_2 receptor antagonist ranitidine or the long-acting H_2 receptor antagonist BL-6341 hydrochloride, hypergastrinemia as well as ECL cell hyperplasia and ECL cell carcinoids were produced. Omeprazole-dependent hypergastrinemia in rats resulted in an increased proportion of ECL cells that incorporated thymidine in preparation for mitosis during the first 10 to 20 weeks of treatment. ECL cell HDC activity, a marker of ECL cell activation by gastrin, was also noted to remain elevated for the duration of treatment (1 year). In addition,

Sequence of Gastrin Effects on ECL Cells

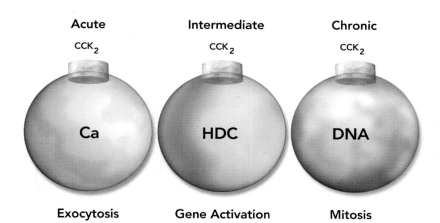

The time of onset of the three major studied effects of gastrin on the ECL cell. Acute = Ca^{2+} signaling and histamine release. Intermediate = upregulation of histidine decarboxylase. Chronic = stimulation of ECL cell replication.

using isolated ECL cell preparations, the presence of a functional gastrin/CCK_2 trophic receptor on the rat ECL cell has been identified. Antrectomy prevented ECL cell changes due to omeprazole administration. Omeprazole and other PPIs were without effect on ECL cell growth *in vitro*.

Gastrin stimulates growth of the oxyntic mucosa, and lack of gastrin is associated with atrophy of the oxyntic mucosa. Thus, the induction of endogenous hypergastrinemia by antral exclusion or by partial removal of the acid-reducing part of the stomach (fundectomy or corporectomy) results in increased ECL cell density. Hypogastrinemia induced by antrectomy has the reverse effect. In rats with uremia, hypergastrinemia is associated with increased stomach weight and parietal and ECL cell density. Gastrin immunoneutralization (gastrin-specific monoclonal antibody) significantly inhibited gastric mucosal thickness; parietal and ECL cell density increased but had no effect on gastric weight or the area of the corpus mucosa. Exogenous hypergastrinemia similarly results in ECL cell hyperplasia after 28 days. *In vitro* rodent studies using ^{3}H-thymidine–labeled DNA demonstrate that ECL cells display a greater labeling index during the night than during the day, which coincides with the time that the rats exhibit a higher circulating gastrin level. Similarly, endogenous hypergastrinemia generated by acid-inhibitory therapy resulted in an eightfold increase in the ECL cell labeling index as well as an increase in ECL cell mitotic figures.

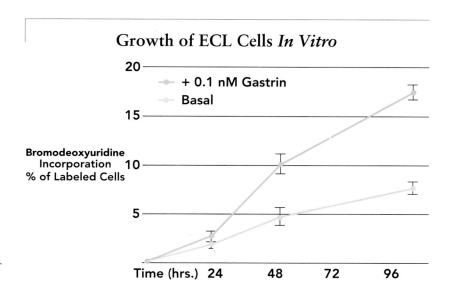

The effect of gastrin on ECL cell DNA replication under *in vitro* culture conditions.

Mature ECL cells are capable of dividing but have a relatively low mitotic activity *in vivo*, with an estimated cell cycle duration of approximately 60 days in mice. Hypergastrinemia activates self-replication of the ECL cells, and there appears to be a direct correlation between the ECL cell proliferation rate and circulating gastrin levels. A recent report suggests that the normal endocrine cells of the human gut have no proliferative capacity, and that, in this cell lineage, population expansion is preceded by differentiation. If the endocrine (ECL) cell is regarded as terminally differentiated and postmitotic, this would suggest that hypergastrinemia acts at the stem cell level rather than on the ECL cells themselves.

ECL cell density thus reflects the circulating gastrin concentration, and hypergastrinemia induced by acid inhibition is responsible for the proliferation of ECL cells. In humans, the results of 10-year treatment with omeprazole show no significant change in the ECL cell population, presumably because there is a lack of effect of gastrin on the stem cell population, and possibly the mature ECL cell is terminally differentiated in people.

The South African rodent *Mastomys* spontaneously develops ECLomas at 12 to 18 months of age, even though it is normogastrinemic. Factors other than gastrin are thus required. This situation appears in some ways more analogous to the human multiple endocrine neoplasia type 1 (MEN-1). Hypergastrinemia, despite increased acid secretion, results in development of fundic gastric ECL cell hyperplasia and gastric carcinoids. This process is significantly accelerated by the introduction of acid-inhibitory treatment. The generation of hypergastrinemia by any acid-inhibiting agent in *Mastomys* results in two- to fourfold elevation of gastrin levels and tumor formation in 3 to 4 months. The more potent the agent in inhibiting acid and increasing gastrin levels, the more effective its ability to generate ECL cell hyperplasia and neoplasia. The administration of octreotide (a somatostatin analog) results in significant lowering of plasma gastrin levels and decrease of ECL cell hyperplasia and neoplasia.

The incorporation of bromodeoxyuridine (BrdU, a thymidine analog incorporated into single-stranded DNA during the S-phase of cell mitosis) has been predominantly used to study the effects of gastrin on the DNA synthesis of cultured rat or *Mastomys* ECL cells. Under short-term culture conditions, gastrin stimulated DNA synthesis in approximately 20% of ECL cells. Isolated ECL cells are not synchronized in their cell cycles. Because mouse ECL cells *in vivo* have a cell cycle of approximately 60 days, and hypergastrinemia causes ECL cell proliferation in 4 to 7 days, the increase noted in labeled ECL cells in culture is comparable with *in vivo* data. It has been suggested that ECL cells in short-term culture exhibit transit with a time delay from a G0 to a G1 state, because the cells are undergoing recovery.

Gastrin directly stimulates DNA synthesis in ECL cells via a gastrin/CCK_2 receptor subtype. It has been demonstrated that gastrin-receptor activation is associated with protein tyrosine kinase activation. During 48 hours of gastrin stimulation, BrdU incorporation increases two- to threefold. The response of BrdU incorporation was significant at low concentrations between 10^{-12} M and 10^{-10} M. These observations correspond to *in vivo* reports of gastrin increasing the ECL cell density two- to fourfold at similar plasma concentrations. Gastrin increased DNA synthesis in ECL cells with an EC_{50} of 1.7×10^{-12} M. This effect was inhibited by L365,260 (IC_{50}, 5×10^{-9} M) and by genistein (10^{-4} M) but was not altered by L364,718 (10^{-8} M). The trophic gastrin effect, as well as the acute secretory effect, is mediated via a gastrin/CCK_2–receptor subtype.

The differential response to gastrin in terms of secretion and DNA synthesis may reflect different intracellular coupling or transduction mechanisms that follow ligand binding. Genistein, a nonselective protein tyrosine kinase inhibitor, inhibits both cytoplasmic and membrane-associated tyrosine kinases. At 10^{-4} M, genistein failed to inhibit histamine secretion but blocked gastrin-stimulated DNA synthesis.

This may reflect differences in the intracellular signal-transduction pathways by which gastrin stimulates the ECL cell. In colonic cell lines, gastrin has been noted to stimulate DNA synthesis via a tyrosine kinase–mediated pathway. It is apparent, however, that the coupling mechanism that stimulates DNA synthesis is not the same as the one regulating histamine secretion. Thus, nonsulfated CCK-8, which is equipotent and equally effective in stimulating histamine release and calcium signaling, is significantly less effective in inducing DNA synthesis. This may be due to decreased stability of nonsulfated CCK-8 due to the presence of endopeptidases or may reflect different receptor binding to the gastrin receptor. *In vivo* infusion of sulfated CCK-8, which has a similar affinity to the CCK_2 receptor as nonsulfated CCK-8, did not induce rat ECL cell hyperplasia at tenfold plasma concentrations but did increase histamine synthesis.

Acid-inhibitory agents, such as the PPIs omeprazole, lansoprazole, and pantoprazole, which are responsible for hypergastrinemia, did not affect BrdU incorporation in isolated ECL cells.

2. Pituitary adenylate cyclase–activating polypeptide

PACAP is widely distributed throughout the fundus and is localized in enteric nerves. In isolated ECL cells, it displays a proliferative effect significantly more potent than gastrin, which has until recently been regarded as the

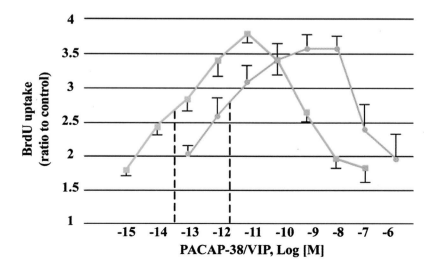

Effects of PACAP and VIP on ECL Cell Proliferation

Gastrin had initially been recognized as the most potent stimulus of ECL cell proliferation (quantified by BrdU uptake). This figure demonstrates that the neurotransmitters PACAP (3×10^{-14} M) and VIP (3×10^{-12} M) are significantly more potent than gastrin (1.7×10^{-12} M). Both PACAP and VIP bind to the PAC-1 receptor for growth stimulation, with VIP having lower potency at this receptor.

primary regulator of ECL cell proliferation. The specificity of this effect was confirmed by the identification of a PACAP receptor on the ECL cell using RT-PCR and Southern blot. The inhibition of the proliferative response with the PACAP-receptor antagonist, PACAP6-38, further established the functional significance of this peptide. VIP, a member of the same family, was significantly less potent (as it was for stimulation of histamine release), and use of specific receptor antagonists confirmed the effects to be mediated via the PACAP receptor.

3. Transforming growth factor-α

The transforming growth factor-α (TGF-α) content of ECL cells also increases significantly as measured by radioimmunoassay, nuclease protection assay, and Northern blot analysis. Similarly, EGF-receptor expression is correspondingly increased with the duration of hypergastrinemia. Thus, gastrin-induced ECL cell proliferation evokes increased ECL cell TGF-α production, which may be responsible for a gastrin-independent phase of ECL cell proliferation.

4. Histamine

The histamine 1 (H_1) receptor agonist (2-[(3-trimethyl)-diphenyl] histamine), although having no measurable effect alone, reversed the inhibitory effect of the H_1 receptor antagonist (terfenadine) on gastrin-driven DNA synthesis. The H_3 receptor subtype agonist, imetit, stimulated gastrin-driven DNA synthesis with an EC_{50} of 10^{-10} M. The H_3 receptor antagonist, thioperamide, inhibited gastrin-stimulated BrdU uptake (IC_{50} 5×10^{-10} M). These data are consistent with potentiation by histamine of gastrin-induced ECL cell proliferation via histamine-receptor subtypes. Sodium cromoglycate, an inhibitor of histamine release in both the mast and the ECL cells, also inhibits ECL cell proliferation (IC_{50} 10^{-11} M).

5. Somatostatin

Somatostatin has been demonstrated to inhibit ECL cell proliferation (IC_{50} 10^{-10} M) under culture conditions and *in vivo*.

6. General

There are apparently different agents involved in stimulation or inhibition of ECL cell division, depending on the stage of transformation of the cell. The primary and most potent acute local regulator may be PACAP, whereas gastrin may function as an endocrine modulator linking ECL cell and acid-secretory activity to cell number. Autocrine regulation may be involved, particularly when the cell is moving toward a neoplastic phenotype. In this respect, TGF-α appears to exert an important influence. Somatostatin is the predominant inhibitory regulator of proliferation, acting via a somatostatin 2–receptor subtype.

A cartoon of an isolated ECL cell (electron micrograph) demonstrating the variety of peptide agonists that regulate ECL cell DNA synthesis. Somatostatin (SST) has been demonstrated to inhibit each of these. TGF-α may, in the transformed ECL cell, exert an autoregulatory effect.

G cells

General

In the adult, gastrin occurs mainly in the G cells of the gastric antrum and duodenum, but small amounts have been identified in the pituitary and some vagal nerve fibers. In early life, the fetal and neonatal pancreas produces gastrin, which may be the source of neonatal hypergastrinemia. After birth, gastrin production in the periphery is due to the G cell in the antral mucosa. In the circulation, the predominant form of gastrin is a heptadecapeptide, G17, although both shorter and longer forms have been identified. Gastrin contains a COOH terminal amide resulting from the posttranslational amidation of a glycine-extended precursor. Gastrin shares an identical pentapeptide amide with CCK, which results in relatively similar binding to the CCK_2 receptor. CCK contains a tyrosine residue in the seventh position from the COOH terminal that is always sulfated, whereas gastrin has a tyrosine in the sixth position that may or may not be sulfated. The position and sulfation of the tyrosine residue appear to be critical for recognition by the CCK_1–subtype receptor. Structural differences between the two peptides result in receptor-subtype selectivity and thereby determine selective biologic activity.

Because the G cells of the gastric antrum are of the "open" type, with their apical surfaces reaching the glandular lumen, luminal contents (protons, amino acids, NH_3) may be able to directly modulate G cell activity and the release of gastrin generated by the urease of *H. pylori*. Intracellular granules containing gastrin are abundant in the basal portion of the cells, and on stimulation, gastrin is released by an exocytotic process into the extracellular fluid, from which it diffuses into the circulation and travels to the gastric fundus. Gastrin thus meets Hardy's archetypal criteria of a true hormone.

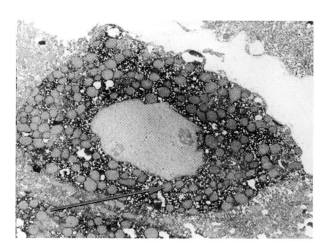

An electron micrograph of a gastrin cell showing the dense granules containing gastrin (red arrow).

Regulation of the G cell

The primary event responsible for the physiologic release of gastrin from the antral G cells is the presence of food in the stomach. The mechanism involved in this process comprises at least three stimulatory pathways that include central neural activation, distention of the antrum, and specific chemical components in the food. At the cellular level, these pathways regulate gastrin release through the actions of ACh, GRP, somatostatin, and the direct chemical effects of H^+ and aromatic amino acids. It is likely that other cellular effectors, such as adenosine, galanin, and epinephrine, play a role, but their physiologic significance is dubious.

Vagal influences

Because gastrin is released in response to oropharyngeal and central stimuli via the vagus nerve, selective antral vagotomy abolishes both sham feeding and hypoglycemia-stimulated release. Given the observation that selective fun-

A model of stimulation of gastrin release by aromatic amino acids in the antral lumen or by pH elevation and by ACh and GRP on the basal surface. The apical surface has been drawn to emphasize and illustrate the luminal connection. There are probably receptors for tryptophan, tyrosine, and phenylalanine on the apical surface of the G cell exposed to the lumen of the antral gland, and perhaps also receptors for protons. The basal lateral surface contains receptors for gastrin-releasing peptide (GRP) and acetylcholine as activating receptors. The cell also expressed the pH regulator Na^+/H^+ exchanger. Gastrin is illustrated as being exocytosed from the basal surface of the G cell.

Elevation of pH_{in} and Gastrin Release

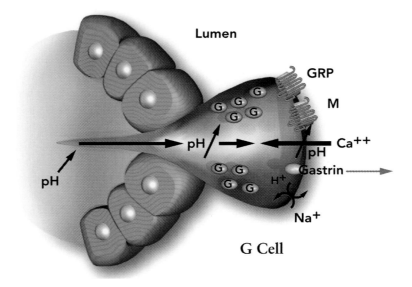

dic vagotomy leads to an enhanced vagal release of gastrin, it is likely that the vagus also initiates an inhibitory action mediated by the fundus. Because atropine inhibits both the antral release and the fundic inhibitory reflex, it is evident that muscarinic synapses are involved in both pathways. Peripheral mechanisms are primarily stimulatory for gastrin release, and the major central influence appears to be inhibition, because bilateral truncal vagotomy leads to a sustained elevation of serum gastrin levels. It seems likely that the inhibitory tone exerted by M_2 or M_4 receptors on the D cell is removed with a decrease of somatostatin release.

The presence of food in the stomach activates peripheral pathways that include mechanisms associated both with gastric distention and the chemical composition of the gastric lumen. The study of peripheral mechanisms in the intact animal and *in vitro* often yields conflicting results, given the presence or absence of different components of the regulatory system in a specific model. To more precisely define these interactions, we have opted to focus on the cellular mechanisms participating in the peripheral pathway.

Enhanced release of gastrin follows significant distention of the antral portion of the stomach, whereas distention of the fundus alone tends to inhibit gastrin secretion. This phenomenon of distention-induced gastrin release is reported to be either inhibited or enhanced by atropine, depending on the dose. Such *in vivo* results suggest that the distention responses are mediated by local neural reflexes. *In vitro* studies that attempt to mimic the local reflex by field stimulation or application of nicotinic agonists have indicated that ACh stimulates gastrin release from the G cell but also inhibits somatostatin release from antral D cells, thus providing a partial explanation for the contradictory actions of atropine. Accordingly, low doses of atropine would suppress somatostatin release, relieving tonic inhibition of the G cell by somatostatin, whereas higher doses would inhibit the G cell directly.

Acid

There are a number of specific chemical components of antral contents that modulate the release of gastrin. The most effective and well studied of these is the pH of the antral lumen, which at values of less than 3.0 completely suppresses gastrin release. This serves to terminate gastric digestion, and, if the antral luminal pH remains elevated in the presence of continuing stimulation, hypergastrinemia results.

Amino acids and amines

The presence of aromatic amino acids is responsible for luminal initiation of the release of gastrin. Intact protein fails to increase gastrin secretion, whereas the ingestion of peptone, a partially digested protein mix, is a powerful stimulant. In this respect, the preferential stimulation by aromatic amino acids is consistent with the preferred cleavage sites for the major gastric protease pepsin. The effect of amino acids on gastrin release represents a direct action on the G cell, because it can be reproduced *in vitro* and is not blocked by atropine or other inhibitors of neural transmission. Given the fact that the G cell is open to the gastric lumen, chemical effectors can bind to the apical membrane or become internalized by the G cells to influence gastrin secretion.

This is thought to mimic the digestive processes occurring normally and, thus, to be a physiologic mechanism for gastrin release. On the other hand, release of gastrin by amines may be an artifact of high concentration and simply due to the general action of these agents as weak bases. These would then elevate G cell pH, which per se can result in the release of gastrin or sensitize the system to GRP or Ach.

Gastrin-releasing peptide

Because a significant component of the neural release of gastrin, whether initiated locally by distention or through the vagus, was known to be atropine resistant, a mediator of this phenomenon was sought. The identification of GRP, a neurocrine peptide in the brain, spinal cord, and enteric nerve fibers of the gut, prompted suspicion that it might fulfill this role. GRP was initially defined as the mammalian counterpart to the amphibian peptide bombesin, because the two peptides share nine of ten COOH terminal amino acids. Both GRP and receptors for GRP are widely distributed in the body, including fetal and neonatal bronchial epithelium. The last location is of considerable clinical relevance, because GRP acts as an autocrine growth factor for human tumors, including small-cell lung cancer. Although GRP-like peptides are now well documented as mitogens, their initial biologic assays measured the release of gastrin and, as a result, this name has persisted. GRP is localized to enteric gastric nerve fibers, where it is responsible for gastrin release, and in the fundus, where it may be related to GRP regulation of motility. Administration of GRP does not influence acid secretion in the absence of an intact antrum. Antral GRP is released from enteric nerves, at least in part, through nonmuscarinic cholinergic (nicotinic) pathways. Because atropine blocks most of the vagal release of gastrin, it is uncertain which portion of the response is mediated by GRP. Similarly, the role of endogenous GRP in mediating the release of gastrin due to distention or chemical components of food remains uncertain. A substantial role for GRP in gastrin release appears certain.

In studies using isolated G cells, GRP and its analogs affect direct stimulation of gastrin by activation of phospholipase C, leading to liberation of diacylglycerol (DAG) and elevation of Ca^{2+}. In addition, the calcium ionophore, A 23187, was found to be a potent stimulus for gastrin release, as were phorbol esters that mimic the action of DAG in activating protein kinase C. These actions are consistent with the finding that the GRP receptor belongs to the G protein–coupled superfamily and appears to be coupled to phospholipase C activation in other cells. Because cAMP analogs and forskolin also stimulate gastrin release, it appears that both cAMP and Ca^{2+} serve as intracellular coupling agents in the G cell. The G cell ligand that activates G_s and, hence, elevates cAMP is not known.

Somatostatin

An important factor in the regulation of gastrin release is inhibition of the G cell by somatostatin, but the infusion of somatostatin at doses sufficient to inhibit acid secretion failed to inhibit gastrin secretion. Presumably, the effect of somatostatin on the ECL cell occurs more readily than on the G cell when infused. Immunoneutralization of somatostatin enhances basal and stimulated gastrin release, showing that local release of the peptide is exerting a direct effect on the G cell. Somatostatin, therefore, acts only as a paracrine agent to suppress gastrin secretion, and any action on antral G cells is not due to circulating somatostatin. There are five known subtypes of somatostatin receptor, and the receptor subtype on the G cell is probably type 2. A model of the G cell is shown in the figure below.

Model of G Cell Function

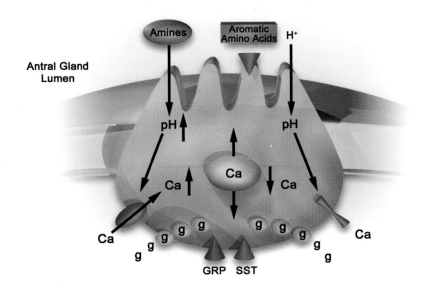

A model of the antral G cell exposed to both serosal and luminal factors for its regulation by modification of cell calcium and pH. Gastrin (g) is depicted as being released into the paracellular spaces from the basolateral domain of the G cell. The entry of amines on the left elevates intracellular pH as the primary effect, resulting in calcium entry and gastrin release. Aromatic amino acids stimulate Ca^{2+} signaling via receptors and again gastrin release. Acidic pH results, as shown on the right, with decrease of intracellular pH and inhibition of calcium signaling.

D cells

General

D cells are present both in the fundus and antrum and contain somatostatin. The D cells of the antrum exhibit elongated processes that extend to the basal portions of G cells and are more frequent here than in the fundus. These cells also extend processes to the lumen of the antral gland. The fundic D cells are relatively sparse and have no contact with the lumen of the fundic gland.

As for the G cell, the D cells contain a large number of secretory granules and are somewhat larger than the ECL cell and denser, because they do not have hollow vacuoles.

Regulation

Gastrin and CCK

The release of somatostatin from antral D cells, like the release of gastrin from G cells, is regulated by a complex set of mechanisms, not all of which are defined clearly.

Because somatostatin is so widespread in its distribution, there is some difficulty in assigning an origin for somatostatin released into the circulation. Gastrin and CCK both stimulate somatostatin release from isolated D cells, and this cell type has both CCK_1 and CCK_2 receptors.

Because CCK stimulates acid secretion *in vitro* through release of histamine from ECL cells but inhibits acid secretion *in vivo*, it is likely that the inhibitory action *in vivo* is due to somatostatin release driven by CCK_1 activation.

Gastrin also stimulates the D cell, providing a negative feedback mechanism for both G and ECL cell function by the CCK_2 receptor.

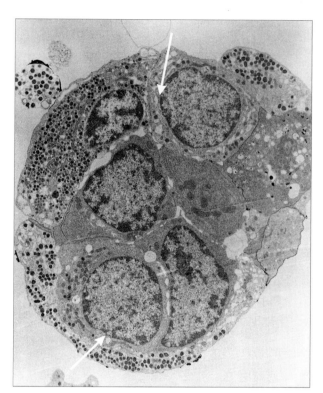

An electron micrograph of antral D cells showing the luminal extension folded onto the surface of the cell and the electron-dense somatostatin-containing granules.

Secretin/VIP

Peptides of the secretin/VIP family stimulate somatostatin release, and the consequent suppression of gastrin release may account for at least some of the ability of such peptides to inhibit acid secretion *in vivo*. PACAP, when injected *in vivo*, inhibits gastrin-stimulated acid secretion; this is probably due to stimulation of the fundic D cell at a VIP receptor. When somatostatin-neutralizing antibody is given along with PACAP, acid secretion ensues due to the effect of PACAP on the ECL cell being revealed.

Acetylcholine

In contrast to the other cells in the gastric mucosa, the D cell has inhibitory muscarinic receptors of either the M_2 or M_4 subtype, allowing the conclusion that vagal stimulation of acid secretion inhibits somatostatin release.

Acid

Antral D cells, unlike those of the fundus, project to the gastric lumen and, thus, are capable of detecting chemical components of food. Of particular interest in this regard is the observation that antral somatostatin is released in response to acidification of the gastric lumen. This may represent a mechanism for suppression of gastrin release at low intraluminal pH, a critical factor in the physiologic regulation of gastric acidity. The G and D cells of the antrum both therefore have sensing mechanisms of conditions in the lumen of the antral gland. A simple model would place the amino acid sensor on the G cell and the acid sensor on the D cell. Presumably, aromatic amino acids elevate $[Ca^{2+}]_i$ in the G cell, and reduction of pH to less than 3.0 elevates the same second messenger in the D cell.

Knockout models

Novel insight into the regulation of gastric mucosal architecture, cell census, and acid regulation has recently become available from studies of transgenic mice receptor knockouts (KNOs) and the examination of rats with naturally occurring double mutants. Although such models have limitations, the information derived provides useful alternative interpretations of previously held concepts regarding acid-secretory regulation derived from more standard experimental models.

H_2 receptor knockout (KNO) mice

Histamine H_2 receptor–deficient mice have been generated by gene targeting, and the homozygous mutant mice are viable and fertile, without apparent abnormalities. An examination of the gastric morphology demonstrates that the oxyntic mucosa in these KNO mice exhibited a marked hypertrophy, with enlarged folds in gastric mucosa. Immunohistochemical analysis has revealed increased numbers of parietal cells. Despite this hypertrophy, parietal cells are significantly smaller than in wild-type (WT) mice and contained enlarged secretory canaliculi with a lower density of microvilli and few typical tubulovesicles in the narrow cytoplasm. Immunohistochemical analysis has also revealed increased numbers of ECL cells, and the histamine levels of the gastric mucosa are elevated approximately 300% in KNO animals. Although the distribution of other endocrine cells was not examined, an elevated serum gastrin level (approximately 400%) was noted in the transgenics. Acid secretion has been examined in KNO mice, which showed normal basal gastric pH. However, induction of gastric acid secretion by histamine or gastrin was completely abolished. In contrast, the M_1 muscarinic receptor agonist, carbachol, was able to induce acid secretion to levels similar to that in WT mice. This study

Abnormal functional and morphological regulation of the gastric mucosa in histamine H2 receptor–deficient mice

Takashi Kobayashi,[1] Shunsuke Tonai,[2] Yasunobu Ishihara,[3] Ritsuko Koga,[1] Susumu Okabe,[2] and Takeshi Watanabe[1]

[1]Department of Molecular Immunology, Medical Institute of Bioregulation, Kyushu University, Fukuoka, Japan
[2]Department of Applied Pharmacology, Kyoto Pharmaceutical University, Kyoto, Japan
[3]Developmental Research Laboratories, Shionogi & Co., Osaka, Japan

Address correspondence to: Takeshi Watanabe, Medical Institute of Bioregulation, Kyushu University, 3-1-1 Maidashi, Higashi-ku, Fukuoka 812-8582, Japan. Phone: 81-92-642-6835; Fax: 81-92-632-1499; E-mail: watanabe@bioreg.kyushu-u.ac.jp.

Received for publication January 25, 2000, and accepted in revised form May 2, 2000.

Takeshi Watanabe's group from Kyushu and collaborators generated H_2 receptor–deficient mice (top) and were able to detail the abnormalities in gastric function. The central panel demonstrates the targeted deletion of the mouse H_2 gene, while the bottom panel confirms the mutation (lane 3). Despite normal basal gastric pH, these mice exhibited mucosal hypertrophy and elevated serum gastrin levels. Acid secretion in these animals was mediated by the neural reflex.

demonstrates that a functional H_2 receptor is required for cellular homeostasis of the gastric mucosa and normally formed secretory membranes in parietal cells. Interestingly, impaired acid secretion due to the absence of the H_2 receptor could be completely overcome by activation of cholinergic receptors.

CCK receptor 2 transgenic mice

To elucidate the contribution of the CCK_2 receptor to gastric trophic and secretory factors, mice that lack this receptor have been generated by targeted gene disruption and inactivation of both alleles. The resultant homozygous mutant mice are viable and fertile, and their overall appearance and behavior are indistinguishable from their WT littermates. Overall, these KNO mice appear grossly normal into adulthood. In the stomach, the gastric oxyntic mucosal weight and thickness are significantly decreased (approximately 50%) in KNO mice. Parietal cell numbers are decreased (32%), and the proportion of active acid-secreting cells is also reduced by approximately 70%. In the KNO mice, ECL cell numbers are decreased (52%), HDC activity is below the level of detection, and the histamine content of the gastric mucosa is only a fraction of that in the WT mice. Interestingly, although there are similar numbers of pancreastatin- and $VMAT_2$-immunoreactive cells in both WT and KNO mice, only WT mice have histamine-immunoreactive ECL cells. An electron microscopy study has revealed numerous "ECL-like" cells in KNO animals—cells characterized by a lack of secretory vesicles (a hallmark feature of normal ECL cells) and the presence of dense-core granules and microvesicles. In the antrum of these animals, an increase in the G cell number and a decrease in somatostatin cell density are observed, and the ratio of gastrin to somatostatin cells is markedly elevated (approximately 200%), consistent with the concomitant elevation in circulating gastrin (approximately 1,000%). The KNO mice exhibit a marked increase in basal gastric pH (from 3.2 to 5.2) compared with WT controls. In comparison to the WT mice, KNO mice failed to respond to food stimulation, with an increased gastric acid output after pyloric ligation. These findings demonstrate that the deficiency of a single gene product (CCK_2 receptor) can disrupt the intricate balance of normal cellular composition and function of the gastric mucosa. In addition, congenital absence of this receptor alters the differentiation and function of the ECL cells.

CCK receptor 1

A naturally occurring CCK_1 receptor gene KNO exists. This is the Otsuka Long-Evans Tokushima fatty (OLETF) rat. Histologic examination of the gastric mucosa in OTLEF rats reveals thickening of the fundic mucosa, and the "wet" stomach weight of these animals is increased compared to controls. Hyperplasia and hypertrophy of parietal cells is noted in OLETF rats, and plasma levels of histamine are elevated (approximately twofold) in these animals. Immunohistochemistry of gastrin and somatostatin has revealed no significant difference in cell numbers in the OLETF compared to control rats. This observation is supported by the finding that plasma gastrin levels are not significantly different from those noted in control rats. Somatostatin levels are, however, decreased. Interestingly, plasma concentrations of CCK are higher in these animals. Basal acid output in OLETF rats is significantly higher than that in control rats. In addition, gastric acid secretion stimulated by gastrin, CCK, or histamine is enhanced in the OTLEF rats. CCK_2 receptor antagonists reduced both basal acid outputs and completely suppressed CCK-stimulated acid secretion to similar levels in both strains. Interestingly, CCK was able to enhance the gastrin-stimulated gastric acid output in OLETF rats but not in control rats. These results in the CCK_1 receptor–deficient rats confirmed that CCK stimulates acid secretion by binding to CCK_2 receptors but at the same time inhibits acid responses by stimulating the paracrine secretion of somatostatin from D cells in the gastric mucosa.

Both the H_2 receptor and the CCK_2 receptor are critical for the correct development of gastric mucosal architecture and cell census. In addition, alterations in these receptors are associated with profound changes in acid secretion, particularly in stimulated-acid release. Interestingly, a functional acid response can be elicited in the absence of an H_2 receptor, suggesting that a direct neurally mediated acid-release pathway that is as effective as the paracrine/hormonal pathways exists. In addition, it is clear that the major gastrin-elicited acid effect is via the ECL cell and not through the parietal cell. CCK may stimulate acid secretion directly and indirectly by binding to the CCK_2 receptor, but at the same time, CCK inhibits acid responses by stimulating the paracrine secretion of somatostatin from D cells and thereby exerts a tonic inhibition on the parietal cells.

CHAPTER 3
THE PARIETAL CELL

It has been more than 100 years since it was suggested that the secretory canaliculus of the parietal cell was the site of gastric acid secretion by Camillo Golgi. The pump responsible for acid secretion was identified some 20 years ago, and, recently, the high-resolution crystals of the SERCA ATPase have rationalized many of the structure-function studies on this enzyme. However, analysis of the complexity of the processes that regulate acid secretion by the parietal cell in terms of signaling pathways that alter cell morphology, the regulation of trafficking of the pump to the apical membrane, and activation of the necessary KCl conductance is only now becoming possible with the advent of modern cell and molecular biology and genomics and proteomics. Much remains to be discovered.

Early work on understanding parietal cell biology was based on data derived from the exteriorized dog flap in a hemi-chamber. More exact physiologic data were obtained on isolated amphibian mucosae in Ussing chambers. The major technical breakthrough in defining the stimulatory pathways in the mammalian parietal cell was the development of the rabbit gastric gland preparation with measurement of acid secretion by uptake of the weak-base ^{14}C-aminopyrine.

Isolated Rabbit Gastric Glands

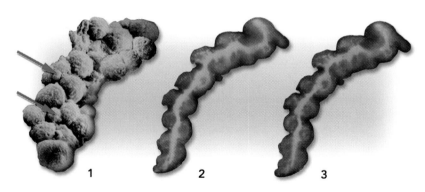

1   2   3

The gastric gland model of acid secretion. In the left of the figure (1), a scanning electron micrograph of a gland is shown, with the large parietal cells prominent on the surface of the gland. Two small cells, shown by arrows, inserted between four parietal cells, are enterochromaffin-like cells that release histamine in the immediate environment of the secreting cell. In the middle (2) is a gastric gland in the presence of acridine orange that is not stimulated, showing green fluorescence only. To the right (3) is the same gland after stimulation. The red fluorescence corresponds to accumulation of the weak base—acridine orange—with stacking and a metachromatic shift to red emission. The red shift shows the presence and location of acid in the secretory canaliculus and the lumen of the gastric gland.

In amphibia and birds, the acid-secreting cell is called the *oxyntic cell*; in mammals it is the *parietal cell*. These are epithelial cells, characterized by a difference between their mucosal or apical surface and their serosal or basolateral surface. These two domains are separated by a specialized region of the membrane, the tight junction.

The major function of the parietal cell at the neck of the gastric gland is the polarized secretion of HCl across its mucosal surface; in some species, this cell also secretes intrinsic factor, a protein vital for the absorption of cyanocobalamin. More mature parietal cells closer to the base of the gastric gland are also able to secrete Cl⁻, resulting in water flow by coupling this Cl⁻ flux to Na⁺ flux across the tight junction. This secretion of water independent of acid may be useful in flushing out secreted pepsinogen from the lumen of the gland in this region.

As has been discussed, acid secretion is a regulated process, and the target for this regulation is the parietal cell, with a variety of receptors on its cell surface. But beyond this cellular target is the proton pump itself, the H,K ATPase. All natural stimuli and inhibitors converge to activate or inhibit this P-type ATPase. The parietal cell has developed extraordinary measures to be able to regulate the act of acid secretion. Regulation of acid secretion at the cellular level involves three stages: activation of receptors on the basolateral surface, cytoplasmic signaling events consequent to ligand interaction with these receptors, and thence regulation of the H,K ATPase itself and a pathway enabling KCl efflux into the secretory canaliculus.

Development of the parietal cell

The parietal cell is an epithelial cell derived from stem cells in the isthmus of the gastric gland. These cells give rise to progenitor cells, which differentiate into parietal cells, forming three helical chains spiraling down to the base of the gland. Markers of parietal cell differentiation are an abundance of mitochondria and the presence of the H,K ATPase. Although the parietal cell itself is a terminally differentiated cell, there are differences between the parietal cells in the neck of the gland and in the lower part of the gland.

For example, stimulation of acid secretion affects the superficial cells more than the deeper cells. Also, the deeper cells, although having similar levels of the gastric H,K ATPase, also express the $NaKCl_2$ cotransporter ($NKCC_2$), which the more superficial cells do not. This finding implies that the deeper cells can act as Cl^- secreting cells as well as HCl secreting cells. Perhaps there is a need for fluid secretion, independent of acid, for elution of secreted pepsinogen.

Morphology of the parietal cell

The morphology of the parietal cell is unique. It is conical, with a small apical and large basolateral membrane. Thirty-four percent of cell volume is occupied by mitochondria dedicated to the synthesis of ATP as an energy source for acid secretion. A large percentage of resting cell volume is also occupied by smooth-surfaced membranes called *tubulovesicles* that, when observed by freeze-smash electron microscopy, are actually elongated tubules. Also, there is a small infolding even in the resting cell of the apical membrane named the *secretory canaliculus*.

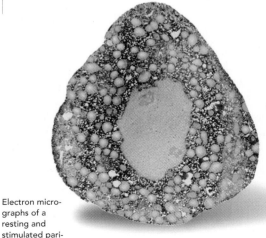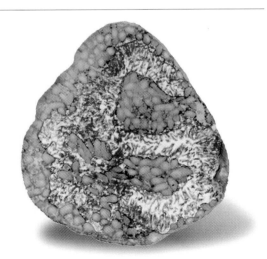

Electron micrographs of a resting and stimulated parietal cell showing the conversion of the cytoplasmic tubulovesicles to the microvilli of the secretory canaliculus.

On stimulation, the tubules decrease in number and transform into microvilli, decorating the secretory canaliculus, which expands in surface area and volume as acid is secreted into the canalicular space. The microvilli contain actin fibers that have moved from the cytoplasm, as shown by phallucidin staining. However, the ratio of globular (G) to filamentous (F) actin stays approximately the same, suggesting that eversion of the tubules is by a process of addition of actin at the growing tip and removal of actin from the base of the tubule.

These morphologic events in the parietal cell reflect stimulation-secretion coupling in the parietal cell; much of this chapter will be devoted to a discussion of the mechanisms underlying activation of acid secretion.

Receptors

The parietal cell appears to possess a variety of receptors for both stimulatory and inhibitory ligands. The majority of these have been defined functionally. Because most of the evidence for the action of modulating agents has been obtained in preparations that are heterogeneous with respect to cell type, some caution must be exercised in concluding that the effects are direct rather than indirect. There are few studies reported using specific receptor antibodies or *in situ* probes.

With the advent of viable isolated gastric gland preparations that can be stimulated or inhibited under superfusion, direct evidence has been obtained for the presence or absence of a specific receptor on the basolateral surface of the parietal cell. Because the gastric gland is composed of several cell layers, confocal microscopy provides a means of determining the presence or absence of a Ca^{2+} signal after addition of a ligand. An alternative approach in the case of isolated, dispersed cells is the use of single-cell video-imaging techniques when direct visualization can provide positive identification of parietal cells and assure that cells are sufficiently well separated to dilute any substances that might be released by potentially intervening cell types. The stimulatory receptors all belong to the seven transmembrane segment trimeric G protein type of receptor, as illustrated in the figure. These receptors function by releasing the bound trimeric G protein after ligand binding, resulting in a lower-affinity state of the receptor. The three subunits, α with GDP bound, β, and γ, are bound to the receptor or to a member of the RGS protein family.

After ligand binding, the α subunit releases GDP and binds GTP. The GTP-liganded trimer dissociates into α monomers and β–γ dimers. The α-GTP monomer then hydrolyzes GTP to GDP, enabling reassociation of the trimer and termination of the signal. These trimer G proteins are responsible for the effects of ligand binding to the receptor. The nature of the protein constituents of the trimeric G protein determines whether there is activation of adenylate cyclase or phospholipase C or inhibition of these enzymes. This determines whether there is an increase of cAMP-dependent protein kinase A activity, an elevation of intracellular Ca, or an inhibition of cell responses.

Most receptors are promiscuous in terms of which G proteins are bound. Antagonists of these receptors can be divided into pure antagonists that can only displace agonist or inverse agonists that are able to affect the conformation of the receptor in the absence of agonist. The latter class can therefore affect cell function in the absence of ligand.

Parietal Cell

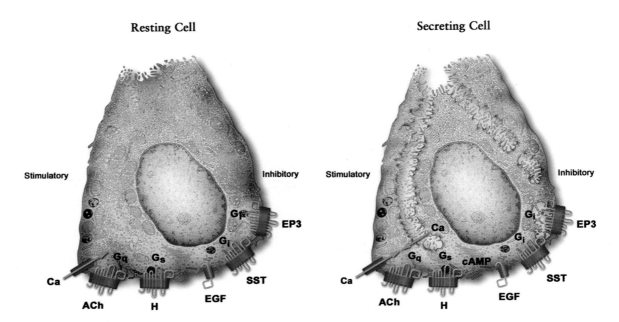

Resting Cell

Secreting Cell

The morphologic transformation of the parietal cell moving from a resting state, or low basal acid secretory state, to a stimulated, or high acid secretory state, based on the activation of stimulatory receptors on its basolateral surface. These receptors are the muscarinic receptor, stimulated by acetylcholine, and the histamine-2 receptor, stimulated by histamine released from the ECL cell. The gastric receptor on the parietal cell is of doubtful significance in direct stimulation of the parietal cell. The somatostatin (SST) receptor, the prostaglandin EP$_3$-receptor subtype, and the epidermal growth factor (EGF) receptor are able to inhibit acid secretion stimulated by histamine or acetylcholine (ACh). The independent pathways for muscarinic and histaminergic stimulation explain why histamine-2 receptor antagonists are not able to fully inhibit neural stimulation of acid secretion.

The majority of receptors affecting acid secretion belong to the G7 (seven transmembrane segments) class of receptors (H$_2$, muscarinic, CCK$_2$, somatostatin, prostaglandin). The EGF/TGF-α receptor, which also inhibits acid secretion, is a tyrosine kinase receptor (single transmembrane segment with an intracellular ATP kinase domain).

In receptors such as the β-adrenergic receptor or others that bind biogenic amines, such as histamine, an aspartyl residue in the third transmembrane domain is thought to bind the positive charge of the ligand, and two serines in the fifth transmembrane domain (TM5) bind the aromatic residue. A phenylalanine residue in TM6 is also conserved in the biogenic amine–responsive G protein–coupled receptors. Antagonists may bind in different regions of the receptor, such as that close to the seventh transmembrane domain. Peptide agonists have a larger binding domain, which includes the second transmembrane segment. Nonpeptide antagonists at the peptide receptor bind at the top of TM5 and 6.

Histamine 2 receptor

The stimulatory action of histamine is mediated by the H$_2$-subtype receptor. Histamine stimulation of acid secretion is inhibited competitively by selective H$_2$ receptor antagonists but is not inhibited by agents acting at other receptors, indicating that histamine acts directly on the parietal cell. The cellular localization of H$_2$ receptors using both *in situ* hybridization and autoradiographic localization of H$_2$-receptor antagonist binding (^{125}I-aminopotentidine) shows that the H$_2$ receptor is located on the parietal cell. Also, elevation of intracellular Ca^{2+} can be observed directly in the parietal cell on addition of histamine to the superfusion medium.

H$_2$ receptor antagonists inhibit gastrin stimulation fully but not that induced by carbachol (cholinomimetic), showing that the former, but not the latter, stim-

Activation of the H₂ Receptor

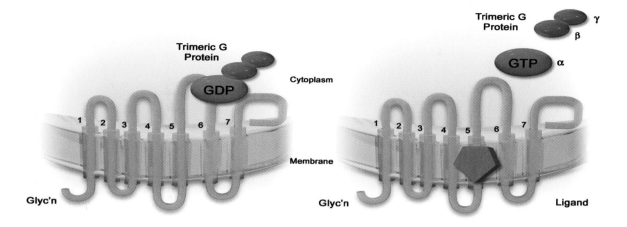

A model of a G7 receptor showing the transmembrane topography, with the N terminus outside and the C terminus inside the cell. The trimeric G protein is bound mainly to the third intracellular loop and also to the C-terminal domain. Charged small-molecule ligands bind in the membrane domain in the region of the third and fifth transmembrane segment, and a conformational change is transmitted to the cytoplasmic domain, illustrated by the red pentagon in the image on the right, releasing the trimeric G protein. GDP is then converted to GTP, allowing dissociation of the α subunit from the β–γ dimer. The former activates PK-A and the latter phospholipase C, in the case of the histamine-2 receptor. Numbers indicate transmembrane segments.

ulant depends on histamine release from the ECL cell. Histamine may be permissive for gastrin, and removal of this permissive action may also be responsible but to a lesser extent for the inhibition of gastrin stimulation by H₂ antagonists. The histamine H₂ receptor has been cloned and expressed, and the cDNA-derived amino acid sequence shows typical features of a G protein–coupled receptor with seven transmembrane segments. The quantitative correlation between stimulation of acid secretion, activation of adenylyl cyclase, and accumulation of cAMP, shown by a variety of H₂ receptor agonists, provides strong evidence that the H₂ receptor is coupled to activation of adenylate cyclase via phosphokinase A (PKA). The nature of the G trimeric proteins coupled to this receptor has not been determined. Addition of histamine also generates Ca^{2+} signals in the parietal cell. Perhaps both cAMP and Ca pathways must be activated for generation of the morphologic transformation essential for acid secretion.

Acetylcholine receptor

Extracts of belladonna have been used to treat dyspepsia since the Roman Empire, and its major component, atropine, was a primary medical treatment for peptic ulcer before development of the H₂ receptor antagonists. Because atropine is a nonselective muscarinic antagonist, it is not possible, based solely on *in vivo* inhibition, to conclude that the parietal cell contains a cholinergic receptor. *In vitro*, particularly in the presence of H₂ receptor antagonists, cholinergic stimulation of acid secretion is weak and often transient. That portion of the cholinergic stimulation that is not inhibited by H₂ receptor antagonists is blocked by atropine. These results suggest that there is indeed direct action of ACh on the parietal cell in addition to the observed interaction with histamine. Inhibition of acid secretion by atropine indicates that ACh acts through a muscarinic-type cholinergic receptor but does not define the specific subtype of muscarinic receptor involved. To date, five muscarinic receptor subtypes

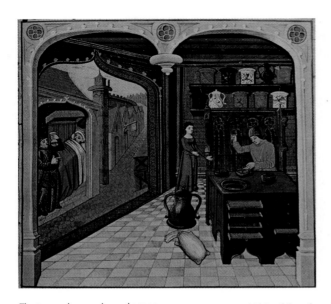

The terms *pharmacology, pharmacy,* and *pharmaceutical* are all originally derived from the Greek word *pharmakon,* which was used indiscriminately by Homer to describe a drug, whether healing or noxious in nature. Subsequently, experiments with roots, leaves, and applied ointments lead to the development of infusions, decoctions, and ointments and the evolution of pharmacology.

have been cloned and sequenced. All are G-protein coupled and exhibit structural similarities, although they couple to different intracellular signaling mechanisms. The M_1, M_3, and M_5 receptors are activated via enhancement of intracellular Ca^{2+}. The M_2 and M_4 receptors are inhibitory. Pharmacologic characterization of cholinergic stimulation of acid secretion *in vitro* indicates that the parietal cell contains an M_3-subtype muscarinic receptor. Accordingly, carbachol stimulation of acid formation by isolated gastric glands is found to be inhibited by subtype-selective antagonists with a potency order of 4-DAMP followed by pirenzepine followed by AF-DX 116. An identical order of potency was found also for displacement of N-methyl scopolamine binding and elevation of intracellular calcium. This is the same order of potency exhibited by the cloned M_3 receptor. The presence of an M_3-subtype receptor on the parietal cell was further evidenced by detection of mRNA encoding the M_3 receptor in parietal cells, whereas no evidence was found for expression of M_1 or M_2 subtypes. Thus, the direct action of ACh on the parietal cell appears to be mediated by an M_3 muscarinic receptor. The M_1 antagonist, pirenzepine, is an effective inhibitor of acid secretion. Presumably this occurs at a site in the peripheral regulatory pathway before convergence of stimuli on the parietal cell.

Gastrin receptor

The function of a receptor for gastrin on the parietal cell has been the subject of controversy. The central observation is the total absence or marginal stimulation of acid secretion by gastrin in the presence of H_2 receptor antagonists. This has led most investigators to conclude that gastrin acts indirectly on the parietal cell by stimulation of histamine release from ECL cells. Favoring a direct action of gastrin on the parietal cell are reports indicating the presence of gastrin-binding sites on gastric mucosal membranes and enriched preparations of parietal cells. These binding sites are characterized as gastrin or CCK_2-type sites in that they show equal affinity for gastrin and sulfated CCK. The presence of gastrin receptors on the parietal cell received further support by the cloning and expression of a CCK_2-type receptor from a cDNA library derived from purified parietal cell mRNA.

Single-cell video imaging has provided direct evidence for a functional CCK_2 receptor on the parietal cell. In particular, gastrin has been shown to produce an elevation of intracellular calcium in individual parietal cells, which is blocked by the CCK_2 antagonist, L365,260. The pattern of intracellular calcium increase, consisting of a biphasic response, indicates a direct action of gastrin on the parietal cell, as opposed to mediation by histamine. Although parallel responses of acid secretion were observed, most of these experiments were not done in the presence of H_2 receptor antagonists, and, therefore, one cannot rule out a permissive effect of H_2 receptor activity on either the secretory or the cell calcium

Analysis of Signaling Between ECL and Parietal Cells

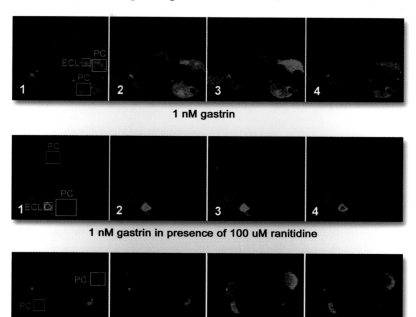

1 nM gastrin

1 nM gastrin in presence of 100 uM ranitidine

10 nM gastrin in presence of 100 uM ranitidine

The figure shows a confocal image of a gastric gland, illustrating the location of the parietal and ECL cells that have been loaded with a calcium-sensing dye, fluo 3. The top image shows the response of both the ECL cells and parietal cells to gastrin at 1 nM in the perfusate. The second image shows the continued response of the ECL cell and the absence of responses in parietal cells when 1 nM gastrin is added in the presence of 100 µM ranitidine. The bottom figure shows the response of parietal cells reappearing in the presence of 100 µM of ranitidine when 10 nM of gastrin is added to the perfusate. Parietal cells and ECL cells of interest are shown inside rectangles. The increase of red coloration indicates an increase in intracellular Ca^{2+} due to action of gastrin.

response. Using confocal imaging, it was then shown that H_2 receptor antagonists did not block the action of gastrin on ECL cells in rabbit or rat gastric glands but blocked the action of gastrin on parietal cell Ca^{2+}. Further experiments showed that, whereas physiologic levels of gastrin stimulated Ca signaling in ECL cells and then parietal cells, the latter also blocked by H_2 receptor antagonists, supraphysiologic levels of gastrin were able to elicit Ca signals in the parietal cells of the gastric gland. This suggests that there is a low-affinity gastrin response in the parietal cell, but this may not be to the presence of a CCK_2 receptor.

Miscellaneous receptors

A variety of agents has been reported to stimulate or inhibit acid secretion by a direct action on the parietal cell. Many of these (e.g., cAMP derivatives, forskolin) do not act through cellular receptors, whereas others are suggested to reflect the presence of parietal cell receptors. Although no direct evidence for a parietal cell location exists, the ability of some substances to inhibit histamine stimulation of acid secretion argues for the presence of a parietal cell receptor, because the action of histamine is direct. Even in these cases, caution is necessary to interpret the inhibition as being direct rather than due to the release of another inhibitor. With this caveat in mind, the parietal cell appears to contain inhibitory receptors for somatostatin, prostaglandins (PG, EP_3), and EGF. Each of these has been shown to inhibit histamine stimulation of acid formation by isolated cell preparations.

Somatostatin is thought to act through an inhibitory G protein to interfere with receptor-mediated second messenger production, explaining the inhibition of histamine stimulation. In the case of EGF, the inhibition appears to occur at a site beyond the H_2 receptor, because EGF also inhibits dibutyryl cAMP stimulation of acid formation. The PG EP_3 receptor has been shown to reduce cAMP levels, and, presumably, bonding to this receptor by relatively nonselective PGE_2 compounds accounts for their inhibition of acid secretion.

The physiologic significance of inhibitory receptors on the parietal cell is not at all clear. A possible role for fundic or circulating somatostatin in con-

A model showing both activated (left) and inhibitory (right) receptors of the parietal cell. The presence or absence of these receptors is discussed in the text.

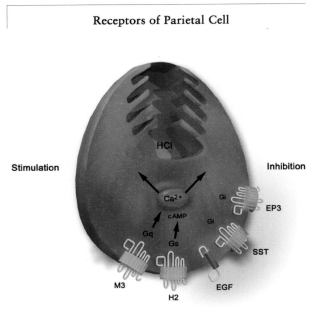

Receptors of Parietal Cell

trolling gastric acidity is discussed above, but this function could be served fully by the action of somatostatin on histamine release from ECL cells. Because the putative direct action of somatostatin on the parietal cell is selective for histamine stimulation, dual inhibition of ECL and parietal cells would seem redundant. In the case of EGF and prostaglandins, it may be speculated that these inhibitors, which are known mediators of wound healing, act only during periods of mucosal injury to reduce acidity and allow more rapid healing. A model showing these receptors on the parietal cell is shown in the figure.

Intracellular signals

Intracellular messengers

The gastric histamine H_2 receptor is coupled to the formation of cAMP, whereas activation of the parietal cell M_3 cholinergic receptor or the putative CCK_2 receptor on the parietal cell leads to an elevation of intracellular calcium. The elevation of cAMP by the H_2 receptor appears to result from a direct coupling, via a G protein, to adenylate cyclase; the elevation of $[Ca]_{in}$ proceeds by a more complex mechanism. The stimulation of a G_q-coupled receptor results in dissociation of the trimeric protein. Thus, there is activation of phospholipase C with breakdown of phosphatidylinositol 4,5-biphosphate (PIP_2) to inositol 1,4,5-triphosphate (IP_3) and diacylglycerol. The former results in the release of Ca from intracellular stores, perhaps aided by binding of the β–γ complex. The latter activates protein C kinase. Stimulants of C kinase, such as the phorbol esters, do not activate acid secretion in gastric glands. Activation of Ca entry accompanies release from intracellular stores, perhaps due to the interaction of the IP_3 receptor with a membrane-located calcium channel.

Using fluorescent indicators with single-cell video imaging, the $[Ca]_{in}$ responses of individual parietal cells are typically found to be biphasic, consisting of an initial peak elevation that rapidly declines to a sustained steady-state elevation. This pattern of $[Ca]_{in}$ response is seen in many cell types and is interpreted to result from an initial release of calcium from intracellular storage sites followed by a sustained influx of calcium from the extracellular fluid via a receptor-operated Ca channel. Similar mechanisms appear to be involved in the agonist-induced elevation of $[Ca]_{in}$ of parietal cells. Accordingly, removal of extracellular calcium or blockade of influx with La^{3+} abolishes the steady-state elevation but not the initial peak response.

In analogy with other cells, it is assumed that the intracellular pool of calcium is stored in specialized regions of the endoplasmic reticulum (ER), where it is released through calcium channels and resequestered by a calcium pump in the ER. Thapsigargin, an inhibitor of the ER calcium pump binding to the cytoplasmic loop between TM4 and TM5, raises $[Ca]_{in}$ in parietal cells, indicating that a typical calcium pump is involved in maintaining the intracellular pool. The release of $[Ca]_{in}$ appears to occur via a regulated calcium channel, two types of which have been identified. In muscle, the ER calcium channel binds ryanodine and is regulated by voltage and possibly by various ligands. In nonexcitable cells, presumably including the parietal cell, the predominant ER calcium channel appears to be one regulated by IP_3.

The observations that cholinergic agonists elevate IP_3 levels in gastric cells and that IP_3 releases calcium from internal stores in permeabilized parietal cells provide evidence that the initial peak response of $[Ca]_{in}$ is due to activation of IP_3 receptor–activated Ca^{2+} channels. This is consistent also with the finding that the cloned M_3 receptor mediates phosphoinositide hydrolysis. The agonist-dependent formation of IP_3 is likely due to activation of phospholipase C. There are various isoforms of this enzyme. The exact mechanism for calcium influx that results in the steady-state elevation of Ca_i remains unidentified. The influx pathway is not a voltage-dependent channel, because it is not blocked by dihydropyridine-type channel blockers.

There is ignorance as to the target of $[Ca]_{in}$ as a coupling signal. The initial observation that removal of external calcium blocked the acid-secretory response to cholinergic agonists suggested that the calcium influx was necessary for secretion. It was argued, however, that removal of calcium depleted the intracellular pool, which was the true second messenger, and acid secretion could be related to the peak $[Ca]_{in}$ response. Recent studies in which the peak and steady-state phases of the $[Ca]_{in}$ response to carbachol could be distinguished by antagonist sensitivity demonstrated that the steady state, but not the peak elevation, is necessary for stimulating acid secretion. Interestingly, elevation of $[Ca]_{in}$, to the same extent as seen in the steady-state response to carbachol, with ionomycin or arachidonic acid failed to induce a secretory response. Similarly, elevation of $[Ca]_{in}$ by thapsigargin mimics steady-state calcium response to carbachol but not the secretory response. The acid-secretory response to cholinergic stimulation requires the steady-state elevation of $[Ca]_{in}$, but this alone is not sufficient.

Although the parietal cell CCK_2 receptor has not been studied in as much detail as the M_3 receptor, it is reasonable to assume that the general mechanisms involved in the $[Ca]_{in}$ response apply to both receptor types. However, it is not clear why the CCK_2 response may require cAMP and that of the M_3 receptor does not.

The long-standing observation that cholinergic and gastrin stimulation of acid secretion is potentiated by histamine or agents such as phosphodiesterase inhibitors, which elevate cAMP, suggests that cAMP and Ca_i interact at some level. Thus, histamine, which acts primarily to elevate cAMP, has been shown to produce a small, transient elevation of $[Ca]_{in}$ in parietal cells. Further, buffering $[Ca]_{in}$ below basal levels inhibits secretory responses to histamine. Accordingly, it may be that both cAMP and elevated $[Ca]_{in}$ are necessary for an optimal secretory response to the extent that a permissive level of one second messenger is required for a full response to the other. A summary of the intracellular M_3 signaling systems is shown in the figure. Similar coupling mechanisms exist for the other G_q-linked receptors.

Signal transduction

The intracellular reactions that ensue from the elevation of $[Ca]_{in}$ and cAMP are unclear. Indeed, this aspect of stimulus-secretion coupling probably represents the single greatest challenge to our understanding of the mechanisms that regulate gastric acid secretion. Based on their known action in a variety of tissues, it is most probable that the intracellular second messengers, particularly in the case of cAMP, serve to activate protein phosphokinases, with subsequent phosphorylation of specific target proteins. With a few notable exceptions, the target proteins for parietal cell protein kinases have not been identified. Two general approaches have been used in attempting to identify the intermediate reactions of stimulus-secretion coupling in parietal cells: The most popular and seemingly straightforward approach, based on the assumption that activation of protein kinases represents the initial step, has been to attempt identification of stimulation-associated phosphoproteins. This approach has been frustrated thus far by technical and conceptual difficulties and has yielded few positive results. A second, recently initiated, approach involves attempts to first identify components associated with the proton pump and then to assess possible modulations related to activation of secretory activity. Perhaps the most significant result from any of these studies is the recognition that the H,K ATPase itself is not the final target for covalent regulatory modification.

The only known action of cAMP is to activate the cAMP-dependent protein kinase (PK-A). In the case of the parietal cell, histamine has been reported to selectively activate a soluble type I PK-A, as indicated by the presence of free catalytic subunit. Type II PK-A appears also to be activated, but in this case, the regulatory subunit and much of the catalytic subunit remain associated with the particulate fraction. This is consistent with the finding that PK-A–binding proteins associated with membranes are selective for the type II regulatory subunit. This selectivity may indicate a preferential location of the target proteins for the type II kinase.

Several protein kinases are known to be dependent on or activated by calcium, including the isoforms of phospholipid-dependent protein kinase, PK-C, and several calcium-calmodulin–dependent protein kinases (CaM kinases). A

M3 Receptor Coupling

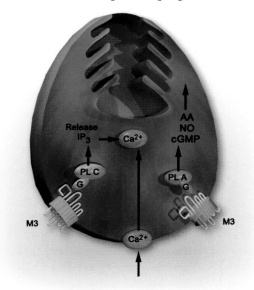

This figure shows the coupling of the M_3 Ca^{2+}-signaling receptors to various intracellular signaling systems. PLC releases IP_3 from phospholipids, and PLA releases arachidonic acid (AA), with stimulation of cGMP and NO.

potential role for PK-C is suggested by the activation of this enzyme by DAG. The latter is a product of the cholinergic activation of phospholipase C. However, exogenous activators of PK-C (e.g., phorbol esters) inhibit acid secretion rather than stimulate it. The presence of a type II CaM kinase has been demonstrated in gastric cells, where both parietal and chief cells appear to express the γ and δ subtypes. A potential role for CaM kinase II in cholinergic stimulation of acid secretion has been proposed, because the CaM kinase II selective inhibitor, KN-62, inhibits carbachol but not histamine stimulation. An interesting example of a putative direct action of calcium is the activation of the cytoskeletal-associated protease, calpain, which has been proposed to be involved in the cytoskeletal rearrangements associated with activation of the parietal cell.

A variety of experimental approaches have been used in attempts to identify the specific target proteins of the protein kinases postulated to be activated during stimulation of acid secretion. The general experimental paradigms have included both *in vitro* (i.e., with cell fractions) and *in situ* (i.e., intact cells) phosphorylation, followed by isolation and identification of phosphoproteins.

With either approach, the typical result is that a great many proteins appear to undergo protein kinase–dependent phosphorylation. The complex patterns of phosphorylation have impeded prohibited identification of specific target proteins. Separation of individual phosphoproteins by one-dimensional SDS gel electrophoresis has usually been inadequate to allow sequence identification of the protein, whereas two-dimensional separations have generally yielded insufficient quantities of single proteins to permit sequence analysis. Because many proteins appear to undergo phosphorylation, it is not clear which, if any, of them is a true intermediate in the stimulation of acid secretion as opposed to parallel events, such as metabolic activation or transcriptional regulation.

The single exception to the negative results has been the identification of the cytoskeletal linking protein, ezrin, as a potential intermediate in parietal cell activation. Initially discovered as a stimulation-related phosphoprotein localized to the apical plasma membrane of the parietal cell, this 80-kDa protein was identified as ezrin. Ezrin is a member of a gene family related to the erythrocyte band 4.1 protein. These proteins, including radixin, moesin, and talin, act as end-capping actin-modifying proteins, which serve to link cytoskeletal elements to the plasma membrane. Although the members of this family of proteins are structurally and functionally homologous, they tend to be preferentially localized in different cells and, thus, serve distinct cellular functions. Ezrin is thought to be associated with cytoskeletal elements at the apical pole of epithelial cells, where it is involved in the organization of microvilli. In cultured cells, ezrin is found to insert into membrane ruffles and become phosphorylated on tyrosine and serine residues in response to EGF. A similar role for ezrin has been proposed in the parietal cell, although in this cell type, ezrin does not appear to change location with stimulation, nor is there phosphorylation of tyrosine. It may be that the tyrosine phosphorylation observed in other systems associated with growth-factor stimulation may be required for translocation, whereas serine phosphorylation is sufficient for actin interactions. Because the formation of microvilli at the canalicular surface is part of the parietal cell response to stimulation, the phosphorylation of ezrin is considered to be a direct intermediate in the coupling reactions. However, as discussed below, the two critical events in activation of the proton pump are the translocation of H,K ATPase to the canalicular membrane and the association or activation of a KCl permeability pathway. Neither of these events has been related to ezrin as yet. There is also the presence of dynamin associated with the actin microfilaments. Dynamin is a GTPase often involved in endocytosis.

An alternate approach to identifying intermediates in the stimulus-secretion coupling events is based on the assumption that cellular components associated with the H,K ATPase undergo regulatory modification with parietal cell stimulation. Accordingly, substantial effort has been made to identify proteins associated with the H,K ATPase–containing membranes, with a long-term view to define which of these may serve a regulatory function.

This approach has yielded limited but promising results. In particular, it has been found that low-molecular-weight GTP-binding (LMWG) proteins are associated with the cytoplasmic vesicles in parietal cells. The LMWG proteins constitute a large group of monomeric peptides with molecular masses in the range of 20 to 30 kDa. These peptides share structural homology with the oncogenic peptide, Ras, and appear to function as intermediates in a wide range of regulatory functions, including growth and secretion.

The LMWG proteins associated with the parietal cell membranes appear to belong to the Rab (Ras-related rat brain) subgroup. Rab peptides, particularly Rab 3a, have been implicated in synaptic vesicle exocytosis, release of histamine

Mechanisms of Parietal Cell Transformation

Fusion

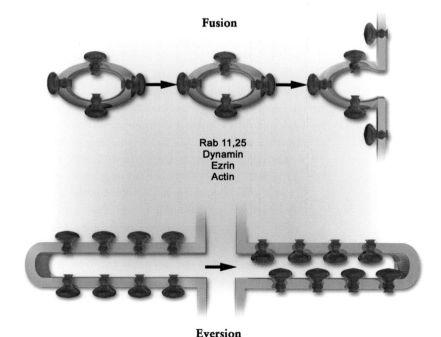

Rab 11,25
Dynamin
Ezrin
Actin

Eversion

A conceptual model showing eversion of cytoplasmic tubules to form the secretory microvilli along an actin filament where ezrin is a major coupling protein. At least two of the small G protein–binding molecules, Rab 11 and 25, are also associated with activation/deactivation of the microvilli. The ATPase molecules are shown in red, with the inside face (sphere) facing the cytoplasm. Two models are shown: on the top, fusion with the membrane of the secretory canaliculus or eversion (bottom of figure). The proteins associated with these events are dynamin, ezrin, and actin.

from mast cells, and exocytosis in pancreatic acinar and adrenal chromaffin cells. Accordingly, it has been suggested that Rab peptides may be involved in the fusion of cytoplasmic membrane tubules with the secretory canaliculus, which is a central event in the activation of the proton pump.

The extent and exact nature of Rab involvement in pump activation are under investigation and hold promise for defining further the events linking second messengers to acid secretion. Whereas Rab 3 proteins are not found in the parietal cell, Rab 11a is present. However, it remains associated with membranes in both the resting and stimulated states. Similar data have been observed for Rab 25.

A schematic model of these activation events is shown in the following figure. Two possible models are envisaged: expansion or fusion. The fusion model is the dominant hypothesis in the field. In assessing the evidence, the finding that the ATPase is present in tubules, not vesicles, suggests that fusion is restricted to the tips of the tubules and does not really resemble exocytosis in the strict sense. After fusion, there must be eversion of the tubules to form the microvilli. Presumably, the KCl pathway is at the base of the microvilli to allow effective reabsorption of K.

Activation of the H,K ATPase

Acid secretion is a regulated process whose rate is determined by its necessity after a meal. Consequently, the eventual result of the complex mechanisms for regulation of secretion described in previous sections is to activate the H,K ATPase. In contrast to the regulation of many other enzymes, there is no evidence for any chemical factors that directly influence the activity of the H,K ATPase, other than the availability of the necessary substrates MgATP, H^+, and K^+. Because within the parietal cell the availability of protons and MgATP is not likely to be rate limiting, it follows that the major, if not the only, factor that controls proton transport is the availability of K^+ at the extracytosolic surface of the H,K ATPase. Substantial evidence has accumulated to indicate that this is indeed the case, and that activation of the proton pump results from association of the H,K ATPase with a K^+ and Cl^- permeability in the membrane of the secretory canaliculus.

When gastric membrane vesicles are isolated from unstimulated tissues, essentially all the H,K ATPase requires addition of a K^+ ionophore to exhibit enzymatic or transport activity. When isolated from stimulated tissues, the H,K ATPase is able to transport protons in the absence of ionophore, indicating that the membrane vesicle now contains an endogenous K^+ permeability. Similarly, in permeabilized parietal cells, the proportion of ATPase and transport activity that requires ionophore decreases with cell stimulation, indicating that more of the H,K ATPase is associated with an endogenous K^+ permeability. When intact cells are incubated with NH_4^+, a membrane-permeable K^+ substitute, the H,K ATPase becomes activated. NH_4^+ gains access to the extracytosolic exchange site of the H,K ATPase as the permeable gas NH_3 acquires a proton to form the exchangeable species, NH_4^+, which is recycled back to the cytosolic surface. Accordingly, although NH_4^+ activates the proton pump, no acid actually accumulates under this condition, and the enzyme activity is measured as ATP hydrolysis or some index of metabolic turnover. These findings show that association of the H,K

A model of activation of acid secretion by the parietal cell. On the left is the resting cell, with most of the pumps (in red) present in the cytoplasmic tubules. On the right, after stimulation either by histamine or acetylcholine (ACh), the pump is now associated with the microvilli of the expanded secretory canaliculus that also contains conductances for K+ and Cl−. Both Ca and cAMP signaling systems are involved.

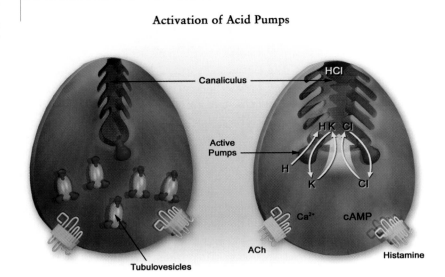

Activation of Acid Pumps

ATPase with an endogenous K+ permeability is necessary and sufficient for activation of the proton pump in the parietal cell. However, for K+ to efflux by itself would result in a large membrane potential hindering acid secretion; thus, the exit of K+ through a K channel is accompanied by the efflux of Cl− through a Cl− channel. Several different channels have been claimed to be associated with the secretory canaliculus, but the means whereby they are activated along with translocation of the ATPase remain unknown.

The exact mechanism by which the H,K ATPase associates with a K+ Cl− permeability remains controversial. It has been known for some time that stimulation of the parietal cell leads to a change in the morphology of the cell, involving a disappearance of cytoplasmic tubules and the development of the secretory canaliculus. This was the basis on which Golgi proposed the parietal cell as the site for acid secretion more than 100 years ago. It now is accepted generally that the canaliculus forms as a result of incorporation of cytoplasmic tubules into the apical surface of the parietal cell. Additionally, there is a reorganization of the cytoskeleton to form microvilli at the canalicular surface. Likely, it is within the events of cytoskeletal reorganization that the membrane cytoskeletal linker, ezrin, contributes to the stimulus-secretion coupling pathway. Although there still is controversy concerning the mechanism for incorporation of tubule membrane into the canaliculus, a clear consequence of this event is the translocation of H,K ATPase molecules from the tubules to the canalicular microvilli. When present in the cytoplasmic tubules, the H,K ATPase is inactive as a proton pump due to the lack of K+ access to the interior (extracytosolic) of the tubule. It should be noted that if K+ access is provided exogenously, the proton pump can be activated even in the tubules. Translocation of the H,K ATPase from the tubules to the canaliculus results in activation of the proton pump, because the canaliculus now contains a K+ and Cl− permeability.

Regardless of the nature of the K+ pathway, it must be argued that most of the K+ permeability is lost from the apical membrane in the unstimulated parietal cell. If this were not the case, the gastric mucosa would continuously secrete KCl in substantial quantities. Thus, the molecules representing the K⁺ permeability must be inactivated, removed from the surface, or both during the transition from a secreting to a nonsecreting parietal cell.

Assembly and trafficking of the H,K ATPase

The two subunits of the ATPase are synthesized in the ER of the parietal cell. The only other location of the pump is in the intercalated cells of the collecting duct of the kidney. Formation of transmembrane segments requires interaction of hydrophobic sequences during translation with the interior surface of the translocon. A sequence that determines membrane insertion with its N-terminal cytoplasmic and C-terminal extracytoplasmic is termed a *signal anchor sequence*. A sequence that returns the translating protein back to the cytoplasm and, thus, with its N-terminal extracytoplasmic, is named a *stop transfer sequence*.

The process of assembly of the transmembrane domain of the α subunit involves cotranslational insertion of the first four transmembrane segments as sequential signal anchor/stop transfer sequences. Insertion of the fifth, sixth, seventh, and eighth transmembrane segments appears to occur as a bundle with protein-protein interaction of the fifth and sixth segments more significant than protein-membrane lipid interaction. The ninth and tenth segments then insert as signal anchor and stop transfer sequences, respectively. The single transmembrane domain of the β subunit is efficiently inserted as a signal anchor sequence, and the remaining 200 amino acids are located extracytoplasmically. All six or seven N-glycosylation consensus sequences are used and are core glycosylated in the ER and then processed in the Golgi to form the mature subunit.

The β subunit is required for stabilization of the α subunit and is sorted to the plasma membrane in transfected cells. The strong interaction between the TM7/TM8 loop of the α subunit and the two regions of the β subunit discussed in the chapter on the structure of the H,K ATPase thus not only stabilizes but sorts the α subunit to the plasma membrane.

In the parietal cell, the Na,K ATPase is sorted to the basolateral surface and the H,K ATPase to the cytoplasmic tubules destined for insertion into the canalicular membrane with stimulation of secretion. The basis for this selective sorting is not well defined. Part of the sorting signal may be due to the β subunit. Recent work has shown that mutation of Tyr 19 of the β subunit in transgenic mice results in retention of the ATPase in the canalicular membrane, suggesting that perhaps phosphorylation of this residue is important in the stimulatory cycle of the enzyme. However, this event is subsequent to the cellular sorting of the two pumps.

Synthesis and turnover of the H,K ATPase

Biosynthesis of the two subunits of the ATPase takes place in the ER of the parietal cell. It appears that there is a need for coassembly of the two pump subunits for stabilization of the α subunit and for targeting of the dimer to the post-Golgi membrane compartment and the plasma membrane. Upstream

Life Cycle of the Acid Pump

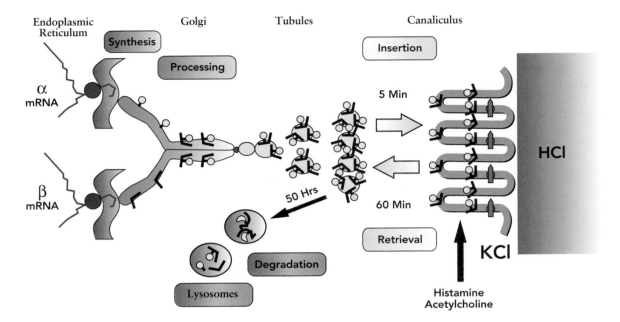

A model depicting turnover and biosynthesis of the H,K ATPase is shown in the figure. The two subunits of the ATPase are synthesized and coassembled in the endoplasmic reticulum and proceed to the trans-Golgi. From there, tubules are budded off. The turnover of the protein in the cytoplasmic tubules is relatively slow compared to when the protein is present in the membrane of the secretory canaliculus, where it is subject to endocytosis. On the right is shown the synthesis of the two subunits followed by processing in the Golgi. The mature pump subunits are inserted into the tubulovesicles. Stimulation of acid secretion by histamine or acetylcholine results in rapid movement to the secretory canaliculus ($t_{1/2}$ = 5 minutes). Return from the canaliculus to the tubulovesicles has a $t_{1/2}$ of 60 minutes. The half-life of the pump protein is approximately 50 hours.

sequences have been identified by gel retardation assay on both the α and β genes that bind gastric nuclear proteins selectively, but the role of these particular proteins has not been identified.

Activation of the H_2 receptor by histamine injection or by elevation of histamine release by gastrin results in a transient increase in mRNA for the α subunit. H_2 receptor antagonists prevent the gastrin- or histamine-dependent elevation of mRNA and appear to reduce mRNA to slightly below basal levels. These data were obtained in the rat, and the ATPase genes of this species possess cAMP- and Ca-responsive elements upstream of the coding sequence.

The half-life of the α subunit has usually been inferred rather than directly measured. Treatment of rats with cycloheximide resulted in a loss of ATPase activity, with a half-life of 72 hours. Recovery from inhibition with the covalent inhibitor, omeprazole, showed a half-life of 30 hours in the same series of experiments. Other workers have claimed a half-life of recovery as short as 15 hours. Direct measurement of the half-life of the ATPase in the rat gave a value of 54 hours. Treatment with omeprazole did not change this value, whereas treatment with the H_2 receptor antagonist, ranitidine, gave a value of 125 hours, a statistically significant increase. In these experiments, H,K ATPase activity recovered also, with a half-life of 15 hours. From these data showing a more rapid recovery of acid secretion than anticipated from protein turnover, it may be that reversal of PPI inhibition is due not only to *de novo* pump biosynthesis, but also to removal of the bound inhibitor, due either to chemical instability of the S-S (disulfide) bridge or, more likely, to access of glutathione (GSH) as the pump cycles between canalicular and tubular compartments.

The determinants of pump turnover are not well understood. From the above data, binding of the covalent inhibitor, omeprazole, evidently does not affect turnover, whereas inhibition of cell stimulation slows turnover. A hypothesis that would explain these observations is that pump turnover depends mainly on endocytosis of the pump from the canalicular membrane. Stimulation of acid secretion, which results in more pump being present in that membrane, would increase turnover; inhibition of acid secretion by reducing stimulation, which results in less pump being present in the canaliculus, will slow turnover. Neutral events, such as inhibition of the pump itself by omeprazole, if there is no change in the amount of pump in the canalicular membrane, will result in a rate of turnover similar to that found in untreated individuals.

Parietal cell homeostasis

The secretion of 160 mM of HCl across the canalicular membrane of the parietal cell represents a significant challenge to the cell's ability to maintain pH and electrolyte balance. In the steady state, transporters located in the basolateral membrane must respond to this challenge by replacing the secreted Cl^- and removing the accumulated excess base. A general model depicting the components involved in maintaining parietal cell homeostasis is presented. The existence of the various transporters shown has been demonstrated experimentally, although the quantitative role of each component still is subject to some speculation.

Activity of the H,K ATPase results in a primary secretion of 160 mM of HCl into the secretory canaliculus. Because the H,K ATPase is electroneutral, it is necessary that the KCl permeability pathway associated with the canaliculus transfer a minimum of 160 mmol of KCl for each liter of acidic fluid secreted. This is true whether the KCl pathway consists of conductive or electroneutral transporters. It is likely, in fact, that the KCl pathway allows transfer of a slight excess of KCl over the minimum required for the production of HCl. This is suggested both by the observation that gastric secretions contain a low but significant concentration of KCl and by the likelihood that the H,K ATPase is not fully efficient at recovering K^+ from the canalicular fluid. In the absence of other mechanisms, the combined activity of the transporters at the apical pole of the parietal cell would lead to alkalinization of the cell and depletion of cellular Cl^- and K^+. The potential disturbances in electrolyte balance are prevented by the activity of transporters at the basolateral membrane. These include an anion exchanger (AE, HCO_3^-/Cl^-), a sodium/proton exchanger (NHE), and the Na,K ATPase.

Basolateral transporters

The existence of a basolateral AE in the parietal cell was postulated because the conductance of the parietal cell for H^+, OH^-, and HCO_3^- was insufficient to account for the removal of intracellular base. A mechanism in erythrocyte membranes that exchanges HCO_3^- for Cl^- led to the proposal that such a mechanism in the parietal cell could account both for the extrusion of base and for the replacement of secreted Cl^-. Cloning and sequencing of AE proteins indicate that there is a family of band 3–related proteins that exhibit differential tissue expression. The AE isoforms appear to have conserved C-terminal regions containing the membrane-spanning domains and variable N-terminal sequences. The isoform designated AE_2 appears to be the predominant transporter of the parietal cell.

The presence of an NHE in parietal cells is demonstrated by the finding that recovery of intracellular pH (pH_i) from an acid load is dependent on sodium in the medium and blocked by high concentrations of amiloride (Na/H exchange inhibitor). As with the AE, the NHEs are known to be a family of proteins. In contrast to the AE isoforms, however, the NHE isoforms exhibit a variable C-terminal region and a conserved N-terminal region that contains the membrane-spanning domains. It is suggested that isoform NHE-1 is the primary transporter in gastric chief cells and mucous cells, whereas NHE-4 may be the basolateral transporter of the parietal cell. The significance of differential cellular expression of the isoforms is unclear, although it may relate to differential sensitivity of the isoforms to regulatory factors. Most of the consensus sequences for covalent modification by protein kinases are located in the isoform-specific C-terminal regions.

The two exchangers, together with the Na,K ATPase, appear to be the primary transporters responsible for maintaining parietal cell homeostasis. An additional transporter, an $NaHCO_3$ cotransporter, has been reported to be present in the parietal cell, but its functional significance has not been defined.

The basolateral membrane of the parietal cell also contains conductive channels for both K^+ and Cl^-, because these two ions dominate the membrane potential.

The presence of a basolateral K^+ conductance has been confirmed by direct electrophysiologic measurements, whereas the Cl^- conductance has not as of yet. The contribution of the conductances to the net fluxes of K^+ or Cl^- have not been determined but likely are small relative to those of the Na pump and AE.

In addition, it has recently been shown that older parietal cells express the Na-K-2Cl cotransporter, which suggests that these cells secrete Cl ion, because Cl is maintained above equilibrium by the coupling of basolateral Na,K and 2Cl entry across the transporter to activity of the basolateral Na,K ATPase. This Cl-secretion model applies to other epithelia, such as intestine and kidney, and is responsible for the secretion of water in those organs. In the gastric fundic gland, perhaps this water secretion occurring at the bottom of the glands is used to propel the pepsinogen secreted by the chief cells towards the lumen.

Homeostatic responses

Under nonsecreting conditions, as with most cells, the parietal cell most likely maintains its electrolyte balance through activity of the Na pump and regulatory responses of the NHE and AE to incidental perturbations of pH_i.

On activation of the proton pump, it would be anticipated that the parietal cell becomes more alkaline, because for each proton secreted, an equivalent OH^-, rapidly converted to HCO_3^- by carbonic anhydrase, is accumulated within the cell. However, experimental measurements during stimulation of acid secretion indicate only a small or no change in pH_i compared to the nonstimulated state.

Only changes of pH_{in} on the order of 0.1 pH units were observed for individual parietal cells. Although somewhat larger changes were reported for populations of isolated parietal cells, most of this response was not blocked by inhibition of the H,K ATPase with SCH28080. It is noted that the small responses of pH_i were monophasic, with a relatively slow onset, indicating that there is no transient alkalinization followed by recovery to a new steady-state value.

The minimal responses of pH_i to stimulation initially could reflect intracellular buffering but in the steady state require that the AE, which is primarily responsible for base excretion, be activated coordinately with the H,K ATPase. The simplest explanation for the increase in AE activity is that the slight increase of intracellular HCO_3^- (indicated by a small rise of pH_{in}) combined with a decrease of intracellular Cl^- is sufficient to increase the rate of anion exchange by the observed three- to fivefold. NHE activity is inhibited during steady-state secretion, and this also is attributed to the small rise of pH_{in}.

Alternatively, it has been proposed that the second messengers (i.e., cAMP and Ca_{in}, which activate the proton pump) may modulate the pH_i regulatory transporters directly by altering their pH setpoint. Accordingly, stimulation of parietal cells was observed to result in an elevated pH_i, which occurred before detectable acid secretion and which was blocked by amiloride, suggesting a direct activation of the NHE.

Further, it was suggested that an initial rise of pH_i due to activation of the NHE could result in an anticipatory activation of the AE and thus prevent any significant transient alkalinization of the parietal cell.

Although it is reasonable to expect that the NHE and AE interact, insofar as both are required for normal pH_i regulation and are inversely affected by changes in pH_i, it is unclear whether such interactions include a cause-and-effect response to stimulation.

Apart from a role in regulating pH_i in the resting parietal cell, the NHE may serve indirectly to supply K^+, which is lost into the gastric secretions. Although the NHE activity is inhibited during secretion, it is not abolished. The exchange of cellular protons for Na^+ by the NHE would lead to uptake of K^+ by the Na,K ATPase and thus replace any net loss of K^+ across the apical membrane. Perhaps the observed initial activation of the NHE is more critical for K^+ conservation than it is for AE activation and regulation of pH_{in}. This would be the case if any decrease in intracellular K^+ due to secretion were insufficient to stimulate Na pump activity directly. Despite the apparent complexity of interactions, it appears that the responses of the AE, NHE, and Na pump are qualitatively sufficient to account for electrolyte balance in both the resting and the secreting parietal cells. A representation of the homeostatic mechanisms available to the parietal cell is shown in the figure.

The parietal cell is a remarkable example of the product of evolution, dedicating an epithelial cell to the production of HCl by providing ATP via a large number of mitochondria, a specialized ion pump, regulatory receptors, and an intrinsic intelligence, enabling secretion of 160 mm HCl without damage to itself.

Ion Transport Homeostasis

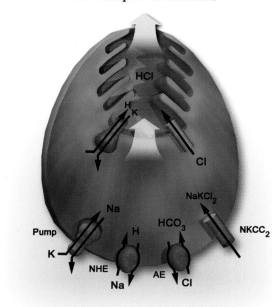

Different ion transporters in the parietal cell, showing the presence of the Na/H exchanger (NHE), the Cl/HCO₃ exchanger (AE), and, in older parietal cells, the NaKCl₂ cotransporter (NKCC₂). The Na,K ATPase is expressed only on the basolateral surface and the H,K ATPase only in the apical membrane. The basolateral transporters maintain intracellular pH and supply K and Cl to the KCl conductance in the canaliculus. The AE removes HCO₃ and supplies Cl. Efflux of KCl and recycling of K by the H,K ATPase result in secretion of an isotonic solution of HCl.

SUGGESTED READING

Adams H, Card W, Riddell M, et al. Dose-response curves for effect of histamine on acid secretion in man. *Br J Pharmacol* 1954;9:329–334.

Altman R. *Die elementarorganismen und ihre beziehung zu den zellen*. Leipzig: Veit and Co, 1894.

Alvarez W. Sixty years of vagotomy: a review of some 200 articles. *Gastroenterology* 1948;10:413–441.

Andersson K, Chen D, Hakanson R, et al. Enterochromaffin-like cells in the rat stomach: effect of alpha-fluoromethylhistidine evoked histamine depletion. *Cell Tissue Res* 1992;270:7–13.

Ash A, Schild H. Receptors mediating some of the actions of histamine. *Br J Pharmacol* 1966;27:427–439.

Barger G, Dale H. The presence in ergot and physiological action of B-imidazolylethylamine. *J Physiol Lond* 1910;40:38–40.

Bayliss W, Starling E. Preliminary communication on the causation of the so-called "peripheral reflex secretion" of the pancreas. *Lancet* 1902;2:810–813.

Bayliss W. *Principles of general physiology*. London: Longmans, Green, 1915:700–706.

Beaumont W. Experiments and observations on the gastric juice and physiology of digestion. Plattsburgh, New York: A.P. Allen. Facsimile of the original edition of 1833 together with a biographical essay, A Pioneer American Physiologist, by Sir William Osler. Cambridge, Massachusetts: Harvard University Press, 1929.

Beaumont W. Further experiments on the case of Alexis St. Martin, who was wounded in the stomach by a load of buckshot, detailed in the Recorder for 1825. *Med Recorder* 1826;9:94–97.

Bertaccini G, Coruzzi G. Control of gastric acid secretion by histamine H_2 receptor antagonists and anticholinergics. *Pharmacol Res* 1989;21:339.

Best C, McHenry E. The inactivation of histamine. *J Physiol Lond* 1930;70:349–372.

Black JW, Duncan WAM, Durant CJ, et al. Definition and antagonism of histamine H_2 receptors. *Nature* 1972;236:385.

Brillat-Savarin JA. *The physiology of taste (meditation on transcendental gastronomy)*. San Francisco, CA: Northpoint Press, 1986.

Brimblecombe RW, Duncan WAM, Durant GJ, et al. Characterization and development of cimetidine as a histamine H_2-receptor antagonist. *Gastroenterology* 1978;74:339.

Brodie B. Experiments and observations on the influence of the nerves of the eighth pair on the secretion of the stomach. In: *Abstracts of the papers printed in the philosophical transactions of the Royal Society of London, 1800–1814*. London: Taylor, Red Lion, Court, Fleet Street, 1832:102–106.

Capella C, Vassallo G, Solcia E. Light and electron microscopic identification of the histamine-storing argyrophil (ECL) cell in murine stomach and of its equivalent in other mammals. *Zeitschrift Zellforschung* 1971;118:68.

Card W, Marks I. The relationship between the acid output of the stomach following "maximal" histamine stimulation and the parietal cell mass. *Clin Sci* 1960;19:147–163.

Carter DC, Forrest J, Werner W, et al. Effect of histamine H_2-receptor blockade on vagally induced gastric acid secretion in man. *Br Med J* 1974;3:554.

Chen D, Zhao CM, Al-Haider W, et al. Differentiation of gastric ECL cells is altered in CCK(2) receptor-deficient mice. *Gastroenterology* 2002;123(2):577–585.

Chew CS, Hersey SJ, Sachs G, et al. Histamine responsiveness of isolated gastric glands. *Am J Physiol* 1980;238:G312.

Code C. Histamine and gastric secretion. In: Wolstenholme G, O'Connor C, eds. *Histamine*. Boston: Little, Brown and Company, 1956:189–219.

Code C. The role of gastric juice in experimental production of peptic ulcer. *Surg Clin North Am* 1943;23:1091–1101.

Costa M, Furness JB, Llewellyn-Smith IJ. Histochemistry of the enteric nervous system. In: Johnson LR, ed. *Physiology of the gastrointestinal tract*, 2nd ed., vol. 1. New York: Raven Press, 1987:1.

Dale H. *Adventures in physiology*. London: Pergamon Press, 1953.

Debas HT, Lloyd KCK. Peripheral regulation of gastric acid secretion. In: Johnson LR, ed. *Physiology of the gastrointestinal tract*, 3rd ed., vol 2. New York: Raven Press, 1994:1185.

Dohlman HG, Thorner J, Caron MG, et al. G-proteins. *Ann Rev Biochem* 1991;60:653.

Dolinsky J. Etudes sur l'excitabilité sécrétoire specifique de la muqueuse du canal digestif, l'acide, comme stimulant de la secretion pancreatique. *Arch Soc Biol St. Petersbourg* 1895;3:399–427.

Dragstedt L. Section of the vagus nerves to the stomach in the treatment of peptic ulcer. *Ann Surg* 1947;126:687–708.

Edkins J. The chemical mechanism of gastric secretion. *J Physiol Lond* 1906;34:133–144.

Fujita T, Kobayashi S. Structure and function of gut endocrine cells. *Int Rev Cytol* 1977;6:187.

Gantz I, Schaeffer M, Del Valle J, et al. Molecular cloning of a gene encoding the histamine H_2-receptor. *Proc Natl Acad Sci U S A* 1991;488:429.

Gerber JG, Payne NA. The role of gastric secretagogues in regulating gastric histamine release in vivo. *Gastroenterology* 1992;102:403.

Gregory R, Tracey H. The preparation and properties of gastrin. *J Physiol Lond* 1959;149:70–71.

Hakanson R, Owman CH, Sporong B, et al. Electron microscopic identification of the histamine-storing argyrophil (enterochromaffin-like) cells in the rat stomach. *Z Zellforschung Mikroskop Anatomie* 1971;122:460.

Hakanson R, Boettcher G, Ekblad F, et al. Histamine in endocrine cells in the stomach. *Histochemistry* 1986;86:5.

Hanzel D, Reggio H, Bretscher A, et al. The secretion-stimulated 80K phosphoprotein of parietal cells is ezrin, and has properties of a membrane cytoskeletal linker in the induced apical microvilli [published erratum appears in *EMBO J* 1991;10(12):3978–3981]. *EMBO J* 1991;10:2363–2373.

Heidenhain, R. Untersuchungen über den Bau der Labdrusen. *Arch Mikro Anat* 1870;6:368–406.

Hirschowitz B. Neural and hormonal control of gastric secretion. In: *Handbook of physiology, section 6: The gastrointestinal tract*, vol. 3, New York: Oxford University Press, 1989:127.

Hoffman HH, Schnitzlein NN. The number of vagus fibers in man. *Anat Rec* 1969;139:429.

Home E. Hints on the subject of animal secretions. In: *Abstracts of the papers printed in the philosophical transactions of the Royal Society of London, 1800–1814*. London: Taylor, Red Lion, Court, Fleet Street, 1832.

Hunter J. *Essays and observations on natural history, anatomy, physiology, psychology and geology, vols. 1 and 2*. London: J. Va. Vooret, 1861.

Johnson RG, Carty SE, Scarpa A. Coupling of H^+ gradients to catecholamine transport in chromaffin granules. *Ann N Y Acad Sci* 1985;456:254.

Kahlson G, Rosengren E, Svann D, et al. Mobilization and formation of histamine in the gastric mucosa as related to acid secretion. *J Physiol Lond* 1964;174:400–416.

Kajimura M, Reuben M, Sachs G. The muscarinic receptor gene expressed in rabbit parietal cells is the M3 subtype. *Gastroenterology* 1992;103:870.

Kanagawa K, Nakamura H, Murata, et al. Increased gastric acid secretion in cholecystokinin-1 receptor-deficient Otsuka Long-Evans Tokushima fatty rats. *Scand J Gastroenterol* 2002;37(1):9–16.

Kobayashi R, Tonai S, Ishihara Y, et al. Abnormal functional and morphological regulation of the gastric mucosa in histamine H_2 receptor-deficient mice. *J Clin Invest* 2000;105(12):1741–1749.

Komarov S. Gastrin. *Proc Soc Exp Biol Med* 1938;38:514–516.

Kopin AS, Lee YM, McBride EW, et al. Expression cloning and characterization of the canine parietal cell gastrin receptor. *Proc Natl Acad Sci U S A* 1992;89:3605–3609.

Langhans N, Rindi G, Chiu M, et al. Abnormal gastric histology and decreased acid production in cholecystokinin-B/gastrin receptor-deficient mice. *Gastroenterology* 1997;112(1):280–286.

Larsson H, Golterman N, De Magistris L, et al. Somatostatin cell processes as pathways for paracrine secretion. *Science* 1979;205:1393.

Lewin MJM. The somatostatin receptor in the GI tract. *Ann Rev Physiol* 1992;54;455.

Lichtenberger LM. Importance of food in the regulation of gastrin release and formation. *Am J Physiol* 1982;243:G429.

Major RH. Jean Cruveilhier. In: *Classic description of disease*. Springfield, IL: Charles C. Thomas, 1932:593–596.

Miyasaka K, Kanai S, Ohta M, et al. Overexpression of cholecystokinin-B/gastrin receptor gene in the stomach of naturally occurring cholecystokinin-A receptor gene knock-out rats. *Digestion* 1998;59(1):26–32.

Modlin IM, Waisbren SJ. Pavlov in the U.S.A. *Gastro Int* 1993;6(1):48–53.

Montegre AJ. *Expériences sur la digestion dans l'homme. Presentées a la première classe de l'Institut de France, le 8 Septembre 1812*. Paris: Le Normant Colas, 1814.

Müller E. Über der Fundusdrusen des Magens. *Z Wissensch Zool* 1898;64:624–647.

Nwokolo CU, Smith JT, Sawyerr AM, et al. Rebound intragastric hyperacidity after abrupt withdrawal of histamine H_2 receptor blockade. *Gut* 1991;32:1455.

Padfield PJ, Balch WE, Jamieson JD. A synthetic peptide of the Rab3a effector domain stimulates amylase release from permeabilized pancreatic acini. *Proc Natl Acad Sci U S A* 1992;89:1656–1660.

Prinz C, Kajimura M, Scott DR, et al. Histamine secretion from rat enterochromaffin-like cells. *Gastroenterology* 1993;105:449.

Prinz C, Sachs G, Walsh J, et al. The somatostatin receptor subtype on rat enterochromaffin-like cells. *Gastroenterology* 1994;107:1067.

Rangachari PK. Histamine, mercurial messenger in the gut. *Am J Physiol* 1992;262:G1.

Schepp W, Prinz C, Hakanson R, et al. Effects of bombesin-like peptides on isolated rat gastric G-cells. *Regul Pept* 1990;28:241.

Schubert ML, Makhlouf GM. Regulation of gastrin and somatostatin secretion by intramural neurons: effect of nicotinic receptor stimulation with dimethyl-phenylpiperazinium. *Gastroenterology* 1982;83:626–632.

Seal AM, Yamada T, Debas HT. Somatostatin 14 and 28, clearance and potency on gastric function in dogs. *Am J Physiol* 1982;143:G97.

Simonsson M, Eriksson S, Hakanson R, et al. Endocrine cells in the human oxyntic mucosa. *Scand J Gastroenterol* 1988;23:1089.

Tache Y. Central nervous system regulation of acid secretion. In: Johnson LR, ed. *Physiology of the gastrointestinal tract*, 2nd ed., vol. 2. New York: Raven Press, 1987:911.

Thomas HA, Machen TE. Regulation of Cl/HCO_3 exchange in gastric parietal cells. *Cell Regul* 1991;2:727–737.

Vesalius A. *De humani corporis fabrica*. Basel, 1543:327–330.

Walsh JH. Gastrointestinal hormones. In: Johnson LR, ed. *Physiology of the gastrointestinal tract*, 3rd ed., vol. 1, New York: Raven Press, 1994:181–254.

Wilkes JM, Kajimura M, Scott DR, et al. Muscarinic responses of gastric parietal cells. *J Membr Biol* 1991;122:97.

Wood JD. Physiology of the enteric nervous system. In: Johnson LR, ed. *Physiology of the gastrointestinal tract*, 3rd ed., vol. 1. New York: Raven Press, 1994:23.

Yao X, Forte JG. Cell biology of acid secretion by the parietal cell. *Annu Rev Physiol* 2003;65:103–131.

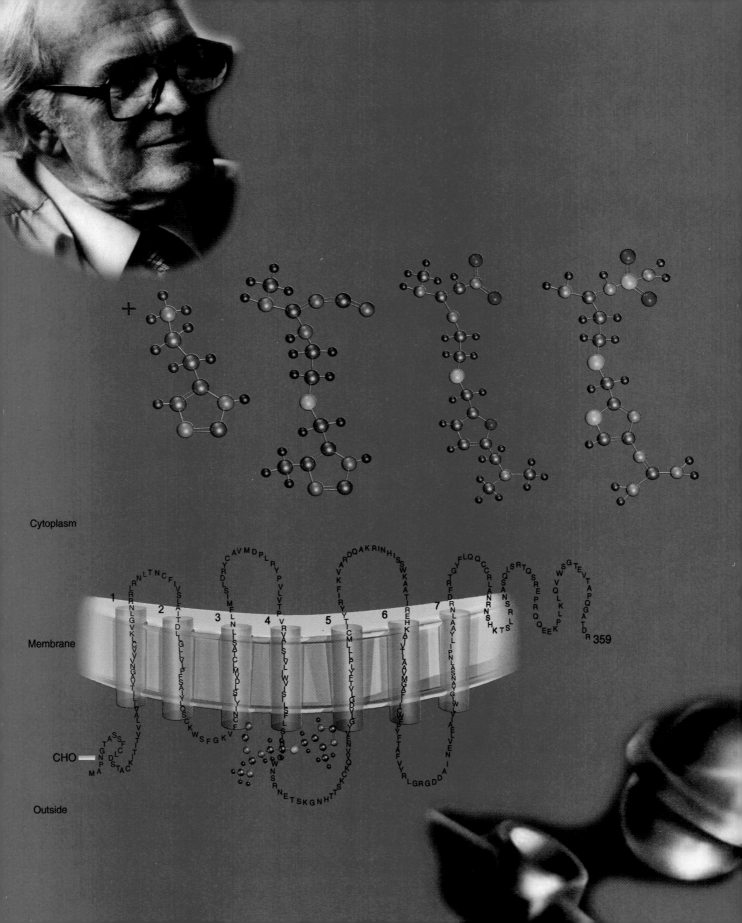

Cytoplasm

Membrane

CHO

Outside

PHARMACOLOGY OF ACID SECRETION

CHAPTER 1
HISTORY OF THERAPEUTIC APPROACHES TO ACID RELATED DISEASES

The evolution of therapy

Prout initially identified gastric acid as hydrochloric acid in 1823. However, it was only in the late nineteenth century that hyperchlorhydria was recognized as contributing to ulcer generation. For centuries, treatment had not changed. Only as pathogenesis and stimulatory pathways became recognized did surgical and then medical therapy become more focused and more effective.

Diet

In 1915, Dr. Bertram Sippy advocated hourly feedings of milk, eggs, and purees from 7:00 a.m. to 8:00 p.m. Between these hourly feedings, and every half hour for $2^{1}/_{2}$ hours after the last feeding, Sippy powder (calcium and sodium bicarbonate) was administered. In addition, to relieve dyspepsia, the patient's stomach was aspirated at regular intervals each night. This regimen provided a challenge both for the patient and for the nursing staff.

An alternative dietary therapy developed by Richard Doll involved the use for up to 3 weeks of continuous milk drips through a nasogastric tube, with or

Dr. Bertram Sippy of Chicago (left) devised a complex dietary regimen of bland food that included hourly feedings of milk, eggs, and puree as well as the administration of large quantities of calcium and sodium bicarbonate. In addition, he proposed that particularly severe nocturnal dyspepsia could be relieved by regular gastric aspiration. Although cumbersome and likely to generate obsessive-compulsive disorders, this strict regimen was of some benefit and particularly efficacious when compared with the outcome of current surgical intervention for acid peptic disease. Many physicians (bottom) enthusiastically attended lectures by Sippy to learn more of his novel therapeutic techniques. An alternative dietary therapy developed by Richard Doll proposed hospital admission for up to 3 weeks with continuous nasogastric milk infusion with and without alkali (top right). Although this therapy promoted ulcer healing and relieved pain, the prolonged hospitalization and use of resources, as well as loss of productive work time, generated a less than optimal solution for the management of acid peptic disease. Cynics proposed that the excessive use of milk accelerated coronary artery disease, and that any putative therapeutic benefit was actually derived from the bed rest, the charm of the nursing staff, and the Freudian benefits of the acquisition of milk. This treatment soon fell into disregard except among unusual sects of medical practice.

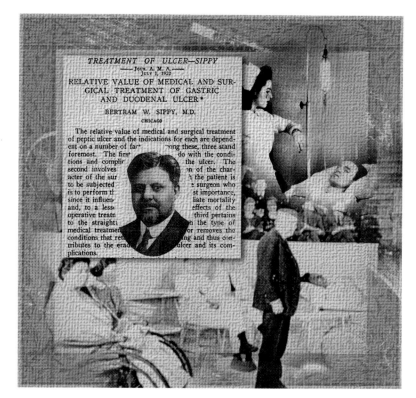

TREATMENT OF ULCER—SIPPY
—— JOUR. A. M. A. ——
JULY 1, 1922
RELATIVE VALUE OF MEDICAL AND SURGICAL TREATMENT OF GASTRIC AND DUODENAL ULCER*

BERTRAM W. SIPPY, M.D.
CHICAGO

The relative value of medical and surgical treatment of peptic ulcer and the indications for each are dependent on a number of fac...

without alkali. Although this therapeutic strategy seemed to improve the nutritional status of his patients, the obsessive need for dietary management and regulation of alkali intake so interfered with the lifestyle of patients and so often failed to prevent complications from developing that even surgery became a reasonable option.

Surgery

The first dedicated operation was a gastrectomy, but the high morbidity and mortality engendered a degree of caution in both patient and physician alike. Subsequently, vagotomy, which had been initiated in France by Raymond Latarjet and then reactivated in North America by Lester Dragstedt, provided a better alternative for management. Dragstedt's observations that gastric acid output was decreased by vagotomy were widely cited in favor of this operation. Initial postoperative problems due to decreased gastric emptying were subsequently obviated by the construction of a variety of pyloroplasties to facilitate drainage. Recurrence of peptic ulcer disease and the long-term side effects of the surgery itself show that this therapy option was suboptimal.

Andre Latarjet (1877–1947) (top left) was born in Dijon and studied medicine in Lyons. In collaboration with Pierre Wertheimer, he defined the neural innervation of the stomach in detail and recognized that the vagal nerve supply to the lesser curve was critical in the regulation of gastric acid secretion (top). In 1923, he published the results of a series of operations (right) in which he had severed the vagal nerves to the stomach and demonstrated not only a decrease in gastric acid secretion but also a resolution of acid peptic disease (bottom). A rigorous scientific thinker, he documented the associated significant delay in gastric emptying consequent on vagal denervation and described the need to add a drainage procedure to the operation. Lester Dragstedt introduced the vogue for vagotomy in the United States on January 14, 1943, in Chicago, at the Merritt Billings Hospital. As a transmogrified physiologist, Dragstedt was able to provide experimental evidence that gastric denervation decreased acid secretion and facilitated ulcer healing and relief of pain. It has taken almost 50 years for the surgical community to recognize that Latarjet's original decision to abandon the operation was well founded on scientific fact. The long-lasting dramatic postvagotomy symptomatology consequent on denervating large portions of the gastrointestinal tract far outweighed the modest advantages achieved by a 20% to 30% decrease in acid secretion. Further debate on the merits and demerits of the innumerable permutations and commutations of vagotomy were swept away by the introduction of H_2 receptor antagonists in 1976. The subsequent availability of PPI therapy considerably decreased the use of vagal resection, which should now only be considered in rare clinical circumstances.

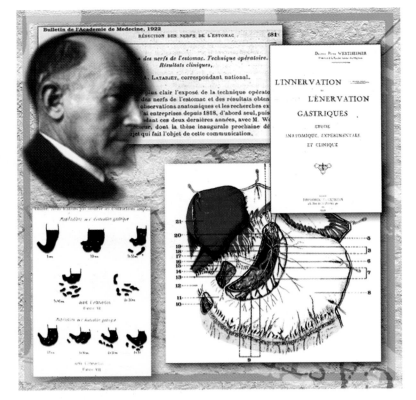

Gastroprotection

The evolving trend to use less invasive methodology in the management of peptic ulcer disease resulted in a significant interest in the use of antacids in association with both diet modification and bed rest.

Numerous preparations with different concentrations of alkali or buffers were developed to remove the pain of peptic ulceration and to facilitate healing. Their widespread availability and relative safety resulted in broad popular acceptance.

Such agents required four to six daily administrations and resulted in a high frequency of side effects that included constipation, diarrhea, and decreased absorption of concomitantly administered medications. Large doses of baking soda even led to gastric rupture!

Glycyrrhetinic acid is a constituent of licorice that had been used in folk remedies for peptic ulcer disease. For some time, this compound, in the form of carbenoxolone, was tried as a means of peptic ulcer treatment, but its renal toxicity prevented its introduction.

A sulfated polysaccharide, sucralfate, was introduced to the market as a protective agent and has had some following for treatment of peptic ulcer disease. It is claimed to enhance the gastric barrier. However, the large number of patients needed to show efficacy indicates its weak effect.

As it became recognized that acid secretion depended on stimulation by a variety of ligands, such as ACh, gastrin, and histamine, a more logical approach to pharmacotherapy could be taken.

liquiritia.

Namre. c 7 b. teperare melio: er ca. no nimis grosa nec mihi tr nuus 7 mtenus crocea humametis ardori urine aspirati pectoris. 7ftu nocumeti. finascitur interia cretosa 7 oura . 7 remotio nocumiti. tranfplatata intera fabulofa.

The licorice plant was regarded as an important component of many early herbal remedies.

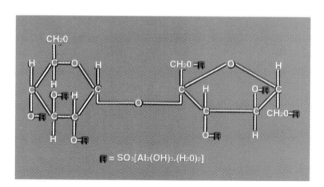

$R = SO_3[Al_2(OH)_5.(H_2O)_2]$

Sucralfate chemical structure. The development of complex surfactant agents to neutralize and protect the ulcerated mucosa resulted in effective healing rates and avoided some side effects of other agents. Of particular interest has been the ability of such compounds to promote ulcer healing by the proposed mechanism of growth-factor delivery to the ulcer site itself.

Receptor pharmacology

Muscarinic agents

Extract of belladonna began to be used toward the latter half of the nineteenth century for treatment of peptic ulcer disease. The active principle, atropine, is a nonselective muscarinic antagonist able to block transmission in the enteric nervous system. This medication was administered 1 hour before each meal and at bedtime, but to ensure effectiveness, the evening dosage had to be sufficiently high to control symptoms throughout the night. The widespread distribution of muscarinic receptors results in unpleasant and often intolerable side effects, such as blurred vision, dry mouth, and bladder dysfunction. A possible solution was to develop more selective muscarinic antagonists. One such was pirenzepine, a relatively selective muscarinic M_1 receptor antagonist. There were still side effects and relatively low efficacy. A higher-affinity M_1 antagonist, telenzepine, arrived too late to make any impact on ulcer treatment. Peculiarly, although these are M_1-selective antagonists, the parietal cell has M_3 receptors and the ECL cell has no stimulatory muscarinic receptors. Hence, these compounds must act on neurons of the myenteric plexus that then relay to the parietal cell without the intervention of the ECL cell, because H_2 antagonists do little to block cholinergic stimulation of acid secretion.

Prostaglandins

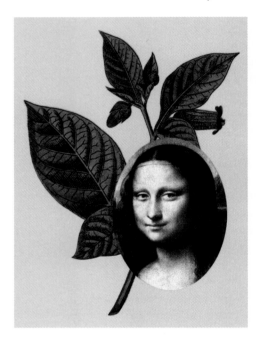

Atropine-like derivatives of plants, including deadly Nightshade (*belladonna*) were used for their cosmetic influence on women's eyes as well as their acid-inhibiting properties.

The prostaglandins are natural products discovered in the 1960s. They are derived from arachidonic acid, which is released from phospholipids or diacylglycerol by the action of phospholipase A_2. There are two enzyme cascades responsible for prostaglandin generation, based on cox I (constitutive) and cox II (regulated).

After the initial conversion of arachidonic acid into the prostaglandin core structure, several modifications generate various prostaglandins with specific affinities to different prostaglandin receptors. Prostaglandins of the E_3 class are potent inhibitors of acid secretion by action at a G_i-coupled EP_3 receptor. These were therefore natural lead compounds for development of antiulcer agents. The natural prostaglandins have a short half-life, and before subtypes of the receptors were recognized, the concept driving development of these compounds was prolongation of their half-life. The compound that is now on the market, misoprostil, is not particularly receptor subtype selective and results in stimulation of intestinal secretion and diarrhea in at least 20% of treated individuals. No PG E_3 subtype-selective agent has been introduced, and misoprostil is suggested for cotreatment with cox-I inhibitors and not as a general antiulcer drug.

Hence, this compound was introduced as therapy for NSAID-based gastric damage, based on replacement of natural prostaglandins depleted by administration of cox I inhibitors, such as aspirin or indomethacin. The introduction of selective cox II inhibitors has diminished the necessity for prostaglandin replacement therapy in NSAID treatment.

The physiologic role of PG receptors in gastric physiology is nevertheless important in that there is not only regulation of acid secretion, but also of bicarbonate secretion and mucosal blood flow; these latter regulations may not be via the EP$_3$ receptor.

Histamine-2 receptor antagonists

The first series of H$_2$ receptor antagonists was synthesized in Welwyn Garden City, at the site of a stately home occupied by Smith, Kline & French (SK&F). This house had been used for development of diving gear during World War II, because there was a very deep pond on the property. Cimetidine reformed the treatment of acid related diseases by introducing effective pharmacotherapy that was free of significant side effects and largely negligible adverse events. Peculiarly, James Black, the project leader, Bill Duncan, the site director, and Bryce Douglas, the head of research at SK&F (based then in Philadelphia), were all Glaswegian Scots. As Welwyn was working on the receptor antagonist, Philadelphia began working on pump inhibitors.

During the 1980s, the H$_2$ receptor antagonists became first-line therapy in peptic ulcer disease and led to effective treatment and an improvement in quality of life for a large number of patients. It was found to be superior to any other form of medication at the time, giving good inhibition of nighttime secretion and lesser inhibition of daytime acid secretion.

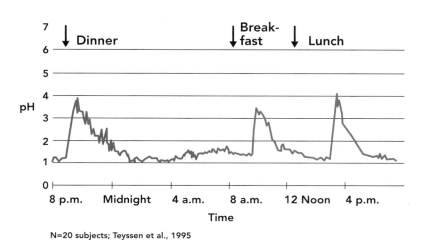

Intragastric pHmetry Profile Without Treatment

N=20 subjects; Teyssen et al., 1995

Typical profile for intragastric pH for untreated healthy individuals. Intragastric pH is approximately 1.0 in the absence of the buffering action of food. The rise in pH at 8 p.m., 8 a.m., and after 12 noon is due to dinner, breakfast, and lunch at those times.

The introduction of H$_2$ receptor antagonists was associated with an exponential decrease in hospital admissions, although duodenal ulcer patient numbers were already declining. It should be noted that, while the incidence of duodenal ulcer is declining in the Western world, this is not the case in the Third World, where the incidence of infection with *H. pylori* remains high. Of particular note is the observation that, while both the frequency and the severity of the disease may be decreasing (as judged by the decline in hospital admission rates), the complications of duodenal ulceration (hemorrhage and perforation) are declining less. (CHPA, Commission on Professional and Hospital Activities; NCHS, National Center for Health Statistics.)

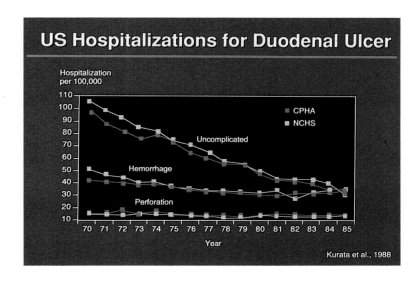

US Hospitalizations for Duodenal Ulcer

Kurata et al., 1988

Whereas the introduction of the H_2 receptor antagonist class of agents revolutionized the management of acid peptic-related disease, it became apparent that further improvement in the regulation of the acid-secretory process would yield better clinical results. This was especially true of erosive esophagitis. The identification of the proton pump as the final step in the pathway of parietal cell acid secretion provided a unique opportunity for better control of parietal cell secretion. Also, it was realized that without continuous treatment, peptic ulcer disease returned after healing the ulcer.

Gastrin antagonists

The central role of gastrin in stimulation of ECL cell release of histamine has resulted in some significant effort being applied to the development of gastrin antagonists. For many years after the definition of the structure of gastrin, gastrin antagonists were sought in the form of peptide analogs of pentagastrin, but without success. More recently, nonpeptide antagonists of both the CCK_1 and CCK_2 receptors have been synthesized based on a benzodiazepine core structure. Some of the more recent compounds are potent and highly selective for their receptor subtype and may be introduced clinically, although it would be surprising if they proved superior to H_2 receptor antagonists.

Proton pump inhibitors

The concept that drove the development of alternatives to H_2 receptor antagonists was the recognition that these would have limited efficacy given the multiplicity of secretory inhibitors. It seemed that inhibition of the pump itself would be a more effective way of controlling acid secretion. Work toward this end began at SK&F in Philadelphia but was terminated with the launch of cimetidine. As will be discussed in the section on inhibition of the H,K ATPase, the synthesis of timoprazole heralded not only a novel therapeutic approach to acid control but also an entirely novel principle of drug mechanism.

The PPIs have a unique mode of action, being acid-activated prodrugs. They covalently inhibit the gastric H,K ATPase. First, as weak bases, they accumulate in the acid space generated in the secretory canaliculus of the stimulated parietal cell. This accumulation is followed by acid-dependent conversion to the active compound, a cationic thiophilic reagent. The active species binds covalently to one or more cysteines accessible from the luminal face of the pump; hence, there is covalent inhibition of the proton pump by these PPIs. Their inhibitory effect is prolonged as compared to their dwell time in the blood.

The introduction of this class of drug produced a conflict between companies marketing H_2 receptor antagonists and those marketing PPIs that could form the basis for a course in pharmaceutical company strategies and even ethics. At this time, PPIs have largely superseded H_2 receptor antagonists in most countries as prescriptions for acid related disease.

Acid pump antagonists

Whereas the PPIs have a unique targeting and covalent inhibitory action on the proton pump based on their chemistry and the biology of the parietal cell, another class of compounds—acid pump antagonists—have a structural specificity for their target region on the pump—close to the K$^+$ binding region of the H,K ATPase—and are K$^+$ competitive and, hence, dissociate from the pump when their blood concentration falls. Although they have been actively pursued for almost 15 years, thus far none of these compounds has reached the marketplace. They promise a more rapid onset of inhibition than the PPIs and an inherent chemical stability that will allow design of more flexible formulations, such as timed-release formulations and intravenous formulations that do not require addition of buffer to the dry powder immediately before administration.

The targets for inhibition of acid secretion are shown below.

Pharmacological Control of Acid Secretion

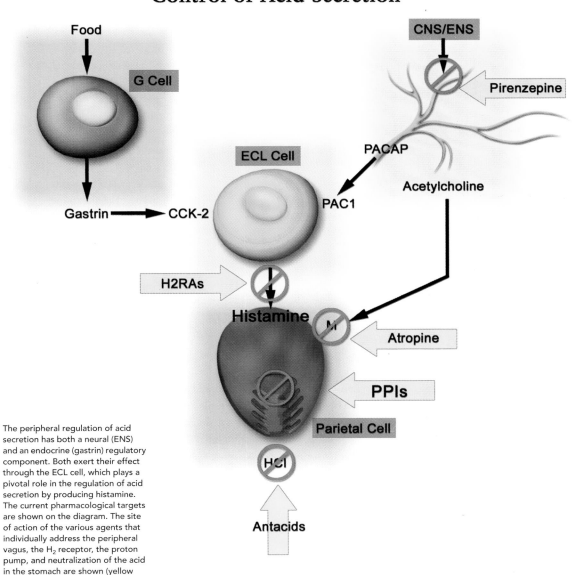

The peripheral regulation of acid secretion has both a neural (ENS) and an endocrine (gastrin) regulatory component. Both exert their effect through the ECL cell, which plays a pivotal role in the regulation of acid secretion by producing histamine. The current pharmacological targets are shown on the diagram. The site of action of the various agents that individually address the peripheral vagus, the H$_2$ receptor, the proton pump, and neutralization of the acid in the stomach are shown (yellow arrows).

CHAPTER 2
INHIBITION OF THE HISTAMINE-2 RECEPTOR

Histamine antagonists

The pharmaceutical industry had long recognized the importance of peptic ulcer disease, and many companies had intensive programs searching for a treatment. In most cases, they used an animal model, such as the pylorus-ligated rat, measuring the change in ulceration given by compounds in their chemical libraries. This approach was unsuccessful, because the real target was acid secretion, not the number of ulcers found in these rat stomachs.

Histamine-1 receptor antagonists were first synthesized by Bovet in the 1940s. Most of these structures were derived by the modification of the imidazole ring of histamine, leaving the ethylamine side chain of the molecule untouched.

These antagonists often penetrate the CNS, resulting in drowsiness. The recognition of the presence of a different subtype of a histamine receptor in the stomach by Keir led to an intensive program for the development of an antagonist selective for what became the H_2 receptor. At that time, the histamine-3

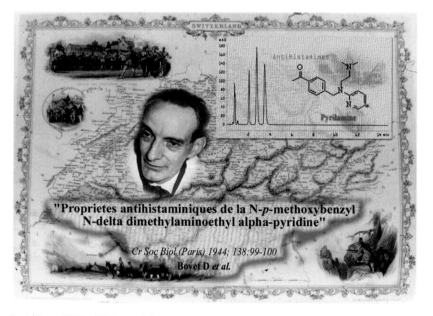

"Proprietes antihistaminiques de la N-*p*-methoxybenzyl N-delta dimethylaminoethyl alpha-pyridine"

Cr Soc Biol (Paris) 1944; 138:99-100
Bovet D *et al.*

Daniel Bovet (1907–1992) (center left) was a Swiss-born Italian pharmacologist who received the 1957 Nobel Prize for Physiology or Medicine for his discoveries of a number of clinically important chemotherapeutic agents (including histamine and curare). While the head of the therapeutic chemistry laboratory at the Pasteur Institute, he discovered pyrilamine (mepyramine) (top right), the first antihistamine agent, in 1944 (bottom), which has become an effective therapy against allergic reactions.

receptor had not been discovered, although now it has been cloned. It appears to play an important role in the brain but not in the periphery.

The H_2 receptor is found on the parietal cell of the gastric mucosa, where it plays a dominant role in stimulation of acid secretion by binding the histamine released from the ECL cell due to gastrin and PACAP. It is also found in the uterus and in the heart but does not appear to play a medically significant role in these tissues, because these organs remain unaffected by these drugs.

Success in treatment with a receptor antagonist depends on several factors. The expression of several subtypes of receptors for the same ligand differently in different tissues allows the development of receptor- and organ-selective agonists and antagonists. Selectivity is, of course, a paramount requirement for therapy free of side effects.

Lack of side effects depends largely on the distribution of the receptor and its role in the different organs where it is found. Lack of toxicity depends on the nature of the molecule, its metabolism, and its metabolites. Adverse events are idiosyncratic happenings not predictable from preclinical profiles of the

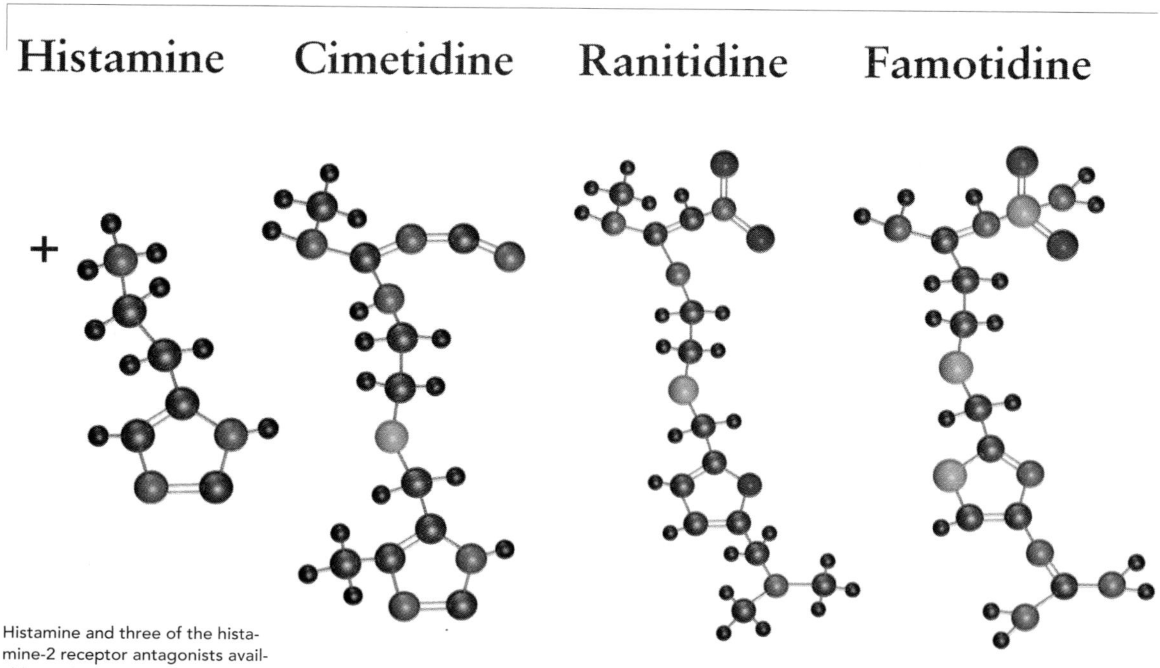

Histamine Cimetidine Ranitidine Famotidine

Histamine and three of the histamine-2 receptor antagonists available on the market. All of these have a positive charge, as does histamine, and there is conservation of a five-membered ring and a variable side chain. The histamine-1 receptor antagonists generally retain the ethylamine side chain of histamine but change the structure of the ring system. The histamine-2 receptor antagonists retain a five-membered ring and modify the ethylamine side chain.

compound; side effects result from lack of target uniqueness and structural problems in the drug.

Black and his colleagues, after many attempts to modify the imidazole ring to create an H_2 receptor–selective antagonist, turned their attention to the side chain and, fairly rapidly thereafter, generated the first H_2 receptor antagonist, burimamide. The screen used by this group was inhibition of histamine-induced acid secretion in the perfused rat stomach in the Gosh-Schild preparation, an eminently suitable screen for the discovery of a gastric-targeted antihistaminic! Metiamide and cimetidine followed this first success, and cimetidine was introduced for treatment of acid related diseases in 1977.

The perception of the SK&F research team that the imidazole ring was essential for H_2 antagonism allowed relatively simple bypass of the SK&F patent by a group of chemists working at Allen and Hanbury, led by David Jack, also from Glasgow.

The imidazole ring was exchanged for a furan, a small side-chain modification was made, and then ranitidine was announced to the world. Ranitidine (Zantac) became the world's leading medication for many years. Thereafter, the most potent of the H_2 receptor antagonists was introduced: famotidine with a thiazole ring; this was followed by nizatidine. Famotidine is the largest selling antiulcer medication in Japan. The structures of some of these molecules are shown in the figure.

After the first flush of success with the short-acting H_2 receptor antagonists, considerable effort was expended on finding compounds that were longer acting—hence, relatively irreversible or insurmountable—to improve the acid-inhibitory profile of this class of drug. For reasons still not understood, so far all of these, such as loxtidine, have produced toxicities, such as generation of adenocarcinomata of the gastric epithelium. However, they have provided excellent acid control in animals.

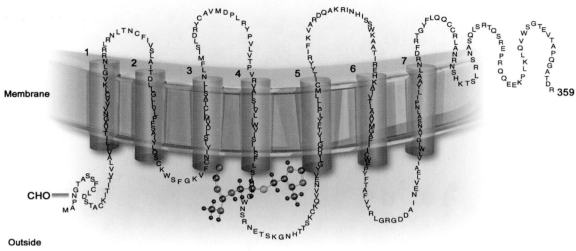

Histamine 2 Receptor

The amino acid sequence of the H₂ receptor, with the transmembrane domains and the glycosylation site on the outside. The seven transmembrane segments (TM1–7) are shown, as well as a histamine antagonist (colored chemical molecule) binding between TM3 and TM5.

The histamine-2 receptor

The H_2 receptor is a member of the trimeric G-coupled protein-receptor family. These have seven transmembrane segments, with the N-terminal exposed on the cell surface, with one or more N-linked glycosylation sites. There are three intracellular loops and a C-terminal cytoplasmic domain. The third loop is thought to be the region mainly responsible for coupling to the alpha subunit of the heterotrimeric G proteins, such as G_s, G_q, or G_i. However, the C-terminal region also determines the relative affinity of coupling to a panoply of G proteins present in almost every mammalian cell. The coupling to the G proteins and some other aspects are also discussed in more depth in the section on parietal cell stimulation.

Cloning and expression of the H_2 receptor showed that it was indeed a seven transmembrane–segment protein with N-terminal glycosylation and its C-terminus in the cytoplasm, as shown in the figure above.

The understanding of the structure of these receptors has not enabled improved design of the original H_2 receptor antagonists, but knowledge of the amino acid sequence and protein–protein interactions should be able to explain many of the idiosyncrasies of their effects, such as tolerance.

Binding of histamine and its antagonists is thought to involve the cytoplasmic loop between TM-4 and -5 and the inner surface of the transmembrane segments 3 and 5, similar to concepts evolving for the β-adrenergic receptor. For example, the aspartyl group (D) in the middle of TM3 is thought essential for the binding of the $^-NH_3^+$ of the ethylamine side chain of histamine and for the positive charge at the corresponding end of all the H_2 receptor antagonists.

Binding of histamine results in activation of adenylate cyclase by interaction with a G_s trimeric G protein and also a Ca^{2+} signal due to interaction with a G_q

trimeric G protein. The reason for the presence of both signals may be that the cAMP cascade is necessary for pump activation, and that elevation of intracellular calcium is necessary for redistribution of the pump to the microvilli of the secretory canaliculus.

Pharmacology of the receptor

The availability of these selective antagonists was instrumental in establishing that histamine was a direct mediator of stimulation of acid secretion. Concomitantly, the role of gastrin was relegated largely to the release of histamine from ECL cells while maintaining its standing as a trophic factor for the gastric fundic epithelium. When initially introduced, cimetidine was prescribed four times a day, because it was recognized that its duration of action was relatively short. When ranitidine was launched, it was slightly more potent and was recommended twice a day. Recently, however, the prescribing recommendation has fallen to once at night. This is because, with general use of these medications in combination with intragastric pHmetry, it was found that there was remarkably little effect on daytime acidity but a large effect on nocturnal acid output. The reason for the failure to control daytime pH adequately is still not understood, because insurmountable H_2 antagonists, such as loxtidine, were effective over a 24-hour period. However, it should be remembered that intragastric pH does not fully predict the volume of acid secretion, and that these drugs probably do reduce the volume of daytime acid secretion.

These drugs were the first to be effective in treatment of duodenal ulcer disease; they are less effective in gastric ulcer treatment and more or less ineffective in treatment of erosive esophagitis but quite effective in the treatment of nonerosive esophagitis. They are all available over the counter (OTC) and, hence, are no longer the mainstay for prescriptions for acid related diseases. They are still prescribed for dyspepsia or other relatively vague upper gastrointestinal disturbances. Their effect on healing was carefully analyzed in a series of metaanalyses of duration and magnitude of elevation of intragastric pH as a predictor of optimization of healing, as shown in the figure below.

The degree of approach to optimal treatment of duodenal ulcer, GERD, and *H. pylori* eradication given by b.i.d. ranitidine. The results of a metaanalysis of approximately 300 clinical trials where the presumed intragastric pH was correlating with the healing of duodenal ulcer, esophagitis, and efficiency or eradication of gastric infection by *H. pylori*. It was calculated that pH control should be greater than 3.0 for rapid healing of gastric ulcer, above 4.0 for healing of GERD, and above 5.0 for eradication of *H. pylori* for at least 16 hours per day. Under placebo conditions (C), control of pH to this level is minimal, and with ranitidine treatment (R), 10 hours per day is above pH 3.0 and only 5 hours per day is at pH above 4.0. Hence, ranitidine and other H_2 receptor antagonists are effective for healing of gastroduodenal ulcer.

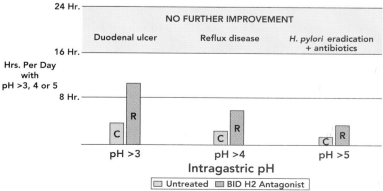

Level and Duration of Intragastric pH Elevation Achieved for Optimal Treatment of:

A typical profile of intragastric pH using nighttime H_2 receptor antagonists, showing initially good inhibition at night, but then, with continued usage, significant tolerance, resulting in loss of efficacy. Daytime administration does not provide daytime acid control. On the first night of dosage, there is excellent nocturnal pH control, but this is less evident during the day. After 7 days of treatment, nocturnal acid pH control is blunted due to tolerance to these drugs.

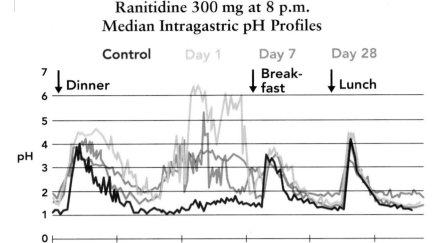

Ranitidine 300 mg at 8 p.m.
Median Intragastric pH Profiles

N=20 subjects; Teyssen et al., 1995

Treatment of duodenal ulcer requires elevation to a pH greater than 3.0 for 18 hours per day. It can be seen that, whereas the H_2 receptor antagonist ranitidine twice a day shows very significant improvement over placebo, the benefits fall far below the target of pH greater than 4.0 for 18 hours per day for reflux disease; their benefit in eradication therapy for *H. pylori* is found only in combination with bismuth subcitrate and two antibiotics.

H_2 receptor blockade displays rapid tolerance during therapy. In pHmetric studies with H_2 receptor antagonists, a 50% loss of efficacy is found relative to the beginning of treatment after 7 days of drug administration, and the effect becomes even more pronounced after 4 weeks of therapy. This tolerance does not depend on upregulation of the H_2 receptor, because increasing the dose of H_2 antagonist several-fold does not reverse the tolerance. No change in gastrin levels was noted either, denying the possibility that changes in gastrin could account for the tolerance. It may be that there is upregulation of other pathways, elevating cAMP in the parietal cell, or upregulation of cholinergic stimulation via the M_3 receptor on the parietal cell. It appears that there are no changes in cAMP levels during tolerance, making the last explanation the only likely one.

A typical set of intragastric pHmetric curves vividly illustrates the tolerance experienced with H_2 receptor antagonists and their lack of effect on pH during the day as compared to their good effect at night.

Upregulation of the H_2 receptor on the parietal cell is thought to account in part for the acid rebound found after withdrawal of H_2 receptor antagonists. Upregulation of this receptor would sensitize the parietal cell to the normal levels of histamine released from the ECL cell. Another factor that should be considered is the delay in pump turnover induced by H_2 receptor antagonists, leading to more pumps per parietal cell. Both factors could result in acid hypersecretion after withdrawal of H_2 antagonist therapy. These shortcomings have enabled the successful introduction of significantly more effective agents, the PPIs.

CHAPTER 3
INHIBITION OF THE GASTRIC ACID PUMP

H^+ transport by the gastric ATPase is the final step in acid secretion. It follows that inhibition of the ATPase would be an effective means of regulating acid secretion and cannot be surmounted by alteration of stimulatory pathways. There are various parameters that need to be considered when designing a drug for inhibition of this process by inhibiting the ATPase.

There has to be a large therapeutic index. The acid related diseases are in general not life threatening, and, although theoretically less effective, there are several H_2 receptor antagonists available, both as generics and OTC in most countries in the world. These latter drugs have a large margin of safety, and compounds that treat acid related diseases by inhibition of the gastric acid pump have to have at least an equal margin of safety. There are several P-type ATPases, and a gastric drug needs to be selective for the gastric ATPase. The ATPase is a member of the P_2-type ATPase family, with homology to the Na,K ATPases and the colonic H,K ATPase. Hence, inhibitors of the H,K ATPase must not interfere with functioning of other ATPases and also should affect as few other targets as possible.

Whereas design of small-ligand antagonists is not easy, at least the structure of the natural ligand provides a template for such molecules. In the case of the ATPase, the natural ligands are ATP and the hydronium ion, H_3O^+, on the cytoplasmic side and K^+ on the luminal surface. A compound competing with ATP in cell cytoplasm would obviously be nonspecific, inhibiting all other ATP-dependent processes. Design of molecules to act as H_3O^+ surrogates would have to take advantage of a special structure in the pump able to bind hydronium ion without affecting other such binding sites. Similar considerations would apply to design of compounds substituting for K^+ on the outside surface. Clearly, such compounds could not be designed based on the structure of the transported cations.

An advantage accrues in drug design from the specialized location of the functioning ATPase. In the actively secreting parietal cell, the active pumps are present in the microvilli of the secretory canaliculus and produce a pH gradient by far the most acidic space in the body. It is approximately 1,000-fold more acidic than anywhere else. Protonatable weak bases will accumulate selectively in the canalicular space as a function of their pK_a. This is because the protonated positively charged form is significantly less permeable than the uncharged species. Because this is the only space in the body with a pH of less than 4.0, weak bases with a pK_a of 4.0 or less will accumulate only in the canaliculus of active parietal cells. The unprotonated form will permeate the basal-lateral and canalicular membrane of the parietal cell; the protonated form, being relatively membrane impermeable, will concentrate in the canaliculus. In the fully active cell, the pH of the canalicular lumen is approximately 1.0; therefore, a compound with a pK_a of 4.0 will accumulate approximately 1,000-fold in this space and gain a significant therapeutic advantage if presented to the parietal cell in the serosal space. The acidity of the space could also confer a chemical advantage if such weak bases are inactive but are also acid labile. These would then convert more rapidly in the acidic secretory canaliculus to compounds able to inhibit the ATPase. As will be seen, this prodrug concept has played a vital role in the development of the current drugs used to control acid secretion by covalent pump inhibition.

P₂-type ATPases

There are several mammalian P ATPases, and each has several isoforms, but there are sufficient differences in amino acid sequence to enable specificity of inhibitory agents. For example, the cardioglycosides, such as digoxin, have only one known target, the Na,K ATPase. Similarly, thapsigargin targets the sarcoplasmic and endoplasmic reticular but not the plasma membrane Ca ATPase. Bafilomycin targets only the V-type ATPases and oligomycin, largely the F_1F_0 ATPase. There is, therefore, good reason to expect that drugs targeted against the gastric H,K ATPase will have strict specificity if properly designed.

Targets of the PPIs

The three-dimensional structure of the gastric acid pump is based on the structure of the SR Ca ATPase, and there is sufficient difference in detail that this structure, although highly informative as to mechanism, cannot provide a template for design of specific inhibitory ligands. Design of the PPIs does not depend on details of molecular structure, because these are chemical in concept, rather than biologic.

It is possible to define the amino acids in proteins that are able to react under biologic conditions. Whereas relatively harsh conditions are used for chemical reactions with carboxylic acids, histidines, lysines, arginines, and tyrosines, the most reactive amino acids under biologic conditions are cysteines by virtue of the higher reactivity of the ⁻SH group. Given that an ⁻SH-reactive group has to be generated in the canalicular space, it is the cysteines accessible from the luminal space that are potential specific targets for thiol-reactive (thiophilic) prodrugs. Obviously, the conversion of the prodrug to the cysteine-reactive thiophilic compound should occur predominantly in the acidic-secretory canaliculus of the active parietal cell. If it were formed elsewhere, rapid reaction with other proteins and glutathione would be found, inactivating the drug and possibly causing side effects.

It is, therefore, pertinent to inquire as to which of the 28 cysteines in the catalytic subunit of the pump and which of the nine cysteines of the beta subunit are available for stable derivatization. From the analysis of the structure of the membrane domain of the catalytic subunit, there are at least five possible cysteines that are accessible from the luminal side of the pump to a fairly bulky cationic organic molecule: the cysteines at positions 321, 813, 822, 892, and 981 in or between the third, fifth, and sixth membrane segments, in the loop between TM7 and TM8, and at the luminal end of TM9, respectively. Because the cysteines in the beta subunit are in disulfide linkage, either they are not attacked or they reform after reaction.

The substituted pyridal methylsulfinyl benzimidazoles

Discovery of PPIs

The development of the first of this series of drugs is due to a combination of serendipity, analysis of mechanism, and conviction that the ATPase was the best target for control of acid secretion. A compound, pyridine-2-acetamide, had been purchased by a company (Hässle in Göteborg, Sweden) for possible use as an antiviral agent. This compound was found ineffective but had some antisecretory activity. It was modified to pyridine-2-thioacetamide to improve its antiviral efficacy, but this did not happen, although it retained its antisecretory activity. In 1973, SK&F announced the development of cimetidine, the world's first H_2 receptor antagonist. Based on the structure of cimetidine, a benzimidazole ring was added to the antisecretory pyridine-2-thioacetamide, with the hope that the mechanism of action of these forerunners was H_2 antagonism. Antisecretory activity was retained. Finally, the sulfide was modified for stabilization to a sulfoxide, and timoprazole was born.

This compound had rather remarkable antisecretory properties: it inhibited gastric acid secretion, whatever the stimulus; it inhibited secretion in isolated gastric glands, whatever the stimulus, but was relatively acid unstable and showed inhibition of iodide uptake by the thyroid and was thymotoxic.

The first polyclonal antibody against the H,K ATPase reacted with the stomach, of course, but also mysteriously with the thyroid and thymus. This suggested that perhaps the ATPase was the target of timoprazole. By 1977, a

Chemical Development of Omeprazole

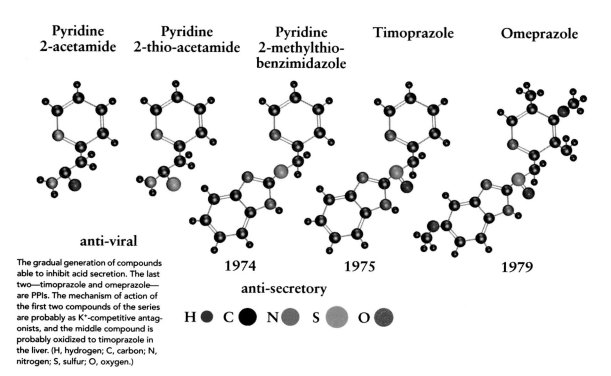

| Pyridine 2-acetamide | Pyridine 2-thio-acetamide | Pyridine 2-methylthio-benzimidazole | Timoprazole | Omeprazole |

anti-viral

1974   1975   1979

anti-secretory

H ● C ● N ● S ● O ●

The gradual generation of compounds able to inhibit acid secretion. The last two—timoprazole and omeprazole—are PPIs. The mechanism of action of the first two compounds of the series are probably as K⁺-competitive antagonists, and the middle compound is probably oxidized to timoprazole in the liver. (H, hydrogen; C, carbon; N, nitrogen; S, sulfur; O, oxygen.)

compound, picoprazole, had been made, retaining the core structure of timoprazole. It was shown that this compound and timoprazole did inhibit the gastric ATPase only when the ATPase was making acid, and that there was a lag phase of inhibition of transport activity. Because the compound was a weak base, the steps that were thought to result in inhibition of ATPase activity and acid secretion involved accumulation of the compound in the acid space of the isolated gastric vesicle during H^+ transport (or the parietal cell canaliculus), followed by acid-dependent conversion to an active compound. It was postulated that this class of compound acted as a prodrug that only reacted with the ATPase after this acid catalyzed conversion to an active form, perhaps the sulfenic acid. Later, it was proven that the active form in solution was a rearranged planar tetracyclic compound containing a highly reactive sulfenamide group. To optimize the acid stability of the parent compound and to generate absolute selectivity for accumulation in the acid space of the parietal cell, omeprazole was synthesized in 1979 and became the compound that was launched in 1988 at the Rome World Congress of Gastroenterology.

The name coined for this class of drug was *proton pump inhibitor* (PPI). After publication in 1981 of the first of a series of papers on the mechanism of action of these drugs, a variety of derivatives were synthesized that also led to the introduction of other drugs with generally similar properties to omeprazole.

The core structure of all currently marketed benzimidazoles, with points of substitution, is shown in the figure.

Mechanism of action

Chemistry

The key steps are (a) acid gradient–dependent accumulation of the prodrugs and (b) an acid- or enzyme surface–catalyzed conversion of the prodrugs to a sulfenic acid and then to a tetracyclic, planar sulfenamide. A detailed mechanistic analysis of the chemistry behind the substituted benzimidazoles was published recently. Recent findings may suggest that the pump itself may play a role in its own inhibition in that perhaps the sulfenic acid is formed on the surface of the pump, and this is the reactive intermediate binding to the relevant cysteines.

The structure of four examples of these drugs is given in the illustration. It can be seen that they all share the same backbone, a 2-pyridyl methylsulfinyl benzimidazole with various substitutions on the pyridine or benzimidazole moieties, which are added to modify solution reactivity or to decrease toxicity.

Design criteria

1. pK_a

Biologic accumulation of weakly basic compounds depends on a pH gradient between solution or cytoplasm and a membrane-bounded or enclosed compart-

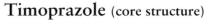

Timoprazole (core structure)

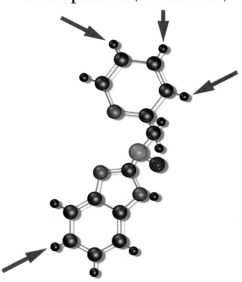

The core structure of all the clinically approved PPIs is timoprazole. Although effective as an acid-suppressive agent, this molecule was unstable at neutral pH, as well as exhibited thyrotoxic and thymotoxic effects. This led to the development of similar chemical moieties that were not only stable at neutral pH, but also exhibited no organ toxicity. The arrows show the position of substitution of different groups to produce the different PPIs now on the market. The initial substitutions designed for omeprazole resulted in the loss of the side effects of timoprazole.

Current Proton Pump Inhibitors

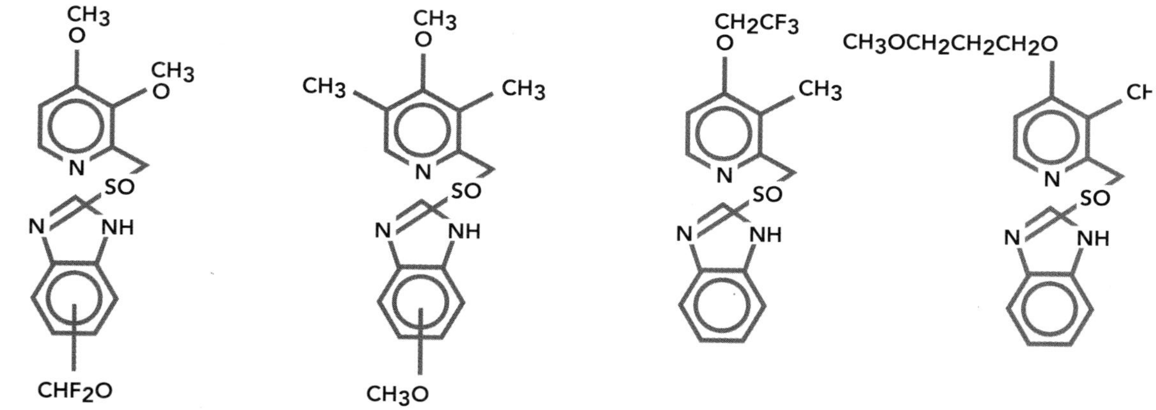

Pantoprazole

Omeprazole
S-Omeprazole

Lansoprazole

Rabeprazole

The current proton pump inhibitors, pantoprazole, omeprazole, lansoprazole, and rabeprazole. The 2D structure of esomeprazole is the same as omeprazole, but the 3D structure differs in the orientation of the S→O group.

ment of lower pH. The protonated form of the weak base is relatively membrane impermeable, and, therefore, the chemical accumulates in acidic compartments, depending on the gradient and the pK_a of the chemical. There are various acidic compartments, such as lysosomes, neurosecretory granules, and endosomes, that have a pH_i of approximately 4.5 to 5.0. The active secretory canaliculus of a fully stimulated parietal cell has a pH_{ni} of close to 0.8. Therefore, to target only the acidic compartment of the parietal cell, the pK_a of a PPI must be 4.5 or less to avoid accumulation in lysosomes or neurosecretory granules. The accumulation of these drugs preferentially in the acid space of the secreting parietal cell gives them an excellent therapeutic index, or margin of safety.

2. Membrane permeability

Because the compound accesses this compartment by crossing both the plasma membrane and the canalicular membrane, it also has to be membrane permeable, requiring a log P of between −3 and 0. Too high a log P drives the chemical into the hydrophobic domain of the membrane bilayer, perhaps decreasing access to the target or generating an inappropriate target site; too low a log P reduces membrane permeability and access to the acid space.

3. Acid activation

The prodrug forms, as shown, are ampholytic, with three N atoms able to accept or donate protons. The important site of protonation for accumulation of these drugs is the pyridine N, with a pK_a of 4.0 or thereabout. This pK_a ensures that accumulation of the prodrug will occur only in the secreting parietal cell canaliculus. Acid activation depends on protonation of the benzimidazole N followed by reaction of the 2C with the unprotonated pyridine N.

Mechanism of Pump Inhibition

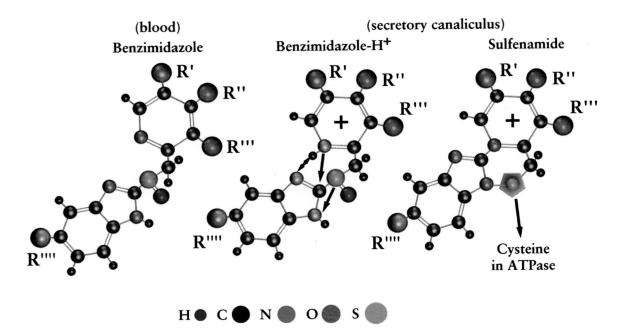

(blood)	(secretory canaliculus)	
Benzimidazole	Benzimidazole-H$^+$	Sulfenamide

Cysteine in ATPase

H ● C ● N ● O ● S ●

Mechanism of action of the PPIs, showing acidity-dependent accumulation, conversion to the sulfenamide, and reaction with the H,K ATPase. The acid space–dependent accumulation of the PPIs gives them a large margin of safety, and the acid-catalyzed conversion to the cationic SH-reactive sulfenamide produces the long-lasting covalent inhibition of the acid pump. The R moieties represent different substituents at these positions.

The pyridine of timoprazole, the core structure, has a pK$_a$ value of 2.9. Although this would seem appropriate for acid-space targeting, this lead compound was unstable at neutral pH due to the higher nucleophilic reactivity of the pyridine N, an undesirable property when considering either biologic targeting or formulation stability, because the sulfenamide would form spontaneously at neutral pH.

The compounds undergo an acid-catalyzed conversion to a relatively acid-stable sulfenamide. This is probably the active compound in free solution, because methylation of the benzimidazole N inactivates the drugs. The molecular rearrangement depends on the presence of a deprotonated pyridine N and a protonated benzimidazole N. The reaction involves a nucleophilic attack by the unprotonated pyridine N on the 2C of the benzimidazole; therefore, an increase of the electrophilicity of this 2C is also required. This is achieved by protonation of the benzimidazole N. The figure illustrates the general chemical mechanism of all current PPIs. The property of acid activation of the PPIs that occurs rapidly at pH of less than 4.0 adds to the safety margin of these drugs.

An alkoxy group at the pyridine 4 (green R") position flanked by a substituent at the 3 position is the substitution pattern common to all the PPI drugs giving the best combination of efficacy and selectivity. A decrease in the nucleophilicity of the pyridine N (a lower pK$_a$) was able to increase neutral pH stability. In the case of omeprazole, this was achieved by the addition of a methyl group at the 5 position; in lansoprazole, the fluorination of the ethoxy moiety also contributes to this decreased nucleophilicity, and in pantoprazole this was performed by the addition of a second methoxy substitution in the 3

Benzimidazole Inhibition of Acid Secretion

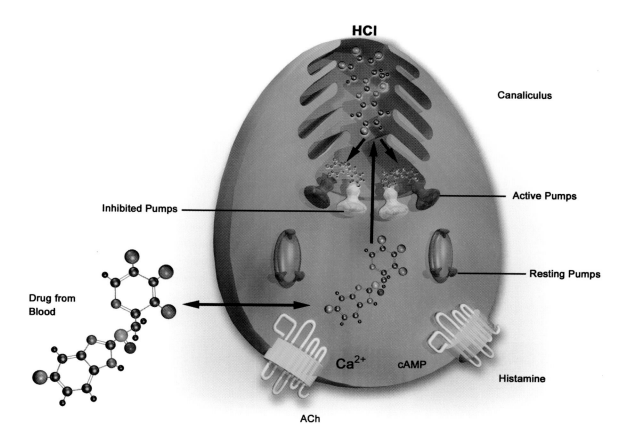

This illustrates the general mechanism for benzimidazole inhibition of gastric acid secretion. The PPI is absorbed from the duodenum and passes via the blood into the parietal cell. If the cell is secreting acid, the prodrug accumulates in the canaliculus and undergoes acid-catalyzed conversion to the sulfenamide, whereon it reacts with cysteines in the active H,K ATPase molecules.

position. This substitution also increases the polarity in this region of the molecule, which may play a role in the cysteine selectivity of this particular drug (see below). The substitution in rabeprazole results in a pK of 4.9, which may contribute to its neutral pH instability but will increase the accumulation in the parietal cell canaliculus.

The rate-limiting step in the formation of the sulfenamide in solution is the formation of the spiro intermediate, which requires folding of the prodrug to allow approach of the pyridine N to the benzimidazole N with perhaps intramolecular proton transfer. This is followed by an attack of the pyridine N on the 2C of the benzimidazole. Access to the transition state is also important. For example, the 3 CH_3 substitution favors a folding and interaction of the two ring systems, whereas a 6 CH_3 substitution appears to hinder folding and, hence, activation. This latter reactivity can be modified by substitution in the benzimidazole moiety, but this is less important than substitution in the pyridine ring. The difluoromethoxy substitution used in pantoprazole reduces the pK_a of the benzimidazole N, explaining the greater neutral pH stability of this compound relative to the other PPIs.

The pH activation curve for the four compounds differs significantly. They are all rapidly converted to the sulfenamide below a pH of 2.0. However, the half-maximal rate of activation is found at a pH of 3.0 for pantoprazole, a pH of 4.0 for omeprazole and lansoprazole, and a pH of 5.0 for rabeprazole. Protein binding of these drugs may markedly alter the rate of conversion to the sulfenamide, resulting in an unexpected efficacy of pH-unstable compounds.

The sulfenamide that is formed from all of these drugs is a permanent cation. This is of benefit because the compound retains its membrane impermeability even after acid secretion into the canaliculus has been inhibited. It is unlikely, therefore, that the active compound can get to the parietal cell cytosol *in vivo*, adding to the safety profile of these compounds.

This property also ensures targeting only to those SH groups accessible from the luminal or extracytoplasmic surface of the gastric acid pump. The sulfenamide is stable in the absence of SH groups and in acidic medium and is very unstable at neutral pH. This property allowed isolation of the omeprazole sulfenamide in solution, and it also adds to the safety profile of the drugs in that, were the sulfenamide to enter the cytoplasm of a cell, it would have a half-life in the millisecond range.

The reaction of the sulfenamide with SH groups in solution is diffusion limited. However, this does not necessarily extend to the situation *in vivo*, where the compact structure of the membrane and extracytosolic domains of the H,K ATPase have to be taken into account. This three-dimensional structure of the ATPase could, in principle, dictate derivatization of cysteines that are easily reached from acidic solution and those that are not.

Biologic mechanism of PPIs

1. Cellular

The chemistry of the PPIs dictates reaction with electrophilic groups in amino acids after acid-catalyzed conversion of the prodrug. The reactive group is the free −SH of cysteine, which can then form a disulfide bond with the sulfenic acid or sulfenamide derivative of the PPI. In principle, cysteine disulfides can also react, but reformation of the native disulfide would eliminate the bound drug.

There are five potentially reactive cysteines in the catalytic subunit and three disulfide bonds in the beta subunit. After development of omeprazole and knowledge of its chemistry, it was important to show that the mechanism deduced from its chemistry applied to the biologic situation.

Whole-body autoradiography of a mouse injected intravenously with tritiated omeprazole showed general labeling after 5 minutes, but after some hours, labeling was found only in the stomach. Higher magnification showed that labeling was present only in the parietal cell. This means that not only was there highly targeted accumulation of the drug, but also that the binding in the parietal cell was covalent, because it remained for several hours.

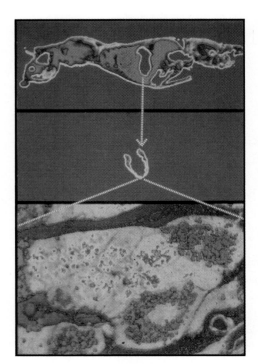

Whole-body autoradiography of a mouse after administration of labeled omeprazole, showing initially a general distribution, but then, at a later time, labeling is confined to the stomach and therein to the parietal cell, demonstrating the remarkable specificity of PPIs.

Reaction of omeprazole with isolated gastric glands results in inhibition of acid secretion. Treatment with thiol-reducing agents reversed the inhibition in the parietal cell. Omeprazole therefore depends on formation of disulfide bonds for its inhibitory action on gastric acid secretion, as deduced from its chemistry.

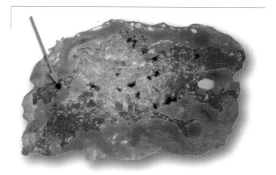

A high-resolution micrograph of a stimulated parietal cell after inhibition by radioactive omeprazole, showing the localization of the binding of this PPI exclusively to the active secretory canaliculus. The dark grains indicate the covalent binding of acid-activated omeprazole to the pump in the secretory canaliculus.

Both cysteine and glutathione were effective, and glutathione depletion increased the efficacy of omeprazole.

Treatment of isolated gastric glands with tritiated omeprazole under nonsecreting and acid-secreting conditions allowed analysis of the distribution of the drug as a function of time. The drug showed labeling mainly under acid-secreting conditions and initially labeled only the canalicular compartment, as illustrated in the figure.

In the unstimulated state, there is no labeling of the canaliculus until approximately 30 minutes after introduction of omeprazole. This is due to a basal level of acid secretion. With stimulation, there is rapid labeling of the canaliculus, with a reaction half-time ($t_{1/2}$) of approximately 10 minutes. The tubules are not labeled until approximately 30 minutes. Hence, omeprazole reacts only with the pump in the membrane of the acidic canaliculus. Labeling of the cytoplasmic tubules depends on retrieval of the pump from the canalicular membrane.

The mechanism of inhibition of the gastric H,K ATPase *in vivo* that results from these experimental data suggests that the drug, provided it is given in a gastric acid–protected form, reaches the cytoplasm of the cell via the circulation. It then is accumulated in the canaliculus only if the cell is secreting and then reacts only with the active pumps present in the membrane lining the canaliculus, as illustrated.

2. Enzymic

Treatment of a rabbit with radioactive omeprazole, isolation of gastric membranes, and separation using SDS PAGE, showed that only the catalytic subunit of the H,K ATPase was labeled. Hence, the drug is specific for the alpha subunit of the pump. The general mechanism of pump inhibition by these compounds is illustrated. The drug is accumulated on the luminal face of the pump, where it undergoes acid conversion to the sulfenamide, which then reacts with one or more exposed cysteines on the luminal surface of the enzyme.

The morphologic sites in the parietal cell that bind omeprazole after stimulation of acid secretion. Binding is first found only in the secretory canaliculus and then, as the pump is retrieved into the tubules, the labeling is found there as well. The acid space–dependent accumulation of the PPIs gives them a large margin of safety, and the acid-catalyzed conversion to the cationic SH-reactive sulfonamide produces the long-lasting covalent inhibition of the acid pump. Grains are the precipitates formed on the emulsion due to the radioactive disintegration of the ^{14}C in omeprazole.

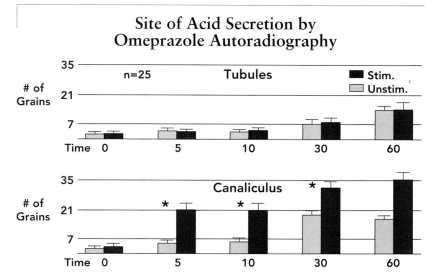

Site of Acid Secretion by Omeprazole Autoradiography

Reaction of PPIs with the isolated ATPase resulted in inhibition of the ATPase only under acid-transporting conditions. This was found for all of the PPIs. Inhibition by omeprazole was reversed by mercaptoethanol or dithiothreitol, also showing that disulfide formation was responsible for inhibition of the gastric acid pump.

The PPIs inhibit ATPase activity or acid transport at different rates *in vitro*. The order of reactivity was rabeprazole, followed by omeprazole and lansoprazole,

Site of Action

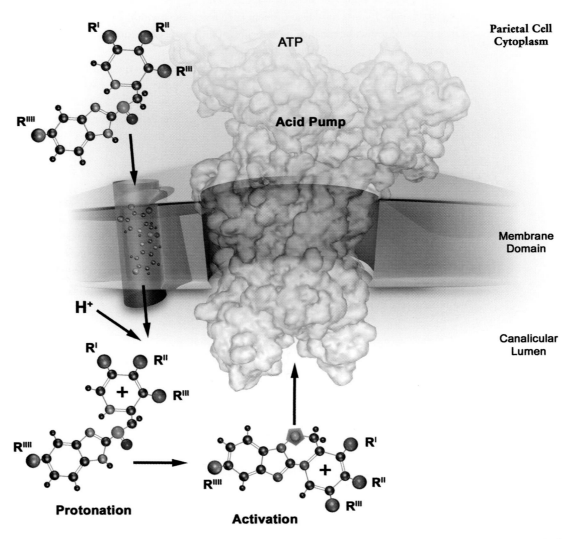

General reaction mechanism of the PPIs with the H,K ATPase in the membrane of the parietal cell canaliculus, showing passive diffusion across the canalicular membrane, accumulation of the protonated form, conversion to the sulfenamide, and reaction with one or more cysteines in the catalytic subunit of the H,K ATPase. The outline of the pump structure illustrates the vestibule of the pump on its outside surface where binding of the PPIs results in inhibition of acid secretion correlated with inhibition of ATPase activity.

and then pantoprazole, consistent with the order of acid stability. This is explained by the relatively weak acidification in gastric vesicles, allowing a measurable separation of inhibition based on the relative rates of activation of the compounds.

The location of the site of binding of the radioactive PPIs on the pump under acid-transporting conditions identifies the cysteine(s) critical for inhibition of enzyme activity. Labeling at essentially full inhibition showed that lansoprazole labeled cysteine 321 and 813. A similar set of cysteines was labeled by rabeprazole. Omeprazole labeled cysteine 813 and cysteine 892, whereas pantoprazole labeled both cysteine 813 and 822 and no other cysteine. Cysteine 321 is at the end of TM3, cysteine 813 and 822 are in the TM5/TM6 domain, and cysteine 892 is in the large outside loop between TM7 and TM8. This is illustrated in the figure showing the general mechanism.

When the time course of labeling was compared to the time course of inhibition for all of the PPIs, labeling of the cysteines in the TM5/TM6 region (either cysteine 813 or 822) correlated with inhibition. Definition of which of these two cysteines was labeled was done by using labeled omeprazole under trans-

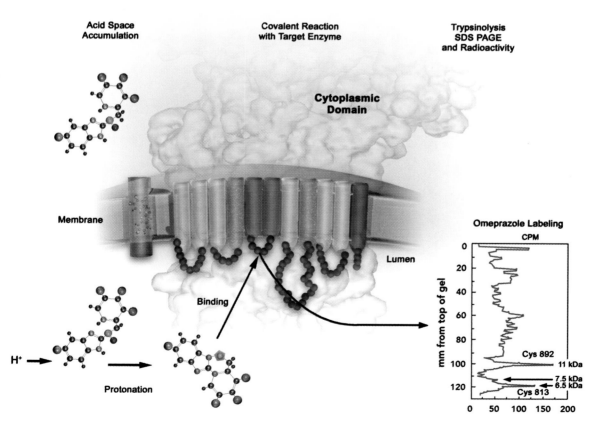

The Reaction of Omeprazole with the H,K ATPase

The mechanism of action of the PPIs, showing the target region and the labeling of M5/6 by omeprazole. Isolation of the radioactive band and redigestion with thermolysin showed that all of the label in M5/6 was at cysteine 813 in the case of omeprazole. Pantoprazole also labels cysteine 822.

port conditions, tryptic digestion, isolation of the labeled peak by SDS-tricine gradient PAGE, redigestion with thermolysin, and sequencing of the peak, retaining the label. It was deduced that cysteine 813 was labeled in the M5/M6 domain. Because the sulfenamide is a bulky cation, this placed cysteine 813 in the loop between M5 and M6, a supposition confirmed by the crystal structure of the SR Ca ATPase. A model for the PPI binding sites is shown in the figure when cysteine 813 is placed in the loop between M5 and M6, cysteine 321 at the other side of the luminal vestibule, and cysteine 822 much deeper in the membrane domain. Cysteine 892 is in the large exocytoplasmic loop between M7 and M8 and does not participate at all in inhibition of acid transport.

Different Cysteine Targets in Membrane Domain

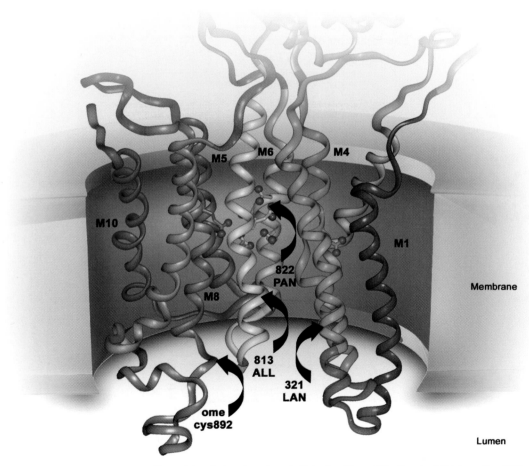

The cysteines that are bound covalently by the different PPIs. Cysteine 813 is bound by all PPIs, cysteine 321 by lansoprazole, and cysteine 892 by omeprazole and lansoprazole. Cysteine 822 is unique for pantoprazole. The sites in the vestibule and in the membrane domain are responsible for the covalent inhibition of acid transport. The cytoplasmic domain has been removed, and only the membrane and exoplasmic domain are shown. The binding of the PPIs is to the major transport domain of the pump, in particular M5/M6 at cysteine 813 (all PPIs) and cysteine 822 (pantoprazole only).

Reversal of acid-secretory inhibition

Measurement of protein turnover in the rat showed that the alpha subunit of the pump had a half-life of 54 hours, and that this was unaffected by proton pump inhibition. It was prolonged to approximately 120 hours, however, by treatment with H_2 receptor antagonists. This is explained by the finding that PPI treatment does not affect recycling of the pump between cytoplasmic tubules and canalicular membrane microvilli, whereas H_2 receptor antagonists return all the pumps to cytoplasmic tubules, thus abolishing recycling and proteolysis after membrane endocytosis. Surprisingly, however, acid secretion and H,K-ATPase activity returned with a half-life of only 15 hours in this species, approximately three times faster than anticipated if only protein turnover were responsible for recovery of acid secretion. After treatment of people with PPIs, acid secretion also returns faster than expected from protein turnover for omeprazole or lansoprazole (approximately 20 hours). Only pantoprazole has a duration of action compatible with recovery due only to pump biosynthesis (approximately 47 hours). Pantoprazole is unique in being able to access both cysteine 813 and 822, and the latter is deeper within the membrane domain as compared to the other cysteines that react with the PPIs.

Rats were treated with the different PPIs *in vivo*, namely, omeprazole, esomeprazole, lansoprazole, rabeprazole, and pantoprazole to provide identical inhibition of acid secretion. The pump was isolated and incubated for different lengths of time with glutathione, the natural reducing agent in the parietal cell. Measurement of the reversal of inhibition of the pump by glutathione showed that inhibition by all the PPIs was reversed after 60 minutes of incubation, except for inhibition by pantoprazole, for which there was no reversal. This is consistent with cysteine 822 being inaccessible to this reducing agent and, thus, making inhibition by pantoprazole, *ex* or *in vivo* reversible only by *de novo* pump synthesis. This is consistent with the shielded position of cysteine 822 in the membrane domain, in contrast to cysteines 321 and 813. This observation also predicts a longer duration of inhibition by pantoprazole than for other PPIs. This is illustrated explicitly in the model of PPI binding sites.

Improvement of PPI profile

The limitation of benefit of PPIs is determined by their plasma half-life or their dwell time on the pump. Much effort has been and is being expended on modifying these properties to obtain even better levels of acid inhibition extending into nighttime regulation of pH and volume.

Reversal of inhibition of the acid pump depends both on protein turnover and on reversal of inhibitor binding. For example, it appears that the duration of action of omeprazole and lansoprazole on acid secretion is shorter than expected from the 54-hour half-life of the protein of the pump. Measurement of the half-life of labeled omeprazole on the pump gives a value of approximately 15 hours, similar to the half-life of the return of ATPase activity after 7 days of inhibition with omeprazole. The half-life of pantoprazole is approximately twice as much, perhaps due to its binding to cysteine 822, a position less accessible to the natural reducing agent, glutathione.

On the right is the plasma level profile of 20 mg omeprazole and 40 mg S-omeprazole after 5 days of dosage. It can be seen that there is an increase in the maximal concentration and dwell time of 40 mg S-omeprazole. The benefit of esomeprazole is due to slower metabolism and therefore longer plasma half-life of this enantiomer.

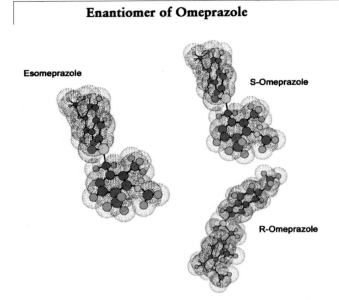

Enantiomer of Omeprazole

Omeprazole vs. Esomeprazole

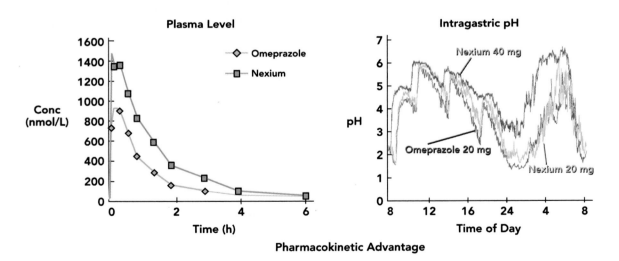

Pharmacokinetic Advantage

Another approach is to increase the plasma dwell time of the PPI. All PPIs have a chiral center and thus have two enantiomers. These may have different properties before activation. Once activated to the sulfenamide, the chiral properties are lost.

To achieve a longer plasma half-life, an enantiomer of omeprazole has been introduced: S-omeprazole, esomeprazole. These structures are shown in the figure. This has a slower metabolism than the R-enantiomer and therefore appears to have a longer dwell time in the blood. At 40-mg dosage, there appears to be improvement in pH control as compared to omeprazole as shown in the figure.

Apart from a better pH profile, it is also important to reduce acid output in terms of improvement of symptom relief and healing.

Therapy with PPIs

When these compounds were introduced clinically, there was not only some degree of confusion as to the inhibition of acid secretion obtained, but there were also intentional marketing attacks by competitors on what has proven to be the most effective and safest means of controlling acid secretion. It is interesting to analyze the consequences of covalent inhibition of the gastric H,K ATPase, which also depends on acid secretion being present for inhibition to occur.

The PPIs, because they are acid labile, must be formulated so as to pass through the stomach without exposure to acid. In the case of omeprazole, this was achieved by microencapsulation, providing a coating that was acid resistant and dissolved only at a pH greater than 6.1. Because acid secretion should be present, the drug is given 30 minutes after breakfast, usually once a day. However, even after a meal, not all parietal cells, let alone all pumps, are active. Therefore, the first dose of the drug will inhibit only those pumps present in the canalicular membrane while the drug is present in the blood. The half-life of these compounds is between 60 and 90 minutes. As inactive pumps are recruited, acid secretion will reappear at the same intragastric pH, albeit at reduced volume.

On the second dose, more pumps will have been recruited during the dwell time of the drug in the blood, and these will be inhibited; hence, inhibition will be more effective on the second day. On the third day, an additional fraction of pumps have been recruited, and further inhibition of acid secretion may be expected.

However, new pumps are also being synthesized. The half-life that was experimentally determined in the rat of pump protein is approximately 54 hours. Therefore, if recovery of acid secretion depended solely on pump synthesis, recovery after cessation of PPI administration should also have a half-life of 48 hours. ATPase activity and acid secretion, however, were restored with a half-life of approximately 15 hours in the rat and approximately 13 hours in humans after lansoprazole administration for 14 days and 27 hours for omeprazole. Recovery, therefore, also involves reversal of the disulfide

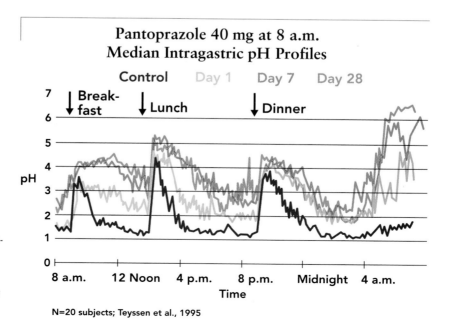

Pantoprazole 40 mg at 8 a.m.
Median Intragastric pH Profiles

Control   Day 1   Day 7   Day 28

N=20 subjects; Teyssen et al., 1995

A typical pHmetric response to once-a-day dosing with pantoprazole, showing inhibition on the first dose but increase of inhibition by days 3 to 7 and maintained elevation of intragastric pH even after 28 days of dosing.

linkage of the drug to the pump, as discussed above. Only pantoprazole shows a recovery of acid secretion compatible with protein turnover. This is due to the inaccessibility of the cysteine 822 labeling position to a reducing agent, such as glutathione.

Steady-state inhibition on once-a-day dosing is reached at approximately the third dose. At steady state in humans, once-a-day dosing results in 66% inhibition of maximal acid output after 5 days of drug administration. This is the degree of inhibition expected with a 24-hour half-life of pump recovery and 75% active pumps at the time of drug administration.

The following chart illustrates the percentage of pumps compared to control available for inhibition immediately before drug administration on each day, assuming that 80% of the pumps are active during the presence of the drug ($t_{1/2}$ = 90 minutes in blood), the percentage of pumps remaining without covalently bound inhibitor after administration, and the percentage of time that intragastric pH is greater than 4.0.

It can be seen that the combination of *de novo* biosynthesis and reversal of disulfide linkage results in approximately 50% of pump capacity inhibited 24 hours after the first dose, approximately 38% 48 hours after the first dose, and 30% 72 hours after the first dose, for omeprazole. The duration of action of pantoprazole is longer, because there is no reversal of the disulfide bond.

It can be seen that steady-state inhibition of stimulated acid output is expected by day 3, as is stabilization of intragastric pH and the degree of inhibition immediately after drug administration. The latter parameter is the most rapidly affected, still providing better acid control than H_2 receptor antagonists. To improve the response of acid secretion, because the lag is due to the maximal number of pumps active during the dwell time of the drug in blood, the dose should be divided rather than increased.

The PPIs as a class have a plasma half-life of approximately 60 to 90 minutes. Their covalent mechanism allows inhibition of secretion to persist long after effective levels of the drug have disappeared from the circulation. The bioavailability of the different PPIs varies either as a function of their metabolism or of the particular formulation developed for their administration. Further, if there is some acid instability of the formulation, bioavailability will increase as a function of duration of administration and the degree of acid inhibition achieved.

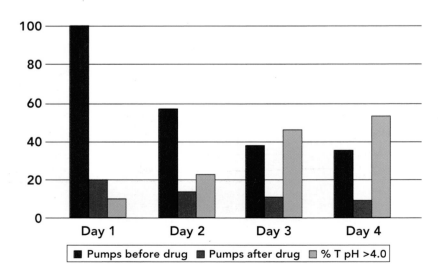

Increased Efficacy of PPIs with QD Dosing

■ Pumps before drug ■ Pumps after drug □ % T pH >4.0

A plot of the time course of inhibition by q.d. dosing of a PPI, illustrating the decline in the number of pumps available for acid secretion (red) with successive doses and the progressive increase in median intragastric pH.

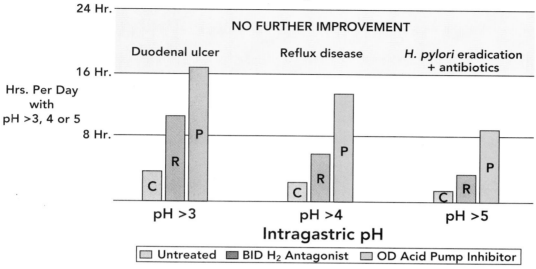

Level and Duration of Intragastric pH Elevation Achieved for Optimal Treatment of:

The control of intragastric pH comparing ranitidine and a PPI, showing that PPIs reach optimal pH control for healing of duodenal ulcer and are superior to H₂ receptor antagonists, especially in GERD and eradication of *H. pylori*. These data are derived from a meta-analysis of pH control by PPIs (P) as compared to ranitidine (R) and placebo (C). The time above pH >3 for more than 16 hours results in optimal healing of duodenal ulcer and is achieved by current PPIs. The optimal pH of >4 for 16 hours is approached by current PPIs, but optimal pH of 5.0 for eradication of *H. pylori* is not.

Because this is covalent inhibition, the efficacy of inhibition is related not to the maximal level of prodrug but to the total exposure of the active parietal cell to above-threshold levels of the PPI, which is most easily related to the area under the curve of plasma levels. Analysis of pHmetric curves shows that steady state is achieved by day 3 and that, in contrast to H_2 receptor antagonists, there is effective inhibition of daytime acid secretion and no tolerance.

The metaanalysis of efficacy of H_2 receptor antagonists presented earlier to analyze pH elevation as a function of once-a-day dosing with PPIs may be extended to provide the data shown in the figure. Elevation to a pH greater than 3.0 and optimization of healing of duodenal ulcer is indeed achieved by once-a-day doses. Treatment of gastroesophageal reflux disease (GERD) by elevation of gastric pH to greater than 4.0 is also reached for most patients, and the pH is also elevated sufficiently to synergize with amoxicillin and clarithromycin in eradication of *H. pylori*.

For consistent inhibition of acid secretion, there must be coincidence of plasma levels of the drug and the state of activation of the pumps. There seems to be considerable interindividual variability in this timing and also variability in the effectiveness of a given PPI. To avoid this, methods need to be developed that produce a longer half-life for the PPI.

Mechanism of acid pump antagonists

There are several protonatable tertiary amines that have been synthesized that are capable of K-competitively inhibiting the ATPase. This class of drug has been called *acid pump antagonists* (APAs). In contrast to the PPIs, they are able to inhibit the pump without acid activation, but because they are also weak bases, they are accumulated in the parietal cell canaliculus and their potency is increased as a function of their pK_a.

The original lead structure, SCH28080 (3-cyanomethyl-2-methyl-8-[phenyl-methoxy] imidazo[1,2α]pyridine), binds to the enzyme largely in its protonated form and to a site accessed from the luminal surface of the pump. A photoaffinity analog, MeDAZIP⁺, after photolysis binds within the membrane domain in the region of TM1 and TM2. Its inhibition constant (K_i), calculating for the protonated form, is in the region of 10 nM. It does not inhibit the Na,K ATPase, as ouabain does not inhibit the H,K ATPase.

K⁺-competitive acid pump antagonists showing the core SCH28080 and the photoaffinity-derivative thereof, MeDAZIP⁺, and the quinoline MDPQ. SCH28080 was the first of its class to be identified as an acid pump antagonist, and MeDAZIP⁺ was an analog enabling labeling of the site to which SCH28080 bound. MDPQ is a fluorescent acid pump antagonist that showed conformational changes in the pump.

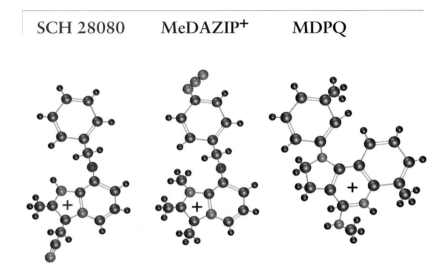

SCH 28080   MeDAZIP⁺   MDPQ

Derivatives of the SCH28080 structure, such as BY 841, are also K competitive, and its effect has been studied in people. This compound produces rapid (within 30 minutes) full inhibition of acid secretion and in principle could be used as a therapeutic antacid with the speed of symptom relief of an antacid and the healing properties of a PPI. A different series of chemical structures, the arylquinolines, has also been developed as therapeutic agents, and this type of structure is illustrated also as MDPQ. This particular compound is fluorescent, and its fluorescence is enhanced on binding to the enzyme and with addition of ATP. This latter reaction suggests that the conformation of the ion "out" site changes with phosphorylation, such that it is probably deeper within the membrane. Their kinetic mechanism involves binding either to the free enzyme or to the phosphoenzyme form, as illustrated in the ion "out" or E_2 configuration.

The K⁺-competitive APAs, such as the imidazopyridines, bind noncovalently, and their specific site of attachment is much harder to predict, because the region of the protein that binds K⁺ or whose conformation prevents K⁺ binding is not known.

The site of ouabain inhibition of the Na pump has been studied in some detail using site-specific and random-site mutagenesis. Ouabain binds to the outside surface of the pump in a partially K⁺-competitive manner. It was well known that rat Na,K ATPase was relatively resistant to ouabain compared to other species. When various Na pumps were sequenced, it was found that the

BY 841

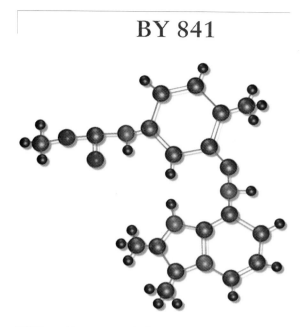

BY 841, an acid pump antagonist that has been shown to be an effective antisecretory agent in humans, providing an intragastric pH of approximately 6.0, 1 hour after administration.

luminal-boundary amino acids of the rat were arg and asp, as compared to gln and asn in other species, at the end of TM1 and the beginning of TM2, respectively. Mutation of rat enzyme to the more usual amino acids resulted in an ouabain-sensitive form of the enzyme. Hence, one ouabain-binding site is in the region of the loop between TM1 and TM2. This finding enabled a series of studies on Na pump expression by transfecting cell lines expressing ouabain-sensitive pumps with rat enzyme. Random mutagenesis also provided evidence for interaction of ouabain with the TM5 and TM6 domain using ouabain binding as a marker. Hence, there are at least two binding regions for this inhibitor.

The gastric H,K ATPase is not inhibited by ouabain, and chimers of the Na,K and H,K ATPases are ouabain sensitive when the N terminal of the chimer is Na,K ATPase and the C terminal is H,K but ouabain resistant when the N-terminal half is the H,K ATPase. This shows that ouabain binds to the N-terminal half of the sodium pump but not to the N-terminal half of the acid pump.

A series of inhibitors has been found for the H,K ATPase that are K^+-competitive inhibitors of enzyme activity. The most potent of these are heterocyclic imidazopyridines, but other heterocyclics, such as arylquinolines or aza-indoles, and many other structures are also effective. In general, these have much lower affinity for the Na,K ATPase.

Analysis of their mechanism of action showed that the protonated form of an inhibitor such as SCH28080 was more effective, and that their reaction was with the external surface of the enzyme. This conclusion was reached because the quaternary form generated by methylation of the pyridine N of SCH28080 was ineffective in intact right-side-out vesicles of the H,K ATPase; also, their K_i decreased with decreasing pH.

Because these inhibitors are noncovalent, the site of binding can be investigated by mutational analysis or by generating photoaffinity derivatives of, for example, SCH28080, an imidazo-1,2α pyridine. The azido form of the methylated imidazopyridine, MeDAZIP$^+$ was shown to be K-competitive and, after photolysis, was covalently bound to the TM1/TM2 domain of the H,K ATPase. Substitution in the loop between TM1 and TM2 did not affect inhibition, resulting in the conclusion that inhibition depends on interaction of the inhibitor with the TM1/TM2 membrane domain itself rather than with the connecting loop. Construction of a chimer between TM1 and TM2 of the H,K and the fungal H ATPase resulted in an SCH28080-sensitive ATPase, again confirming the site of inhibition by these compounds.

A series of mutations has also shown that the loop between M5 and M6 is an important determinant of binding of SCH28080 and has also shown that the binding sites for K^+ and the inhibitor are different and that competitive kinetics arise from mutual exclusion of binding.

A model of their binding site is shown in the figure.

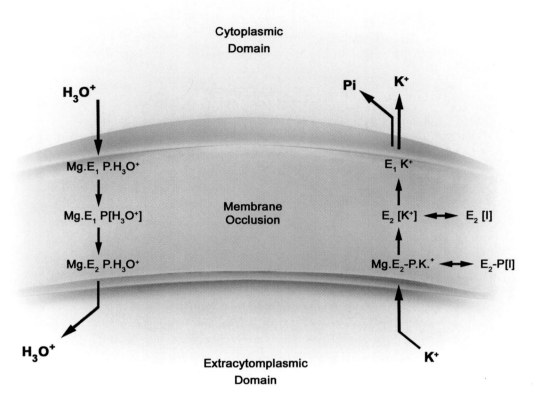

The reaction scheme for the H,K ATPase, showing the step of inhibition by the APAs forming either E_2 [I] or E_2-P[I].

In contrast to PPIs, the action of APAs is independent of the secretory status, and there is no lag time expected. These are, therefore, fast-acting compounds able to abolish acid secretion during their presence in the blood. Their efficacy will be related more to peak levels than area under the curve, unless time-release formulations are developed. If these compounds have a plasma half-life similar to that of the PPIs, a pH greater than 5.0 will be found for approximately 4 hours, but acid-secretory capacity will be restored fully after two half-lives, namely within 4 to 6 hours of administration.

These drugs, if introduced into clinical practice, will be therapeutic antacids, allowing on-demand dosage, but they will not have the extended inhibitory characteristics of PPIs. It remains to be seen whether they will achieve the same healing rates of GERD as PPIs although they are predicted to markedly improve the onset of symptom relief.

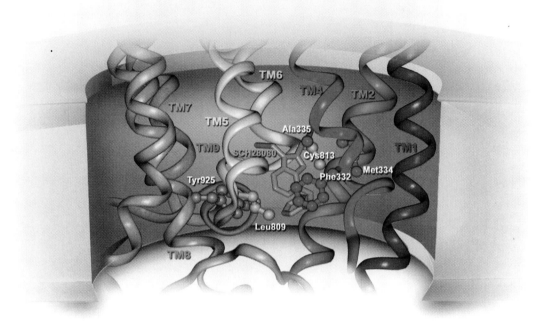

An illustration of the binding site of acid pump antagonists such as the imidazopyridine, SCH28080, with the transmembrane segments numbered and the amino acids to which this compound binds emphasized as ball-and-stick forms and named. By comparing this to the binding site for PPIs, it can be seen that there is overlap of this binding site with that of omeprazole and other PPIs.

SUGGESTED READING

Bell NJ, Burget D, Howden CW, et al. Appropriate acid suppression for the management of gastro-oesophageal reflux disease. *Digestion* 1992;51(Suppl 1):59–67.

Bertaccini G, Coruzzi G. Control of gastric acid secretion by histamine H_2 receptor antagonists and anticholinergics. *Pharmacol Res* 1989;21:339.

Besancon M, Shin JM, Mercier F, et al. Membrane topology and omeprazole labelling of the gastric H+,K+-adenosine triphosphatase. *Biochemistry* 1993;32:2345–2355.

Besancon M, Simon A, Sachs G, et al. Sites of reaction of the gastric H,K-ATPase with extracytoplasmic thiol reagents. *J Biol Chem* 1997;272:22438–22446.

Black JW, Duncan WAM, Durant CJ, et al. Definition and antagonism of histamine H_2 receptors. *Nature* 1972;236:385–390.

Brimblecombe RW, Duncan WAM, Durant GJ, et al. Characterization and development of cimetidine as a histamine H_2-receptor antagonist. *Gastroenterology* 1978;74:339.

Brandstrom A, Lindberg P, Bergman N-A, et al. Chemical reactions of omeprazole and omeprazole analogues. I. A survey of the chemical transformations of omeprazole and its analogues. *Acta Chem Scand* 1989;43:536–548.

Brandstrom A, Bergman N-A, Lindberg P, et al. Chemical reactions of omeprazole and omeprazole analogues. II. Kinetics of the reaction of omeprazole in the presence of 2-mercaptoethanol. *Acta Chem Scand* 1989;43:559–568.

Brandstrom A, Bergman N-A, Grundevik I, et al. Chemical reactions of omeprazole and omeprazole analogues. III. Protolytic behaviour of compounds in the omeprazole system. *Acta Chem Scand* 1989;43:569–576.

Brandstrom A, Lindberg P, Bergman N-A, et al. Chemical reactions of omeprazole and omeprazole analogues. IV. Reactions of compounds of the omeprazole system with 2-mercaptoethanol. *Acta Chem Scand* 1989;43:577–586.

Brandstrom A, Lindberg P, Bergman N-A, et al. Chemical reactions of omeprazole and omeprazole analogues. V. The reaction of N-alkylated derivatives of omeprazole analogues with 2-mercaptoethanol. *Acta Chem Scand* 1989;43:587–595.

Brandstrom A, Lindberg P, Bergman N-A, et al. Chemical reactions of omeprazole and omeprazole analogues. VI. The reaction of omeprazole in the absence of 2-mercaptoethanol. *Acta Chem Scand* 1989;43:595–611.

Burget DW, Chiverton SG, Hunt RH. Is there an optimal degree of acid suppression for healing of duodenal ulcers? A model of the relationship between ulcer healing and acid suppression. *Gastroenterology* 1990;99:345–351.

Carter DC, Forrest J, Werner W, et al. Effect of histamine H_2-receptor blockade on vagally induced gastric acid secretion in man. *Br Med J* 1974;3:554.

Code CF. Histamine and gastric secretion: a later look, 1955–1965. *Federation Proc* 1965;24:1311–1321.

Davenport HA. *History of gastric secretion and digestion.* New York: Oxford University Press, 1992:320–321.

Feldman M. Inhibition of gastric acid secretion by selective and nonselective anticholinergics. *Gastroenterology* 1984;86:361.

Feldman M, Burton ME. Histamine H_2 receptor antagonists. *N Engl J Med* 1990;323:1672.

Feldman M, Burton ME. Histamine H_2 receptor antagonists. Part two. *N Engl J Med* 1990;323:1749.

Fellenius E, Berglindh T, Sachs G, et al. Substituted benzimidazoles inhibit gastric acid secretion by blocking ($H^+ + K^+$)ATPase. *Nature* 1981;290:159–161.

Figala V, Klemm K, Kohl B, et al. Acid activation of H^+-K^+-ATPase inhibiting 2-(2-Pyridylmethylsulphinyl) benzimidazoles: isolation and characterization of the thiophilic 'active principle' and its reactions. *J Chem Soc Chem Commun* 1986:125–127.

Fitton A, Wiseman L. Pantoprazole, a review of its pharmacology and therapeutic use in acid-related disorders. *Drugs* 1996;51:460–482.

Forte JG, Ganser A, Beesley R, et al. Unique enzymes of purified microsomes from pig fundic mucosa. *Gastroenterology* 1975;69:175–189.

Fryklund J, Gedda K, Wallmark B. Specific labelling of gastric H^+,K^+-ATPase by omeprazole. *Biochem Pharmacol* 1988;37:2543–2549.

Gantz I, Schaffer M, Del Valle J, et al. Molecular cloning of a gene encoding the histamine H_2 receptor. *Proc Natl Acad Sci U S A* 1991;88:5937.

Gedda K, Scott D, Besancon M, et al. The turnover of the gastric H,K ATPase alpha subunit and its effect on inhibition of rat gastric acid secretion. *Gastroenterology* 1995;109:1134–1141.

Havu N. Enterochromaffin-like cell carcinoids of the gastric mucosa after life-long inhibition of gastric secretion. *Digestion* 1986;35:42.

Hawkey CJ, Long RG, Bardhan KD, et al. Improved symptom relief and duodenal ulcer healing with lansoprazole, a new proton pump inhibitor, compared with ranitidine. *Gut* 1993;34;1458–1462.

Helander HF, Ramsay CH, Regardh CG. Localization of omeprazole and metabolites in the mouse. *Scand J Gastroenterol* 1985;20(Suppl 108):95–104.

Herzog P, Grendahl T, Linden J, et al. Adverse effects of high dose antacid regimen. Results of a randomized, double-blind trial. *Gastroenterology* 1980;80:1173.

Hollender LF, Bahnini J. Jules Emile Péan. In: Nyhus LM, Wastrell C, eds. *Surgery of the stomach and the duodenum.* Boston: Little, Brown and Company, 1986:39–41.

Im WB, Blakeman DP, Davis JP. Irreversible inactivation of rat gastric (H^+-K^+)-ATPase *in vivo* by omeprazole. *Biochem Biophys Res Commun* 1985;126:78–82.

Im WB, Blakeman DP, Sachs G. Reversal of antisecretory activity of omeprazole by sulfhydryl compounds in isolated rabbit gastric glands. *Biochim Biophys Acta* 1985;845:54–59.

Jaup BH, Bloomstrand CH. Cerebro-spinal fluid concentration of pirenzepine after therapeutic dosage. *Scand J Gastroenterol* 1980;15:35.

Keeling DJ, Fallowfield C, Underwood AH. The specificity of omeprazole as an $(H^+ + K^+)$-ATPase inhibitor depends upon the means of its activation. *Biochem Pharmacol* 1987;36:339–344.

Keeling DJ, Laing SM, Senn Bilfinger J. SCH 28080 is a lumenally acting, K^+-site inhibitor of the gastric $(H^+ + K^+)$-ATPase. *Biochem Pharmacol* 1988;37:2231–2236.

Koop H, Schepp W, Damman HG, et al. Comparative trial of pantoprazole and ranitidine in the treatment of reflux esophagitis: results of a German multicenter study. *J Clin Gastroenterol* 1995;20:192–195.

Lamberts R, Creutzfeldt W, Strueber HG, et al. Long-term omeprazole therapy in peptic ulcer disease. Gastrin, endocrine cell growth, and gastritis. *Gastroenterology* 1993;104:1356.

Lambrecht N, Corbett Z, Bayle D, et al. Identification of the site of inhibition by omeprazole of a α-β fusion protein of the HK-ATPase using site-directed mutagenesis. *J Biol Chem* 1998;273:13719–13728.

Lanzon-Miller S, Pounder, RE, Hamilton MR, et al. Twenty-four-hour intragastric acidity and plasma gastrin concentration before and during treatment with either ranitidine or omeprazole. *Aliment Pharmacol Ther* 1987;1:239–251.

Larsson H, Carlsson E, Jinggren U, et al. Inhibition of gastric acid secretion by omeprazole in the dog and rat. *Gastroenterology* 1983;85:900–907.

Larsson H, Carlsson E, Mattsson H. Plasma gastrin in gastric enterochromaffin-like cell activation and proliferation: studies with omeprazole and ranitidine in intact and antrectomized rats. *Gastroenterology* 1986;90:391–399.

Larsson H, Carlsson E, Mattson H, et al. Plasma gastrin concentrations and gastric enterochromaffin-like cell activation and proliferation. *Gastroenterology* 1986;90:391.

Latarjet A. Preliminaire sur l'innervation et l'enervation de l'estomac. *Lyon Med* 1921;130:160–166.

Latarjet A. Resection des nerfs de l'estomac; technique operatoire; resultats cliniques. *Bull Acad Natl Med Paris* 1922;87:681–691.

Levine RA, Kohen KR, Schwartzel EH Jr. Prostaglandin E2-histamine in interactions on cAMP, cGMP, and acid production in isolated fundic glands. *Am J Physiol* 1982;242:G21–G26.

Lind T, Cederberg C, Ekenved G. Effect of omeprazole—a gastric proton pump inhibitor—on pentagastrin stimulated acid secretion in man. *Gut* 1983;24:270–276.

Lind T, Cederberg C, Ekenved G, et al. Inhibition of basal and betazole- and sham-feeding-induced acid secretion by omeprazole in man. *Scand J Gastroenterol* 1986;21:1004–1010.

Lindberg P, Nordberg P, Alminger T, et al. The mechanism of action of the gastric acid secretion inhibitor omeprazole. *J Med Chem* 1986;29:1327–1329.

Lindberg P, Brandstrom A, Wallmark B, et al. Omeprazole: the first proton pump inhibitor. *Med Res Rev* 1990;10:1–54.

Lorentzon P, Jackson R, Wallmark B, et al. Inhibition of $(H^+ + K^+)$-ATPase by omeprazole in isolated gastric vesicles requires proton transport. *Biochim Biophys Acta* 1987;897:41–51.

Maton PN. Omeprazole. *N Engl J Med* 1991;324:965.

Mattson H, Havu N, Braeutigam J, et al. Partial gastric corpectomy results in hypergastrinemia and development of gastric enterochromaffin-like carcinoids in the rat. *Gastroenterology* 1991;100:311.

McTavish D, Buckley MMT, Heel RC. Omeprazole. An updated review of its pharmacology and therapeutic use in acid-related disorders. *Drugs* 1991;42:138.

Modlin IM, Waisbren SJ, Lester R. Dragstedt and his role in the evolution of therapeutic vagotomy in the United States. *Am J Surg* 1994;167:344–359.

Morii M, Takeguchi N. Different biochemical modes of action of two irreversible $H^+,K^{(+)}$-ATPase inhibitors, omeprazole and E3810. *J Biol Chem* 1993;268:21553–21559.

Munson KB, Gutierrez C, Balaji VN, et al. Identification of an extracytoplasmic region of H^+,K^+-ATPase labelled by a K^+-competitive photoaffinity inhibitor. *J Biol Chem* 1991;266:18976–18988.

Munson KB, Sachs G. Inactivation of H^+,K^+-ATPase by a K^+-competitive photoaffinity inhibitor. *Biochemistry* 1988;27:3932–3938.

Naesdal J, Bodemar G, Walan A. Effect of omeprazole, a substituted benzimidazole on 24 hr intragastric acidity in patients with peptic ulcer disease. *Scand J Gastroenterol* 1984;19:916–922.

Nwokolo CU, Smith JT, Gavey C, et al. Tolerance during 29 days of conventional dosing with cimetidine, nizatidine, famotidine or ranitidine. *Aliment Pharmacol Ther* 1990;4(Suppl 1):29–45.

Nwokolo CU, Smith JT, Sawyerr AM, et al. Rebound intragastric hyperacidity after abrupt withdrawal of histamine H_2 receptor blockade. *Gut* 1991;32:1455.

Prinz C, Scott DR, Hurwitz D, et al. Gastrin effects on isolated rat enterochromaffin-like cells in primary culture. *Am J Physiol* 1994;267:G663.

Pue MA, Laroche J, Meineke I, et al. Pharmacokinetics of pantoprazole following single intravenous and oral administration to healthy male subjects. *Eur J Clin Pharmacol* 1993;44:575–578.

Rabon E, Sachs G, Bassilian S, et al. A K^+-competitive fluorescent inhibitor of the H,K-ATPase. *J Biol Chem* 1991;266:12395–12401.

Regardh CG, Gabrielsson M, Hoffman KJ, et al. Pharmacokinetics and metabolism of omeprazole in animals and man. *Scand J Gastroenterol* 1985;20:79–94.

Ryberg B, Tielemanns Y, Axelson J, et al. Gastrin stimulates the self-replication of enterochromaffin-like cells in the rat stomach. *Gastroenterology* 1990;99:935.

Ryberg B, Axelson J, Hakanson R, et al. Trophic effects of continuous infusion of [Leu15]-gastrin-17 in the rat. *Gastroenterology* 1990;98:33.

Sachs G, Shin JM, Briving C, et al. Pharmacology of gastric H,K ATPase. *Annu Rev Pharmacol Toxicol* 1995;35:277–305.

Sachs G, Carlsson E, Lindberg P, et al. Gastric H,K-ATPase as therapeutic target. *Annu Rev Pharmacol Toxicol* 1988;28:269–284.

Sachs G, Shin JM, Besancon M, et al. The continuing development of gastric acid pump inhibitors (Lansoprazole). *Aliment Pharmacol Ther* 1993;7(Suppl 1):4–12.

Schepp W, Heim HK, Ruoff HJ. Comparison of the effect of PGE2 and somatostatin on histamine stimulated 14C-aminopyrine uptake and cyclic AMP formation in isolated rat gastric mucosal cells. *Agents Actions* 1983;13:200–206.

Scott D, Besancon M, Sachs G, et al. The effect of antisecretory drugs on parietal cell structure and H/K ATPase levels in rabbit gastric mucosa in vivo. *Dig Dis Sci* 1994;39:2118.

Senn-Bilfinger J, Kruger U, Sturm E, et al. (H^+-K^+)-ATPase Inhibiting 2-[(2-Pyridylmethyl)sulfinyl]benzimidazoles. 2. The reaction cascade induced by treatment with acids. formation of 5H-pyrido[1',2':4,5][1,2,4]thiadiazino[2,3-α]benzimidazol-13-ium salts and their reactions with thiols. *J Org Chem* 1987;52:4582–4592.

Shin JM, Besancon M, Simon A, et al. The site of action of pantoprazole in the gastric H^+/K^+-ATPase. *Biochim Biophys Acta* 1993;1148:223–233.

Shin JM, Sachs G. Restoration of acid secretion following treatment with proton pump inhibitors. *Gastroenterology* 2002;123:1588–1597.

Simon B, Muller P, Marinis E, et al. Effect of repeated oral administration of BY1023/SK&F96022—a new substituted benzimidazole derivative—on pentagastrin-stimulated gastric acid secretion and pharmacokinetics in man. *Aliment Pharmacol Ther* 1990;4:373–379.

Smallwood RA, Berlin RG, Castagnoli N, et al. Safety of acid suppressing drugs. *Dig Dis Sci* 1994;40(Suppl):63–80.

Sturm E, Kruger U, Senn-Bilfinger J, et al. (H^+-K^+)-ATPase inhibiting 2-[(2-pyridylmethyl)sulfinyl]benzimidazoles. 1. Their reaction with thiols under acidic conditions. disulfide containing 2-pyridinio-benzimidazolides as mimics for the inhibited enzyme. *J Org Chem* 1987;52:4573–4581.

Tielemanns Y, Hakanson R, Sundler F, et al. Proliferation of enterochromaffin-like cells in omeprazole treated hypergastrinemic rats. *Gastroenterology* 1989;96:723.

Tielemanns Y, Axelson J, Sundler F, et al. Serum gastrin affects the self-replication rate of enterochromaffin-like cells in the rat stomach. *Gut* 1990;31:274.

Vagin O, Denevich S, Munson KB, et al. SCH28080, a K^+-competitive inhibitor of the gastric H,K-ATPase, binds near the M5-6 luminal loop, preventing K^+ access to the ion binding domain. *Biochemistry* 2002;41:12755–12762.

Wallmark B, Skaenberg I, Mattson H, et al. Effects of 20 weeks ranitidine treatment on plasma gastrin levels and gastric enterochromaffin-like cell density in the rat. *Digestion* 1990;45:181.

Wallmark B, Brandstrom A, Larsson H. Evidence for acid-induced transformation of omeprazole into an active inhibitor of ($H^+ + K^+$)-ATPase within the parietal cell. *Biochim Biophys Acta* 1984;778:549–558.

Wallmark B, Briving C, Fryklund J, et al. Inhibition of gastric H^+,K^+-ATPase and acid secretion by SCH 28080, a substituted pyridyl(1,2α)imidazole. *J Biol Chem* 1987;262:2077–2084.

Wallmark B, Larsson H, Humble L. The relationship between gastric acid secretion and gastric H^+, K^+-ATPase activity. *J Biol Chem* 1985;260:13681–13684.

Wangensteen O. *The rise of surgery*. Minneapolis: University of Minnesota Press, 1978:154.

Wolfe MM, Sachs G. Acid suppression: optimizing therapy for gastroduodenal ulcer healing, gastroesophageal reflux disease, and stress-related erosive syndrome. *Gastroenterology* 2000;118:S9–S31.

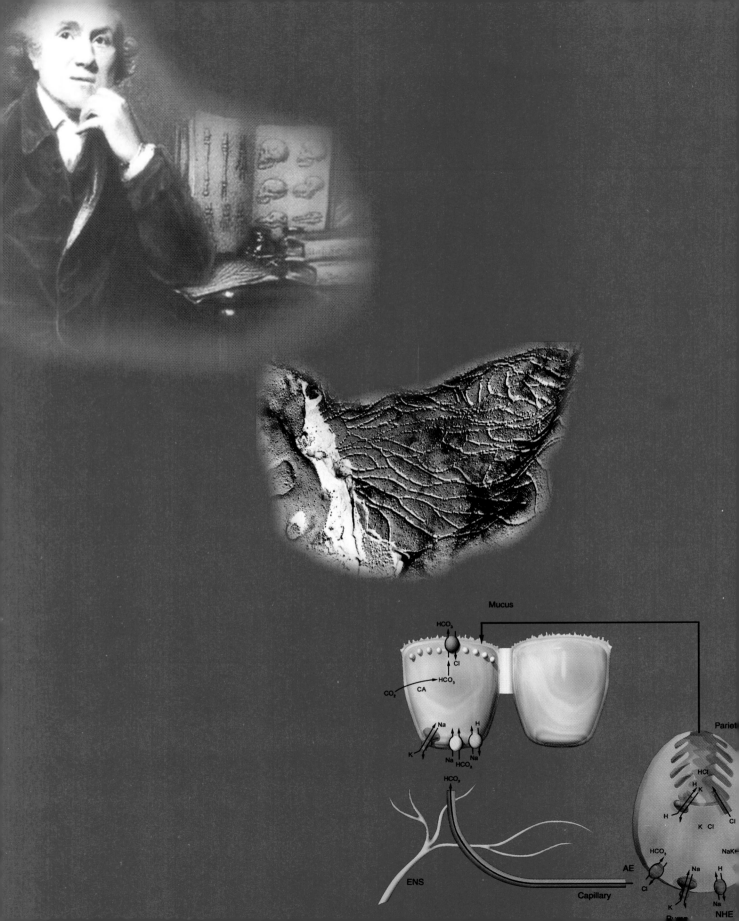

THE BIOLOGY OF ACID RELATED DISEASE

CHAPTER 1
THE BARRIERS OF THE UPPER GASTROINTESTINAL TRACT

Introduction

The common acid related diseases of the upper gastrointestinal tract can be considered as primarily due to a defect in barrier function of the esophageal epithelium or primarily the lower esophageal sphincter in the case of GERD or of the gastric mucosal or duodenal epithelium in the case of gastric or duodenal ulcers. The defect may be natural or induced, for example, by infection with *H. pylori*. In rarer situations, such as Zollinger-Ellison syndrome, the extraordinary levels of acid may overwhelm otherwise normal barriers. The lower esophageal sphincter will be discussed in some detail in the section on GERD, and this introduction to acid related diseases will focus on the acid-resistance properties of the esophageal, gastric, and duodenal epithelia.

Historical aspects

Once it had become apparent that digestion was an active process involving acid and pepsin that was initiated in the stomach, a further fundamental question arose. Why did the stomach not digest itself? This problem had long been pondered, and Archibald Pitcairn, the great Iatromathematician, had himself questioned the Iatrochemists rigorously on this issue: "...*Why on the digestion of food on the stomach, which is as easily digestible as the food, yet the stomach itself should not be dissolved?*" No reasonable answer was forthcoming, and the pundits, such as John Hunter, could only perseverate on the existence of a putative vital force that maintained the gastric wall intact under the circumstances of digestion. Issues such as the existence of a "*locus minoris resist-*

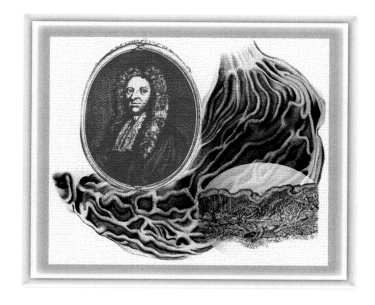

Archibald Pitcairn (top left), the noted Iatromathematician, questioned why the stomach (background) failed to ingest itself. A number of thoughtful scientists of the time, including John Hunter, pondered why the digestive agents present in the lumen had no effect on the stomach itself. Their speculations in this regard included the presence of a "vital force" that might protect the organ from the process of digestion and internal dissolution. It was, however, apparent that with death this vital spirit dissipated, as did blood flow, and it was anticipated, although unproven, that the two events were related. An intact gastric mucosa demonstrating viable arterial and venous blood supplies is indicated (bottom right).

The apparatus and graphic information used by T. Teorell (left) to determine H⁺ back diffusion.

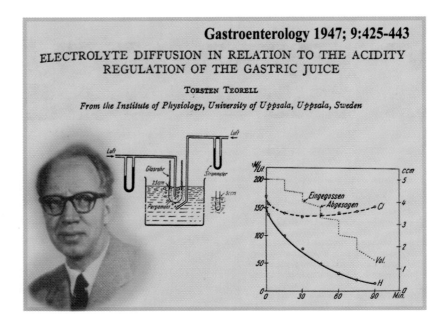

Gastroenterology 1947; 9:425-443

ELECTROLYTE DIFFUSION IN RELATION TO THE ACIDITY REGULATION OF THE GASTRIC JUICE

TORSTEN TEORELL

From the Institute of Physiology, University of Uppsala, Uppsala, Sweden

entia" were entertained to explain ulceration and embrace the concept that this was indeed local digestion of the stomach mucosa.

Nevertheless, it seemed difficult to understand why food in the lumen of the stomach would be broken up whereas the wall of the stomach remained intact. The invocation of "vital spirit" was of little satisfaction and represented a regression to archaic views on the nature of digestion. Further reflection on the matter resulted in the recognition that the stomach wall itself must harbor an intrinsic "force" capable of resisting digestion. Indeed, the attractive concept that a breakdown of such an intrinsic mechanism might be responsible for the development of ulcers or even neoplasia became a source of considerable speculation. Nevertheless, little evidence existed to delineate the specific nature of the mechanism responsible for the generation of mucosal protection from acid, pepsin, and even noxious agents that might be ingested.

In the early 1930s, Torsten Teorell had begun to examine the permeability characteristics of gastric mucosa by suggesting that H⁺ diffused back through the mucosa in exchange for Na⁺. Thus, issues had arisen as to whether acid was neutralized within the lumen or after diffusion into the mucosa in the interstitial fluid. An alternative hypothesis had been that the bicarbonate content of gastric secretion might be responsible for some of the acid that was neutralized. Nevertheless, the ability of the stomach to retain the acid it secreted under normal circumstances without digesting itself once again raised the concept of the existence of a "gastric mucosal barrier." Teorell began the delineation of the barrier properties by demonstrating that unionized organic acids, but not ionized mineral acids, would disappear rapidly from the gastric contents by diffusing into the mucosa. Although not fully resolving the issue, his concept of a diffusion process in the mucosa had by 1947 initiated the formal evaluation of the intrinsic mechanisms available to deal with back diffusion of acid into the interstitium of the stomach.

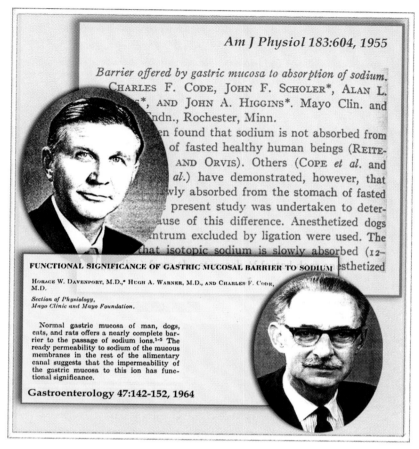

Am J Physiol 183:604, 1955

Barrier offered by gastric mucosa to absorption of sodium.
CHARLES F. CODE, JOHN F. SCHOLER*, ALAN L.
s*, AND JOHN A. HIGGINS*. Mayo Clin. and
ndn., Rochester, Minn.

n found that sodium is not absorbed from
of fasted healthy human beings (REITE-
AND ORVIS). Others (COPE *et al.* and
al.) have demonstrated, however, that
wly absorbed from the stomach of fasted
present study was undertaken to deter-
use of this difference. Anesthetized dogs
ntrum excluded by ligation were used. The
that isotopic sodium is slowly absorbed (12-
esthetized

FUNCTIONAL SIGNIFICANCE OF GASTRIC MUCOSAL BARRIER TO SODIUM

HORACE W. DAVENPORT, M.D.,* HUGH A. WARNER, M.D., AND CHARLES F. CODE,
M.D.

*Section of Physiology,
Mayo Clinic and Mayo Foundation.*

Normal gastric mucosa of man, dogs,
cats, and rats offers a nearly complete barrier to the passage of sodium ions.[1-5] The
ready permeability to sodium of the mucous
membranes in the rest of the alimentary
canal suggests that the impermeability of
the gastric mucosa to this ion has functional significance.

Gastroenterology 47:142-152, 1964

Charles Code (top left), who was an initial proponent of the critical role of histamine in acid secretion, also proposed the existence of a gastric mucosal barrier. H. Davenport (bottom right), in collaboration with Code, sought the pathophysiologic basis for mucosal permeability to ions.

In 1955, Davenport and Code published a series of experiments under the title *The Functional Significance of Gastric Mucosal Barrier to Sodium* and thus initiated the first formal usage of the term *barrier*. They described the results of the relative rates of disappearance of radiolabeled $^{42}K^+$, $^{22}Na^+$, thiocyanate, or $^{3}H_2O$ from solutions in contact with oxyntic mucosa. They observed that when the gastric contents were neutral, $^{3}H_2O$ disappeared rapidly but $^{42}K^+$ slowly and $^{22}Na^+$ at an intermediate rate. However, when the gastric contents were acid, or gastric secretion was stimulated by histamine, the rates of disappearance of THO and $^{42}K^+$ were unaffected, whereas the rates of disappearance of $^{22}Na^+$ fell to zero. In recognition of the significance of this observation, Code commented presciently on this subject in the manuscript entitled *The Barrier Offered by the Gastric Mucosa to Sodium*.

Further experiments in this area were designed to identify the site of this zone and resulted in proposals that it was mucus that construed the barrier function. Proof for this, however, was difficult to obtain, and a reconfiguration of this proposal by others resulted in the hypothesis that bicarbonate secreted by the gastric mucosa neutralized acid and thus created a biochemical barrier. Further elaboration of this line of work generated much discussion about the "unstirred layer" and held that the modest concentration of bicarbonate held in this would produce a barrier of both functional and physical significance to acid. In a fashion reminiscent of the determination of the physical aura produced by plants, the size of this barrier was then measured and its certain presence fixed in the minds of the believers. Davenport in later work further explored the concept of the gastric mucosal barrier by seeking to damage it with various agents including eugenol, fatty acids, and alcohol, and was able to prove that back diffusion into the mucosa of acid occurred under such conditions. These observations were substantiated by anatomic evidence of increased mucosal permeability by demonstrating damage to the surface epithelial cells and underlying tissues, including vessels. Some support was thus provided for the important association of barrier breaking and its relationship to acute mucosal ulceration and stress bleeding.

An immense body of work was then undertaken by diverse investigators to identify the effects of hypoxia, acid, bile salts, aspirin, nonsteroidal antiinflammatory drugs (NSAIDs), prostaglandins, etc., on the integrity of the barrier. The commutations and permutations of these studies achieved little except to further document the existence of the mucosal barrier and the ability of a variety of agents to break it. Unfortunately, this did little to identify the precise site and mechanism of the phenomenon. The summation of much work established that the barrier represented a generalized function common to a polarized epithelial cell system and that acids in an unionized state and fat-solubilizing agents were capable of acting as barrier-breaking agents. Breaking the barrier in itself was not sufficient but represented an initial step in the process of mucosal injury. A subsequent cascade of physiologic events involving back diffusion of acid with liberation of histamine and the activation of pepsinogen was involved.

The exploration of the multiplicity of associated phenomena provided further complex information regarding the fact that the barrier might not be a single entity but represent a multiplicity of physiologic protective mechanisms. The more recent use of sophisticated techniques to investigate cell function has determined the relevance of tight junctions and identified the specific property of the apical membrane of the gastric mucosal cells as being of vital importance in maintaining barrier function.

Davenport and Code thus deserve credit for extending the word *barrier* to include the property of the mucosa governing its permeability to H+. In subsequent years, the word would become a term broadly used to designate permeability of the mucosa in general. Fromm, in an evaluation of the entire subject, was to later remark that *barrier* and *barrier breakers* were simply catch phrases that, "*while novel and clever, reflect our ignorance.*" Davenport himself, in summarizing his accomplishments in the area, published them in a book whimsically entitled *The Gastric Mucosal Barrier: A Swan Song.*

The esophageal epithelium

Malfunction of the lower esophageal sphincter results in acid reflux into the esophagus. The acid load presented to the esophagus is likely to be the major determinant of heartburn or erosion. Reflux is mainly episodic, so that the esophagus is not often presented with a continuous acid load. Expulsion of the refluxate back into the stomach shortens the time of exposure.

The volume of reflux is also an important parameter for estimation of the acid load on the esophageal epithelium. Finally, the pH of the gastric contents that are refluxed into the esophagus also determines the possible damage. Intraesophageal pH monitoring provides an approximate measure of the acid load to the lower esophagus in terms of the pH of refluxate and dwell time of the acid solution and is probably the most useful semiquantitative measure of the degree of exposure of the esophageal epithelium.

The human esophageal epithelium is a multilayered, stratified squamous epithelium. Afferent nerves are present, reaching into the superficial layers of the epithelium. With incompetence of the lower esophageal sphincter (LES), acid reflux results with consequently the possibility of pain and damage to the epi-

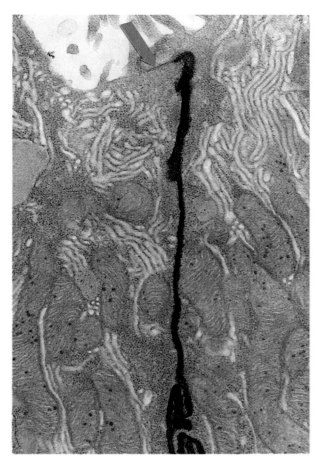

The use of lanthanum to define the tight junctions of the gastric mucosa. The electron-dense lanthanum fails to pass the "tight" junction at the apex of the mucosal cells. The arrow indicates the tight junction, and below is the basolateral space penetrated by lanthanum added to the outside surface.

thelium, depending on the pH of the refluxate. Rather than being protected by a continuous tight junction, this epithelium has largely regional cell-to-cell contact via desmosomes. There is some evidence for the presence of tight junctions in the first layer of the epithelium, but the very few strands seen on EM freeze fracture show that these at best are "leaky" tight junctions. This epithelium, being multilayered, provides a winding path for proton diffusion into the deeper layers of the epithelium. It is significantly more acid sensitive than the gastric epithelium, which is provided with "tight" tight junctions.

The thresholds of acidity for damage and pain may be different. A higher acidity is likely needed for damage to the epithelial cells compared to the acidity required for stimulation of the pain fibers. This is probably because the epithelial cells have acid-recovery mechanisms (such as Na^+/H^+ or anion exchange) mostly absent in the pain fibers. Also, pain fibers contain acid-sensitive ion channels (ASICs) that respond to environmental acidity. Depending on the location of the pain fibers and access thereto of H^+, individuals have different sensitivities to luminal acidity. The therapeutic aims of acid control may vary, being elevation of mean diurnal pH for healing of erosions or prevention of acidic excursions for symptom relief, or both.

Esophageal healing

Given the absence of continuous tight junctions or only leaky tight junctions, the lower esophageal epithelium is an inviting target for acid back diffusion. Mucus is an aqueous gel and is unlikely to provide a significant barrier to acid. In water, protons can move faster than other cations due to their ability to jump from water molecule to water molecule, and there are continuous chains of water in aqueous gels.

Resistance to acid may therefore depend more on the ability of the esophageal epithelium to neutralize an acid load than on restriction of entry of acid between the cells. Neutralization of acid occurs at the surface due to net HCO_3^- secretion and also diffusion across the paracellular pathway, because the epithelial cells can produce, buffer, or absorb H^+. However, once damage has occurred, this paracellular pathway is shorter or more open and the lesion consequently more sensitive to acid than the normal epithelium. The measured average net flux of bicarbonate is approximately 78 μmol per 30 minutes per 10 cm in the human esophagus. It appears to be subject to regulation by muscarinic receptors, responding to the vagal stimulation of acid secretion by the stomach. It is possible to approximate the pH of unbuffered refluxate that can be neutralized by esophageal surface secretion. If buffering is present, such as that due to amino acids or weak acids, e.g., citrate, the acid load will be greater in the buffering range of gastric contents and reflect not only pH.

With reflux of unbuffered gastric contents at a pH of 4.0, there is a load of acid equivalent to 100 nmol per mL. If 10 mL of gastric contents at that pH is refluxed each minute for 30 minutes and spreads over a length of 10 cm, 30 μmol of acid is presented to this length of the esophagus in that 30-minute time span. This is within the average neutralizing ability of the secreted HCO_3^-. Reflux at a pH of 4.0 should therefore be largely neutralized at or close to the esophageal surface. This calculation may explain the results of a metaanalysis of the ideal pH elevation for the most rapid healing of esophageal lesions, as discussed below.

At a pH of 3.0, there is tenfold more acid, and 300 μmol of acid is presented to the lower esophagus, with 10 mL refluxing each minute. This is beyond the capacity of net HCO_3^- secretion to neutralize the HCl. Acidification of intercellular spaces is likely, which may result in pain in some individuals. Epithelial cell pH may remain within viable limits given adequate Na^+/H^+ or Cl^-/HCO_3^- exchange.

At a pH of 2.0 and below, the limits of the HCO_3^- response are greatly exceeded, and the intercellular spaces will acidify even more and to a deeper level. At this stage, the ability of the epithelial cells to maintain constant intracellular pH may be overcome due to the high acid load, with resultant erosion. As the more superficial cells are eroded, pepsin may also back diffuse, adding proteolytic insult to acid injury.

These calculations, although fraught with assumptions, do predict that elevation to a mean diurnal pH of greater than 4.0 will optimize healing of erosions of the lower esophagus. Gastric contents contain pepsin in addition to acid. Proteolytic activity of pepsin requires a pH less than 3.0, and probably there is adequate neutralization of intercellular pH if the refluxate does not fall much below 3.0. At a refluxate of pH 2.0, because the esophageal surface cannot neutralize this acid load, peptic activity may begin to contribute to esophageal damage. Peptic activity is less likely to contribute directly to pain.

Rationale for treatment of GERD with PPIs

Treatment of reflux esophagitis can be accomplished by improving the response or structure of the LES or by effective inhibition of acid secretion. Currently available compounds targeted to the LES are relatively nonselective compounds and have lower efficacy than acid inhibition. Ideally, control of GERD, in terms of both healing and symptom relief, would not allow gastric pH to fall much below 4.0 at any time.

On once-a-day PPI treatment, the inhibition of maximal acid output is approximately 70%. Steady-state inhibition is found on approximately the third

Predictive Values for Esophagitis Healing

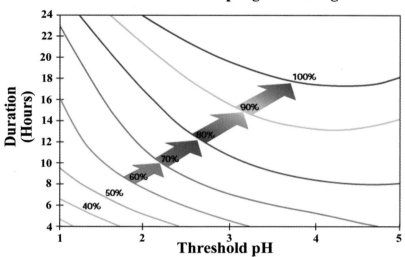

A compilation of metaanalysis data provides evidence that as the threshold pH of the gastric effluent increases toward a putative or idealized goal of pH 4.0, the percentage healing rates of esophagitis similarly heals. Thus, increasing the duration of the elevation of pH values increases the percentage probability of esophagitis healing. Although such information in general is borne out by clinical observation, it assumes that acid is the only or dominant pathogen in engendering esophagitis or maintaining the disease state.

day on once-a-day dosing, because previously resting pumps have to be recruited to respond to the drug. Improvement in effect of PPIs is achieved by divided doses, not by increasing the single dose. On twice-a-day treatment, inhibition of maximal acid output rises to 80%, and steady state is achieved on day 2. Even then, in many individuals, there are still rapid transient periods of relatively high acidity with the possibility of episodic pain.

Metaanalysis of the degree of acid inhibition required for optimization of healing rates for erosive esophagitis has shown that elevation of mean diurnal intragastric pH to at least 4.0 is required for approximately 18 hours per day. This result may reflect the calculated ability of the epithelium and its cells to handle acid reflux. This seems to be achieved in most patients on once-a-day PPI therapy. If eradication of *H. pylori* blunts the effect of PPIs on intragastric acidity, as has been recently suggested, twice-a-day PPI therapy may be required to reach optimal healing pH. Twice-a-day therapy for H_2 receptor antagonists only achieves the required pH for half the time, due mainly to poor daytime pH elevation but good nighttime pH increase. These drugs are therefore more effective for nighttime pain relief but have rather weaker effects on ambulatory reflux, as they are administered at night.

Thus, inhibition to pH greater than 4.0 is sufficient to optimize healing but may be often inadequate for complete symptom control, because intragastric acidity may increase to pH less than 2.0, especially toward the end of digestion of a meal. Short periods of high acidity that may not result in epithelial damage may be sufficient to stimulate esophageal nerves, and the metaanalysis only addresses mean diurnal pH, not periods of high acidity. Rapid symptom control may require more frequent dosing for the first 3 days, until steady-state inhibition is reached, or reformulation of the PPIs. It also may be that there are anatomic variations between patients in terms of access of acid to the nerves, resulting in a more sensitive esophagus. One is left with the paradox that the severe disease is more easily dealt with than the milder symptoms.

The gastric epithelium

The presence of high concentrations of acid in the normal gastric lumen without damage to the epithelium has always puzzled investigators, given that most cells in the body have an exquisite sensitivity to acidic excursions of pH. This has led to the idea that the gastric mucosa has developed specialized mechanisms to protect itself against acid under the collective sobriquet the *gastric barrier*, explicitly enunciated by a gastric physiologist, Horace Davenport, as outlined above.

The function of acid itself is not entirely clear. Evidently, acid secretion is not essential for survival, because patients with total gastrectomy or pernicious anemia do not suffer from consequences of the lack of gastric digestion. It is often thought of as providing a barrier to bacterial infection, but several pathogens have developed mechanisms to resist gastric acid and transit the stomach to their site of infection. Some organisms, such as the gastric *Helicobacter* species, have even adapted so well to gastric acidity that they are able to colonize the gastric mucosa of animals and humans, implying not only survival but growth in gastric acid. Peculiarly, the gastric *Helicobacter* do not survive in the rest of the gut.

Mucous secretion is a prominent feature of gastric-surface epithelial cells. Gastric mucus, as part of the gastric barrier, is considered to restrict back diffusion of acid or to expand the unstirred layer on the gastric surface, enabling maintenance of locally high concentrations of HCO_3^- emanating from the mucosa. Mucus is an aqueous gel and is therefore physically unlikely to provide a significant barrier to acid back diffusion.

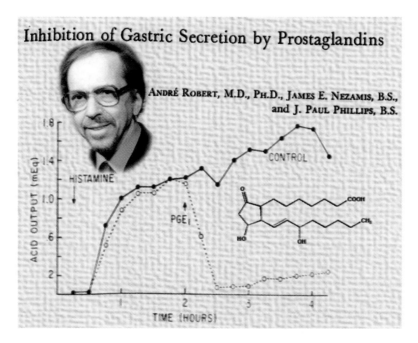

André Robert and colleagues from the Metabolic Diseases Research of the Upjohn Company in Kalamazoo (MI) demonstrated the ability of prostaglandins to inhibit gastric secretion (top). In this series of studies in mongrel dogs with Heidenhain pouches, the authors were able to show that intravenous injection of PGE₁ completely inhibited histamine-mediated acid output (bottom) as well as gastric volume.

Experiments on *in vitro* mucosae have shown that K^+ addition to the mucosal side results in rapid changes in transepithelial potential, indicating that mucus is not a significant barrier to this cation and also suggesting that it would not be a significant barrier to H^+.

HCO_3^- secretion was first shown to occur in *in vitro* preparations of amphibian stomachs (both fundus and antrum). The secretion was found to consist of two components: an active secretion and a passive diffusive component. HCO_3^- secretion was then shown to be an important property of the human stomach. The idea that cells themselves manufacture agents that aid in recovery from or prevention of acid injury came from the area of prostaglandin research. André Robert showed that administration of low doses of a prostaglandin, 16,16-dimethyl prostaglandin E_2, prevented gross damage to rat stomachs after treatment with high levels of alkali, acid, alcohol, or heat. This cytoprotective mechanism replaced acid inhibition as the target of prostaglandins as antiulcer medications.

There are several components of this barrier currently under consideration as contributing to the pathogenesis of acid related disease: the mucous layer, HCO_3^- secretion, and cellular factors providing "cytoprotection," such as prostaglandin biosynthesis or generation of a phospholipid layer similar to lung surfactant. Defects in one or more of these is thought to predispose to ulcer disease in which the defensive factors are overcome by normal aggressive elements. Adequate perfusion of the gastric epithelium by the local blood supply is also a factor often ignored in consideration of pathogenesis of mucosal damage.

The luminal membrane of the epithelial cells and the tight junctions connecting the epithelial cells are a major deterrent to acid back diffusion, and agents that damage either must also render the stomach subject to damage.

Both acid and pepsin contribute to aggressive factors enabling peptic ulcer disease or reflux erosions. The recent implication of *H. pylori* in generation of duodenal and gastric ulcer disease has added an additional element for consideration as an aggressive factor that can result in loss of epithelial integrity.

After damage, several options are open for initiation and completion of the repair process. Restitution, wherein the surface cells migrate to cover the lesion and release mucus to form a mucoid cap, is among the earlier events, and epithelial cell renewal, stimulated by local release of TGF-α, is a later step in the repair process.

The model below summarizes the concepts of the gastric barrier at the level of the surface epithelial cell.

Gastric Barrier

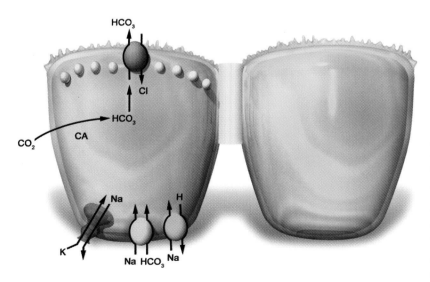

Components of the gastric barrier. Illustrated is a mucous coat, which acts as an unstirred layer, inhibiting fast diffusion of secreted HCO_3^- via an apical anion exchanger. The basal-lateral surface has pH regulatory mechanisms, such as sodium proton exchange or sodium-dependent entry of bicarbonate. The necessary Na^+ gradient is driven by the sodium pump, and bicarbonate is formed by the action of carbonic anhydrase (CA).

Mucous secretion

The gastric mucosa is divided into acid-secreting and non–acid-secreting portions. The fundic area contains the acid-secreting parietal cells in deep invaginations, the fundic glands, which also contain chief or peptic cells. The latter secrete pepsinogen I. The antral region is devoid of parietal cells but still contains peptic cells as well as G and D cells that make luminal contact. The chief cells of the antrum contain pepsinogen II. This region, in contrast to the acid-secretory fundus, is largely absorptive. The transition between fundus and antrum—the transitional zone—contains some parietal cells and a mixed population of chief cells secreting both types of pepsinogen.

Surface cells of the gastrointestinal epithelium secrete mucus by a process of regulated exocytosis. Mucus secretion by the columnar surface cells of the gastric epithelium is especially abundant. The mucus is composed of a complex set of sulfated polysaccharides with several O- or N-linked oligosaccharide cores that create an aqueous gel at the surface of the epithelial cells. In the last several years, cloning of the genes encoding the peptide domain has shown the presence of several genes, each with a signal sequence enabling secretion into the secretory organelle. There is both unregulated basal secretion and regulated secretion by muscarinic and β-adrenergic agonists, prostaglandins, and perhaps secretin. Both cAMP and Ca^{2+} signaling pathways are used. As an aqueous gel, although gastric mucus cannot retard back diffusion of hydrogen ions, it can provide an extended unstirred layer with some retardation of HCO_3^- diffusion. Most likely, its major function is for lubrication of freshly ingested food.

Secretion of HCO_3^-

Secretion of HCO_3^- is mainly the product of gastric surface epithelial cells and is stimulated by acetylcholine released by vagal stimulation showing that there is central regulation. Much is energy dependent *in vitro*, suggesting active secretion. Probably, entry of bicarbonate is via Na^+/HCO_3^- cotransport and efflux by Cl^-/HCO_3^- exchange. Gastric acid is also a powerful stimulant of HCO_3^- secretion when the pH is less than 2.0. It seems that HCO_3^- secretion is enhanced with stimulation of acid secretion, improving the neutralizing capacity of the gastric surface cells. It may be noted that the HCO_3^- content of the interstitial fluid of the secreting fundic mucosa rises sharply due to HCO_3^- production by the activated parietal cells, providing more intracellular HCO_3^- for secretion across the cell membrane. This anion can also diffuse between the cells via a paracellular pathway, although this pathway is considered to be a minor contributor to bicarbonate secretion in the stomach.

The secretion of HCO_3^- by gastric mucosa is at most 10% of acid output. Assuming that the stomach is secreting 100 mM HCl, 10 mM HCO_3^- can be secreted. Hence, this base is not able to neutralize a gastric solution at a pH of 1.0. However, if the stomach is only secreting 10 mM HCl, this can be neutralized by 10 mM HCO_3^-. Secretion of the base could, in principle, then neutralize an unbuffered solution at a pH of 2.0. However, below a pH of 2.0, the neutralizing capacity of the epithelium is exceeded, and gastric surface pH must become acidic, since there is no real barrier to proton back diffusion.

Gunnar Flemström (above) and George Sachs published an article examining gastric ion transport in the *Necturus* (top) using the Ussing approach (center) for whole mucosal mounts. At the bottom is a representation of the equivalent circuit for the *Necturus* antrum consisting of K^+, Cl^-, HCO_3^-, and Na^+ conductance in the nutrient membrane and Na^+ and HCO_3^- conductance in the secretory membrane.

Cytoprotection

The production of arachidonic acid in the gastric epithelial cells can result in production of prostaglandins via cyclooxygenase and leukotrienes via lipoxygenase. Prostaglandins of the E_2 subtype have been shown to reduce gastric mucosal blood flow and, hence, reduce hemorrhage due to tissue injury. They inhibit acid secretion by binding to an EP_3 receptor in the parietal cell that is linked to G_i, inhibiting cAMP production. Clearly, agents that inhibit the constitutive cyclooxygenase (cox) I are capable of inducing severe gastric damage. Newer agents that inhibit the inducible cox II are less likely to induce gastric damage. It also appears that low doses of misoprostil are able to reduce NSAID-induced damage. Depletion of endogenous prostaglandins does appear to have a deleterious effect on gastric mucosal integrity, although the mechanism of this remains entirely obscure.

Gastric mucosal perfusion

There is a marked change in the blood flow on the stimulation of gastric acid secretion, such that blood is now supplied in large quantities to the gastric epithelium by relaxation of the mucosal arterioles. Histamine, prostaglandins, and NO are some of the factors increasing epithelial perfusion. Limitation of blood flow, such as in hemorrhagic shock, predisposes to gastric ulceration.

Apical cell membrane

For many years after the development of techniques investigating lipid membranes, it was thought that natural bilayers had a high proton permeability. This was based on observations in these artificial membranes, however, that were due to artifacts such as contamination with weak acids and weak bases. More recent findings when these contaminants were removed showed that the permeability of phospholipid bilayers to protons was approximately the same as that to Na^+ or K^+. Further, the lipid composition of the membrane containing the H,K ATPase is similar to that of other membranes, and this enzyme can generate a pH of 0.8 without measurable back leak into the cytoplasm of the parietal cell. For protons to move across membranes, transport proteins must be present that are capable of transporting protons. Hence, because the apical membranes of the gastric epithelial cells do not contain proteins capable of proton transport, they are, per se, acid resistant. In contrast, the basolateral membranes not only contain specific proton pathways, such as Na^+/H^+ or anion exchange, but may also contain proteins that allow passive inward leak of protons. Specific experiments demonstrated that monolayers of isolated peptic cells resist a pH of 2.0 on their apical surface.

Cellular disposal of acid

The gastric surface cell is able to deal with limited amounts of intracellular acidity due to acid extrusion by the Na^+/H^+ exchanger and HCO_3^- entry via Na^+/HCO_3^- cotransport. Given the low permeability of the apical membranes and paracellular pathway, these disposal mechanisms suffice under normal conditions.

Tight junctions

In contrast to the "leaky" tight junctions of intestinal epithelia, the gastric junctions show multiple strands of embedded protein, without visible defect in freeze fracture. These are, therefore, "tight" tight junctions generally resistant to acid back diffusion. The junctions in the fundus are tighter than those in the antrum, where there may be less acid exposure.

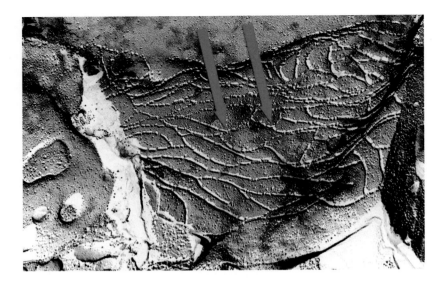

A freeze fracture EM of a "tight" junction between parietal cells of gastric mucosa, showing a belt of approximately 15 strands of protein. Arrows indicate the tight junction strands.

Surfactant

There have been reports that the gastric surface is coated with a phospholipid, which is in principle similar to the surfactant found in the lung. If present as a continuum—and this is difficult to demonstrate—such a phospholipid could prevent access of protons to the gastric surface. In the fundus, under acid secretion, it is unlikely that such a continuous bilayer would persist, but it may do so in the antrum.

Surface pH measurements

Several laboratories have shown the presence of a pH gradient when the surface pH is probed with microelectrodes such that there is measurement of a relatively neutral pH when the luminal pH is 3.0 or greater. These observations have generally been interpreted as showing the barrier function of mucus in combination with HCO_3^- secretion. All of these workers also seem to agree that this pH gradient disappears when the pH in the luminal solution is 2.0. Further, it is claimed that acid secretion from fundic pits (the confluence of five gastric glands in mammals) streams through channels in the mucus and does not diffuse laterally.

These data may be correct, but possible artefacts exist. The pH electrodes used in these studies are usually open-tip microelectrodes with a small volume of aqueous solution at the tip. This is followed by an oil layer containing an electrogenic protonophore and then a KCl solution to make electrical contact with the wire leading to the voltmeter. When a pH gradient exists across the oil, the protonophore moves protons across the oil layer, thereby generating a potential that measures pH. If inward diffusion into the pipette tip is restricted, such as by compressed mucus, the pH in the aqueous solution in the tip would rise, because the protonophore would remove the excess protons. This electrode then would report a higher pH than really existed outside its tip.

One way of eliminating this possible artifact is to calibrate the electrode on the gastric mucosa in strong buffer (e.g., 100 to 200 mM citrate). There is no way that the gastric HCO_3^- secretion could neutralize this level of buffering; therefore,

Acid Resistance of Gastric Mucosa

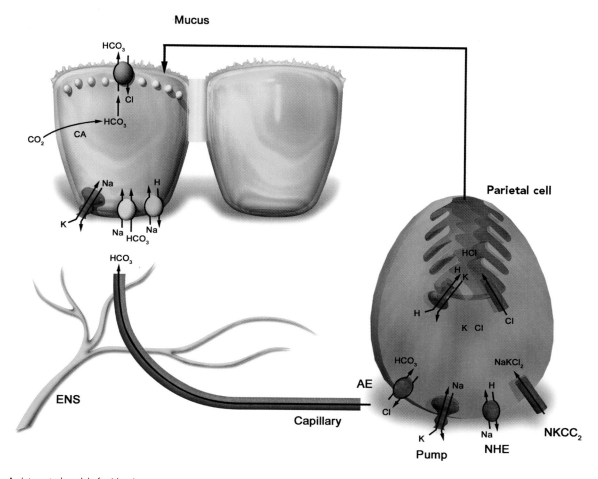

An integrated model of acid resistance of the gastric epithelium, where the surface cell provides neutralization and generally a proton impermeable barrier. The parietal cell extrudes bicarbonate into the serosal side to supply this anion to the surface cell, and acid also appears to stimulate surface cell bicarbonate secretion.

no pH gradient should be measured. However, the pH gradients were the same as those found without buffer. This is suggestive of a tip artefact. Indeed, recent measurements using confocal microscopy argue against the presence of a pH gradient on the surface of an exteriorized mouse stomach at pH 2.0.

H. pylori is an acid-tolerant neutralophile, with most of its urease being internal. This internal urease is acid activated and easily detected *in vivo*, especially after acid stimulation. The bacteria dwell on the mucosal surface and, if this were neutral, only low urease activity would be detected. Further urease activity is toxic to these bacteria at neutral pH, because the enzyme elevates pH to more than 8.0. If the organism is a pH biosensor, it is then reporting on the presence of an acidic pH in its environment on the gastric surface.

Quite recently, it has been claimed that gastric surface pH is neutral even with a luminal pH of 1.0, and in direct opposition, measurements using fluorescent dyes and confocal microscopy have shown the absence of a surface-to-lumen pH gradient at pH 2.0. Indeed, *H. pylori* is not found in the gastric fundic epithelium in an infected rat model, showing that this region is too acidic even for its survival (pH less than 2.5). As discussed in the chapter on *H. pylori*, the urease system is essential for gastric colonization, showing that the bacterial habitat must be acidic.

Agents such as NSAIDs and *H. pylori* decrease the effectiveness of this barrier, leading to the appearance of gastric ulcers. Whether these agents affect the integrity of the cell membrane or of the tight junctions is not known, although at least one of these is a likely target for initiation of epithelial damage. The figure illustrates some of the integrated protective functions of the gastric epithelium.

Duodenal barrier

The duodenum is composed of a monolayer of cells, divided into villus cells with brush borders and deeper crypt cells. The brush border membranes contain a large variety of proteins and are significantly proton permeable. The duodenal tight junctions are significantly leakier than are those of the gastric mucosa. The exact resistance of the mammalian duodenal tight junction is not known but is probably comparable to that of the jejunum, because tissue electrical resistance is low. In the *Necturus* amphibian, the paracellular pathway is approximately tenfold greater than that of the stomach. In some contrast to the stomach, the duodenum, especially the proximal region, is capable of strong HCO_3^- secretion and is also bathed by the alkaline secretion of the pancreas.

The early duodenum is exposed to gastric acid and, therefore, must have properties enabling survival in the face of this high luminal acidity. Much of this is attributed to HCO_3^- secretion by this tissue.

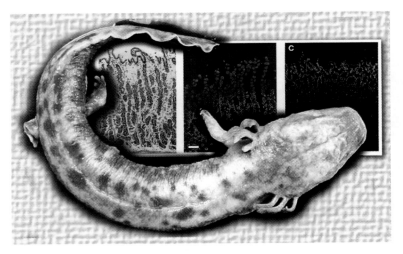

The mud-puppy (*Necturus maculosus*) (bottom) was extensively used for the examination of gastric physiology and particularly bicarbonate secretion. In the background is gastric mucosa that has been stained for chloride transporters (green immunofluorescence).

Both cellular and paracellular pathways contribute to duodenal bicarbonate secretion. The paracellular pathway contributes approximately 40% of net HCO_3^- secretion in this tissue—a much larger fraction than in the gastric mucosa. This is due to the low resistance of the paracellular pathway in this tissue. Cellular secretion is stimulated by various agents, but there is abundant species variation. In humans, CCK, prostaglandins, and VIP stimulate secretion. Intracellular stimulants, such as dibutyryl cAMP (dbcAMP) and forskolin, stimulate secretion in animal models.

Both exchange and conductive pathways seem to be present. The villus cells appear to be major contributors. Carbonic anhydrase inhibitors decrease secretion, as do NSAIDs. Luminal acidity also stimulates HCO_3^- secretion; the threshold, however, is approximately pH of 3.0 in the duodenum as compared to pH of 2.0 in the stomach. It is thought that this response to acid is mediated

Pathways of acid resistance in the duodenum, showing apical bicarbonate secretion by anion exchange and bicarbonate conductance, paracellular bicarbonate secretion and generation of intracellular bicarbonate by carbonic anhydrase, and entry of the anion by sodium cotransport.

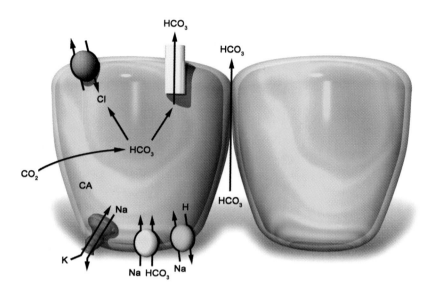

Acid Resistance of the Duodenum

by prostaglandins, and that there are surface pH receptors. Atropine blocks only 30% of duodenal secretion in dogs and is without action in humans. Vagal stimulation of acid secretion in animals seems to be mediated by nicotinic rather than muscarinic receptors in the duodenum, in contrast to the stomach. The figure above illustrates the pathways of alkali secretion by the duodenal villus cell.

It has been repeatedly demonstrated that HCO_3^- secretion is impaired in duodenal ulcer patients. It seems that infection with *H. pylori* must play a role in this inhibition, but whether this is a direct effect of local infection or remote, as a function of the organism's pathogenic effects on the gastric mucosa, is not clear.

CHAPTER 2
INTRAGASTRIC PH

Profound acid suppression has raised several concerns about the possible consequences of long-term acid inhibition. These have included the loss of bactericidal activity of gastric acid with an increase in bacterial overgrowth, with the predisposition either to enteric infection or to the increased production of potentially carcinogenic N-nitrosamines and nitrosamides by colonization of the stomach by nitrate-reducing bacteria. Elevation of plasma gastrin has been associated with ECL cell hyperplasia and the possibility of the development of gastric carcinoids. Long-term pharmacologic suppression of acid secretion has been equated to conditions such as pernicious anemia or to situations analogous to those found after subtotal gastrectomy, for which, after 15 to 20 years, an increased risk of gastric cancer has been proposed. To evaluate both the benefits of acid suppression and some of the issues related to the subsequent prolonged elevation in pH and gastrin levels, the measurement of actual gastric acid secretion in addition to gastric luminal pH needs to be considered.

Hypochlorhydria and achlorhydria

A confusing terminology has grown up around the inability to adequately quantify low levels of gastric acid secretion.

In 1886, Chan and Von Mehring associated pernicious anemia with anacidity. In 1889, Einhorn first used the term *achylia gastrica* to describe the absence of both enzymes and acid in the stomach. *Achlorhydria* was used to denote the absence of free acid as determined by Topfer's reagent. Despite these different terminologies, there was no good agreement as to what they meant; nor did they identify whether the conditions that caused them were reversible or irreversible. In addition, achlorhydria suggested that no acid at all was being secreted, whereas in fact, the presence of some parietal cells secreting acid might be obscured by bicarbonate secretion, and, thus, absence of gastric secretion could not be detected by pH measurement alone. In 1952, Card and Sircus proposed that pH of 6.0 be used to define anacidity. A reasonable definition, therefore, of achlorhydria is the persistent failure of intragastric pH to fall below 6.0 in the presence of any stimulation of gastric acid secretion.

The terms *hypochlorhydria* and *hypoacidity* have not achieved wide acceptance, because the pH electrode does not distinguish between HCl and other inorganic or organic acids, and acid secretion varies widely, depending both on the time of measurement and the methodology used.

An arbitrary maximal acid output (MAO) of less than 5 mmol per hour has been used to define this term. Even in such situations, however, the gastric

18 P   PROCEEDINGS OF THE PHYSIOLOGICAL
            SOCIETY, 23–24 SEPTEMBER 1955

Observations on achlorhydria. By W. I. CARD, I. N. MARKS and
    W. SIRCUS. Gastro-intestinal Unit, Western General Hospital, Edinburgh

W. I. Card (inset), I. N. Marks, and W. Sircus defined the different levels of acid secretion and their chemical relevance.

juice pH may fall below 2.0 and, thus, provide information difficult to interpret using 24-hour pH-measurement techniques.

Quantification of gastric acid secretion

Two approaches have been used to measure gastric acid secretion, one quantitative and the other qualitative. The quantitative measurements have included basal and stimulated acid secretion, nocturnal acid secretion, food-stimulated acid secretion using intragastric titration, and 24-hour acid secretion. The qualitative measurements use 24-hour intragastric acidity. For the most part, quantitative measurements are rarely used today except under experimental circumstances to define physiologic pathways or to evaluate the effect of therapeutic agents on gastric acid secretion. Stimulants include histamine, pentagastrin, insulin, 2-deoxyglucose, or sham feeding. Currently, the use of quantitative acid-secretory measurement is rarely applied except in the diagnosis of the Zollinger-Ellison syndrome and even here has mostly been supplanted by plasma gastrin measurements and the secretin-provocation test.

pHmetric measurement of acid secretion is now the most frequently applied method. This obtains a profile of intragastric acidity and evaluates the state of acid secretion as well as the influence of pharmacologic agents on ulcer healing and symptomatology. Twenty-four-hour intragastric acidity may be evaluated either by repeated rapid sampling of small volumes of gastric juice by aspiration or, alternatively, by continuous recording of intragastric acidity using intragastric pH electrodes. Although the primary agent of interest is acid secretion, the values obtained may also be influenced by bicarbonate secretion, ingested food and fluids, reflux alkaline duodenal juice, and the rate of gastric emptying. Nevertheless, in an individual patient, measurement under such circumstances closely defines the events occurring in that particular stomach.

The measurements obtained have some drawbacks in both qualitative and quantitative groups. Thus, in the aspiration group, pH is measured at fixed time points and fails to define events that might occur in the intervening time. Continuous recording with a pH electrode provides a better overall picture, but the site of the electrode is of critical relevance in determining the pH measurements. Furthermore, because the pH profile varies in different parts of the stomach, not only are sites important, but the maintenance of location throughout the measured period is also important. An advantage of the pH-electrode methodology is its ability to establish the pH in the duodenal bulb, thus quantifying the effects of hypersecretion and the acid load to which the duodenum or a duodenal ulcer is exposed. A critical difficulty in this type of evaluation, however, is stabilizing the pH electrode in the correct position and maintaining it in position for the duration of the study. It has been established, however, that luminal acidity in the duodenal bulb is no higher in ulcer patients than in controls by day or night, and neither fasting nor food produces any difference between these two groups.

In quantitative evaluation of acid secretion, total acid output is the product of the [H^+] (millimoles per liter) and the volume of gastric juice secreted (milliliters

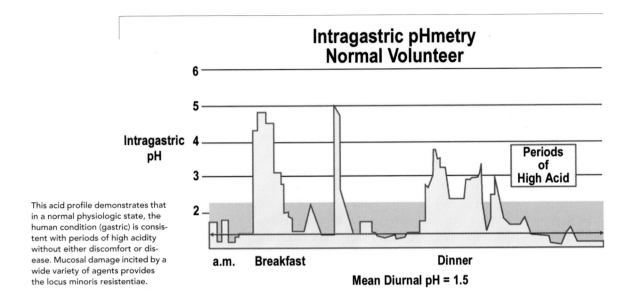

**Intragastric pHmetry
Normal Volunteer**

Intragastric pH

Periods of High Acid

This acid profile demonstrates that in a normal physiologic state, the human condition (gastric) is consistent with periods of high acidity without either discomfort or disease. Mucosal damage incited by a wide variety of agents provides the locus minoris resistentiae.

a.m.   Breakfast   Dinner

Mean Diurnal pH = 1.5

per hour). To evaluate acid secretion, the measurements that have been most commonly used include basal acid output (BAO), peak acid output (PAO), and MAO. BAO represents acid secretion in the absence of stimulation, whereas PAO and MAO are measured in response to stimulation, using pentagastrin at a maximal dose and expressed as millimoles per hour. Alterations in gastric acid secretion may be due either to changes in secretory volume or to changes in the acid concentration of the gastric juice secreted, or to both. There is usually a relationship between the volume of secretion and acid concentration, with concentration increasing in parallel with increased volume.

There is some discussion as to what might be the best methodology for expressing the information provided by pH monitoring. pH is a logarithmic expression of [H$^+$] activity, and therefore, the mean pH is not numerically the same as the mean [H$^+$] converted to pH units. Thus, averages of pH recordings reflect a geometric mean, whereas average concentration-derived data provide only an arithmetic mean. Because the two means do not provide the same value, they are capable of producing different assessments of acid suppression, particularly in the evaluation of acid-suppressive agents.

Thus, reporting that gastric pH may be above or below a particular pH value somewhat marginalizes the information, because an increase in pH of one unit reflects a suppression of acidity of 90%. Similarly, it is difficult to evaluate whether an alteration of pH from 2.0 to 1.0, as opposed to from 4.0 to 3.0, is reasonable, because both are equivalent to 90% acid suppression. Similar problems apply to the expression of the information when using the area under the concentration/time or pH/time curve, and it seems likely that the best compromise may be the use of median pH or hydrogen ion concentration [H$^+$]. Nevertheless, because it is not possible to use all data points, analyses are usually conducted using summary values and particular time points compared to specific activities such as meals, sleeping, and drug ingestion. It should also be remembered that volume of gastric contents is an important parameter in esophageal exposure to acidity if reflux occurs, and that therapy should be designed to maximally reduce volume and acidity.

Factors affecting gastric acid secretion

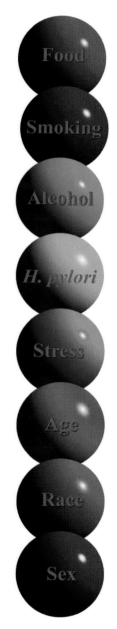

The factors that affect acid secretion range from sex and ethnicity to stress and bacterial infection.

The physiologic regulation of acid secretion is complicated, as has been delineated in Section 2 of this book. A number of other factors, including *H. pylori*, age, smoking, NSAIDs, and mental status, influence both secretory events and the health of the gastric mucosa. In general, acid secretion has been noted to fall with advancing age. To a large extent, this reflects the increasing gastritis in older individuals and is reflected by a decrease in both basal- and histamine-stimulated acid secretion. In individuals who do not exhibit the atrophic gastritis often seen in older persons, basal-, food-stimulated-, and gastrin-17–stimulated-acid secretion may be normal or even higher than in younger subjects, especially women. Overall, it appears that although age is a critical determinant in the decrease of acid secretion, to a large extent this represents the state of the gastric mucosa and the presence or absence of gastritis.

The role of *H. pylori* is a complex one, with gastric acidity appearing to influence its ability to survive as well as its presence influencing gastric acidity itself. A detailed evaluation of this issue appears in Section 7. In brief, however, *H. pylori* is highly susceptible to the pH of its environment and seeks to alkalize its microenvironment as it colonizes the gastric epithelium. Low intragastric acidity is an unwelcome scenario for *H. pylori*, as noted in the low prevalence of infection evident in patients with pernicious anemia. *H. pylori*, by its effect on gastrin and somatostatin cells, similarly alters the gastric acid secretory profile.

The subject of smoking as it relates to peptic ulcer disease has been one of considerable public and medical interest. Overall, smoking increases basal and maximal acid output and pepsin secretion as well as decreasing bicarbonate output, with the result that an increased acid load and a decreased buffering capacity in the duodenum are evident. Such effects are most obvious during the daytime, when cigarette consumption is highest. Overall, they serve to prolong the period during which the duodenal bulb pH falls below 3.5 in both normal subjects and acid hypersecretors. Because duodenal ulcer is more common in individuals who smoke than in nonsmokers, and because relapse is more frequent in smokers, it has been accepted that smoking in an as-yet ill-defined fashion renders the duodenal bulb more prone to ulceration.

Although it is clearly evident that NSAIDs are related to mucosal ulceration, their direct effect on the alteration of gastric acid secretion or pH has not been firmly established. Nevertheless, although there exists clinical evidence to support the fact that acid is of relatively little importance in the development of NSAID-associated gastric ulcers, both duodenal and gastric ulceration in patients receiving NSAIDs heals with antisecretory therapy. It is evident, however, that such healing is augmented if the NSAID is discontinued, suggesting that a direct mucosal effect of the drug is of relevance.

Traditional concepts of mental status influencing acid secretion and peptic ulceration have indicated that stress may result in punitive effects on the gastroduodenal mucosa. The precise effects of stress on acid secretion have been variable, however, and hypnosis has been demonstrated to either increase or decrease gastric secretion, depending on the particular mood induced. Given the critical relevance of the brain and regulation of gut function, it is likely that the CNS effects on acid secretion are of significance; however, they remain to be defined.

Low-acid states

The long-term maintenance of a low-acid state has raised five general concerns: (a) the loss of the primary bactericidal barrier against the ingestion of enteric pathogens, (b) the alteration of the absorption of important nutrients, (c) the alteration of the gastric mucosal morphology, (d) risks of adverse drug effects, and (e) the development of hypergastrinemia and the induction of mucosal hyperplastic changes. These initial theoretic concerns have faded with the widespread long-term use of PPIs (more than 300 million treatments) without evidence of any significant sequelae to treatment.

Definition of a low-acid state

Achlorhydria can be defined as a luminal pH greater than 6.0 that cannot be decreased by stimulation with histamine or pentagastrin. Achlorhydria may be present in pernicious anemia and can be achieved transiently with intravenous PPIs. The existence of a low-acid state might be more operationally defined as a luminal pH above 3.0 or 4.0, because such levels have been demonstrated to be necessary for optimal benefit for patients with duodenal ulcer disease or GERD. Perhaps such a pH could be defined as *hypochlorhydria*. It should be remembered that even at this luminal pH, significant acidity exists at the secretory surface of the mucosa. The output is low, allowing neutralization.

The duration of an achlorhydric or hypochlorhydric state may be life-long in atrophic gastritis, pernicious anemia, and after postsurgical procedures such as vagotomy, with or without antrectomy. In addition, acid suppression may be induced acutely in the management of patients in intensive care units at risk for stress bleeding. Alternatively, acid suppression may be used for longer periods, from 4 weeks to months or even years, in the management of intractable peptic ulcer disease, gastrinoma (Zollinger-Ellison syndrome), or GERD.

Areas of potential concern

Enteric pathogens

The acid milieu of the stomach provides a barrier against the promulgation of ingested pathogens into the lower gastrointestinal tract. In the presence of decreased acid, colonization of the stomach with pathogenic bacteria may occur, and these organisms may even transit the stomach unimpeded by the normal acid barriers. Studies in less-developed countries with poor sanitation do show an increased susceptibility to cholera and shigella in patients with low-acid states. In contrast, no such susceptibility data exist in developed countries where the water supply is more highly regulated. Western travelers using acid-inhibitory therapy probably do not need to be cautioned before making journeys to poor-sanitation areas. The possibility of nosocomial pneumonia developing secondary to gastric bacterial aspiration in ventilator-dependent intensive care unit patients treated with antisecretory therapies has been shown to be virtually nonexistent.

Alteration of nutrient absorption

The presence of gastric acid promotes the absorption of important nutrients by release of minerals, particularly calcium, from their complexed organic forms. However, low-acid states do not appear to predispose to decreased calcium absorption in humans. In contrast, the absorption of ferric iron is decreased in achlorhydric states and in gastrectomized patients. This deficit is related directly to the low solubility of ferric iron at a pH greater than 5.0. Nevertheless, the absorption of heme iron is not compromised, and no evidence exists for a predisposition to iron-deficiency anemia. In the case of vitamin B_{12}, neither PPIs nor H_2 receptor antagonists have been implicated in significant alterations in absorption of this compound.

Progression of chronic atrophic gastritis

This is a dynamic process that progresses with age and is independent for either the antral or oxyntic mucosa. The long-term nature of this process makes it difficult to study the effects of drugs on its development. Nevertheless, concerns have been raised that long-term PPI treatment might be associated with progression of chronic active gastritis. In the few studies published, there does appear to be a small (less than 1.5%) increase in its incidence in these patients. This is not, however, associated with alterations in cell lineage or the development of intestinal metaplasia, apart from the occasional occurrence of type I metaplasia with no evidence of dysplasia.

Inhibition of cytochrome P450, risk of adverse toxic drug interactions, and putative genotoxicity

Metabolism of polycyclic compounds by the hepatic cytochrome P450 systems is a critical step in drug metabolism. Of the various PPIs currently available, pantoprazole appears to have the cleanest profile, with no significant effects with regards to drug interaction. None of the PPIs has been shown to have clinically significant drug interactions, however. In addition, PPIs induce the P450-1A isozyme, which initially raised concerns of compounding tumorigenesis, because this P450 may result in carcinogen formation from other compounds. However, no evidence exists for either the induction of the isozyme *in vivo* or an elevated incidence of tumorigenesis by any of the PPIs. Most data indicate that induction (if it occurs) is protective rather than harmful. No genotoxic effects can be ascribed to PPIs.

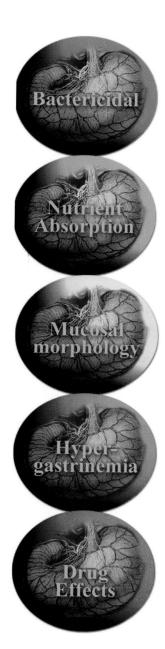

The factors that predispose to low acid (high pH) states in the stomach range from bacterial infection to drug effects.

Hypergastrinemia

The effect of gastrin on the proliferation of the gastric mucosa has been well described. Of particular interest is the more recent appreciation of its ability to stimulate ECL cell proliferation and its putative influence on the development of gastrointestinal neoplasia. Normal fasting levels vary but range between 50 and 100 pg per mL. Short-term treatment courses of antisecretory therapies seldom result in significant elevations of gastrin levels. Nevertheless, in long-term studies, these therapies raise serum gastrin above normal (usually in the range of 200 to 300 pg per mL) but do not achieve the levels noted in pernicious anemia (2,000 pg per mL), which are an order of magnitude higher and sustained throughout the day.

Chronic active gastritis and pernicious anemia

Although differences in both populations and environment certainly modulate the risks of the development of gastric neoplasms, data from a number of studies suggest that patients with pernicious anemia and chronic active gastritis are at a higher risk for specific types of gastric carcinomas. Such patients may require long-term, careful endoscopic follow-up to ensure that these diseases do not manifest. Other reports indicate that in addition to a long-term risk of gastric carcinoma, patients with chronic active gastritis and pernicious anemia may be at risk for developing gastric endocrine cell hyperplasia and carcinoids.

Colonic neoplasia

Apart from the stomach, the trophic effect of gastrin on other gastrointestinal organs is less well accepted. Overall, the experimental data (in cell lines and animal models) are equivocal and are not uniform in supporting a role for gastrin in growth regulation in the colon. Clinical observations also fail to support a direct relationship between gastrin and colonic cancer. No evidence supporting a direct relationship between plasma gastrin levels and the evolution of colonic neoplasia in humans exists.

Gastric adenocarcinoma

Although achlorhydria has been linked to an increased incidence of gastric adenocarcinoma, the mechanism for this is probably not related to hypergastrinemia. A number of studies instead have demonstrated associations between gastric tumors and hypo- or normogastrinemia, which argues against a role for gastrin. It is probable that the development of neoplasia may be related to alterations initiated by the concomitant presence of *H. pylori* and its effects on T- and B-cell function. This issue is dealt with in detail in the section on MALT lymphoma in Section 7. However, the increasing prevalence of chronic active gastritis and colonic polyps in elderly patients may correlate with hypergastrinemia.

ECL cell hyperplasia/carcinoids

It has been established that gastrin is a potent proliferative stimulus for the ECL cell system in rats. Initially, the ECL cell hyperplasia is modest, but over a 2-year period, it may progress and eventually become dysplastic and even

The effects of acid suppression and hypergastrinemia on ECL cell proliferation in rats. This figure shows chromogranin staining of gastric fundic ECL cells in rat mucosa. Left: normal. Center: mild hyperplasia (6 months). Right: severe hyperplasia (12 months).

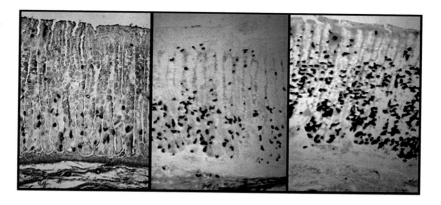

exhibit microcarcinoid formation. The progression to an autonomous carcinoid lesion has not been demonstrated in humans taking PPIs for periods as long as 10 to 15 years, unless the patient has multiple endocrine neoplasia syndrome. The issue of ECL cell proliferation is dealt with in detail in Section 5.

Gastric fundic polyps

Gastric fundic polyps have been described in normal mucosae but may be seen more frequently in association with high-dose PPIs taken for 2 years or longer. They seem more frequent in cases with accompanying hepatic cirrhosis.

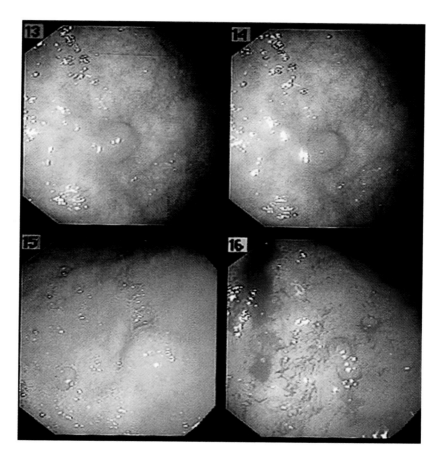

Small, sessile gastric fundic polyps (histologically carcinoid) occurring in a patient with atrophic gastritis.

They are outgrowths or extensions of the gastric epithelium, with all cell types represented, and show no evidence of any cellular transformation. There is some degree of parietal cell hyperplasia. Their etiology is obscure but may come from inhibition of acid secretion without accompanying inhibition of pepsinogen secretion, resulting in a hypertonic gland lumen. This, in combination with gastric hypertension due to liver cirrhosis, may predispose to benign polyp formation. Another possibility is local effects of ECL cell stimulation by gastrin to produce a preponderance of fundic polyps as compared to areas where there are fewer ECL cells. The factor released by ECL cells may be the REG protein.

| **Clinical relevance of gastrin levels and PPI therapy** | Current opinion on hypergastrinemia and its consequences reflects a substantial decrease of concern in this area. Only in cases in which long-term therapy is contemplated should there even be a thought about measuring gastrin levels. In long-term therapy, in which reflux disease is the therapeutic concern, it is safe to assume that occasional symptoms indicate a level of acidity sufficient to inhibit the G cell appropriately. It is only when the patient responds with achlorhydria that consideration may be given to determining the degree of elevation of gastrin. No data, however, have been advanced in clinical studies to indicate that even a considerable elevation of gastrin is of concern. |

CHAPTER 3
PEPSIN

History of pepsinogen

Pepsinogen is a potent digestive enzyme secreted by the chief cell of the gastric gland into the lumen of the stomach. This agent is likely to play a significant role in the pathogenesis of peptic ulcer disease. Although abnormalities in this protein have been epidemiologically linked to gastric carcinoma and its precursors, no specific pathogenic role exists for this potent enzyme.

The story of this poorly understood enzyme began in the Berlin laboratory of J. Müller, where, in 1836, Theodor Schwann described a water-soluble factor in gastric juice that digested egg white. He called it *pepsin*, after the Greek word for digestion.

Schwann had just obtained his MD degree and was continuing as an assistant in Müller's laboratory. His investigation of gastric glands was initiated by the latter, who had asked him to attempt to subject the physiologic properties of either an organ or a tissue to physical measurement. Schwann initially developed a muscle balance and became the first to establish the basics of the tension-length diagram. Thereafter, while successfully measuring secretion from the gastric gland, he stumbled on a proteolytic enzyme whose properties he characterized and soon thereafter published.

Unfortunately for the science of the stomach, this observation became lost in the subsequent spate of diverse investigative work that emanated from the young man. He moved on to fermentation and was the first to demonstrate the importance of oxygen both for alcoholic fermentation in yeast and for putrefaction. His work with yeast led to probably his greatest discovery, which was the assertion of a common cellular basis for all living matter. However, his failure to win a chair at the University of Bonn appeared to have damaged his impetus for scientific investigation—his last useful digestive observation, which appeared 40 years before his death, was the necessity of bile for digestion (and for survival). He had modified a biliary fistula model for these experiments, which also happened to be the last physiologic experiments he would conduct.

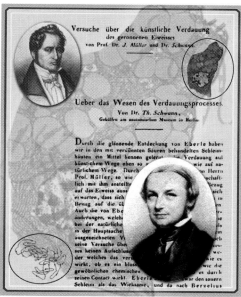

In 1835, Theodor Schwann (bottom right), while working in the laboratory of Johannes Müller (top left), stumbled on a proteolytic enzyme whose properties he characterized and soon thereafter, in 1836, published (right). At the time, they were involved in measuring secretion from the gastric glands (top). Both articles were published sequentially in the same journal; Müller's work was given precedence. It is of interest that the second reference in Müller's work on the artificial digestion of proteins is to William Beaumont's experiments and observations on the gastric juice and physiology of digestion (of 1830). In his studies, Schwann was able to extract a crude preparation of a digestive enzyme from gastric juice, which he demonstrated to have the ability to convert egg-white albumin to peptones *in vitro*. He named this water-soluble factor *pepsin*, after the Greek word for digestion. In the course of his studies, both Müller and Schwann noted that no gas evolved during pepsin digestion of food. These findings were thus able to dispel a notion that had been held for 3 centuries: that digestion was a fermentation-like process. The identification of the cell involved in pepsin secretion (top right) would require another half century, whereas the identification of the prolate ellipsoid structure of pepsinogen (the protein precursor of this enzyme), required an additional 100 years. Despite the identification of pepsin and its properties in 1836, neither the role of this factor in gastric pathology (peptic ulceration) nor its extragastric function has been entirely elucidated.

Rudolf Peter Heidenhain (1834–1897) (left) was the eldest of the 22 children of the physician Heinrich Jacob Heidenhain (1808–1868). Born January 29, 1834, in Marienwerder, East Prussia, he died October 13, 1897, in Breslau, Germany, having revolutionized many spheres of physiology. After completion of his secondary education in his native town at the age of 16 years, he began the study of nature on an estate near his home but soon turned to medicine at the University of Königsberg. He subsequently studied at a number of institutions before undertaking in 1867 a systematic investigation of the physiology of glands and of the secretory and absorption process, which remained his chief field of interest for the rest of his life. Heidenhain noted in the stomach two types of cells in the gastric glands and demonstrated that one produced pepsin and the other hydrochloric acid. By the late nineteenth century, investigators were able to differentiate between these chief cells (*Hauptzellen*, top) and granules from *Belegzellen* (parietal cells), which possessed canaliculi (bottom).

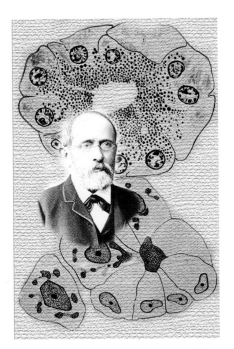

Three years after the initial identification of pepsin by Schwann, Wasmann was able to isolate the protein and thereby establish the premise for protein digestion. In 1846, Claude Bernard wrote extensively on the digestive ferments of the pancreas, whereas the possibility of a proenzyme, pepsinogen, was formally postulated by Epstein and Grutzner in 1854. The first evaluation of the protein products of gastric digestion was described by Meisner in 1859. Heidenhain, while studying the pancreas, was soon thereafter able to describe the secretory mechanisms of proteolytic zymogens. Eight years into his tenure as Professor of Physiology at Breslau, Heidenhain began a systematic study of glands that would occupy him for almost the next 30 years. During this time, his experimental work suggested to him that all secretory phenomena were intracellular rather than mechanical processes. From these, he was able to draw some important conclusions about gastric physiology. First, he concluded that the secretion of saliva was an indicator of blood flow, and second, that there were two kinds of cells in gastric glands: those that secrete hydrochloric acid, which he named *Belegzellen*, and those that secrete pepsin, *Hauptzellen*. His histologic notes also describe a yellow-stained small cell situated adjacent to these cells that 100 years later would be identified as the endocrine ECL cell. His use of a surgical pouch for investigating acid physiology later became the standard model for such investigations.

Heidenhain's observations were followed by those of Kühne, who theorized that because the stomach itself was not digested by pepsin, the gastric ferments must have inactive protein precursors (e.g., pepsinogen). It was Kühne who

The obituary notice of John Newport Langley (1852–1925): "*The main achievements of Langley's research work are familiar to the readers of the* Journal of Physiology *and need little here in the way of description or comment. They stand permanently in their place, not merely as additions here and there to knowledge, but as indispensable stepping stones along which at this point, or that, the progress of knowledge has actually made its way. Each gain he made was a step placed securely and finally, and few indeed of them as the road has become more firmly and widely trodden by others following, have been found wrongly placed. All his chief works keep, and must always keep, their place in the significant history of Animal Physiology. The bare titles of his papers and books deployed there along the years give the plainest testimony to me to his unvarying, unhalting service to science. No single year in all that series, extending well nigh for half a century, from youth to age, appears without its contribution of effective work.*" W. M. Fletcher. J Physiol 1926.

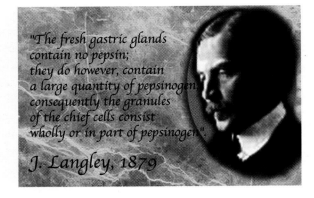

"The fresh gastric glands contain no pepsin; they do however, contain a large quantity of pepsinogen; consequently the granules of the chief cells consist wholly or in part of pepsinogen".

J. Langley, 1879

developed the term *zymogen* for these precursors, as well as the term *enzyme*. He also identified the proteolytic pancreatic enzyme, trypsin, in 1868 and influenced the work of his later English admirers.

However, it remained for Langley at Cambridge in the 1880s to formalize the study of pepsinogen and the mechanisms of its secretion. Langley's introduction to the gastric gland was driven by chance. His mentor, the great physiologist Foster, suggested he study the effects of the drug *jaborandi* (pilocarpine) on the heart. These studies in 1874 led him toward studying its effects on secretion. After an initial prelude in the submaxillary gland, Langley dove into the regulation of secretion in the stomach, which he would pursue for the better part of the next 20 years.

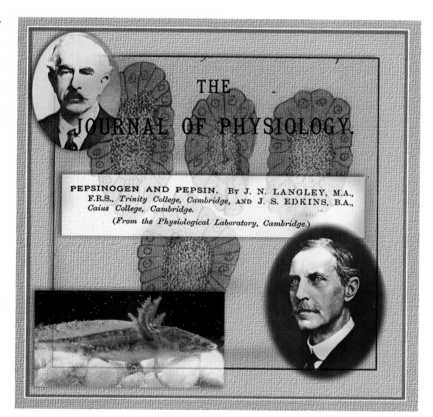

The study of pepsinogen and the mechanisms of its secretion was formalized by John Langley (bottom right) of Cambridge. Langley succeeded Sir Michael Foster (1836–1907) as the editor of the *Journal of Physiology* and trained J. S. Edkins (1863–1940) (top left). His introduction to the gland was by chance, because his initial assignment had been to elucidate the effects of the drug *jaborandi* (pilocarpine) on the heart. In 1874, this work led him toward the investigation of its effects on secretion. After an initial prelude in the submaxillary gland, he began to address the regulation of secretion in the stomach, a field of endeavor that would take him the better part of 20 years. Using the salamander as a model (bottom left), he undertook histologic studies of the gland structure in activity and rest and checked the interpretation of the appearance of killed and stained cells with that of direct observation of living gland cells. He correlated these findings with the effect of nervous influence on the glands and linked these observations to chemical estimations of the changes in the quality of pepsinogen secretion under different circumstances. In the background are esophageal glands of *Rana temporana*. This drawing by Langley (September 1879) shows the end tubes of the esophageal gland of a frog fed with a sponge for 35 hours before it was expelled by vomiting. The animal was killed 10 hours thereafter and the tissue placed in absolute alcohol for 24 hours and then dilute carmine for a further 24 hours. These cells show stained nongranular zones and unstained granular zones. This is consistent with contemporary biologic understanding of apical exocytosis of pepsinogen granules. Indeed, these drawings and sketches, although now more than 100 years old, attest to his clear understanding of the nature of zymogen secretion and the general mechanisms of its stimulation. In addition, Langley was so impressed with Heidenhain's contribution that he was to borrow and translate the former's terms for the cells in the stomach into English as border (*Haupt*) and chief (*Beleg*) cells, respectively, and also coined the term *oxyntic* to identify the role of the acid-secreting cells. In a series of publications between 1879 and 1882, Langley established the basic morphology and secretory characteristics of the pepsin-forming glands of the stomach and esophagus (center) and was, in addition, able to correct Heidenhain by demonstrating that, contrary to previous reports, gland cells became less granular as secretion took place. Langley demonstrated that granules were stored up during rest and discharged during secretion not only in the pancreas, but also in the stomach and salivary glands and that during this event, a chemical change in the zymogen occurred. To quote: "*The fresh gastric glands contain no pepsin; they do however contain a large quantity of pepsinogen; consequently the granules of the chief cells consist wholly or in part of pepsinogen.*" Langley's pupil, Edkins, entered Cambridge University as a scholar of Caius College in 1881. Such was his ability that he was awarded two scholarships, one in mathematics and the other in natural sciences. After Cambridge, he worked with C. S. Sherrington (1857–1952) in Liverpool (who was later to attain a Nobel Prize in Neurophysiology). Edkins taught with great distinction at St. Bartholomew's in London and subsequently became Chairman of Physiology at Bedford College for Women in 1914. In this capacity, he was responsible for training the majority of women physiologists in England between 1914 and 1930. Apart from his fundamental observations in regard to gastrin (he documented the existence of a novel antral stimulant of acid secretion-gastrin in 1905), he investigated the presence of spiral bacteria (*Spirella regaudi*) (*Helicobacter felis*) in the gastric mucosa of cats and their relevance to digestion (1923).

He undertook histologic studies of the gland structure during activity and rest and checked the interpretation of the appearance of killed and stained cells with that of direct observation of living gland cells. He correlated these findings with the effect of nervous influence on the glands and linked these observations to chemical estimations of the changes in the quality of secretion under different circumstances. Indeed, his drawings and sketches, although now more than 100 years old, attest to his clear understanding of the nature of zymogen secretion and some of the mechanisms of its stimulation. In addition, Langley was so impressed with Heidenhain's contribution that he was to borrow and translate his terms for the cells in the stomach into English as *border* and *chief* cells, respectively. Langley also coined the term *oxyntic* to identify the role of the acid-secreting cells. In a series of publications between 1879 and 1882, he established the basic morphology and secretory characteristics of the pepsin-forming glands of the stomach and esophagus. In addition, he was able to correct Heidenhain by showing that contrary to previous reports, gland cells became less granular as secretion took place. He demonstrated that granules were stored up during rest and passed out during secretion in not only the pancreas, but also the stomach and salivary glands. To quote: "*The fresh gastric glands contain no pepsin; they do however contain a large quantity of pepsinogen; consequently the granules of the chief cells consist wholly or in part of pepsinogen.*"

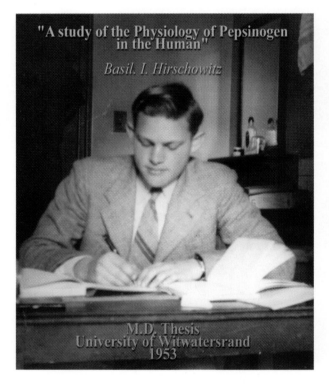

Although Basil Hirschowitz (background—a photograph when he was a freshman) is best known for his seminal contributions to endoscopy, he was also an accomplished gastric physiologist. Prior to his introduction of the fiberoptic endoscope (1957–1961), he had extensively studied pepsinogen. It is noteworthy that when he obtained his medical degree from the University of the Witwaterstrand, he graduated with a thesis on the physiology of human pepsinogen.

Most of Langley's work was conducted in amphibia, and like present-day investigators, he must have struggled with the problem of disappearing peptic granules in the wintertime! Of additional interest is that Langley's pupil, Edkins, would later discover gastrin in 1905. Langley's colorimetric test of digestion of carmine-stained fibrin was so useful that it would only be improved on 50 years later.

The first photographs of pepsinogen granules, from *Salmo salar*, were published in 1898, but it required another 30 years before chemistry had evolved sufficiently to identify that enzymes were, in fact, proteins. Northrop, in 1930, was the first to crystallize pepsin, but further research in this area was initially hindered by the primitive assays for its biologic activities. The description of the colorimetric tyrosine assay for digested hemoglobin in 1932 by Anson and Mirsky allowed for rapid advances thereafter in this field. Indeed, the newly purified pepsin was soon implicated in ulcerogenesis, and Howes, in 1936, reported that although acid alone failed to prevent gastric ulcers in the cat, pepsin and acid together did. Six years later, Schiffrin demonstrated that luminal pepsin was requisite for intestinal ulcer formation in the same animal.

It is of interest that numerous other contributors to this field, after Langley and Schwann, raised many controversial issues, some of which remain unresolved to this day.

Although Brücke, in 1861, first proposed that pepsin was reabsorbed from the gut lumen into the blood and subsequently excreted in the urine, little further understanding of this process has been acquired. Indeed, today there is still controversy as to whether pepsinogen is directly secreted into the blood or whether it represents an ill-understood back-diffusion process. Van Slyke, in 1893, believed that pepsin circulated combined with an inhibitor complex, although alternate ideas ranged from white blood cells to fibrin as carriers. 1912 saw the demonstration of antipepsin: pepsin complexes that were theorized to be set free in the kidney, thus accounting for the existence of urinary pepsinogen. To date, no good explanation for the presence of this proteolytic enzyme in the blood exists, and it has been identified in diverse anatomic sites as far afield as spermatozoa. Its complex role in physiology has been proposed to range from that of a digestive enzyme to a luminal initiator of gut neuroendocrine maturation after weaning. Pepsinogen secretion and pepsin function are still a grey area in the science of gastroenterology. Although their role in pathology has yet to be defined, their relationship to peptic ulcer has received undeservedly scant attention.

Properties of pepsinogen

Pepsinogens are a heterogeneous group of inactive proenzymes, each of which gives rise to a unique pepsin. Pepsinogen consists of the active pepsin plus a variable NH_2-terminal sequence of amino acids acting as a signal peptide. Based on the DNA sequence, pepsinogen is synthesized initially as a pre-pepsinogen containing a 15–amino acid signal sequence at the NH_2-terminus.

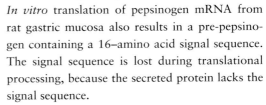

In vitro translation of pepsinogen mRNA from rat gastric mucosa also results in a pre-pepsinogen containing a 16–amino acid signal sequence. The signal sequence is lost during translational processing, because the secreted protein lacks the signal sequence.

Under acidic conditions, pepsinogen is converted to pepsin by autocatalytic (i.e., intramolecular) catalysis, which results in loss of an additional NH_2-terminal sequence. This conversion occurs slowly at pH values of 5 to 6 but very rapidly at pH 2. One of the NH_2-terminal peptides released during the conversion possesses antipepsin activity. This peptide (MW 3,200) and its analogs complex with pepsin at pH values of 5.0 to 6.0 to inhibit catalytic activity. However, at lower pH, the inhibitor dissociates and is digested by pepsin. Thus, it seems unlikely that the inhibitor serves any significant physiologic function, at least in the adult stomach.

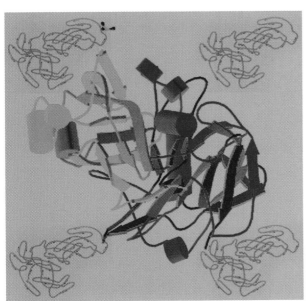

The prolate ellipsoid structure of pepsinogen (the protein precursor of this enzyme).

After the loss of the NH_2-terminal sequence, pepsin undergoes a further conformational change to expose a binding cleft that can accommodate a substrate with approximately eight amino acid residues. The active site contains two

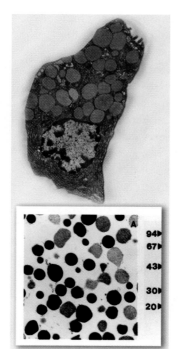

The gastric chief cell involved in pepsin secretion (top) and the precursor pepsinogen granules (bottom). Electron micrograph of isolated pepsinogen granules from rabbit gastric glands. The different size and density of granules represent maturation of pepsinogen.

aspartyl residues, which are found in separate exon coding sequences, suggesting that the pepsinogen gene evolved by duplication of a smaller ancestral gene. Once activated, pepsin may be irreversibly denatured at pH values above 7.2 or temperatures above 65°C. In contrast, pepsinogen is resistant to denaturation by pH values up to 10.0 or temperatures up to boiling. The difference in alkali resistance led Langley to postulate the existence of a proenzyme and provides an operational definition of pepsinogens, as distinct from other acid proteases.

The catalytic activity of pepsin is described in general as *acid-active proteolysis*. The pH optimum for hydrolysis of hemoglobin is 1.5 to 2.5, but the pH optimum is quite broad and depends on the isozyme and specific substrate (e.g., milk clotting exhibits an optimum at pH 5.5). Pepsin acts on a wide variety of peptide bonds, including acidic residues. Part of the broad specificity range may reflect the existence of several isozymes.

Mammalian gastric pepsinogen can be separated electrophoretically into multiple bands. There are at least seven distinct pepsinogens, designated as Pg 1 to 7 in order of decreasing electronegativity. The seven pepsinogens have been divided into two major groups—pepsinogen I and pepsinogen II (PGI and PGII)—based on immunologic reactivity using specific, non-cross-reacting antibodies. PGI contains Pg 1 to 5, and PGII contains Pg 6 and 7. Apart from immunologic reactivity, the two pepsinogen groups display interesting differences. The pH optimum for PGI is 1.5 to 2.0, whereas PGII exhibits an optimum at pH 3.2. PGI is more sensitive to alkali denaturation (pH 7.2 versus 8.0) than is PGII but less sensitive to heat denaturation. The distribution of the two groups also differs. Both groups are found in the body of the stomach, but only PGII is found in the gastric antrum, proximal duodenum, and Brunner's glands. Serum contains both PGI and PGII, but only PGI is found in normal urine (uropepsin), whereas only PGII is found in semen.

In recent years, pepsinogens and pepsins from a number of species have been isolated and characterized. Amino acid sequencing and X-ray crystallographic studies revealed substantial homologies and similar tertiary structures of pepsinogens from different species.

Molecular-weight estimates for pepsinogens from various species, including amphibians, fish, and mammals, range from 29 to 65 kDa. Some of this heterogeneity arises from differences in the NH_2-terminal activation sequence, but significant differences exist in the catalytic peptide as well. Despite such differences, the catalytic site appears to be similar in all species.

Pepsinogen

Pepsinogen possesses no catalytic activity and therefore can be measured only with an immunoassay. Specific radioimmunoassays for PGI and PGII have been developed and used for measurements of pepsinogen in tissues, serum, and urine. This method is very sensitive and highly specific. When a less sensitive assay is adequate, the pepsinogen may be converted to pepsin and the resulting acid protease activity used as a measurement. The classic method of Anson and Mirsky, using hemoglobin substrate at pH 2.0 and read out of the tyrosine released, remains a reliable, inexpensive assay. This assay has been adapted for the autoanalyzer to allow for a large number of samples.

In confirmation of Langley's hypothesis, immunocytochemical studies have identified the gastric chief cell as the major source of pepsinogen in mammals. The chief cells are found primarily in the basal portion of the gastric glands of the body and the fundus of the stomach, but the exact distribution of chief cells varies from species to species. Pepsinogen is found also in the mucous neck cells of fundic glands, and caution is required when attempting to identify chief cells based solely on the presence of pepsinogen. The fundic glands contain both PGI and PGII. The cardiac glands in the gastric cardia and the pyloric glands of the gastric antrum contain pepsinogen, but only PGII has been found in these regions. Because the cardiac and pyloric glands do not contain chief cells, the pepsinogen is thought to be associated with mucous neck cells. PGII, but not PGI, is found in the Brunner's glands of the proximal duodenum and is secreted by the prostate gland into seminal fluid.

Vertebrate species other than mammals do not possess chief cells per se. Instead, a single cell type, the oxyntic cell, is responsible for gastric secretion of both acid and pepsinogen. As with the mammalian chief cell, the oxyntic cells are confined to the fundus or body of the stomach, being absent from the antrum. In certain amphibia (frog and *Necturus*), glands located in the lower esophagus contain peptic-like cells that secrete pepsinogen. The esophageal pepsinogen is unusual in having a low molecular weight, but it has immunologic reactivity and a pH optimum characteristic of the PGI group.

Regulation of secretion

General considerations

Secretion of pepsinogen by the gastric chief cells involves a sequence of events leading to the appearance of this proenzyme in the gastric juice. Studies of both intact animals and *in vitro* preparations have identified a wide variety of agents that stimulate pepsinogen secretion. Some of these agents are naturally occurring and are believed to mimic endogenous regulatory mechanisms. Other stimuli, although found endogenously, have not been identified with a normal regulatory process. Still other stimuli are believed to act purely as pharmacologic agents. To provide some organization, the stimuli and agents related to them are grouped into three categories: neurotransmitters, peptide hormones, and miscellaneous agents.

Both cAMP and intracellular calcium are used as second messengers by this cell. The former mediates adrenergic and histamine-induced secretion, the latter CCK and cholinergic (M_3) stimulation.

Neurotransmitters

The least controversial of the stimuli for pepsinogen secretion are cholinergic agents. ACh and its analogs stimulate pepsinogen secretion in intact animals, gastric glands, and monolayer cultures. The stimulation is antagonized by atropine, indicating a muscarinic receptor. The receptor, at least in the dog and the mouse, appears to be of the M_1 type (i.e., having a high affinity for pirenzepine). The efficacy of cholinergic agonists differs between species, but responses have been observed in all systems examined, from humans to amphibians. Cholinergic stimulation is believed to reflect an endogenous neural control mechanism mediated either by the internal plexi or by vagal innervation of the gastric mucosa. Atropine inhibits the pepsin secretion elicited by direct stimulation of the vagus or by the vagally mediated hypoglycemic response. However, the results of *in vitro* studies showing a direct cholinergic stimulation of pepsinogen secretion indicate that at least part of the response to vagal stimulation is due to a direct action on the chief cells.

A somewhat novel finding from *in vitro* studies is that the β-adrenergic agonist isoproterenol stimulates pepsinogen secretion by rabbit isolated gastric glands. The adrenergic stimulation was found to be inhibited by propranolol but not by atropine or cimetidine, indicating a direct action on the chief cell. Moreover, the stimulation appears to be specific for pepsinogen secretion, because isoproterenol does not stimulate acid secretion by the parietal cells.

As with other β-adrenergic systems, stimulation of pepsinogen secretion by isoproterenol is associated with activation of adenylate cyclase and an increase in cellular cAMP.

Histamine stimulates pepsinogen secretion in the human and several other species, as judged by *in vivo* results. These responses are mediated by an H_2 type of histamine receptor. Stimulation of pepsinogen secretion by histamine *in vivo* has been the subject of controversy, because the dose-response curve shows reduced secretion at high doses of histamine. This observation led to the suggestion that histamine leads to pepsin output by stimulating electrolyte, (i.e., HCl) and water secretion, which "washes out" presecreted pepsinogen, and not by directly stimulating pepsinogen secretion. This argument might hold for experiments using a cumulative dose-response method, but because a similar pattern is seen with dose-response curves constructed from individual doses, the "washout" explanation seems unlikely. Both actions of histamine are postulated to be mediated by H_2 receptors having different affinities. The combined possibilities of "washout," acid activation, and species differences indicate that extreme caution is needed in the interpretation of results concerning the stimulation of chief cells by histamine.

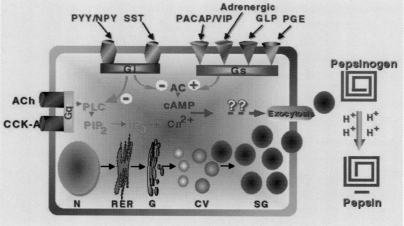

A cartoon depicting the ligands and the transduction mechanisms activating the chief cell to secrete pepsinogen. Under acidic conditions, cleavage of the N-terminal sequence of pepsinogen results in autocatalytic catalysis and activation to pepsin.

Peptide hormones

Gastrin and pentagastrin stimulate pepsinogen secretion by intact animals. The interpretation of this finding is complicated by the observation that gastrin stimulation is inhibited by atropine or histamine H_2 receptor antagonists. Thus, a direct stimulation of the chief cell cannot be demonstrated. In the case of acid secretion by parietal cells, similar observations have led to the recognition that gastrin releases histamine, which is essential for the full response to this peptide. In the case of pepsinogen secretion, the release of histamine by gastrin could lead to an indirect stimulation of the chief cell via histamine in sensitive species or via the consequent increase in acid secretion. Studies using *in vitro* preparations indicate that gastrin does not stimulate pepsinogen secretion by a direct action. Thus, gastric glands isolated from rabbit secrete pepsinogen in response to gastrin, but only at doses well above that required to stimulate acid secretion; pentagastrin does not stimulate pepsinogen secretion by either canine chief cells or frog esophagus. At present, therefore, the evidence does not favor direct activation of chief cells by gastrin as a physiologic mechanism for stimulating pepsinogen secretion.

In contrast to the results with gastrin, *in vitro* studies have shown a potent stimulation of pepsinogen secretion by CCK-like peptides. Stimulation by the C-terminal octapeptide of CCK (CCK-8) appears to be a direct action on the chief cell, because it is not inhibited by atropine, propranolol, or cimetidine but is antagonized competitively by dibutyryl cyclic GMP. The latter observation is significant, because stimulation of acid secretion in gastric glands by CCK-8 is not inhibited by dibutyryl cyclic GMP. Monolayer cultures of canine chief cells also respond to CCK-8 but not to pentagastrin. These results indicate that the mammalian chief cell is able to distinguish between gastrin and CCK, despite the structural similarity of the active C-terminal portions of these peptides. Potency sequences for CCK-related peptides indicate that one crucial feature for chief cell activation is sulfation of the tyrosine residue. This does not appear to be the case for parietal cells, because gastrin-I (nonsulfated) and gastrin-II (sulfated) are equipotent for stimulation of acid secretion. The exact position of the sulfated tyrosine also appears to be important for stimulating pepsinogen secretion, because gastrin-II (tyrosine at the sixth position from the C-terminal) is much less potent than CCK-8 (tyrosine at the seventh position from the C-terminal) and only slightly more potent than gastrin-I.

The difference in potencies of CCK and gastrin analogs for acid versus pepsinogen secretion suggests that parietal and chief cells may possess different peptide receptors. This concept is supported by the results of radiolabeled ligand-binding studies. The combined results of secretion and ligand-binding studies implicate a CCK-like peptide as a stimulus for pepsinogen secretion. However, CCK is not known as a potent stimulus *in vivo*, and the concentrations of CCK required to stimulate secretion *in vitro* appear to be somewhat higher than normal blood levels. Thus, to postulate a physiologic role for a CCK-like peptide, it may be necessary to show that the peptide is released locally, perhaps from nerve terminals or endocrine cells, at a high concentration. Whatever future studies on CCK may reveal, it is reasonably clear that gastrin does not act by direct stimulation of the chief cell.

Secretin has been reported to stimulate pepsinogen secretion in the intact animal and human. The dose of secretin required to elevate pepsinogen secretion appears to be within the normal range, indicating that this hormone may play a physiologic role. Because secretin inhibits acid secretion, the stimulation of pepsinogen output is not due to a washout of presecreted pepsinogen or acidification of the gastric lumen. Based on *in vitro* studies, it is likely that VIP shares a common receptor mechanism with secretin, but a physiologic role for VIP in regulating pepsinogen secretion has not been demonstrated as yet.

Additional peptide hormones have been implicated as modulators of pepsinogen secretion, such as bombesin, glucagon, and somatostatin. Bombesin, or a bombesin-like peptide, stimulates pepsinogen secretion by frog esophageal glands through a direct action, but in mammals, this peptide is thought to act indirectly by modulating gastrin release. Glucagon, which is structurally similar to secretin, is reported to inhibit both acid and pepsinogen secretion. The interpretation of these findings is complicated, because glucagon has several actions in the intact animal, including elevation of blood glucose and reduction in gastric volume secretion. Somatostatin, which is found throughout the gastrointestinal tract, has been shown to inhibit pepsinogen secretion elicited by several stimuli in the intact animal.

Miscellaneous agents

A variety of agents have been found to alter pepsinogen secretion *in vitro*. Most of these agents cannot be used for *in vivo* studies because of solubility or toxicity problems. Many of the compounds do not occur naturally, or at least not in the extracellular environment, and thus do not represent normal physiologic mechanisms. The best-characterized group of agents is the cyclic nucleotides and compounds that alter cyclic nucleotide metabolism. cAMP and its derivatives stimulate pepsinogen secretion in all of the *in vitro* preparations examined. Thus, the present evidence indicates that intracellular cAMP is an effective mediator of pepsinogen secretion.

Several agents have been reported to alter pepsinogen secretion either directly or by influencing responses to other stimuli. In general, the mechanism of action of these agents is unknown. The exact mechanisms by which these factors influence pepsinogen secretion have not been identified. One observation that seems of particular interest is that a variety of weak bases will stimulate pepsinogen secretion or potentiate the action of other stimuli. This is of interest for two reasons: First, identifying the mechanism of action could provide important clues regarding pepsinogen secretion. Second, many agents that are reported to alter pepsinogen secretion are weak bases or weak acids, and caution is urged in distinguishing between a specific action and the possibility that these agents are merely acting as weak acids or bases.

Significance of pepsinogen

Physiologic

The function of pepsin is the initiation of protein digestion. Although this role of pepsin has been recognized for over a century, there is little information available on the quantitative contribution of pepsin versus pancreatic enzymes to the overall digestive process. Because pepsin is highly active on collagen, it is more important for digestion of meat than for vegetable protein. In addition, pepsin is likely to be more important in species in which mastication is limited or absent. Although pepsin can release small peptides and free amino acids, relatively large peptides normally enter the intestine before peptic digestion is complete. Apart from a primary role in protein digestion, pepsin also acts as a milk-clotting factor. This action occurs at a higher pH than does proteolysis and may be more significant in the neonate than in the adult.

A second major physiologic role of pepsin is its contribution to the overall regulation of the digestive process. This regulatory role has received less attention than the enzymatic activity but is no less important. The digestion of proteins by pepsin leads to the formation of peptides that serve as signals for the release of various hormones, including gastrin and CCK. In turn, these hormones serve as the major regulators of the digestive process. Thus, pepsin can initiate a coordinated set of responses that lead to the digestion and absorption of protein.

Clinical

Several studies have shown that instillation into the stomach of HCl alone does not cause ulceration, but inclusion of gastric juice or pepsin with the acid results in ulcer formation. In duodenal ulcer patients, both basal and stimulated pepsin secretions, like acid secretion, are greater than in normal controls. This evidence suggests that pepsin may be a necessary, or at least contributing, factor in ulcer formation. A possible specific role for antral or duodenal pepsinogen in ulcer formation also has been considered. Serious efforts to treat or prevent ulcers by inhibiting pepsinogen secretion or pepsin activity have not been made, despite the probable involvement of pepsin in these diseases. The lack of interest in antipepsin treatment is due, in part, to the success of antacid therapy, particularly the histamine H_2 receptor antagonists. Because acid-secretory inhibitors also suppress pepsinogen secretion and maintain a higher luminal pH, their efficacy may be due partly to a reduced pepsin activity. Development of specific antipepsin agents could provide an alternative approach, which likely would avoid the hypergastrinemia associated with many antacid treatments.

The demonstration of pepsinogen in plasma and urine suggested the possible use of such measurements for diagnosis or prediction of ulcer disease. This has not proven to be of clinical value. The diagnosis of ulcer disease is performed more easily and more definitively with endoscopy. Although correlations have been obtained between serum pepsinogen and such diseases as pernicious anemia and Zollinger-Ellison syndrome, the plasma values likely reflect changes in gastric mucosal mass that accompany the disease and, therefore, are of little value in early detection. Attempts have been made to correlate serum pepsinogen with susceptibility to ulcer formation and gastric cancer, but thus far, no firm basis for prediction has been established.

CHAPTER 4
INTRINSIC FACTOR

Historical issues

Although pernicious anemia was clearly recognized by Addison in 1855, this fatal anemia did not have any effective treatment until 1926, when Minot and Murphy documented satisfactory management with the ingestion of large amounts of raw liver. A debt of gratitude is owed to Castle, who proposed that impaired gastric function was responsible for the disease and successfully proved his hypothesis. Thus, neither beef (200 g daily) nor normal human gastric juice (150 mL) administered by stomach tube produced a hematopoietic response. Nevertheless, simultaneous administration of both resulted in a positive response as effective as that induced by liver alone. It subsequently became apparent that liver contained high levels of cobalamin, and because intrinsic factor was not needed for the nonspecific diffusion of the vitamin across the mucosal membranes, cure resulted—albeit in an inefficient fashion. The availability of isotopically labeled cyanocobalamin in 1950 allowed for the full understanding of the role of intrinsic factor in the absorption of cobalamin. Further studies enabled the localization of the site of intrinsic factor production to the parietal cell and identified two distinct functional sites on the intrinsic factor molecule. The further identification of ileal membrane receptors for intrinsic factor–bound cobalamin demonstrated a role for the pancreas as well as the stomach in normal cobalamin absorption. In addition to intrinsic factor, it also became apparent that there were other cobalamin-binding proteins involved in the normal transport of the vitamin.

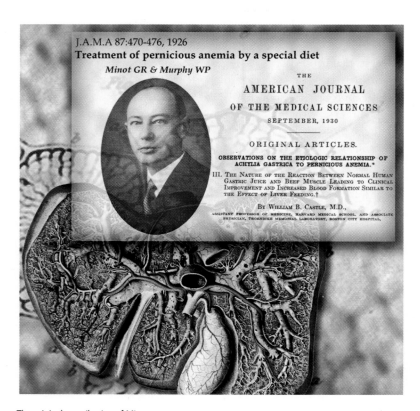

J.A.M.A 87:470-476, 1926
Treatment of pernicious anemia by a special diet
Minot GR & Murphy WP

THE
AMERICAN JOURNAL
OF THE MEDICAL SCIENCES
SEPTEMBER, 1930

ORIGINAL ARTICLES.

OBSERVATIONS ON THE ETIOLOGIC RELATIONSHIP OF ACHYLIA GASTRICA TO PERNICIOUS ANEMIA.*

III. THE NATURE OF THE REACTION BETWEEN NORMAL HUMAN GASTRIC JUICE AND BEEF MUSCLE LEADING TO CLINICAL IMPROVEMENT AND INCREASED BLOOD FORMATION SIMILAR TO THE EFFECT OF LIVER FEEDING.†

BY WILLIAM B. CASTLE, M.D.,

ASSISTANT PROFESSOR OF MEDICINE, HARVARD MEDICAL SCHOOL, AND ASSOCIATE PHYSICIAN, THORNDIKE MEMORIAL LABORATORY, BOSTON CITY HOSPITAL.

The original contribution of Minot facilitated the identification by W. Castle of the critical role of the stomach in pernicious anemia.

Cobalamin

Initial confusion in the nomenclature of the cyanocobalamin reflected the fact that the vitamin exists as hydroxycobalamin, methylcobalamin, and adenosylcobalamin. Given the fact that all of the above compounds have the biologic activity formally attributed to vitamin B_{12}, the general term *cobalamin* is now used.

The structure of adenosylcobalamin is a single cobalt atom in the nucleus of a molecule coordinated in the center of a planer corrin ring by the nitrogens of four pyrroline rings. Cobalamin cannot be synthesized by mammalian tissues—only by microorganisms. Thus, a wide variety of bacteria and protozoa are capable of production of cobalamin, and microbial synthesis of the vitamin serves as the ultimate source for the mammalian organism. Mammalian tissues are capable of efficiently converting hydroxycobalamin to the coenzymes methyl-cobalamin and adenosylcobalamin. It is of considerable importance that the mammalian organism exhibits absolute dependence on the vitamin for normal cellular replication. Despite the fact that the vitamin is crucial for tissue viability, mammalian organisms are not effectively able to assimilate cobalamin by a simple passive process. The relatively large molecule has a radius far in excess of the "effective pore size" of intestinal absorptive membranes. By virtue of its structure, however, it is highly soluble in water and virtually insoluble in most organic solvents. This bulky, polar, water-soluble, lipid-insoluble molecule, therefore, is not easily able to pass the lipid bilayer of biologic membranes and requires a highly specialized membrane-transport system for assimilation and use. Because only 10 to 15 μg per day of cobalamin is available in a diet, the membrane-transport process requires precise identification of the molecule and an effective extraction process. Similarly, transport needs to be specific to avoid absorption of cobalamin-like molecules, which are either inactive or possibly harmful.

Cobalamin-binding transport proteins

There exist three distinct transport proteins for high-affinity binding of the cobalamin molecule: R proteins, transcobalamin II, and intrinsic factor. The last is secreted by the stomach, whereas transcobalamin II is present in the plasma, and the R proteins are a family of glycoproteins found in plasma, granulocytes, and several glandular secretions. All three binding proteins bind cobalamin in a macromolecular complex that involves a single cobalamin-binding site per protein molecule. The affinity of cobalamin for its transport proteins is extremely high, and the association constants are in the picomolar range. Of the three binding proteins, intrinsic factor is by far the most selective. Transcobalamin II is somewhat less specific, and the R proteins are non-specific, binding a wide variety of cobamides. Each cobalamin-binding transport protein has highly specific membrane receptors present on the surface of functionally relevant cells. Thus, receptors for intrinsic factor are present on microvillous membranes of ileal absorptive cells, whereas a wide variety of dividing cells contain receptors for transcobalamin II. Hepatocytes are the only cells that possess receptors specific for R proteins.

Intrinsic factor

The oxyntic mucosa of the body and fundus of the human stomach are the sites of intrinsic factor secretion. Total gastrectomy is associated with cobalamin malabsorption, and unless the vitamin is administered, cobalamin deficiency will occur within 3 to 5 years. The gastric parietal cell is the source of intrinsic factor in almost all species, including humans. The protein is present

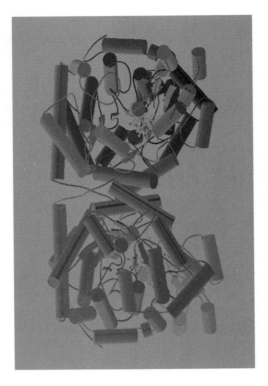

Two views of the structure of the coenzyme B_{12}–dependent enzyme glutamate mutase from *Clostridium cochlearium*, demonstrating binding with methyl–cobalamin (center of each molecule).

on the membranes of the perinuclear envelope, rough endoplasmic reticulum, Golgi apparatus, and tubulovesicular membrane system of the parietal cell. It is of interest that intrinsic factor is found in the chief cell of the mouse and the rat, whereas in the pig, intrinsic factor is located in the mucous cells of the duodenum and pyloric area of the stomach.

Far more intrinsic factor is secreted than is needed to bind and assimilate dietary cobalamin. Thus, in a 60-minute period, the stimulated human stomach secretes enough intrinsic factor to bind all cobalamin ingested in a 24-hour period. Intrinsic factor secretion appears to be stimulated by all agents that stimulate acid secretion. It is thus secreted under stimulation by histamine, pentagastrin, and cholinergic agents and is similarly inhibited by cimetidine. The pattern of intrinsic factor secretion, however, differs from that of acid secretion. Exposure to an agonist results in a rapid stimulation, with peak levels of intrinsic factor within 15 to 30 minutes, whereas acid increases over a far slower period. When acid secretion is at a maximum level, intrinsic factor secretion has returned to control levels.

This phenomenon was initially attributed to a washout of preformed intrinsic factor, but repetition of the stimulus results in secretion of additional intrin-

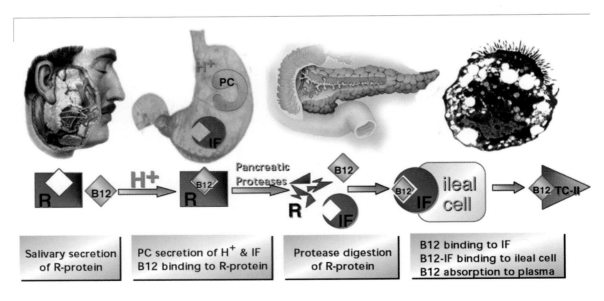

A schematic representation of the physiologic events necessary to enable absorption of vitamin B_{12}.

sic factor, and a continuous infusion of an agonist results in steady-state intrinsic factor secretion for prolonged periods. The cellular mechanism of intrinsic factor secretion appears to be related to cAMP. Morphologic observations of human gastric mucosa suggest that the parietal cell secretes intrinsic factor by membrane translocation. In those species in which intrinsic factor is in chief cells, the protein is secreted in parallel with pepsinogen.

Intrinsic factor is a globular glycoprotein that contains approximately 15% carbohydrate. It has a molecular weight of 44,000 Da and consists of a single polypeptide chain. Intrinsic factor binds cobalamin at a ratio of 30 µg per milligram of intrinsic factor protein, suggesting that each molecule of intrinsic factor binds one molecule of cobalamin. The macromolecular complex exhibits tight binding with a high affinity for the protein and occurs virtually instantly on exposure of the two substances to each other. Although the bond that is formed between intrinsic factor and cobalamin is extremely strong under physiologic conditions, it is readily disrupted above a pH of 12.6, and below a pH of 3.0, the affinity is markedly reduced. In an acid environment, the binding of cobalamin to R protein is greatly favored over binding to intrinsic factor. Once the intrinsic factor molecule binds to cobalamin, it becomes more compact, with a 10% to 15% decrease in its calculated Stokes radius and apparent molecular weight. The cobalamin-bound intrinsic factor complex is resistant to destruction by protease to a far greater degree than is free intrinsic factor itself.

Cobalamin absorption

Only 1 to 2 µg daily of cobalamin is required to maintain normal stores. Almost all sources of animal protein, such as liver, kidney, fish, milk, and eggs, contain substantial quantities of cobalamin, and the average dietary intake is usually 10 to 20 µg per day. Vegetarian diets lack adequate cobalamin to avoid deficiency disease. In the case of herbivores who do not have access to meat, they depend on either rumen bacteria or regular access to microbial products by coprophagy to obtain adequate cobalamin. Under normal circumstances, healthy subjects absorb 30% to 60% of an oral dose of 1 µg of cyanocobalamin. Assimilation of the vitamin occurs by two almost completely different processes. Thus, in small quantities, absorption is quite efficient, whereas in the ingestion of large quantities of cobalamin, much is lost. Although the process is efficient, the absorption of physiologic amounts of the vitamin is extremely slow and occurs almost entirely from the ileum. In the face of large quantities of cobalamin, absorption is by nonspecific diffusion across the entire alimentary canal. The distal half of the ileum is the major site of cobalamin absorption, and resection of this area leads to malabsorption. The colon is not able to assimilate the bound vitamin.

Efficient absorption of cobalamin requires that the vitamin form a macromolecular complex with the glycoprotein secreted by the stomach. In patients with pancreatic insufficiency, cobalamin absorption is poor, suggesting that pancreatic proteases are necessary for this process, although the mechanism responsible has not yet been identified. For efficient absorption, the distal small bowel must be intact, and in its absence, the absorption of cobalamin is limited. Within the ileal mucosa, the assimilation process is extremely slow, which presumably reflects a series of molecular-processing events that have not yet been fully delineated.

Absorption sequence

On the ingestion of a physiologic quantity of cobalamin, a series of specific events occur in a sequential fashion to ensure appropriate and adequate absorption. First, cobalamin is released from dietary proteins, whereon the salivary R proteins ensure intragastric binding of the substance. Thereafter, intraduodenal digestion of the R protein cobalamin complexes occurs, particularly by pancreatic proteases, which are responsible for the release of cobalamin. Once cobalamin is free within the duodenum or upper small bowel, binding of the vitamin by intrinsic factor occurs before its transport to the lower ileum. At this point, the intrinsic factor–bound cobalamin is attached to the apical membrane of the ileum cells, and absorption via specific receptor-mediated pathways occurs. The transcellular transport of cobalamin in the ileal mucosa is a slow process and presumably involves endocytosis. The vitamin is thereafter released into the portal circulation and passes to the liver for processing.

The stomach and duodenum are of considerable importance in the absorption of cobalamin. Because the dietary proteins that bind cobalamin are largely apoenzymes, an acidic environment in the stomach is necessary to ensure rapid release of cobalamin from such proteins. This step does not require pepsin and is not a rate-limiting step for absorption. It is, however, evident that individuals with achlorhydria do not effectively extract and absorb dietary vitamin, even though they may secrete adequate amounts of intrinsic factor and are capable of normal absorption of cobalamin. The free cobalamin within the stomach binds almost exclusively to R proteins that have been secreted by the salivary glands. The cobalamin bound to such R protein is released immediately on entering the proximal small intestine by the action of pancreatic proteases, which are responsible for a rapid degradation of the R proteins. Once the cobalamin is released from the R protein, it rapidly combines with intrinsic factor to generate the stable macromolecular complex previously described. This complex of cobalamin and intrinsic factor is extremely stable and not digestible by proteolytic enzymes of the pancreas or upper bowel. In addition, the binding to intrinsic factor protects the vitamin from bacterial use within the small bowel while the macromolecular complex is being transported to the ileum.

Although much attention has been focused on the regulation of acid secretion and pepsinogen, the mechanisms responsible for the secretion of intrinsic factor and its subsequent role in the absorption of cobalamin are vital to the organism. Indeed, it might be said that without adequate intrinsic factor secretion or cobalamin ingestion, all other secretory processes of the stomach would be defunct within a 3- to 5-year period as the organism perished.

CHAPTER 5
REGULATION OF GROWTH OF GASTRIC EPITHELIUM

Introduction

Disease occurs because of disruption or malfunction of the different barriers of the upper gastrointestinal tract. Recovery from damage depends on the properties of the epithelial cells and their ability to repair injury.

The gastric mucosa contains several cell types, each programmed to undergo cell division at a specific rate and to equal this rate of cell division by an equal rate of apoptosis. Increased apoptosis without change in cell division results in atrophy; increased cell division without change in apoptosis results in hyperplasia. It is an exquisitely modeled epithelium with distinct regions containing specific cell types. Clearly, maintenance of differentiation to generate the normal epithelium is quite specific and requires a precise programming of growth, differentiation, and apoptotic factors.

The cells of the gastric fundic epithelium that appear clinically relevant are the surface epithelial cells, the neck cells, the parietal and chief cells, and the endocrine cells, mainly the ECL and D cells. In the antrum, there are the surface cells, the neck and gland cells, the D and G cells, and a chief cell that secretes a different isoform of pepsinogen. The neck region of the glands contains the progenitor cells for the surface, parietal, and peptic cells.

Rather little attention was paid to growth regulation of many of these cell types until the development of modern knowledge of gastrin. Gastrin was originally considered only of relevance in terms of stimulation of acid secretion, but Rusty Johnson showed in the early 1970s that gastrin was trophic for the fundic, but not the antral, epithelium. Since then, much effort has been expended into a better definition of the mechanism of action of gastrin, at first on the ECL cell and later on the parietal/peptic cells. Several other trophic factors have now been shown to be present or induced after epithelial damage, but it is far too early to even begin to define the program that allows expression of the mature gastric epithelium with its multiple cell types in the right place at the right time.

Cell growth in the stomach

The rat stomach has formed the primary *in vivo* model for studies of the growth regulation of the epithelium, usually by measurement of DNA synthesis (^{3}H thymidine or BrdU incorporation).

Starvation for 24 or 48 hours results first in a degree of fundic atrophy. Refeeding then produces a large increase in DNA synthesis in the neck cells of the fundic glands, which contain the progenitor cells for the surface and the glandular structures. There is also incorporation of these markers into ECL cells scattered throughout the fundus. Refeeding is several-fold more effective than gastrin, showing that gastrin is overshadowed by other factors in this particular model.

The transit time of surface epithelial cells is approximately 72 hours, whereas that of parietal and chief cells is approximately 90 to 120 days.

There is detailed knowledge of cell lineage and growth in the intestinal mucosa not matched by knowledge of these properties of the gastric mucosa.

There are stem cells, very few in number, that divide slowly to provide daughter cells. One of these two cells is destined to remain a stem cell; the other divides to form preprogenitor cells that, in turn, divide to form progenitor cells, which then form cell-type precursors and finally the mature cell type. This program is held within the cells and outside the cells by external factors generated by other cell types. The stem cells of the gastric mucosa are pluripotent.

The generation of parietal cells is in the neck region, and it is possible to recognize preparietal or progenitor cells, which then differentiate to form a triple helix chain of cells down the length of the gastric gland. Parietal cells are recognizable by their large mitochondrial content (34% cell volume) as well as by expression of the gastric acid pump and of the histamine-2 and CCK_2 receptors. They are end cells and have not been shown capable of cell division.

Chief cells are found generally deeper in the fundic gland, mostly in the bottom third. They are recognizable because of their high content of pepsinogen and expression of the CCK_1 receptor subtype. They appear to have some residual capacity for division. There is currently no explanation for their anatomic localization. A slower generation time than that of the parietal cells would enable deeper localization of these cells.

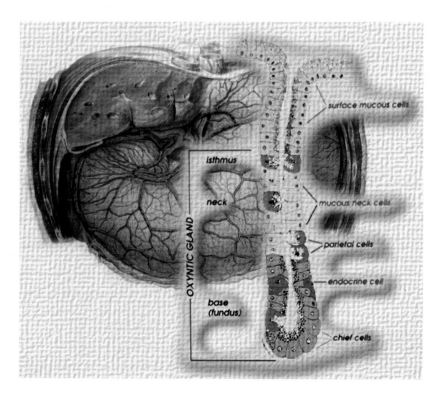

A cartoon of the fundic gastric gland (lower right) demonstrating the location and relationship of the different cell types within the stomach (background).

ECL cells are the major endocrine cells of the fundic mucosa and are found toward the lower third of the gastric fundic gland. In animals, these cells are clearly capable of cell division. Some claim that the ECL cell in the human mucosa is also an end cell like the parietal cell, but it is unusual to find a wide gap between humans and other mammals in something as fundamental as capacity for cell division.

In recent years, the ECL cell has achieved prominence as the target for gastrin's hyperplastic effect on the endocrine cell population in the stomach. ECL cells are easily identified due to their histamine, acidic vacuole, and HDC content.

Growth receptors in gastric mucosa

A large number of factors have been shown to stimulate gastric cell replication *in vivo* and in gastric cell lines *in vitro*. Surely, a well-conducted orchestra of these factors is necessary for the generation and regeneration of a normal gastric epithelium. How the integration of all these factors enables replacement of the mature epithelium remains a challenge for the future, as it does in all organ biology.

Gastrin

This is the best studied of the various factors influencing growth in the fundus of the stomach. Recent investigations using CCK_2 receptor KNO mice have confirmed the critical role of gastrin/CCK in mucosal growth. Although capable of stimulating ECL cell replication, it is less effective than many other factors in driving gastric cell replication. On the other hand, the hypergastrinemia induced by treatment with PPIs can result, in animals and in some patients, in parietal and chief cell hyperplasia as well as ECL cell hyperplasia.

It has been repeatedly demonstrated, however, that these are without clinical consequence in the 15 years that maintenance omeprazole studies have been present. An even longer period of surveillance of selective or highly selective vagotomy patients, in whom hypergastrinemia results with approximately the same elevation found in maintenance PPI therapy, has shown no unexpected changes in gastric mucosal cells. The apparent affinity for the growth receptor on the ECL cell appears to be approximately 50-fold higher than the affinity for the receptor activating histamine release from the same cell type. Neutralizing antibodies to gastrin result in at least 50% inhibition of the feeding response on gastric DNA synthesis, arguing for a continuing important role of this hormone in gastric growth regulation.

Why there is not a trophic action of gastrin on the antrum is completely unknown. As discussed elsewhere, gastrin also regulates HDC expression in ECL cells.

Epidermal growth factor and transforming growth factor-α

EGF and TGF-α are peptide hormones that are potent stimuli for cell division in the gastric mucosa and also potent inhibitors of gastric acid secretion. The former action is undoubtedly due to a tyrosine kinase action, and the latter is due to extracellular signal-regulated kinases (ERKs) 1 and 2 activation.

The inhibition of acid secretion that occurs at the same time as stimulation of growth suggests that the presence of acid secretion is inimical to growth. TGF-α is upregulated in the vicinity of gastric ulcers, suggesting a real physiologic role for this peptide and its receptor in ulcer healing.

Hepatocyte growth factor

Hepatocyte growth factor (HGF) is also a potent mitogen, acting at a c-met receptor. It stimulates expression of the vascular endothelial growth factor (VEGF) receptor for endothelial cell growth and permeability. It is implicated as one of the mediators in mucosal repair.

Keratinocyte growth factor

Keratinocyte growth factor (KGF) is a peptide that also significantly stimulates division of gastric cells *in vivo* and *in vitro*, although its site of production in the gastric mucosal vicinity has not been established.

Transforming growth factor-β1, -2, and -3

TGF-β1, -2, and -3, in general, inhibit cell division in the gastric mucosa and show differential regulation among the different cell types. TGF-β1 is localized exclusively to the parietal cells, β2 is found in chief cells, and β3 in parietal, chief, and mucous cells. Their role in ulcerogenesis is unclear.

Cytokines

Increased expression of a variety of interleukins has been found in gastric mucosa subsequent to infection by *H. pylori*, such as interleukin (IL)-1β and IL-8. The former has clearly been shown to inhibit cell growth in the stomach. Which of these plays a role in the ulcerating damage caused by the organism is not entirely clear.

Ammonia (NH$_3$)

H. pylori produces large quantities of NH$_3$ from urea, especially during periods of acid secretion. *In vitro*, NH$_3$ has been shown to inhibit cell growth, induce alkalinization of the cell interior, and increase intracellular Ca^{2+}. This product of infection may exert pleiotropic negative effects on the gastric mucosa. The action of NH$_3$ entry into cells is alkalinization of the cell interior. This leads to unloading of calcium stores that are IP$_3$-sensitive but also leads to partial unloading of other stores, such as those in mitochondria. This latter event may be proapoptotic.

Epithelial restitution

The term *epithelial restitution* describes the finding that surface epithelial cells migrate over the surface of a gastric wound without undergoing cell division. HGF is a stimulant of restitution, which is the result of the changed expression of a variety of integrins. The targeting scaffold on which restitution rests is an important but as-yet unexplored area of gastric biology.

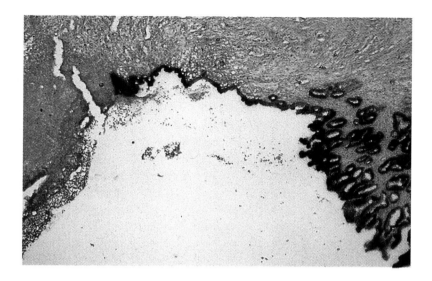

An *in situ* hybridization preparation of an experimental gastric ulcer, demonstrating the expression of the "growth factor" pS_2 in the advancing surface epithelium as well as glands.

Mucosal healing and trefoil peptides

The mucosal lining of the stomach, and the epithelial cells in particular, undergoes constant renewal. Thus, new cells are created from precursors in the proliferative zone and under the influence of "growth factors" undergo maturation and differentiation over the course of a 5- to 7-day period while they move toward the luminal surface. At this site, they perish, not necessarily by passive shedding into the lumen, but by an active process of cell death termed *apoptosis*. Indeed, this may be considered the ultimate terminal-differentiation event. In the gastric mucosa, cells also move downward (at a much slower rate) from the proliferative zone at the base of the gastric crypts into the glands. This constant and rapid turnover of the stomach mucosa is well suited to the prompt restoration of mucosal integrity after damage that may occur during acid peptic disease.

After the establishment of a mucosal breach or ulcer, three main healing events have been defined. The first is a rapid phase of epithelial restitution during which existing viable epithelial cells at the ulcer edge migrate inward to close the gap. Second, over the next few days, new cells are formed by proliferation to repopulate the mucosal gap. Third, new matrix is laid down as nonepithelial cells in the lamina propria replace inflammatory cells. This remodeling is accompanied by angiogenesis. The migrating epithelial cells are not merely undifferentiated and immature but instead have a specialized and polarized phenotype uniquely adapted to movement. The precise differentiation of this migratory phenotype is influenced by a number of factors, including at least the extracellular matrix, peptides, and the more classic growth factors. It has been established that a chronic and repetitive mucosal insult, as opposed to an acute event, significantly influences epithelial restitution. Thus, an acceleration of restitution may occur as an adaptive response, as compared to that found in "unconditioned" mucosa, and is associated with a widening of the proliferative zone.

This process also appears to involve a decrease in parietal and gastrin-secreting cells and a tendency to increase somatostatin-secreting cell numbers. A further change is the generation of a new population of "vesiculated" cells, some of which have features of immature mucous neck cells. These are present in the lower third of the gastric gland in an area previously populated by parietal cells. Such vesiculated cells may represent a distinct lineage of cells ideally located to promote proliferation and healing through the local secretion of mucosal repair proteins. The relationship between this observation and the reports of an ulcer-associated cell lineage (UACL) by Wright and his colleagues may be an important issue in the elucidation of mucosal repair in the upper gastrointestinal tract.

Of considerable importance is the identification of the molecules, which are critical to the regulation of mucosal repair. In more recent times, a number of key mucosal-repair peptides have been identified and classified according to their function. EGF is capable of performing many of the functions essential for good repair and is considered an example of a luminal-surveillance peptide. Although secreted into both serosal and luminal sides, it is only able to bind to its receptor located on the basolateral surface of the epithelial cell when mucosal integrity is breached. On the other hand, pancreatic secretory trypsin inhibitor and TGF-α are considered mucosal-integrity peptides, ensuring normal barrier function.

The third group, the trefoil factors, appears to act as rapid-response molecules upregulated at times of injury. Of particular relevance to the healing process is a distinct glandular constituent—the UACL—that produces several repair peptides, including trefoil peptides and EGF, as well as mucus. It has therefore been suggested that these cells act as a "first-aid kit," pouring healing agents onto the ulcer base. The UACL is present only at the site of chronic mucosal injury and probably arises from the duct region of metaplastic epithelium, such as intestinal metaplasia in the stomach.

The trefoil peptides are a highly conserved group of molecules that are widely distributed in the gastrointestinal tissues, although they have been demonstrated elsewhere in sites as disparate as the breast and lung. It is likely that their primary role, however, is in the gastrointestinal tract. The group takes its title from the characteristic trefoil motif, a three-loop structure secured by disulfide bonds based on cysteine residues. The super-secondary structure of the trefoil motif has been examined by three-dimensional nuclear magnetic resonance, demonstrating that it consists of a seven-residue length of alpha helix followed by a short antiparallel β sheet formed from two strands of four amino acids each. This novel structure clearly identifies the trefoil motif as a new class of module dis-

Three-dimensional magnetic resonance image (center) of a trefoil peptide motif growth factor. The ribbon images of this molecule (pS$_2$) are depicted (top right, bottom left), while the Ramachandran plots (which inform the mainchain torsion angles of the protein) are provided (top left, bottom right). Evaluation of peptides with growth-factor activity has been of value in understanding the regulation of ulcer healing.

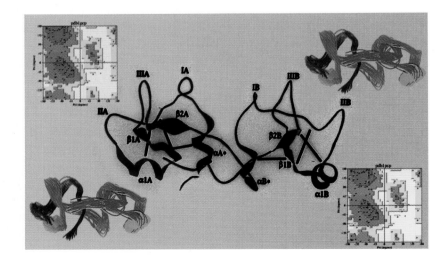

A schematic representation (left) of the development of the "ulcer-associated cell lineage" evident in the photo micrograph (right).

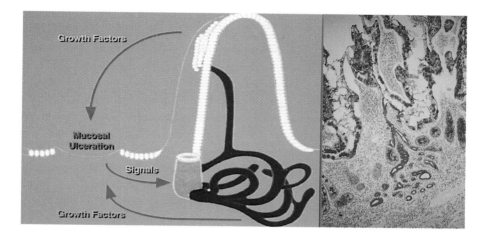

tinct from other types of highly disulfide cross-linked domains, such as those found in EGF and insulin-like growth factor-1 (IGF-1).

pS_2 was the first molecule characterized and consists of a 60–amino acid peptide with a 24–amino acid signal peptide and is homologous with pancreatic spasmolytic polypeptide (PSP). Although found in abundance in human breast cancers, the predominant pS_2 gene expression is most evident in the surface and foveolar cells of the stomach. pS_2 is found in normal gastric juice and is secreted by the surface and foveolar cells. Human SP is coexpressed with pS_2 in gastric foveolar cells and is also expressed abundantly by the basal antral glands. Both these peptides have been demonstrated to be widely expressed in gastrointestinal tissues during disease states, particularly those related to chronic ulcerative conditions. More recently, studies have demonstrated that what was previously regarded as pyloric metaplasia in chronic gastrointestinal ulceration is, in fact, a differentiating cell lineage.

This buds initially from the bases of intestinal crypts adjacent to the ulcer, and its tubules ramify in the lamina propria before emerging from the mucosal surface through a newly formed duct, which in the small intestine grows upward through the core of an adjacent villus to emerge through a pore in its side. The newly formed gland thus passes its secretion to the surface, and cells from the lineage pass out through the pore to displace the indigenous cell lineage and then close the villus surface. As the cells migrate through the tubular system, they acquire differentiation antigens and also develop a proliferative zone within the duct itself.

The glandular portion of this UACL secretes immunoreactive EGF/urogastrone that is then available to combine with its receptors and to stimulate mucosal healing. It is likely that this process or variations of it represent a basic template whereby mucosal healing of the gastrointestinal tract mucosa occurs.

Presumably, site-specific variations take place, particularly at the junctional zones of the gastroesophageal area and the pyloroduodenal area. Because the majority of gastric ulcers occurs close to the junctional zone between the fundus and the antrum, the zones of junctional instability presumably possess mechanisms important for determination of cell lineage and phenotype.

The exact role of the individual trefoils in ulcer healing is unclear. Experimentally, the use of human spasmolytic peptide has been shown to result in a moderate reduction in gastric damage induced by indomethacin. EGF has similar effects but appears to be more potent. It seems likely that each region of the gut may have a particular trefoil peptide, as has been demonstrated for the mucin genes. Indeed, trefoil expression and mucin genes are linked geographically and, in some lower animals, are even encoded by the same gene, providing an explanation for their coexpression in mammals. It is probable that, under normal circumstances, the secretion of trefoils and mucin is probably coordinately regulated. During disease states, they may become uncoupled or produced at a site remote from where they are usually evident, providing a state of *molecular metaplasia*, in the terminology originally proposed by Podolsky.

The UACL expresses both the hSP and pS_2 genes in a site-specific manner. Thus, the surface cells and the upper duct cells of the UACL express abundant pS_2, whereas hSP is found only in the lower duct and glandular area. Thus, the UACL secretes pS_2 and hSP, together with EGF/urogastrone, into the local microenvironment around the ulcer, indicating that trefoil peptides may be of considerable importance in mucosal healing and possibly even cytoprotection. Thus, as cells migrate through the UACL, they also sequentially change the pattern of peptide-gene expression, with EGF/urogastrone being found in the basal acini, hSP in the acini and ducts, and pS_2 in the upper duct and surface cells. Of interest is the fact that adjacent mucosal cells express EGF receptors, and that the normal cell lineage in the mucosa adjacent to the UACL also expresses pS_2. Local mucin-secreting cells express pS_2, which is copackaged by the Golgi apparatus into the mucous granules and secreted into the viscoelastic layer covering the mucosa. Of particular interest is the fact that pS_2 is also copackaged into neurosecretory granules of neuroendocrine cells bordering the UACL.

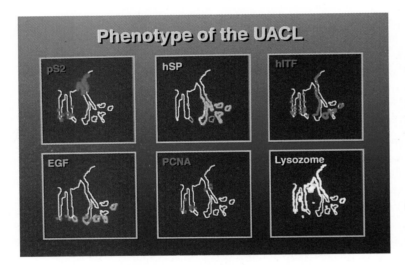

A cartoon depicting the location in the UACL of cells producing specific growth regulators.

The situation is unusual in that the same peptide is copackaged into secretory granules that are released in different ways—the mucous granules in an apocrine manner from the apical surface into the lumen and the neuroendocrine granules through the basolateral surface—in which the contained peptides can act in a paracrine fashion on other local cells. Whether this represents a common-denominator factor whereby neuroendocrine cells regulate not only physiologic responses but are also important in the modulation of repair of damaged mucosa is not known. Of particular interest is the observation that, in damaged mucosa, goblet cells can be demonstrated to produce not only trefoil peptides but also neuroendocrine products. Indeed, the novel concept must now be considered whereby enterocytes, mucous cells, and neuroendocrine cells are linked in a common system to regulate the repair of damaged mucosa.

Thus, the focus of the management of acid peptic–induced mucosal disease by targeting the noxious agents of acid and pepsin may well one day be supported by agents capable of upregulating the healing response. In this respect, a further

An immunohistochemical preparation demonstrating the colocalization of chromogranin-staining material in goblet cells coproducing trefoil peptides in healing mucosa. This provides evidence that phenotype alterations may be of considerable relevance in the healing mucosa. Growth factors and neuroendocrine regulatory agents are critical.

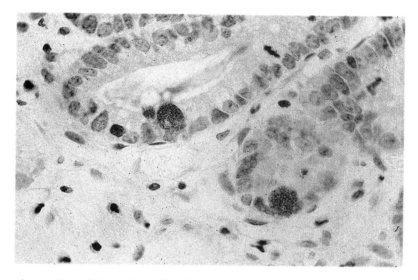

understanding of the goblet cell and its products may be of considerable scientific relevance. Rat intestinal goblet cells have been reported to produce mucin and intestinal trefoil factor as well as the trefoil peptide, spasmolysin. The mucin genes are encoded by a gene family of several members, and MUC 1 is expressed in breast, stomach, salivary gland, and the ulcer-associated cell line tissues, where pS_2 has also been detected. Thus, pS_2 and possibly other trefoil peptides may follow MUC 1 expression. It is thus possible that each mucin type may be cosecreted with its own trefoil peptide, and that trefoil peptides themselves play an important part in the function of mucus, which itself may be an as-yet unrecognized significant modulator of mucosal healing.

What little knowledge of the healing process exists has been mostly directed at the role of epithelial cells in mucosal repair. Nevertheless, the role of nonepithelial cells, particularly in the lamina propria, may be of considerable relevance in areas more complex than simply "filling the gap." In this respect, they may be responsible for producing some of the repair molecules necessary for providing the matrix on which healing can take place. Thus, hepatocyte growth factor has been demonstrated to be produced by gastric fibroblasts in culture and appears to be an extremely potent mitogen as well as a mitogen for epithelial cells. Cell migration is typically accompanied by a reduction in cell–cell interactions, and mucosal repair must also involve alterations in the interaction of cells with the extracellular matrix, which is typically mediated by integrin molecules. In addition, mucosal repair is likely to be dependent on the regulation of matrix protein synthesis as well as its degradation by collagenases and metalloproteinases.

A further important component of the repair process is angiogenesis. The development of a number of agents capable of modulating new vessel formation and thus facilitating mucosal repair is a source of potential considerable scientific and clinical relevance. Basic fibroblast growth factor, which is potently angiogenic as well as being mitogenic to a variety of cell types, accelerates epithelial restitution and has been studied in therapeutic trials. It is possible that agents such as sucralfate, which had always been thought to function as surface protectants, may actually provide some more sophisticated effects by binding agents such as fibroblastic growth factor to breaches in the mucosa.

The fact that mucosal repair occurs after *H. pylori* eradication alone and without acid inhibition suggests that the organism itself must inhibit mucosal repair. Separating the effect of *H. pylori* from the effect of the accompanying inflammatory process is difficult, but it is apparent that epithelial cell function can be modulated by cytokines in many different ways. Because *in vivo* chronic *H. pylori* infection appears to increase epithelial proliferation, the effect of *H. pylori* on restitution, matrix deposition, and angiogenesis remain areas that require evaluation. Similarly, the proteolytic action of pepsin on matrix proteins will delay healing if matrix deposition is involved in mucosal repair. Indeed, one of the most powerful effects of acid suppression may well be to move the median pH outside of the optimum required for activation of pepsinogen.

Gastric stem cells

Although much attention has been focused in the past on the mechanisms of mucosal damage and the pathogenesis of ulceration and carcinogenesis, more recently there has been recognition that the elucidation of the gastric multipotent cell niche may yield considerable biologic information as well as open the door to the identification of areas of therapeutic relevance. In this respect, the question of the nature of stem cell lineage and the identification of the regulators of phenotype expression are important areas that require delineation and elucidation.

Murine gastric stem cells

Mouse gastric glandular epithelium is composed of tubular invaginations termed *gastric units*. In the acid-secreting portion of the stomach, each unit contains three predominant cell lineages: pit, parietal, and zymogenic (chief). The multipotent stem cell and its first incarnation, the undifferentiated granule-free progenitor cell (committed precursor cell), reside in the isthmus of the unit. Within the gastric glands, migration of cell precursors is bidirectional from the neck/isthmus region to form the gastric epithelium. Thus, the pre-pit precursor differentiates into mucus-secreting pit cells as it moves up the isthmus, whereas the pre-neck cell precursor differentiates successively into pepsinogen-producing neck cells and then zymogenic (chief) cells as it migrates downward. In contrast, acid-producing parietal cells differentiate within the isthmus from preparietal cell precursors, which then migrate upward or downward. This precursor cell population—gastric epithelial progenitor cells (which include the multipotent stem cell)—make up approximately 3% of the gastric epithelium in adult mice. It is considered that the antral gastric mucosa, including the endocrine cells, derive from a common stem cell.

Experiments in XX/XY and CH3↔BALB/c chimeric mice have identified the presence of homotypic gastric glands derived from each of the parent strains. This indicates that gastric glands in the mouse are clonally derived. In addition, an examination of the chromosomal complement of the gastrin-producing endocrine cell in the XX/XY chimeras demonstrated that these were or were not Y-positive, depending on whether the gland developed from a Y-containing clone or not. This indicates that at least the gastrin-secreting endocrine cell of the antrum is derived from a common stem cell.

Experiments in X-inactivation mosaic mice expressing the *lacZ* reporter gene that investigated the clonality of gastric glands in the fundic and pyloric regions of

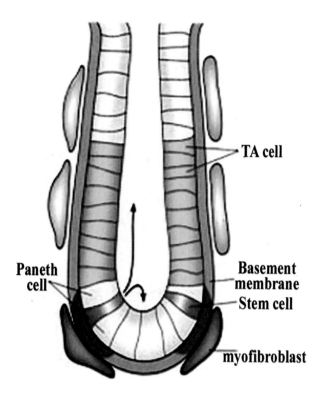

TA cell

Paneth cell

Basement membrane

Stem cell

myofibroblast

A cartoon depicting an intestinal crypt. The stem cells (perhaps a maximum of two in a crypt) are cited adjacent to Paneth's cells. The former divide, differentiate, and migrate up and down the crypt structure, becoming transient amplifying (TA) cells. The proliferative function of the stem cells are regulated by interactions with the basement membrane and messages from myofibroblasts. (Courtesy of N. A. Wright.)

the developing mice demonstrated that, whereas most glands are initially polyclonal with three or four stem cells per gland, they become monoclonal during the first 6 weeks of murine life. This potentially occurs through gland fission or when division of one of the stem cells overrides all other stem cells in the gland. A population of approximately 5% to 10% of mixed, polyclonal glands, however, persists into adulthood. They are potentially derived from glands with reduced fission rates. The significance of these multi–stem cell–containing glands is, however, unknown.

Stem cells within the gastric glands are thought to reside within a niche or group of cells and extracellular substrates, which provides an optimal microenvironment for stem cells to give rise to their differentiated progeny. There are two populations of cell types that may play important roles in this process. It is likely that gastric glands, much like intestinal glands, are enclosed in a protective fenestrated sheath of intestinal subepithelial myofibroblasts (ISEMFs). These cells exist as a syncytial organ that extends throughout the lamina propria and merges with the pericytes of the blood vessels. ISEMFs are closely linked to the gastric epithelium and are believed to play an important role in epithelial-mesenchymal interactions. They secrete HGF, TGF-β, and KGF; the receptors for these growth factors are present on the epithelial cells. Secretion of these growth factors by ISEMFs is thought to play an important role in the regulation of epithelial cell differentiation. In contradistinction, epithelial cells secrete platelet-derived growth factor-α (PDGF-α), which acts by paracrine signaling via its mesenchymal receptor, PDGFR-α, to regulate essential epithelial-mesenchymal interactions during development. Epithelial cells are therefore able to regulate the activity of ISEMFs, and vice versa.

The interstitial cells of Cajal (ICC) represent a second myofibroblast population. These are located close to mural neurones and act as pacemakers for gastrointestinal smooth muscle activity, propagate electrical events, and modulate neurotransmission. Their role in regulating stem cells is unknown but appears likely, given the importance of neural pathways (e.g., PACAP and neuroendocrine ECL cell proliferation) in the gastric mucosa. An increasing number of genes and growth factors expressed by intestinal mesenchymal cells and epithelial cells have, however, also been identified that regulate development, proliferation, and differentiation in adulthood. These include members of the fibroblast growth factor (FGF) family, EGF family, TGF-β, IGF-1 and -2, HGF/scatter factor, sonic and Indian hedgehog, and PDGF-α. Of these, it is clear that the Wnt/β-catenin signaling pathway and downstream molecules, such as APC, Tcf-4, Fkh-6, Cdx-1, and Cdx-2, are vital for normal gastrointestinal function, as mutations at any stage appear to induce tumorigenesis. It has been postulated that these pathways may play an important role in stem cell biology.

A cartoon depicting the interrelation-ships between stem cells, committed progenitor cells, and ISEMFs in the gastric mucosa. This is a bidirectional cross talk that allows the epithelium (and its environment) to affect the fate of stem cells via growth factors and the mesenchyme.

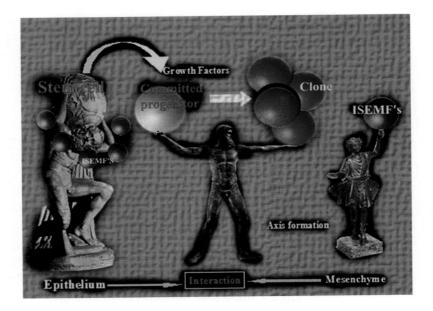

Although gastric multipotent stem cells have not been isolated, the genetic analysis of an enriched mouse gastric epithelial progenitor cell population from the fundus has facilitated the understanding of some of the molecular pathways that regulate this precursor cell proliferation and differentiation in the murine stomach.

Transgenic mice with mutant diphtheria toxin A fragment ablation of parietal cells have an increased number of gastric epithelial cell progenitors (20%, compared to 3% in normal animals). This is increased in transgenic embryonic animals (day 18) to approximately 90%. Gene chip analysis of the epithelial progenitor cell populations derived from intact stomachs from different transgenic mice and normal mice has been performed. The results demonstrate the prominence of growth factor (particularly IGF) response pathways and regulators of protein turnover pathways in these cells. Transcripts encoding products for mRNA processing and cytoplasmic localization were also present in a substantial proportion of genes, as were homologs of genes required for axis formation during oogenesis. This indicates the importance of growth factor signaling and the ability to communicate specifically with different cell types in the epithelial progenitor stem cell niche for the development of different gastric cell types.

Gastric mucosa cells can be derived from cell types other than the gastric epithelial cell progenitor. The adult hematopoietic bone marrow stem cell has a great deal of plasticity and can differentiate into a number of different cell types, including gastric epithelia. Thus, bone marrow–derived epithelial cells in the gastrointestinal tract have been demonstrated in the mouse. In a study that examined the long-term repopulation of hematopoietic stem cells (HSC) in lethally irradiated hosts, female mice received a single labeled male-derived HSC. Five long-term survivors were sacrificed after 11 months, and homing and differentiation of the HSC cell were examined. Donor-derived epithelial cells (cytokeratin-positive) were identified in the gastric pits in the stomach and constituted $0.3 \pm 0.2\%$ of cells. They had differentiated into columnar epithelial cells, appeared to be randomly scattered, and did not appear to be fully functional, because they did not appear to proliferate. This demonstrates that an exogenously applied multipotent stem cell of a very different organ system is capable of contributing to an established, organized glandular system like the gastric mucosa, even in the adult animal.

Human gastric stem cells

Glandular clonality studies in human gastric mucosa using X chromosome–linked inactivation [the phosphoglycerate kinase (PGK) and androgen receptor (HUMARA) genes were used to distinguish the two different X chromosomes] demonstrated that, whereas pyloric glands appear homotypic for either of the loci and are, therefore, monoclonal, approximately 50% of the fundic glands were heterotypic and thus polyclonal. This suggests a more complex situation than in the chimeric mice and suggests both regional and species-specific differences in the development of the gastric mucosa. Unlike in the mouse, however, no technique exists to isolate human gastric stem cells (or epithelial progenitor cell populations), and little is known about the molecular pathways that regulate stem cell proliferation and differentiation in the human stomach.

Ulceration in the stomach is, however, known to induce a novel cell lineage derived from the gastric stem cell (UACL). This cell lineage grows from the bases of existing crypts, ramifies to form a new gland, and ultimately emerges onto the mucosal surface. Cells produce neutral mucin, show a unique lectin-binding profile and immunophenotype, and secrete abundant immunoreactive EGF/urogastrone. It would appear that the production of EGF/urogastrone by the precursor cell stimulates cell proliferation, regeneration, and ultimately ulcer healing under these conditions.

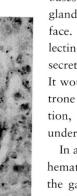

Monoclonal origin of crypts in an X0/XY mosaic individual. Staining using *in situ* hybridization for a Y chromosome–specific probe demonstrates an X0 crypt (left) and an XY crypt (right).

In an analogous fashion to the mouse, multipotent hematopoietic stem cells can also contribute cells to the gastric mucosa. Thus, an *in situ* hybridization study with Y chromosome–specific probes combined with immunohistochemical staining of gastric biopsies was able to demonstrate the presence of mucosal cells (derived from the donor) in the gastric cardia of female patients who had undergone sex-mismatched peripheral blood stem cell transplantation. This suggests the future potential therapeutic possibility of transdifferentiation in the management of gastric and gastrointestinal diseases.

Cells of the gastric mucosa undergo constant renewal, the rate of which varies depending on the demand dictated by the health of the tissue (inflammation, ulceration, carcinogenesis). Each region of the gastric mucosa appears to be morphologically diverse (antral versus fundic), with its own repertoire of cell types and glandular structures. The current evidence suggests that a single stem cell in every gastric gland indirectly gives rise to a clone of differentiated cells by production of committed progenitor cells. It is also this cell (multipotential stem cell) that produces new crypts by crypt fission, repairs entire crypts when damaged, and gives rise to the UACL and gastric carcinomas. It is most likely that this stem cell occupies a niche in the isthmus composed of mesenchymal cells and extracellular matrix factors. This environment regulates the function of the epithelial stem cell via mesenchymal-epithelial cross talk. The molecular events (IGF signaling) that regulate the development of the gastric gland, at least in the mice, are beginning to be understood, but it remains to be determined whether such information will be directly pertinent to the human situation.

Interference with gastric healing

Many factors influence the rate of gastric healing by interfering both with restitution and with cell growth and differentiation. NSAIDs, by inhibiting the constitutive enzyme cox I as one of their targets, deplete cells of prostaglandins. Aspirin can also transport protons into cells as an additional damaging factor. *H. pylori* lyses in the gastric mucus or on its surface and in so doing releases its 1,200 cytoplasmic proteins, such as Vac and Cag, that have been associated with pathogenicity. Inflammatory cells themselves release a host of cytokines that variously and often adversely affect cell homeostasis.

SUGGESTED READING

Allen A, Newton J, Oliver L, et al. Mucus and *H. pylori*. *J Physiol Pharmacol* 1997;48:297–305.

Atherton JC, Cockayne A, Balsitis M, et al. Detection of the intragastric sites at which *Helicobacter pylori* evades treatment with amoxicillin and cimetidine. *Gut* 1995;36:670–674.

Baumgartner A, Koelz HR, Halter F. Indomethacin and turnover of gastric mucosal cells in the rat. *Am J Physiol* 1986;250(6 Pt. 1):G830–G835.

Baumgartner HK, Kirbiyik U, Coskun T, et al. Endogenous cyclo-oxygenase activity regulates mouse gastric surface pH. *J Physiol* 2002;544:871–872.

Brittan M, Wright NA. Gastrointestinal stem cells. *J Pathol* 2002;197:492–509.

Carmel R. Cobalamin, the stomach and ageing. *Am J Clin Nutr* 1997;66:750–759.

Castle WB, Townsend WC, Heath CW. The nature of the reaction between normal gastric juice and beef muscle leading to improvement and increased blood formation similar to the effect of liver feeding. *Am J Med Sci* 1930;180:305–335.

Cavill I. Diagnosis of cobalamin deficiency: the old and the new. *Brit J Haematol* 1997;99:238–239.

Code CF, Scholer JE, Orvis AL, et al. Barrier offered by gastric mucosa to absorption of sodium [abstract]. *Am J Physiol* 1955;183:604.

Davenport HW, Warner HA, Code CF. Functional significance of gastric mucosal barrier to sodium. *Gastroenterology* 1964;47:142–152.

Denker BM, Nigam SK. Molecular structure and assembly of the tight junction. *Am J Physiol* 1998;274(1 Pt. 2):Fl–F9.

De Vault KR. Current management of GERD. *Gastroenterologist* 1996;4:24–32.

Engel E, Garth PH, Nishizaki Y, et al. Barrier function of the gastric mucus gel. *Am J Physiol* 1995;269:G994–G999.

Engel E, Peskoff A, Kauffman GL Jr, et al. Analysis of hydrogen ion concentration in the gastric gel mucus layer. *Am J Physiol* 1984;247:G321–G338.

Flemstrom G. Gastric and duodenal mucosal bicarbonate secretion. In: Johnson LR, Christensen J, Jackson MJ, et al., eds. *Physiology of the gastrointestinal tract*, 2nd ed. New York: Raven Press, 1987:1011–1029.

Flemstrom G, Isenberg JI. Gastroduodenal mucosal alkaline secretion and mucosal protection. *News Physiol Sci* 2001;16:23–28.

Goodlad RA. Acid suppression and claims of genotoxicity. What have we learned? *Drug Safety* 1994;10:413–419.

Heidenhain R. Ueber die Pepsinbildung in den Pylorusdrüsen. *Pflugers Archiv fur die Gesämte Physiologie* 1878;18:169–171.

Heidenhain R. Ueber die Absonderung der Fundusdrüsen des Magens. *Pflugers Archiv fur die Gesämte Physiologie* 1879;19:148–166.

Hein HK, Piller M, Schwede J, et al. Pepsinogen synthesis during long term culture of porcine gastric chief cells. *Biochem Biophys Acta* 1997;1359:35–47.

Hunter J. *Essays and observations on natural history, anatomy, physiology, psychology and geology.* vols 1 and 2. London: J. Va. Vooret, 1861.

Johnson LR. Gastrointestinal hormones and their functions. *Annu Rev Physiol* 1977;39:135–158.

Kimura Y, Shiozaki H, Hirao M, et al. Expression of occludin, tight-junction-associated protein, in human digestive tract. *Am J Pathol* 1997;151:45–54.

Korbling M, Katz RL, Khanna A, et al. Hepatocytes and epithelial cells of donor origin in recipients of peripheral-blood stem cells. *N Engl J Med* 2002;346:738–746.

Krause DS, Thiese ND, Collector MI, et al. Multi-organ, multi-lineage engraftment by a single bone marrow-derived stem cell. *Cell* 2001;105:369–377.

Laboisse C, Jarry A, Branka JE, et al. Recent aspects of the regulation of intestinal mucus secretion. *Proc Nutr Soc* 1996;55:259–264.

Langley JN, Sewall. On the changes in pepsin-forming glands during secretion. *Proc Royal Soc* 1879;XXIX:383–388.

Langley JN, Edkins JS. Pepsinogen and pepsin. *J Physiol* 1886;VII:371–415.

Lehy T, Accary JP, Dubrasquet M, et al. Growth hormone-releasing factor (somatocrinin) stimulates epithelial cell proliferation in the rat digestive tract. *Gastroenterology* 1986;90:646–653.

Logan RPH, Walker MM, Misiewicz JJ, et al. Changes in the intragastric distribution of *Helicobacter pylori* during treatment with omeprazole. *Gut* 1995;36:12–16.

Lozniewski A, de Korwin JD, Muhale E, et al. Gastric diffusion of antibodies used against *H. pylori*. *Int J Antimicrob Agents* 1997;9:181–193.

Ludwig ML, Matthews RG. Structure-based perspectives on B12 dependent enzymes. *Annu Rev Biochem* 1997;66:269–313.

Mills JC, Andersson N, Hong CV, et al. Molecular characterization of mouse gastric epithelial progenitor cells. *Proc Natl Acad Sci* 2002;99:14819–14824.

Modlin IM. To repair the fault or end the acid reign? *Scand J Gastroenterol Suppl* 1995;30(Suppl. 210):1–5.

Modlin IM, Hunt RH. Critical reappraisal of mucosal repair mechanisms. *Scand J Gastroenterol Suppl* 1995;30(Suppl. 210):28–31.

Modlin IM, Kidd M, Sandor A. Perspectives on stem cells and gut growth: tales of a crypt—from the walrus to Wittgenstein. In: *The gut as a model in cell and molecular biology*. Boston: Kluwer Academic Publishers, 1997:121–136.

Modlin IM, Poulsom R. Trefoil peptides: mitogens, motogens or mirages? *J Clin Gastroenterol* 1997;25(Suppl. 1):S94–S100.

Modlin IM, Zhu Z, Tang LH, et al. Evidence for a regulatory role for histamine in gastric enterochromaffin-like cell proliferation induced by hypergastrinemia. *Digestion* 1996;57:310–321.

Montrose MH. Choosing sides in the battle against gastric acid. *J Clin Invest* 2001;108:1743–1744.

Myers CP, Hogan D, Yao B, et al. Inhibition of rabbit duodenal bicarbonate secretion by ulcerogenic agents: histamine-dependent and -independent effects. *Gastroenterology* 1998;114:527–535.

Nomura S, Esumi H, Job C, et al. Lineage and clonal development of gastric glands. *Dev Biol* 1998;204:124–135.

Nomura S, Kaminishi M, Sugiyama K, et al. Clonal analysis of isolated single fundic and pylori gland of the stomach using X-linked polymorphism. *Biochem Biophys Res Commun* 1996;226:385–390.

Orlando RC. The pathogenesis of gastroesophageal reflux disease: the relationship between epithelial defense, dysmotility and acid exposure. *Am J Gastroenterol* 1997;92:35–55.

Patel K, Hanby AM, Ahnen DJ, et al. The kinetic organisation of the ulcer-associated cell lineage (UACL): delineation of a novel putative stem cell. *Epithelial Cell Biol* 1994;3:156–160.

Pitcairn A. A dissertation upon the motion which reduces the aliment in the stomach to a form proper for the supply of blood. In: *The whole works*. London: J. Pemberton, 1727:106–138. Sewell G and Desaguliers JT, translators.

Plebani M. Pepsinogens in health and disease. *Curr Rev Clin Lab Sci* 1993;30:273–328.

Powell DW, Mifflin RC, Valentich JD, et al. Myofibroblasts II. Intestinal subepithelial myofibroblasts. *Am J Physiol* 1999;277:C183–C201.

Quigley EM, Turnberg LA. pH of the microclimate lining human gastric duodenal mucosa in vivo. Studies in control subjects and in duodenal ulcer patients. *Gastroenterology* 1987;92:1876.

Raufmann JP. Gastric chief cells: receptors and signal transduction mechanisms. *Gastroenterology* 1992;102:699–710.

Rondon MR, Trzebiatowski JR, Escalante-Semerena JG. Biochemistry and molecular genetics of cobalamin biosynthesis. *Prog Nucleic Acid Res Mol Biol* 1997;56:347–384.

Sanders MJ, Ayalon A, Roll M, et al. The apical surface of canine chief cell monolayers resists H+ back-diffusion. *Nature* 1985;313:52.

Sanders KM. A case for interstitial cells of Cajal as pacemakers and mediators of neurotransmission in the gastrointestinal tract. *Gastroenterology* 1006;111:492–515.

Sarraf CE, Alison MR, Ansari TW, et al. Subcellular distribution of peptides associated with gastric mucosal healing and neoplasia. *Microsc Res Tech* 1995;31:234–241.

Schade C, Flemstrom G, Holm L. Hydrogen ion concentration in the mucus layer on top of acid-stimulated and -inhibited rat gastric mucosa. *Gastroenterology* 1994;107:180–188.

Schwann T. Ueber das Wesen des Verdauungsprocess. *Arch Anat Physiolwiss Med* 1836:90–138.

Shao JS, Schepp W, Alpers DH. Expression of intrinsic factor and pepsinogen in the rat stomach identifies a subset of parietal cells. *Am J Physiol* 1998;274:G62–G70.

Sharp R, Babyatsky MW, Takagi H, et al. Transforming growth factor alpha disrupts the normal program of cellular differentiation in the gastric mucosa of transgenic mice. *Development* 1995;121:149–161.

Shimizu N, Kaminishi M, Tatematsu M, et al. *Helicobacter pylori* promotes development of pepsinogen-altered pyloric glands, a pre-neoplastic lesion of glandular stomach of BALB/c mice pretreated with N-methyl-N-nitroso urea. *Cancer Lett* 1998;123:63–69.

Silen W. Gastric mucosal defense and repair. In: Johnson LR ed., *Physiology of the gastrointestinal tract*, 2nd ed, vol 2. New York: Raven Press, 1987:1055.

Smout AJ, Geus WP, Mulder PG, et al. GERD in the Netherlands. Results of a multicenter pH study. *Scand J Gastroenterol Suppl* 1996;1218:10–15.

Tatematsu M, Fukami H, Yamamoto M, et al. Clonal analysis of glandular stomach carcinogenesis in C3H/HeN-BALB/c chimeric mice treated with N-methyl-N-nitrosourea. *Cancer Lett* 1994;83:37–42.

Teorell T. On the permeability of the stomach mucosa for acids and some other substances. *J Gen Physiol* 1939;23:263–274.

Teorell T. Electrolyte diffusion in relation to the acidity regulation of the gastric juice. *Gastroenterology* 1947;9:425–443.

Thompson M, Fleming KA, Evans DJ, et al. Gastric endocrine cells share a clonal origin with other gut cell lineages. *Development* 1990;110:477–481.

Tsukita S, Furuse M, Itoh M. Molecular architecture of tight junctions: occludin and ZO-l. *Soc Gen Physiol Ser* 1997;52:69–76.

Verdu EE, Armstrong D, Idstrom JP, et al. Intragastric pH during treatment with omeprazole: role of *H. pylori* and *H. pylori* associated gastritis. *Scand J Gastroenterol Suppl* 1996;31:1151–1156.

Wallace JL, Granger DN. The cellular and molecular basis of gastric mucosal defense. *FASEB J* 1996;10:731–740.

Wetscher GJ, Hinder RA, Perdikis G, et al. Three-dimensional imaging of the lower esophageal sphincter in healthy subjects and gastroesophageal reflux. *Dig Dis Sci* 1992;41:2377–2382.

Williams GR, Wright NA. Trefoil factor family domain peptides. *Virchows Archiv* 1997;431:299–304.

Yasugi S. Regulation of pepsinogen gene expression in epithelial cells of vertebrate stomach during development. *Int J Develop Biol* 1994;38:273–279.

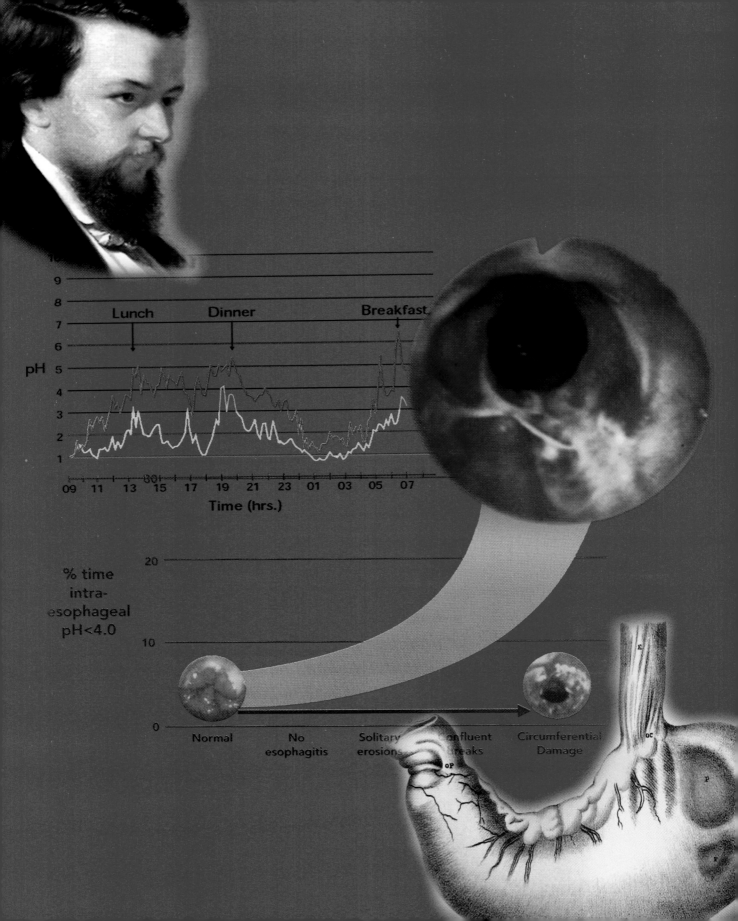

S E C T I O N   5

GASTRIC AND DUODENAL ULCER DISEASE

CHAPTER 1
HISTORY

Introduction

The elucidation of the pathobiology of acid peptic-related disease of the stomach and duodenum has accelerated dramatically in the last 20 years with the advent of scientific techniques that have facilitated the study of the cell biology of the gastric mucosa. The identification of cellular mechanisms has facilitated the development of therapeutic strategies capable of not only ameliorating the mucosal ulceration but also eradicating or abrogating the putative causes. Although acid and pepsin have long been recognized as pathogenic as regards the mucosa, it is only relatively recently that an infective component has been established as being of critical relevance to the etiology of gastric and duodenal ulcer disease.

Early management strategies thus focused briefly on the avoidance of acid-containing foods or substances containing capsaicin-related compounds. The use of bland diets was then augmented with the addition of neutralizing compounds and antacids. Unfortunately, such regimes lead to a significant decline in the quality of life and, in addition, to side effects (diarrhea, milk/alkali syndrome) associated with the use of excessive alkali and cation-containing agents. The development of histamine-2 receptor antagonists and PPIs dramatically altered the efficacy of treatment, whereas the recognition of a bacterial component of the disease and its antibiotic eradication have more recently further amplified therapeutic gains. Within the context of the advance of the knowledge of regulatory mechanisms, various therapeutic strategies have evolved, leading to a substantial change in different types of intervention. In this respect, surgery has for the most part become obsolete as methods of decreasing acid secretion have evolved into more targeted and precise pharmacologic options. Nevertheless, the early surgical remedies were to a certain extent based on a reasonable grasp of the pathophysiology and the recognition of the need to effect relief of the problem of ulceration and its sequelae of pain, bleeding, perforation, and stenosis. The recognition that the ulcer was the crux of the issue led initially to the development of techniques to simply resect the area. Unfortunately, the rapid recurrence of the lesion obviated the use of this technique, and alternative strategies were evaluated to decrease the secretion of acid. The subsequent identification of the regulatory role of the vagus nerves to the stomach inspired a multiplicity of procedures to ensure their severance as well as the development of innumerable methods to overcome the subsequent negative alterations in gastric emptying. Further recognition that the fundus of the stomach contained the acid-secreting cells and the antrum—

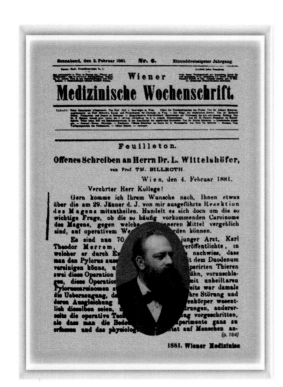

T. Billroth and the first report of a successful gastrectomy, which he undertook in Vienna. The editor noted at the bottom of the page, "and hopefully the last!" Although a pianist and violinist of considerable skill, as well as a music critic of the highest quality, Billroth is best remembered for his contributions to surgery. Although Ludwig Rydigier of Chelmo, Poland, undertook the first gastrectomy in 1880, the patient perished. Thus, when Billroth successfully resected a pyloric tumor a year later, he was credited with having undertaken the first successful gastrectomy.

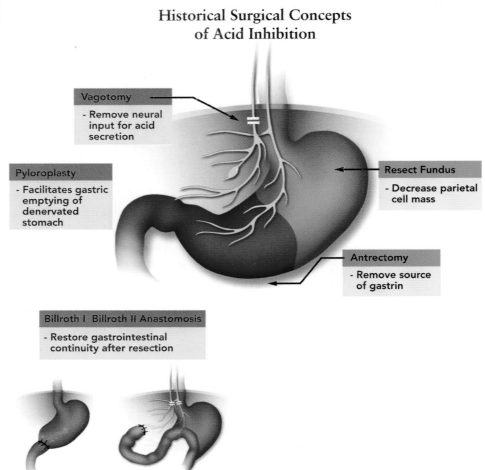

Historical Surgical Concepts of Acid Inhibition

Vagotomy
- Remove neural input for acid secretion

Pyloroplasty
- Facilitates gastric emptying of denervated stomach

Resect Fundus
- Decrease parietal cell mass

Antrectomy
- Remove source of gastrin

Billroth I Billroth II Anastomosis
- Restore gastrointestinal continuity after resection

The principles of gastric surgery for peptic ulcer disease involved vagal nerve severance as well as varying degrees of gastric resection. If vagotomy alone was undertaken, a pyloroplasty was necessary. Gastric resection required construction of a Billroth I or II anastomosis to reestablish continuity of the stomach and intestine. While the surgical targets were appropriate for their times, the more recent elucidation of the cellular events related to the regulation of acid secretion has provided the opportunity to develop a more selective pharmacologic approach to acid suppression. Thus, the mechanical extirpation of the fundic parietal cell mass or the antral source of gastrin has become outmoded by the use of specific acid-suppressive medications that avoid the morbidity and mortality associated with gastric resection, anastomosis, or denervation.

a major component of the regulatory mechanism—led to the development of an extraordinary variety of permutations and combinations of antral and fundic resection. Such operations were devised with the view to variously removing the ulcer, decreasing gastrin stimulation, ablating neural stimulation, and decreasing the parietal cell mass.

Sadly, they not only were plagued by operative morbidity and even mortality but also generated a panoply of symptomatology broadly designated as *postgastrectomy syndromes*, as the gut failed to accommodate the loss of neural innervation, pyloric function, and the severe neuroendocrine aberrations consequent on resective intervention.

At this juncture, it is rare to consider surgical intervention in acid peptic disease for anything less than a major complication; the evolution of the surgical strategies is worthy of consideration, if only to indicate the relative advantages of pharmacologic intervention as opposed to invasive modalities.

Surgical Procedures

Diagnosis	Procedure	Advantage	Disadvantage
Uncomplicated DU, GU	Highly selective vagotomy Vagotomy and pyloroplasty	Laparoscopic Only denervate fundus Rapid	High recurrence rate (up to 15%) Lesser curve necrosis Duodeno-gastric reflux possible Post vagotomy syndrome

Recurrent DU, GU	Vagotomy and antrectomy
	BI reconstruction
	BII reconstruction
		Relatively physiological
		Lower recurrence rate
			BI: stricture 2-5%
			    leakage 3-5%
			BII: Dumping syndrome
			    Duodenal stump blowout
			    Afferent-loop syndromes

Perforated duodenal ulcer	Omental patch	Rapid and safe/laparoscopic	Etiology untreated
Perforated gastric ulcer	Ulcer excision, plication Patch	Rapid, technically easy	Malignancy needs to be excluded Recurrence
MALT lymphoma	Partial/total gastrectomy	70-90% cure	Recurrence if high grade lymphoma
Early gastric carcinoma	Subtotal gastrectomy BII reconstruction	High cure rate (up to 90%)	Aff. Eff. loop syndrome
Extensive gastric carcinoma	Extended/radical or total gastrectomy	Decreases chance of perforation, bleeding, obstruction	Cure uncommon Anastomotic leakage Post gastrectomy syndromes Morbidity 12%, mortality <2%
Zollinger-Ellison syndrome - Pancreatic gastrinoma - Duodenal gastrinoma	? Total gastrectomy ? Pancreatic resection ? Whipple procedure	Most effective ulcer prevention	Nutrient sequelae Tumor recurrence common Altered glucose homeostasis

The advent of H_2RAs and PPIs has virtually abolished the need for peptic ulcer surgery except to deal with complications. For the most part, gastric resections are associated with a morbidity and are therefore avoided unless circumstances absolutely dictate surgical intervention. Gastric resections may be of some benefit in very early neoplastic disease of the stomach.

Early management of peptic ulcer disease

The earliest human texts address issues of the cosmos and the meanings of life, endlessly examining the nature of divinity, pantheism, and the fate of the soul. Throughout these erudite texts runs a common and fundamental issue speculated on both in metaphor and fact. The commonality of food, the stomach, and digestion can be noted in writings as divergent as those of the Sufi mystics, the Sephardic sages, philosophers of the Tang dynasty, or the *Odes* of the Mantuan Bard. Food and its digestion represent a theme of universal interest surpassed only by preoccupation with the ephemeral concept of love. *Homo est quod est*: Man is what he eats. It is therefore no wonder that the subject of digestion has been a matter of concern to doctors and their patients for as long as records exist. Unfortunately, little rational therapeutic intervention was available for the treatment of gastric disorders. Indeed, up until the late nineteenth century, the stomach was often not clearly recognized as a source of symptoms. From the earliest times, chalk, charcoal, and slop diets had been noted to provide symptomatic relief from dyspepsia.

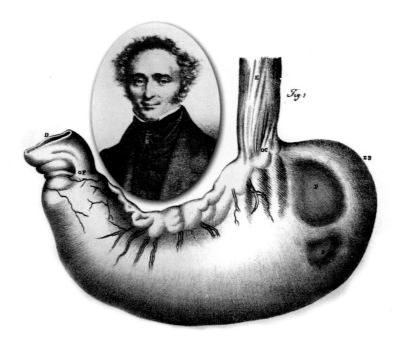

Jean Cruveilhier (1791–1873), a brilliant pupil of Dupuytren and the first incumbent of the chair of pathology in the Paris Faculty. He abjured the use of microscopy but nevertheless produced extraordinarily well-illustrated pathology texts.

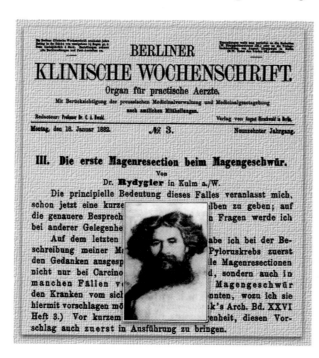

Ludwig Rydiger of Chelmo, on November 16, 1880, performed the second documented gastrectomy. It was unsuccessful!

In the seventeenth century, chalk and pearl juleps were used for infant gastric disorders, but little comment was made about adult problems except by Sydenham, who wrote about gout and dysentery. Jan Heurne, the first proponent of bedside teaching, left a posthumous pamphlet on the diseases of the stomach in 1610. Similarly, Martin Harmes and Ferriol, in 1684 and 1668, respectively, produced books on diseases of the stomach and intestines. In 1664, Swalbe published a long satire on "the quarrels and opprobria of the stomach" (prosopopoia). The favorite theme of the seventeenth-century physicians was the dyspepsia due to gastric atony implicit in the title *De imbecilitate ventriculi*. This term was continued into the eighteenth century, when it was equated with the "hectic stomach" (Arnold, 1743) and later with the term of "*embarras gastrique*," used by the French physicians.

Throughout the eighteenth century, there were various descriptions of gastric and intestinal diseases, but no specific and logical remedies were recorded. The doctrine of acidity was widespread and prevalent, and the general literature of dyspepsia was large. Thus, in 1754, Joseph Black, writing on the subject of carbon dioxide, commented on *De humore acido a cibo orto*. In 1835, in Paris, Cruveilhier had written extensively on the pathology of peptic ulcer, and the condition was referred to as *Cruveilhier's disease*. Yet, in all these tomes, little specific therapy, apart from dietary adjustments or homeopathic remedies, is apparent.

The issue of surgery of the stomach had been confounded for years by the problems related to sepsis and lack of adequate anesthesia. As late as the end of the nineteenth century, Naunyn felt obligated to describe it as "an autopsy *in vivo*." Nevertheless, by 1881, Billroth, Péan, and Rydiger had resected the stomach, and Wölfler had successfully developed the procedure of gastroenterostomy. By the beginning of the twentieth century, Moynihan had transformed the treatment of peptic ulcer disease into a unique surgical discipline.

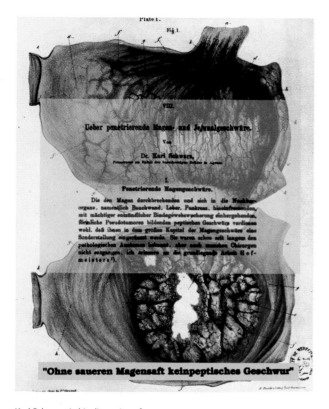

Karl Schwarz, in his discussion of penetrating ulcers of the stomach and intestine, was among the first to note that *"without acid there is no ulcer"* (*"Ohne saueren Magensaft keinpeptisches Geschwur"*).

Unfortunately, the consequences of gastric and vagal surgery produced a generation of patients with either significant postvagotomy problems or postgastrectomy syndrome. The recognition in the first part of the century that the mucosal damage was caused by acid (*"no acid—no ulcer"*) and that this acid could be decreased by luminal neutralization resulted in a wave of enthusiasm for antacid preparations, bland diets, and milk infusion as therapeutic options. The subsequent identification of the histamine-2 receptor subtype and the development of agents specifically capable of blocking acid secretion by antagonism at this receptor revolutionized the management of the disease process and virtually obliterated surgery as a therapeutic option for peptic ulcer, except in cases of emergency.

The more recent identification of the molecular mechanism of acid secretion—the proton pump—resulted in the development of a new class of therapeutic agents, the PPIs.

By defining the pump as the therapeutic target, an almost complete inhibition of acid secretion, with consequent therapeutic efficacy hitherto undreamed of, can be achieved.

Although there is much debate about the initial observations of ulceration of the gastroduodenal mucosa, some of the best original descriptions originated in the work of Jean Cruveilhier (1791–1873). Born in Limoges, France, he subsequently studied with the great surgeon of Paris—Dupuytren—and, having attained the Chair of Pathology in Paris in 1836, subsequently became one of the foremost authorities on stomach ulcers in France. Cruveilhier's interest in the subject of gastric ulcers was substantial, and his knowledge and experience in this area were widely recognized. In France at this time, the management of stomach ulcers became so closely linked with his contributions that the lesions were referred to as *Cruveilhier's disease.* His comments thoughtfully addressed issues such as why an ulcer of the stomach might occur in a single place when the rest of the stomach was *"in the state of perfect integrity."* Cruveilhier care-

"Le Maladie de Cruveilhier." The first autopsy that he witnessed so upset Cruveilhier that he returned to his original desire to become a priest and entered the Seminary Sulpice of St. Sulpice. Cruveilhier pondered why an ulcer of the stomach might occur in a single place when the rest of the stomach was *"in a state of perfect integrity."* Details of the case notes of the management of hematemesis and the autopsy findings are of interest in regard to current therapeutic strategies. In the case of this unfortunate carpenter, on autopsy he noted a deep ulceration *"6 lines in dimension."* Cruveilhier wrote that a stylet introduced into the coronary artery of the stomach pushed a clot out of the center of the ulcer and entered the stomach. The treatment of gastrointestinal bleeding in the nineteenth century involved the use of leeches, brandy, and enemas, but was often of little effect.

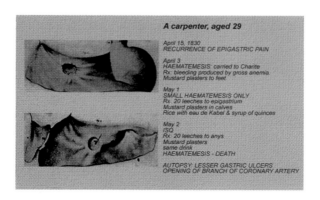

A carpenter, aged 29

April 15, 1830
RECURRENCE OF EPIGASTRIC PAIN

April 3
HAEMATEMESIS: carried to Charite
Rx: bleeding produced by gross anemia
Mustard plasters to feet

May 1
SMALL HAEMATEMESIS ONLY
Rx: 20 leeches to epigastrium
Mustard plasters in calves
Rice with eau de Kabel & syrup of quinces

May 2
ISQ
Rx: 20 leeches to anys
Mustard plasters
same drink
HAEMATEMESIS - DEATH

AUTOPSY: LESSER GASTRIC ULCERS
OPENING OF BRANCH OF CORONARY ARTERY

Lord Berkeley Moynihan (1865–1936) wrote extensively on the surgical management of duodenal ulcer disease. His contributions to the scientific foundation of gastric surgery were internationally recognized. As President of the Royal College of Surgeons of England, he was the prime mover in the introduction of science into surgical training programs.

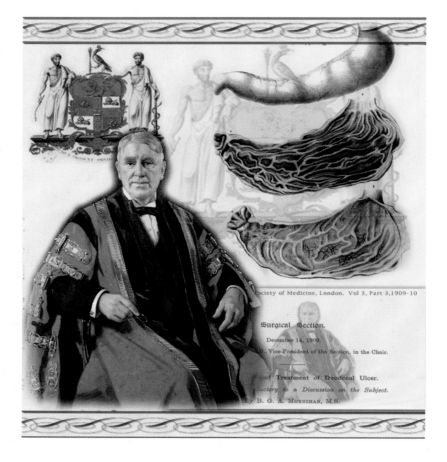

fully documented case histories and autopsies and defined in detail the pathology and sequelae of chronic gastric and duodenal ulceration.

Similarly, contributions to the understanding of the management of peptic ulcer disease were provided by Berkeley Moynihan of Leeds, in England, and so powerful was his effect on prevailing thoughts in this area that British physicians referred to duodenal ulcer as *Moynihan's disease*.

Cruveilhier's great contributions lay mostly in the pathologic description of stomach ulcers. However, the therapy of his time was modest and revolved chiefly around the application of leeches, mustard plasters, bleeding, and various alcoholic concoctions, which presumably allayed anxiety and relieved pain. Moynihan, on the other hand, defined many of the early surgical therapeutic strategies for peptic ulcer and became widely known for his contributions to gastric surgery.

Despite his exaggerated enthusiasm for the surgical management of duodenal ulcer disease, Moynihan is noteworthy for his contribution to the scientific foundation of gastric surgery. As the President of the Royal College of Surgeons of England, he became the prime mover for the first introduction of science into surgical training programs.

The recognition of the association of ulceration of the duodenum with specific circumstances, such as burns, was first attributed to Curling in 1841, who called attention to the connection between cases of burn and acute ulceration of the duodenum. Although it is likely that Dupuytren observed this relationship more than a decade before Curling, the former published little of his work, and his observations were not initially widely known.

Confusion regarding the primacy of this observation was further clouded by the fact that Moynihan claimed that in 1834, James Long of Liverpool had first described duodenal ulcer in two patients with burns.

To date, the precise pathophysiology of the relationship between severe cutaneous burns and the development of peptic ulceration still remains unclear, although the association is important.

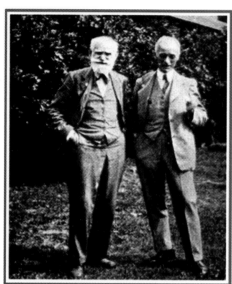

H. Cushing (right) and I. Pavlov (left), circa 1929. Harvey Cushing had defined neurosurgery as a unique discipline after an *"Arbeid"* with Kocher in Berne in 1901. Pavlov's interest in surgery prompted Cushing to let him use the surgical cautery device recently devised by Bovie. He signed his name on a piece of steak still preserved in the Cushing Surgical Collection at Yale University. Cushing was the first to recognize that after posterior cranial fossa surgery, acute duodenal ulcers often occurred.

A further association of duodenal ulceration with surgery of the posterior cranial fossa was noted by Harvey Cushing and initially attributed to alteration in neural pathways regulating gastric physiology. Current investigation is still focused on the central nervous regulation of gastroduodenal physiology, but clear answers in this area are still lacking.

Further correlations between gastroduodenal ulceration and other related conditions noted the association of pancreatic tumors with peptic ulceration. The further elucidation of the neuroendocrine tumor source of gastrin and the consequences of acid hypersecretion led to the resolution of this relationship by Zollinger and Ellison. They identified the existence of a syndrome of pancreatic neuroendocrine tumors associated with a peptic ulcer diathesis. Similar observations in conditions such as basophil leukemia and mastocytosis noted the excessive production of histamine with consequent acid hypersecretion and peptic ulcer disease in such patients.

Associations between the intake of salicylate-containing compounds and peptic ulceration were followed by similar observations in individuals using NSAIDs for the management of joint and muscle disease.

Nevertheless, despite the identification of a number of such associations with gastroduodenal ulceration, the etiology of the disease process was for the most part unrecognized until the identification of *H. pylori* and the elucidation of its relationship to peptic ulcer disease.

Gastric surgery

Until the mid-nineteenth century, the techniques of surgery were mostly confined to the extremities and usually related to the management of trauma. No surgeon would reasonably consider the violation of a body cavity before the introduction of anesthesia and antisepsis. Even under the latter conditions, both the morbidity and mortality were such that incursions into the peritoneal cavity were undertaken with considerable trepidation.

For the most part, the early reports of stomach surgery reflected the consequences of either military action with war wounds or incidental trauma. A therapeutic gastrostomy was reported in 1819 to remove a silver fork that had been "inadvertently" swallowed by a 26-year-old female servant. Jacques-Mathieu Delpech (1777–1832) of Montpellier confirmed the diagnosis of a

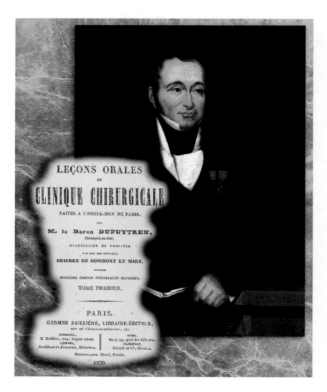

Dupuytren was a technical surgeon of extraordinary dexterity and a medical politician of consummate ruthlessness. Indeed, such was his reputation that he was referred to by his colleagues as "the first of surgeons and the least of men." For his services to the aristocracy, he was in later life awarded a baronetcy. In actuality, he unsuccessfully intervened in an attempt to save the life of an aristocrat who had been stabbed in the chest. His critics maintained that he knew surgery was hopeless but recognized that certain advantages would accrue to him for his effort! Although his surgical experience was extraordinarily rich and his clinical acumen legendary, Dupuytren's written legacy is relatively meager and comprised mostly of a recapitulation of his clinical lectures (inset).

penetrating fork on noting a red inflamed mass on the anterior abdominal wall 5 months after the fork had been ingested. He was a shrewd enough clinician to persuade a colleague, Cayroche of Mende, to remove this foreign body (May 1, 1819) via an anterior abdominal incision. Delpech was subsequently assassinated by a former patient who felt that a varicocele operation had rendered him impotent.

Sedillot subsequently reported the first successful construction of a gastrostomy (November 13, 1849) using a technique not much different from that developed originally by Blondlot to study gastric secretion in dogs. Nevertheless, the principal contributions in surgery at that time emanated from the work of Dupuytren. Few surgeons have evoked more controversy and divergent opinions. He was variously known as "*the first of surgeons and the least of men*" and a "*genius but of unprecedented unkindness and coldness.*" Born on October 5, 1777, to a family of modest means, his extraordinary intelligence was apparent from an early age.

In 1802, at the age of 25, he was appointed to the Hôtel-Dieu, and by 1815 he was chief surgeon, a post he held until his death some 20 years later. Despite the fact that he dressed with appalling taste and that his personal habits left much to be desired, he was highly regarded not only as a teacher but also as a surgeon of extraordinary intellectual and technical proficiency. His workload was extraordinary, and it is reported that at the apogee of his career, he would see some 10,000 private patients a year.

Although Dupuytren's fame as a surgeon and teacher was prodigious, he wrote little, and most of his work is recollected by renditions of his lectures in notebook form. The majority of his teachings were collated in a book entitled *Leçons Orales* and published by his students. His teachings cover a diverse range of conditions ranging from anorectal problems to chronic bleeding, arterial aneurysms, urinary calculi, and cataract management. Among his notable contributions are the following: He classified burns, was the first to remove the mandible, drained brain abscesses, treated torticollis by surgery, and performed cervical excision for uterine cancer. His comments on duodenal ulceration were of critical relevance. Although Curling, in 1841, had called attention to the connection between cases of burn and acute ulceration of the duodenum, it was Dupuytren who had first made this observation. In 1836, he drew attention to the congestion of various mucous membranes in the alimentary canal in the early stages of burns. He described in detail the ulceration and bleeding of the stomach and duodenum consequent on such an event some 5 years before Curling provided the definitive description of duodenal ulceration associated with cutaneous burning.

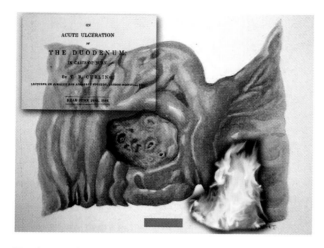

Moynihan stated that it was neither Curling nor Dupuytren but James Long of Liverpool who first described duodenal ulcer in two patients with burns in 1834. More than 150 years later, the nature of the relationship between burns and duodenal ulceration is still unresolved.

Dupuytren's contributions as a leader, surgeon, and teacher of surgery in Paris provided the foundations of the great surgical tradition that would initiate the performance of the first gastrectomy by Jules Emile Péan. Born in 1830 to the family of a miller, in 1855, Péan attended medical school in Paris, and in 1868, after training with Denon Villiers and Nelaton, was awarded a Doctor of Medicine degree in surgery. Péan's reputation as a clinician and a surgeon was prestigious. His day began early at the Augustine's and Frères-St.-Jean de Dieu surgical clinics, followed by surgery at the St. Louis Hospital, and would continue at night until well after dinner. Although his initial contributions to abdominal surgery were in the area of ovarian cystectomy, in 1867, he undertook the first successful splenectomy during a laparotomy for an ovarian cyst in which incidental damage to the spleen had occurred. A further major contribution, in 1868, was the development of a special hemostatic clip made by Gueride that he successfully used for hemostasis.

Doctor Péan operating, painting by Henri Toulouse Lautrec (1891–1892). In 1891, Lautrec shared an apartment with his friend Dr. Henri Bourges and became friendly with other physicians. Gabriel Tape de Celeyran was a cousin of Lautrec and had trained with Péan. It is likely that Lautrec had thus been invited to observe an operation and recorded it (oil on cardboard). Péan is operating on an oral lesion, presumably a forerunner of his epic contribution to gastric surgery (Sterling and Francine Clark Institute, Williamstown, MA). Lautrec's medical interest was not confined to surgery. He used pharmacologic compounds (thujones) contained in high concentration in absinthe to amplify his creativity and color perception.

On April 8, 1879, Péan undertook what was to be his most epic contribution to surgery by resecting a pyloric gastric cancer. The operation lasted $2^{1}/_{2}$ hours, and the patient initially recovered successfully. Unfortunately, over the subsequent 3 days, the patient received two blood transfusions of 50 and 80 mL and died on the fifth postoperative day, before a further transfusion. Although the cause of death is unknown, the recognition of blood groups did not occur until some 40 years later, and it seems likely that either sepsis or transfusion incompatibility may have contributed to this fatality. Nevertheless, to Péan goes the credit for having undertaken the first (albeit unsuccessful) gastrectomy.

On November 16, 1880, Ludwig Rydiger of Chelmo performed the second documented, but also unsuccess-

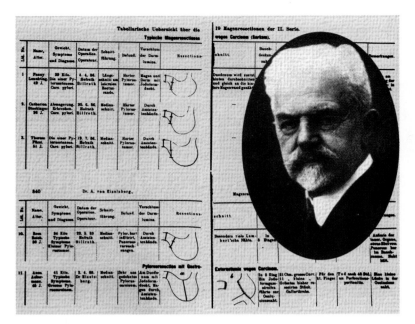

After his training with Billroth, Anton von Eiselberg achieved considerable recognition as a surgical leader and contributed extensively to the technical modifications of gastrectomy.

ful, gastrectomy. Like Péan, he undertook a partial resection of the prepyloric portion of the stomach in a patient with gastric cancer. Some 2 months later, in Vienna, Billroth became the first surgeon to successfully undertake a gastrectomy. The third reported gastrectomy was also for a pyloric tumor, but in this instance, the patient, Theresa Heller, survived to be discharged home 3 weeks postoperatively. The cumulative operative survival from gastrectomy in the 2 decades after Péan's initial operation rarely exceeded 50%.

As a result of the substantial mortality involved in gastrectomy in the preantiseptic era, lesser procedures were usually contemplated in an attempt to deal with diseases of the stomach thought to require surgical intervention.

The most popular operation was the gastroenterostomy, pioneered by Mathieu Jaboulay. Born on July 5, 1860, and educated in the Lyon area, he achieved wide renown as a surgeon of considerable intellectual and technical skill. One of his initial accomplishments had been to remove the vagi, coeliac ganglion, and sympathetic chains of the upper abdomen in an attempt to deal with the discomfort induced by the lightning pains of tabes dorsalis. Jaboulay's later development of the gastroenterostomy procedure to obviate problems generated by the gastric outlet obstruction consequent on vagotomy achieved widespread popularity in Europe.

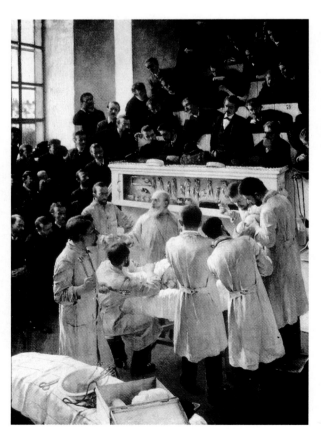

Theodor Billroth in the auditorium of the Allgemeine Krankenhaus in Vienna, by A. F. Seligman, 1889. In 1890, the painting was exhibited at the Society of Artists in Vienna, where it was severely criticized by A. Ilg. In Munich, the work was highly regarded. At the World's Fair in Chicago and Madrid, it received a bronze medal and, in Berlin and London, a gold medal. In 1904, it was purchased by the Ministry of Education and presented to Hochenegg, Chief of the Billroth clinic. Unfortunately, the painting was lost until Karel B. Absolon was able to locate it during a visit to Vienna. Bottcher hands Billroth the scalpel. Josef Winter holds the anesthetized patient's head. To Winter's left is Anton Eiselberg, the anesthetist. Leo Dittel is next to him and, finally, Salzer. The assistant, with the scissors, is Heidenthaller. Sitting is Beck. Left, in the lowest row, is Karl Theodor, the Duke of Bavaria, who commonly attended Billroth's lectures. The painter, A. F. Seligman, is in the first row on the right. The medical student standing in the first row is Alphons Rosthorn, the gynecologist. The patient is an old man suffering from trigeminal neuralgia, who has a neurotomy performed.

The pathologic specimens of the stomach and tumor (resected in 1881 by Billroth) of Theresa Heller, on display at the Josephinum in Vienna. The left bottle is the resection specimen, containing the obstructed pyloric antrum that was successfully resected. The right specimen is of the stomach, recovered at autopsy 3$\frac{1}{2}$ months later, when the patient died of hepatic metastases. The patent gastroduodenal anastomosis is evident. It is worthy of note that more than a century later, the survival of patients with gastric cancer has not improved appreciably since the first intervention by Billroth.

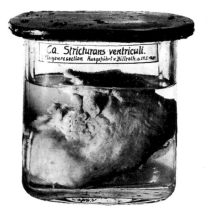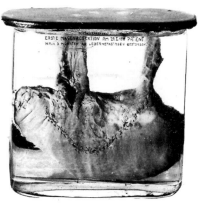

Indeed, gastroenterostomy remained the standard of choice for the first 2 to 3 decades of the twentieth century as the preferred surgical treatment of either peptic ulcer or gastric neoplasia.

Thereafter, better techniques developed to ensure the safety of the anastomosis after gastric resection, and with the advent of Listerian antisepsis, the era of the gastrectomist supervened. The early use of gastrectomy in peptic ulcer disease focused on the management of complications such as obstruction and bleeding. Initial problems related to the leakage of the anastomosis between the duodenum and the gastric remnant led to the widespread acceptance of the gastrojejunal anastomosis known as the *Billroth II*.

The significant disturbances in physiology consequent on this procedure (dumping syndromes, afferent and efferent loop syndromes) were thought tolerable as compared to the invariable mortality associated with a leak from a Billroth I–type anastomosis.

To obviate the development of such symptomatology, a great number of modifications of the procedure, involving the construction of valves or different bowel loop lengths, were introduced, almost to no avail. Similarly, the recognition of the high rates of ulcer recurrence with vagotomy alone led to the amplification of the magnitude of gastric resection in an attempt to decrease the acid-secreting area. The further addition of antrectomy to remove the source of gastrin accentuated the diminution of gastric reservoir size and augmented the difficulties experienced by the patient.

A loss of gastric receptive relaxation engendered by the vagotomy added to the problem of early satiety and, compounded with a variety of postgastrectomy syndromes, served to establish a patient group with an entirely new disease complex initiated by the sequelae of surgical intervention.

Modifications of Gastrectomy

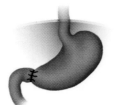

Classic Billroth I
1881

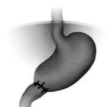

Standard Billroth I

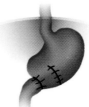

Kocher 1891

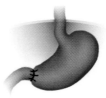

Shoemaker 1911

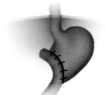

Von Haberer 1922
Finney 1923

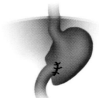

Kutscha-Lissberg 1925

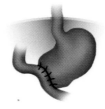

Winklebauer 1927

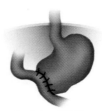

Leriche 1927

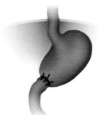

Von Haberer 1933

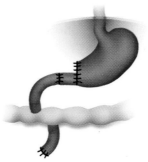

Henley 1952

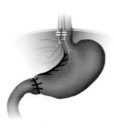

Harkins & Nyhus 1962

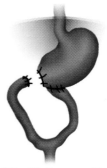

BII with Roux en Y

Some examples of the numerous varieties of gastric resection devised to facilitate safety and ameliorate postoperative symptoms.

Billroth II Gastrectomies

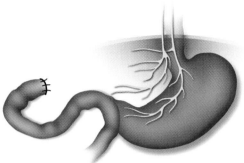

Billroth II Anastomosis

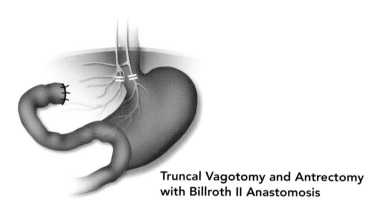

Truncal Vagotomy and Antrectomy with Billroth II Anastomosis

The Billroth II anastomosis was used because it was a safer technical procedure than the Billroth I anastomosis. Although the Billroth I anastomosis often leaked, it more or less reproduced an anatomic likeness, even though the pylorus was absent. On the contrary, while the anastomosis of the jejunum to the stomach (Billroth II) rarely leaked, it produced a substantially different anatomic configuration with consequent major metabolic derangements, collectively referred to as *the postgastrectomy syndrome*. Unless acid-suppressive medication is unavailable, vagotomy is rarely used even if gastric resection is required.

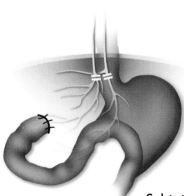

Subtotal Gastrectomy and Vagotomy with Billroth II Anastomosis

Surgery of the vagus

Although investigations of the vagus nerve began as long ago as 2,000 years, it has only been within the last century that its role in the regulation of acid secretion became apparent. Armed with this knowledge, a handful of surgeons appreciated the therapeutic possibilities of interfering with vagal innervation of the stomach. To a large extent, the consideration of such surgery reflected the recent introduction of anesthesia and antisepsis, which enabled body cavities to be entered with some degree of safety. Brodie, early in the nineteenth century, had identified that the vagus played a role in gastric secretion, and by the turn of the century, Pavlov had delineated the neural regulation of gastric secretion.

At almost the same time that Pavlov was experimenting with vagotomy in dogs, other intrepid surgeons were attempting this operation on humans. It seems probable that, in the late nineteenth century, Jaboulay of France performed the first vagotomy on a human patient. Jaboulay excised the celiac plexus of a man suffering from the lightning pains of tabes dorsalis. A few years later, Exner similarly divided the vagi in a number of patients afflicted with tabes but presciently observed that a percentage of these individuals subsequently suffered from the effects of gastric atony.

He later combined vagotomy with a gastrojejunostomy to promote gastric emptying. In time, other surgeons, including Kuttner, Borchers, and Podkaminsky, attempted vagotomies on patients. By 1920, the results of 20 subdiaphragmatic vagotomies for treatment of gastric ptosis were reported by Bircher. He observed decreased acidity and, curiously, improved tonus in 75% of his patients. Alvarez reviewed the work of Bircher and concluded: "*His vagotomies were probably incomplete because, aside from some lowering of acidity, he did not seem to obtain the usual effects of a complete nerve resection.*"

The outcome of these early clinical vagotomies inspired M. A. Latarjet of Lyon to further evaluate the procedure. Latarjet made the most detailed investigations into the anatomy of the vagi to date and applied his findings to the

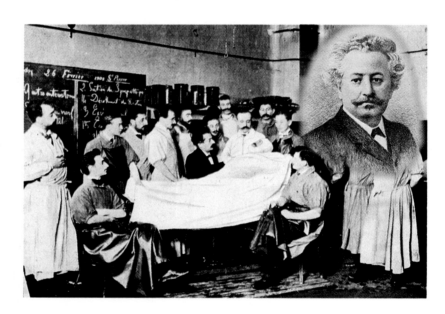

Jaboulay (1901) demonstrating his surgical skills in a picture taken by Harvey Cushing during his tour of French surgical clinics en route to work with T. Kocher in Berne. The lack of masks and gloves and the formal suit of the principal surgeon (M. J.) reflect the current state of surgical antiseptic technique. Inset: A portrait of Mathieu Jaboulay, 1895. Although Anton Wolfler (1850–1917) had introduced gastroenterostomy in 1881, the technique devised by Jaboulay was subsequently most widely used.

M. A. Latarjet of Lyon, in 1922, first described vagotomy for the management of peptic ulcer disease and confirmed that it caused amelioration of symptoms as well as decrease in acid secretion.

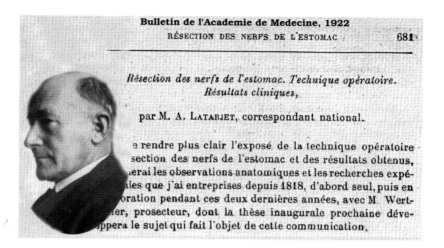

Bulletin de l'Academie de Medecine, 1922
RÉSECTION DES NERFS DE L'ESTOMAC 681

Résection des nerfs de l'estomac. Technique opératoire.
Résultats cliniques,

par M. A. LATARJET, correspondant national.

e rendre plus clair l'exposé de la technique opératoire section des nerfs de l'estomac et des résultats obtenus, erai les observations anatomiques et les recherches expé- les que j'ai entreprises depuis 1818, d'abord seul, puis en oration pendant ces deux dernières années, avec M. Wert- er, prosecteur, dont la thèse inaugurale prochaine déve- ppera le sujet qui fait l'objet de cette communication.

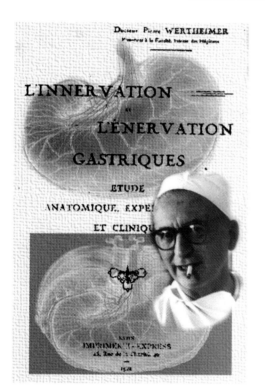

Wertheimer's (right) thesis, De l'Enervation Gastriques, 1921, provided the anatomic information necessary to enable M. Latarjet to successfully undertake vagotomy.

surgical patients he treated. The eponymous attribution of the anterior and posterior vagal nerves of the gastric lesser curve attests to his profound influence and excellent work in this area.

Latarjet was born on August 20, 1877, in Dijon and studied medicine in Lyon. Because of financial pressures, Latarjet was forced to choose between a primary career in surgery or anatomy. The pathway to a practice in surgery was difficult in the hospitals of Lyon, and Latarjet was not financially able to support himself in private practice. He therefore chose a career based principally in anatomy. As an anatomist, he never relinquished his initial dedication to surgery and, together with Raymond Gregoire in Paris, became one of the champions in the field of what was later to become known as *applied anatomy*. His research was directed broadly toward the innervation of the abdominal organs. Thus, over a period of 20 years, he wrote extensively on nerves of the colon, the biliary tract, and the pelvis in both men and women. The detailed study of the hypogastric and sacral plexuses in females resulted in the development of a surgical treatment for dysmenorrhea (*operation de cotte*).

Probably his most important contribution relates to the work undertaken with his colleague Pierre Wertheimer.

In 1921, Wertheimer completed his thesis *De l'Enervation Gastriques*. This study documents both anatomic and experimental work in regard to the vagal innervation of the stomach. Of particular note is the observation that cutting the vagi significantly impaired gastric motility and emptying and resulted in a substantial inhibition of acid secretion. The subsequent publication in 1923 of the surgical studies in which vagotomy and a drainage procedure were used resulted in the international recognition of Latarjet's contributions and his eponymous attribution to the gastric vagi. Some 2 decades later, on January 14, 1943, in Chicago, at the Merrit Billings Hospital, Lester Dragstedt undertook the first truncal vagotomy in North America.

The subsequent enthusiasm for vagotomy as a method of managing duodenal ulcer disease brought further recognition to the contributions of Latarjet in defining the physiologic and therapeutic possibilities of the vagus.

The principal difference between the work of Latarjet and his predecessors was his decision to perform vagotomy in a systematic manner for patients with dyspepsia. His operation, first reported in 1921, entailed denervation of the greater and lesser curvatures and the suprapyloric region, with partial circumcision of the serosa and muscularis down to the level of the submucosa. He designed this operation to sever all the extrinsic nerves to the stomach and pylorus, leaving intact the large branch of the right gastric nerve that accompanies the left gastric artery to the celiac plexus.

In 1922, Latarjet reported his results on 24 patients to the French Academy of Surgery. Like Exner before him, he found delayed gastric emptying in many of these vagotomized patients and later added a gastrojejunostomy to this operation. He explained, *"Indeed, in all of our cases, gastroenteroanastomosis was done at the same time as denervation, either for reasons of promoting mechanical order or to avoid the possibility of an aggravated ulcer evolution as a consequence of the prolonged journey of food in a stomach which has been rendered hypotonic by denervation."* Almost 30 years later, Lester Dragstedt would come to a virtually identical conclusion.

As early as 1927, Charles Mayo was aware that operations not based on sound physiologic principles have no place in the surgical repertoire: *"If anyone should consider removing half of my good stomach to cure a small ulcer in my duodenum, I would run faster than he"* (C. H. Mayo, 1927).

Similarly, surgeons who wish to introduce new procedures must first determine, in the surgical laboratory, the anatomic and physiologic sequelae of their proposed operations. Only when an experimental operation has been shown to be physiologically sound may it be applied for use on patients. The development of the operative procedure known as a *vagotomy* initially followed such a course.

Unfortunately, Latarjet never formally confirmed that vagotomy was a successful therapy for peptic ulcer disease. One theory of ulcerogenesis popular during the 1920s was that ulcers were caused by gastric stasis. Thus, some of his contemporaries proposed that the fine results of his procedure might be attributed to the concomitant gastroenterostomy—not the vagotomy. Indeed, for this reason and possibly because of the provincial location of Lyon, his pioneering work was received with little enthusiasm by his colleagues. Fewer than 100 of these operations were performed before 1940, and Latarjet published nothing further related to his operative procedure after 1923.

At approximately the same time that Latarjet was conducting his studies, E. D'Arcy McCrea of Manchester, England, published an extensive and often-cited review of anatomy, physiology, and surgical treatment of the vagi. McCrea argued that *"operative interference with the nerves of the stomach is*

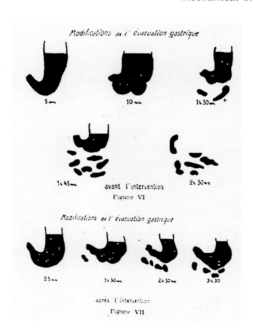

Laterjet's studies of gastric emptying, undertaken in 1922. As a consequence of vagotomy, gastric stasis was noted and then quantified by the use of radio-opaque material and serial radiographic pictures. These investigations documented the need for a surgical drainage procedure of the stomach to be a component of the operation of vagotomy.

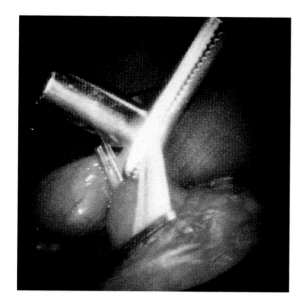

Laparoscopic vagotomy. In recent times, it has been proposed that the advantages of minimally invasive surgery would facilitate the undertaking of acid-inhibitory operations such as vagotomy. The minimal physiologic consequences of surgery without laparotomy, combined with the ability to clearly define vagal anatomy, have been proposed as providing significant advantages for this mode of vagal section. The widespread availability and safety of PPIs have rendered vagotomy, for the most part, an archaic procedure irrespective of the technology used to sever the nerves.

both feasible and in certain instances justifiable." He recognized, however, that physiology of vagal function was, in many instances, not clear.

McCrea claimed that the vagi were either "augmentors" or "inhibitors" of gastric function. In his studies, he noted that the "*vagi regulate both tonus and movement, and moreover, that these may be independent of one another.*" In the resting stomach, the vagi served as augmentors, he argued, but in the actively digesting organ, their work was that of an inhibitor. The theories of McCrea were novel, because he was the first to recognize the vagi as a potential cause of disease: "*A lesion of the gastric or duodenal wall, the result of infection or injury is more likely to become chronic if an irritation of the nerves is set up.*" He further speculated that "*local spasm with resultant anemia is a probable cause of the chronicity of ulcer aided by factors such as retention and infection set up by reflex spasm.*" A lesion in any part of the nerve path, he contended, caused the ulcer to develop.

McCrea, however, was ambiguous. He contradicted himself in relating these nerve lesions and their therapy to acid secretion and its clinical sequelae, and his inconsistencies negated, to a certain extent, his recommendation of a Latarjet operation for peptic ulcer disease. Thus, although the review by McCrea was widely read and generally accepted, it appears to have done little to promote the therapeutic use of vagotomy. In fact, very little was written about and very few operations were performed on the vagus nerves during the next 2 decades. Indeed, the standard antiulcer operation in the first half of the twentieth century was either a partial gastrectomy or gastroenterostomy.

The nerves of Latarjet. The branches of the vagus nerve passing down the lesser curvature supply both the fundus and antrum. Based on the results of denervation at surgery and under experimental conditions, it seems likely that the vagal branches to the fundus are responsible for the regulation of acid secretion and motility, whereas those to the antrum are of importance in regulating gastrin release and gastric emptying. Of more relevance at this time is the role of the central neural mechanisms of secretory regulation in the modulation of mucosal cellular function. It is more likely that the development of specific pharmacologic probes designed to target local neurotransmitters or their receptors will be more effective than neural ablation and its consequent indiscriminate physiologic sequelae.

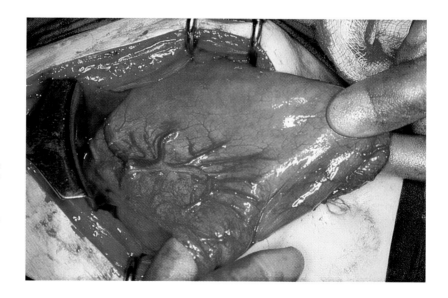

On January 18, 1943, Dragstedt performed a subdiaphragmatic vagal resection on a patient with an active duodenal ulcer and so ushered in the modern era of vagotomy. Dragstedt concentrated his research on the pathogenesis of peptic ulcer disease. He was fascinated by the work of Hunter and Bernard, which showed that normal stomachs do not digest themselves. He recognized that *"pure gastric juice as it is secreted by the fundus of the stomach, has the capacity to destroy and digest various living tissues, including the wall of the jejunum, duodenum, and even the stomach itself. It does not do this under normal conditions because the usual and appropriate stimulus to gastric secretion is ingestion of food. This dilutes and neutralizes the gastric juice and decreases its corrosive powers."* He did not recognize the high acidity that often occurs.

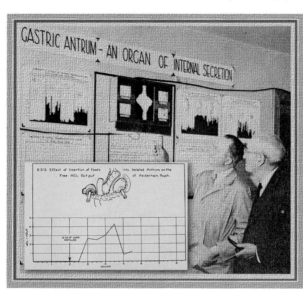

L. Dragstedt and A. Carlson, c. 1950. As a young man, Dragstedt, who came from a small copper-mining town, Anaconda, Montana, had been influenced by Carlson, then Chairman of Physiology at the University of Chicago. Both their families had immigrated from the Göteborg area of Sweden, and this close personal and professional relationship lasted throughout their lives. Carlson was a brilliant and rigorous investigator who had begun his life in America by training as a religious minister. No doubt this background provided grist for his famous comment to all his pupils and at meetings: "What is the evidence?" Apart from his contribution to the neural regulation of acid secretion, Dragstedt confirmed Edkins' original proposal of the existence of an antral regulator (gastrin). The graphic insert demonstrates the effect of food in an antral pouch on HCl output of a Heidenhain pouch. With exquisite surgical technique, Dragstedt designed models to test his physiologic hypotheses. In this study, he confirmed the original hypothesis (50 years previously) of Edkins that antral gastrin would function as a hormone to drive fundic acid secretion.

Dragstedt further postulated that mucosal damage takes place at night, when people do not eat, and that this acid secretion was of nervous origin. He disagreed with his colleagues who speculated that ulcers were caused by diminished mucosal resistance to injury. The key to understanding ulcerogenesis, he reiterated, was acid secretion and, in support of his theory, presented two stimuli of acid hypersecretion: neural and hormonal. In citation of his own experiments, he demonstrated clear evidence that neural stimulation caused increased output of gastric acid. Results of studies from his laboratories of nocturnal output of acid in patients with duodenal ulcers clearly demonstrated levels to be 3 to 20 times that of normal patients. He termed this phenomenon *fasting hypersecretion.* He also noted the clinical success of vagotomy as further evidence of the importance of neural input to acid secretion. Dragstedt recognized that hormonal stimulation could also account for acid hypersecretion. First, he cited the work of Pavlov, in which acid secretion had been elicited in response to food introduced into denervated gastric pouches. Next, he somewhat ungenerously credited Edkins, who had postulated the existence of gastrin, with *"one of the most remarkable guesses in the history of gastrointestinal physiology."* Gastrin, Edkins had said, was secreted into the blood stream by the mucous membrane in the antrum in response to contact with food or the primary products of digestion.

Dragstedt admitted the validity of Edkins' theory only after he conducted his own experiments. In these studies, Dragstedt excised and transplanted the antrum from a denervated stomach of a dog to its abdominal wall and found markedly reduced gastric secretion. When the antrum was reimplanted with the duodenum, normal gastric secretion resumed. With these studies, he not only confirmed the findings of Edkins, but also established a fundamental observation—that gastrin secretion did not take place in an acid environment. Thus, Dragstedt recognized and described the existence of a feedback mechanism dependent on mucosal pH for the control of secretion of gastrin. In so doing, he produced physiologic proof of the antral regulation of acid secretion that could be used to support the rationale for the introduction of the surgical application of antrectomy.

After delineating aspects of the regulation of gastric secretion, Dragstedt sought the mechanism of ulcer formation. He claimed that duodenal ulcers were of nervous origin (a proposal originally made by Rokitansky of Vienna in 1860) and postulated that the pathologic nervous stimuli that resulted in duodenal ulcers were transmitted by the vagi.

Gastric ulcers, he claimed, were caused by abnormal hormonal stimuli. They resulted from gastric stasis, which caused prolonged antral contact with food and, hence, hypersecretion of gastrin.

From this generous theoretical background, Dragstedt set out to provide a surgical cure for patients with peptic ulcer disease. The operation he proposed was a total vagotomy. The first patient to receive a Dragstedt vagotomy was a 35-year-old man who had a bleeding ulcer necessitating multiple blood transfusions despite medical therapy. The young man underwent a bilateral vagotomy by way of a left thoracotomy approach, and his abdominal pain immediately subsided. Dragstedt, always the physiologist, instilled 0.1 normal hydrochloric acid into the stomach of the patient for the next couple of weeks. For the first 8 days, he was able to reproduce the abdominal pain of the patient. On the ninth day, however, acid infusion no longer caused discomfort. Dragstedt took this to indicate that the ulcer had healed.

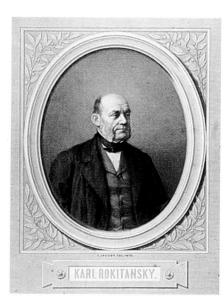

Karl Rokitansky (1804–1878) dissected more than 30,000 cadavers in his lifetime. Although he is best remembered for his studies of defects in the septum of the heart, he was the first to describe acute dilatation of the stomach. In addition, he was of the opinion that ulcer disease was due to abnormal function of the vagus nerve. Apart from his brilliance, and despite the fact that he was a pathologist, Rokitansky was a man possessed of considerable wit. Thus, of his four sons, two of whom were physicians and two singers, he said *"Die Einen heilen, die Anderen heulen."* (One group heals, the other howls.)

Dragstedt went on to perform more than 200 vagotomies during the next 4 years because of its physiologic basis and clinical success. Approximately one-third of these patients had gastric stasis develop that was severe enough to necessitate a gastroenterostomy as a secondary procedure.

To perform these operations simultaneously, an abdominal approach to the vagi was developed. Initially, the drainage procedure of choice was a gastroenterostomy. During the next decade, however, the technique of pyloroplasty was perfected and became the drainage method of choice. Later, as the role of the antrum in the physiology of gastric secretion became better understood, vagotomy combined with antrectomy was the procedure used to reduce the secretion of gastric acid maximally.

Despite the clinical success of Dragstedt and his physiologic arguments favoring vagotomy for peptic ulcer disease, his medical and surgical colleagues in general resisted his methods. Nonetheless, a number of pioneering surgeons dared to try his techniques on patients with difficult ulcers. Such surgeons as Grimson and Ruffin from Duke University, Walters from Rochester, Minnesota, and Moore from Massachusetts General Hospital performed approximately 200 vagotomies. Their findings were presented at the Central Surgical Association meeting in Chicago in February 1947.

By this time, surgeons from the Mayo Clinic, a relatively conservative institution, had performed approximately 80 of these operations. They termed the Dragstedt procedure a *gastric neurectomy* and observed that *"the results are inconstant, variable and in most cases unpredictable"* (Waltman et al., 1947). The most serious complication they encountered was gastric stasis.

Surgical Procedures for Maximal Acid Suppression

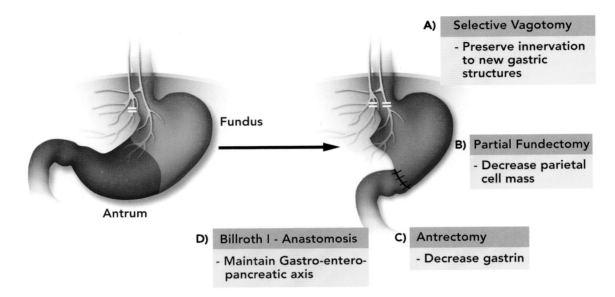

A) Selective Vagotomy
- Preserve innervation to new gastric structures

B) Partial Fundectomy
- Decrease parietal cell mass

C) Antrectomy
- Decrease gastrin

D) Billroth I - Anastomosis
- Maintain Gastro-entero-pancreatic axis

Fundus

Antrum

At least four procedures were proposed as necessary to optimize and maximize acid-suppressive operations for peptic ulcer disease: (a) selective vagotomy; (b) partial fundectomy; (c) antrectomy; and (d) Billroth I anastomosis.

Their conclusions were in contrast with that of Francis Moore of Boston, who reported in the same volume of *Archives of Surgery*. Moore found an 87% success rate and claimed that the complication of gastrostasis was only temporary. But the surgeons from Duke disagreed. "*Complete satisfaction occurred more frequently among the patients with combined vagotomy and gastroenterostomy than among patients with vagotomy alone. Transthoracic vagotomy alone should not be used as a standard treatment of duodenal or gastric ulcer*" (Grimson et al., 1947). In the next year, clinical investigators from around the United States reported conflicting conclusions. Jackson, from Ann Arbor, Michigan, detailed his abdominal approach to vagotomy and suggested that the operation was feasible for residents to perform.

Francis Moore reiterated this positive view and concluded that "*vague resection is not a cure for duodenal ulcer; it is a physiologic procedure which, by removing the majority of the parasympathetic nerves to the upper gastrointestinal tract renders the management of patients with duodenal ulcer a simple rather than a complicated problem.*"

Thus, the practicing surgeons of 1948 had no definite recommendation from their peers in academia. In an attempt to establish a reasonable answer, the American Gastroenterological Association formed the National Committee on Peptic Ulcer in 1952. In a 200 page report, the committee concluded that gastroenterostomy was the operation of choice for peptic ulcer disease and emphasized: "*It should not be concluded from this study that gastro-enterostomy plus vagotomy is superior to gastro-enterostomy alone.*" Fortunately, not all surgeons were persuaded, and the usefulness of vagotomy continued to be investigated.

Gradually, more favorable reports appeared. In 1952, Farmer and Smithwick, from Boston University, recommended that vagotomy be combined with hemigastrectomy for treatment of duodenal ulcer disease. They observed that more than

Gastric Drainage Procedures

A. Heineke-Mikulicz pyloroplasty, B. Finney pyloroplasty,
C. Exclusion pyloroplasty, D. Posterior Gastroenterostomy,
E. Anterior juxtapyloric gastroenterostomy,
F. Pyloric dilation by gastrotomy

Vagotomy, particularly of the truncal variety, often resulted in antral and pyloric motor dysfunction and gastric stasis. A wide variety of drainage procedures was developed to obviate this problem.

80% of the patients they treated who had this operation suffered no serious side effects, and that 93% of these patients had a gastric pH of 3.5 or greater after acid stimulation with either broth or injection with insulin. Refinements in operative technique also yielded better results. By 1956, Weinberg and his colleagues from the Veterans Hospital in Long Beach, California, described an improved single-layer pyloroplasty. The single-layer method contrasted with the double-layer closure of the Heinecke-Mikulicz procedure, which the authors contended could *"cause an infolding of the tissues which constricts the lumen and thus jeopardizes the patency of the canal."* They reported their results using a single-layer pyloroplasty on more than 500 patients and found a 5% recurrence rate and a 5% rate of side effects. They attributed these fine results to the elimination of the retrograde movement of food seen with gastrojejunal anastomoses.

Nevertheless, it was apparent that better methods of preventing gastric stasis were necessary to obviate the side effects of truncal vagotomy. Griffith and Harkins published the theoretic basis for a more selective vagotomy in 1957. They further defined the gastric vagal anatomy and performed a partial vagotomy in ten dogs. They incised the branches of the nerves of Latarjet, which were thought to *"supply clusters of parietal cells."* As a result, they concluded that the cephalic phase of gastric secretion was eliminated, and these dogs experienced minimal to no gastric stasis. Even though they proposed that *"clinical application appears feasible,"* 10 years elapsed before the first selective vagotomy was performed on a human.

Holle and Hart performed the first highly selective vagotomy in 1967. Their procedure was combined with a pyloroplasty. By 1969, it became apparent that a drainage procedure was unnecessary. The technique was further developed to selectively denervate the fundus while retaining antral innervation to facilitate gastric emptying. The term *parietal cell vagotomy* was used to describe operative procedure. Experience from Britain, Scandinavia, and the United States demonstrated only 17 deaths after 5,539 highly successful vagotomies. These reports also documented decreased dumping, gastritis, and duodenal reflux as compared with the more traditional operations. The ulcer recurrence rate after this operation was reported at approximately 5%, a result similar to that after truncal vagotomy and drainage. Subsequent authors, however, reported substantial increases in recurrence rates over time, even after the learning curve for this procedure had been overcome.

Surgical Evolution of Vagotomy

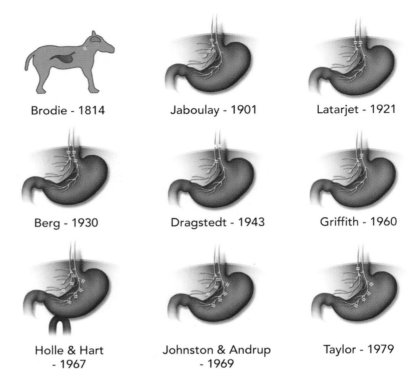

Brodie - 1814

Jaboulay - 1901

Latarjet - 1921

Berg - 1930

Dragstedt - 1943

Griffith - 1960

Holle & Hart
- 1967

Johnston & Andrup
- 1969

Taylor - 1979

In an attempt to minimize the extent of vagal resection, numerous procedures designed to improve selectivity were devised. The objective was to only denervate the parietal cell mass, without interfering with the innervation of the antrum, pylorus, and extragastric organs.

These observations and the technical tedium of the microvagal dissection led to the search for alternative procedures. Taylor of Edinburgh developed a lesser-curve superficial seromyotomy. Initial results from 32 patients revealed no recurrence of ulcer with a short follow-up period. Subsequently, Lygidakis modified the technique of Taylor by performing a posterior truncal vagotomy combined with an anterior superficial seromyotomy. This modification left intact the anterior motor component of the nerve of Latarjet, all that was needed to ensure normal gastric motility. A further putative advantage of the superficial seromyotomy was the fact that it was a far more rapid procedure than the relatively tedious, highly selective vagotomy.

The therapeutic relevance of vagal section has for the most part been overshadowed by the use of acid-inhibitory agents. Indeed, except in conditions of dire emergency, surgical vagotomy should no longer be considered as a means of inhibiting acid secretion.

CHAPTER 2
PEPTIC ULCER DISEASE

General

Although the incidence of peptic ulcer disease has steadily declined in the United States since the turn of the twentieth century, approximately 500,000 new cases and 4 million recurrences annually are reported. In 1990, it was estimated that the annual direct cost related to diagnosis and treatment of peptic ulcer disease in the United States was between 3 and 4 billion dollars, compared to the 2.5 million dollars estimated in 1975.

Duodenal ulcer is the major lesion in Western populations, whereas gastric ulcers are more frequent in Asian countries, particularly Japan. Japanese-Americans develop duodenal ulcers, showing that the frequency of gastric ulcers in Japan is due to environmental factors, not genetic constitution.

Although less prevalent than duodenal ulcer, gastric ulcer (0.1% of the population in developed countries) has a higher associated mortality and a greater morbidity resulting from hemorrhage, perforation, and obstruction. Frequent recurrence after healing has been a major component of the natural history of gastric ulcer, and without therapy, ulcers recur in 35% to 80% of the patients within 6 to 12 months of healing.

The advent of *H. pylori* eradication and appropriate acid-suppressive therapy in recent times has considerably narrowed the gap in therapeutic outcome between gastric and duodenal ulcers. The recognition that two of the major factors in defining gastric ulcer, namely *H. pylori* and NSAIDs, can be therapeutically addressed is mostly responsible for this advance. Therapy, therefore, for gastric ulcers has exhibited a remarkable transition, as PPI therapy combined with *H. pylori* eradication produced healing and recurrence

Despite the fact that *H. pylori* was unrecognized until 1983, it has in the last decade become regarded as the most common cause (85% to 95%) of all duodenal ulcers.

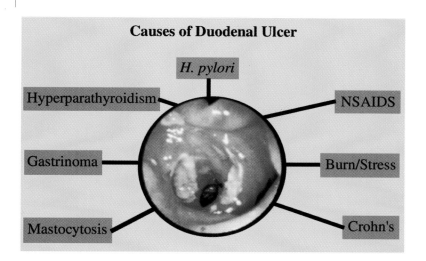

Causes of Duodenal Ulcer

Hyperparathyroidism

H. pylori

NSAIDS

Gastrinoma

Burn/Stress

Mastocytosis

Crohn's

rates quite similar to those obtained with duodenal ulceration. Similarly, the recognition of NSAID involvement and the use of prophylaxis with acid suppressants or prostaglandins or withdrawal of the NSAID has further amplified healing rates. The introduction of curative therapy whereby *H. pylori* may be eradicated has been a further significant advance in eliminating the cause of gastric ulceration. The important caveat is that in all patients with gastric ulceration, an underlying neoplastic process should be considered and eliminated as a possibility. Multiple biopsies of the ulcer margin and rigorous histologic evaluation are critical to ensure that there is no delay in identifying an ulcer of malignant origin. Indeed, the failure of a gastric ulcer to heal in the face of a compliance with a curative regime (PPI therapy and *H. pylori* eradication) should be regarded as an alarm symptom or a sign suggestive of gastric neoplasia.

In this context, the consideration of mucosal-associated lymphoid tumors (MALTs) should not be overlooked. Epidemiologic studies have concluded that *H. pylori* infection is the major cause of gastric cancer worldwide. The infection increases the risk of gastric adenocarcinoma by three to six times, probably by promoting the development of chronic atrophic gastritis. In addition, *H. pylori* increases the likelihood of the development of the primary non-Hodgkin's lymphoma MALT by approximately sixfold. In the majority of circumstances, however, the eradication of *H. pylori* is associated with complete remission of this disease process.

The early introduction of appropriate therapeutic measures once a gastric ulcer has been diagnosed will likely lead to a cure rate in at least 90% of individuals. Ensuring that NSAID therapy is withdrawn and *H. pylori* are eradicated is mandatory in individuals who exhibit recurrence of ulceration. Under such circumstances, however, rigorous endoscopic reassessment by biopsy for the presence of neoplasia should be undertaken. In those individuals who experience a complication, such as hemorrhage, perforation, or obstruction, appropriate surgical intervention is necessary. Although bleeding gastric ulcers may be under-run with a suture, more often than not, they are better managed by appropriate tailored surgical resection. Perforation, which in the past used to mandate resection for management, is currently more often managed by repair of the defect followed by appropriate acid-suppressive and *H. pylori* eradication therapy. In some circumstances, anatomic considerations may mandate resection, particularly in ulcers close to the gastroesophageal junction on the lesser curve.

Chronic gastric obstruction, usually in the juxtapyloric region, usually mandates gastric resection with establishment of a Billroth II anastomosis. Overall, however, the picture of gastric ulcer disease as a difficult problem with a high level of complication often necessitating surgical intervention has declined significantly and has more and more begun to resemble duodenal ulcer as a pathologic process amenable to conservative medical therapy except in complicated circumstances.

Metaanalysis for predicting the degree of acid inhibition (elevation of pH for a given period of the day) showed that a mean intragastric pH of 3.0 for 18 hours per day provided an optimal healing for duodenal ulcer, indicating that

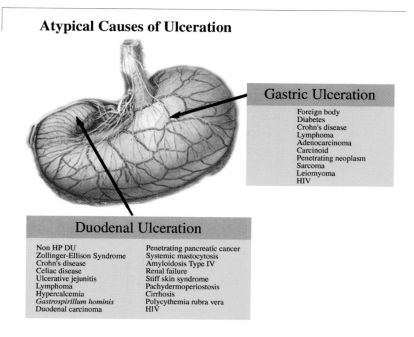

Atypical Causes of Ulceration

Gastric Ulceration

Foreign body
Diabetes
Crohn's disease
Lymphoma
Adenocarcinoma
Carcinoid
Penetrating neoplasm
Sarcoma
Leiomyoma
HIV

Duodenal Ulceration

Non HP DU	Penetrating pancreatic cancer
Zollinger-Ellison Syndrome	Systemic mastocytosis
Crohn's disease	Amyloidosis Type IV
Celiac disease	Renal failure
Ulcerative jejunitis	Stiff skin syndrome
Lymphoma	Pachydermoperiostosis
Hypercalcemia	Cirrhosis
Gastrospirillum hominis	Polycythemia rubra vera
Duodenal carcinoma	HIV

the duodenum was able to handle a significant pH load due to its ability to secrete HCO_3^-. Results of metaanalyses to predict healing of gastric ulcers as a function of pH have not been published. Still, current PPI therapy requires longer administration for healing of gastric, as compared to duodenal, ulcers, presumably because there is still wall acidity in the stomach impeding healing.

Pathogenesis

In the past, considerable attention had been directed to the role of acid in the generation of damage to the mucosa. Innumerable studies have correlated levels of acid secretion with ulceration. Pepsin had been noted as a cofactor in such pathology, but its precise role in the pathogenesis had been largely ignored in favor of a preoccupation with neutralizing or inhibiting acid secretion. Confounding factors, such as cigarette smoking, alcohol ingestion, and spicy foods, had been identified, but their precise involvement in mucosal damage remains controversial. The biology of the mucosa itself was not well understood. Cytoprotection had been proposed as a generic entity, embracing the concept of gastric mucosal defensive mechanisms. In broad terms, these were regarded as preepithelial, epithelial, and subepithelial. Each level was proposed to exhibit specialized properties that allowed the gastric epithelium to protect itself against the many noxious agents it was exposed to. A further philosophic entity entitled the *mucosal barrier* was conceived and variously considered to embrace the mucous bicarbonate barrier, specialized apical ion-transport systems, and tight junctions that provided an anatomic barrier for acid and pepsin diffusion.

The pathogenesis of peptic ulcer may best be viewed as representing a complex scenario involving an imbalance between defensive and aggressive factors, of which the most notable now appears to be *H. pylori*. Although mucosal restitution and the reestablishment of epithelial cell continuity independent of cell proliferation is an important issue closely linked to the expression of growth factors and mucosal integrity, the elucidation of its precise role still remains to be defined. Nevertheless, mucosal integrity as constituted by a variety of mucosal defense mechanisms is an important issue and will be dealt with separately in Section 4, Chapter 1.

Although the subject of *H. pylori* is separately dealt with further on, in Section 7, it is worthy of brief comment at this point in the context of noxious agents affecting the gastric mucosa. Its identification in 90% to 95% of patients with duodenal ulcer and 60% to 80% of patients with gastric ulcer, as compared to 25% to 30% incidences in symptomatic control subjects, confirms its relevance in the genesis of mucosal ulceration. The prevalence of infection increases with age, and infection is more common in those with deprived socioeconomic circumstances. It is apparent that, in some countries, infection is not always involved with peptic ulceration. Such observations have raised the issue as to whether all types of *H. pylori* are of equal pathogenicity. Nevertheless, given the fact that the lifetime prevalence for duodenal ulcer is approximately 10% for men and 5% for women, the importance of *H. pylori* as a component of the disease process is substantial. The recognition that there exists a critical association between gastric metaplasia in the duodenal cap and *H. pylori* that appears to confer a predisposition to ulcer disease has been clearly identified. Similarly, strong evidence has accumulated to demonstrate an association between the eradication of *H. pylori* infection and the cure of peptic ulcer disease.

The production of NH_3 by the urease of the organism may also explain part of the role of *H. pylori* in the generation of duodenal ulcer. It has been established that the majority of the urease activity of the organism is internal and acid activated. Activity reaches maximum at a pH of 6.0 and remains steady until a pH of 2.5. The toxicity of the NH_4^+ depends on entry of NH_3 with a consequent increase in intracellular pH and release of calcium from stores in the endoplasmic reticulum and mitochondria. At gastric pH, the ratio of NH_3 to NH_4^+ is low, but when at the neutral pH of the duodenum, the ratio rapidly rises, providing more NH_3 for entry into duodenal cells. Thus, the load of NH_3 to the duodenal cell may be a contributing factor to the generation of duodenal ulcers. This is discussed in more detail in the section on *H. pylori*.

pH and disease

There is considerable overlap between 24-hour intragastric pH measurements in normal individuals and in those with duodenal ulcer. Nevertheless, there appears to be greater gastric acid secretion in duodenal ulcer patients than normal subjects, particularly at night. Overall, however, the 24-hour pH profile is not predictive of duodenal ulcer in an individual patient. The suppression of nocturnal acid secretion by H_2 receptor antagonists proved effective in downregulating increased nocturnal acid secretion but is not essential to promote healing of a duodenal ulcer. Other factors, particularly duodenal bicarbonate secretion, have been proposed to be implicated in the genesis of duodenal ulceration. For the most part, however, duodenal mucosal bicarbon-

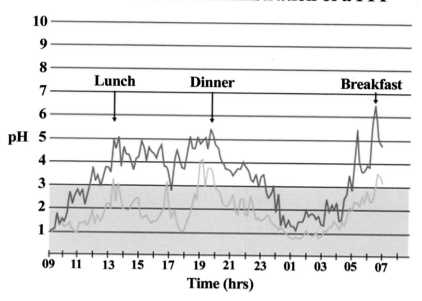

Median 24-hr Intragastric pH Profile Before and After Administration of a PPI

pH

Lunch   Dinner   Breakfast

Time (hrs)

The critical therapeutic ability of the PPIs to increase intragastric pH to above 3.0 for a considerable percentage of a 24-hour period is translated into a significant increase in ulcer healing for this class of drug. This pHmetric curve is generated after at least 3 days of treatment when inhibition of pumps has reached a balance between reactivation of inhibited pumps, de novo pump synthesis, and the action of the PPI after breakfast. The relatively poor acid control at night is due to absence of the drug at night when there are low rates of acid secretion into the unbuffered gastric lumen.

ate effects on luminal pH in the duodenal bulb may only be minor, because the overall secretory rate is in the range of 1 mmol per hour. Given the intermittent release of gastric chyme into the duodenum, a steep pH gradient exists between the terminal part of the pyloric antrum and the first part of the duodenum. When gastric pH values are below 4.0, the correlation between duodenal and gastric pH is linear, but this relationship disappears when the gastric pH is above 4.0; it is not possible to predict intraduodenal pH from intragastric pH during antisecretory therapy. Nevertheless, a series of meta-analytic studies of clinical trials that evaluated duodenal ulcer healing and pharmacodynamic studies of antisecretory drugs and acid suppression have revealed that healing rates for duodenal ulcer correlate with the suppression of gastric secretion. An evaluation of the pH profiles of individuals with ulcers in whom acid-suppressive therapy induced healing revealed three critical determinates predictive of duodenal ulcer healing. These were the degree of acid suppression; the duration of acid suppression within a 24-hour period; and the length of treatment. Thus, the healing rates for duodenal ulcer were demonstrated to be highly correlatable with the degree of acid suppression, and a daily intragastric pH of 3.0 for longer than 18 to 20 hours provided conditions that would achieve maximal healing rates for duodenal ulcers at 4 weeks. It was of interest that increasing acid suppression to an intragastric pH greater than 3.0 did not significantly improve healing. However, increasing the total duration of acid suppression by lengthening treatment or during the individual 24-hour period itself resulted in higher healing rates. It was also evident that the therapeutic effect of H$_2$ receptor antagonists reflected their ability to suppress nocturnal acidity better than daytime acidity.

Diagnosis

The widespread recognition of symptomatology involving epigastric discomfort related to the ingestion of food and broadly grouped under the nomenclature of *dyspepsia* is well accepted as synonymous with evidence of acid peptic disease. Although considerable emphasis in the past had been placed on precise delineation of the symptomatology to determine whether the site of the ulceration is gastric or duodenal, currently, the identification of dyspepsia rapidly leads to upper gastrointestinal endoscopy and the determination of the precise location of the lesion. Of particular relevance in the history should be the determination of alarm symptoms or signs such as weight loss, vomiting, the development of back pain, or failure to relieve symptomatology with acid-inhibitory therapy. Broadly speaking, the presence of such features would suggest either the development of a complicated ulcer (bleeding, penetration, perforation, stenosis, or neoplasia) or that the ulcer may be due to other causes, such as aspirin, NSAID intake, or a gastrinoma. These entities will be discussed separately in further detail.

The establishment of the diagnosis of acid peptic disease requires not only the identification and characterization of the site of the lesion but also the determination of the presence of *H. pylori*. This can be undertaken by a number of techniques, including histologic staining, urease identification in the biopsy material, serology, or breath or stool testing. The sensitivity and specificity of such tests are important criteria, although costs will probably be the dominant issue in determining how the organism should be identified.

Medical management

Duodenal ulcer

Ulcer healing and acid suppression

There is a direct correlation between the healing rate of duodenal ulcers and the degree of suppression of 24-hour intragastric acidity associated with the use of antisecretory agents. Hunt and his colleagues were the first to point out that a primary determinant of duodenal ulcer healing is represented by the fraction of the day for which intragastric pH is maintained above 3.0 as well as the duration of treatment itself. Using metaanalysis, they predicted that all duodenal ulcers could be healed within 4 weeks if intragastric pH were to be maintained above 3.0 for between 18 and 20 hours per day. In this respect, the PPI class of drugs has proved to be superior because they inactivate the H,K ATPase enzyme and produce inhibition of both peripherally and centrally mediated gastric acid secretion. On the contrary, the H_2 receptor antagonists act via competitive antagonism at the H_2 receptor on the basolateral membrane of the parietal cell to inhibit histamine-mediated acid secretion. Such agents are therefore somewhat less effective in controlling food-stimulated gastric acid secretion, because cholinergic-mediated stimulation is not inhibited. Almost every clinical trial has demonstrated the superiority of PPIs over H_2 receptor antagonists in the treatment of both gastric and duodenal ulceration. PPIs thus produce healing in a greater proportion of ulcers than do H_2 receptor antagonists as well as faster healing and more rapid relief of symptoms. Apart from the personal advantages to the patient of the more rapid amelioration of the disease process, both the duration and cost of medical therapy can thus be decreased. A number of comparative studies have demonstrated that omeprazole heals duodenal ulcers faster and more effectively than do H_2 receptor antagonists. Similarly, other studies have demonstrated that pantoprazole (40 mg daily) produces significantly higher rates of duodenal ulcer healing than does ranitidine when compared at both 2 and 4 weeks. In a separate series of studies, lansoprazole (30 mg daily) produced more rapid and effective healing of duodenal ulcers than 300 mg of ranitidine administered at night. Other data have demonstrated that omeprazole (20 mg daily) resulted in significantly less daytime pain than that experienced by patients receiving 300 mg of ranitidine at bedtime. Studies comparing pantoprazole (40 mg daily) with ranitidine (300 mg daily) demonstrated that improvement of pain relief after 2 weeks was greater in patients receiving pantoprazole than in those receiving ranitidine. Similarly, lansoprazole has been shown to decrease ulcer pain more effectively than ranitidine, with a significantly greater percentage of patients free of symptoms after 2 weeks using the PPI as opposed to the H_2 receptor antagonist.

Comparable observations of the use of acid suppression in gastric ulcer patients have been found. Omeprazole (20 mg daily) produced consistently higher rates of healing than did H_2 receptor antagonists. Pantoprazole (40 mg daily) resulted in significantly higher healing rates of gastric ulcers than did ranitidine (300 mg daily) at both 4 and 8 weeks. Lansoprazole (30 mg daily) healed significantly more ulcers than did famotidine (20 mg twice daily). In addition, pantoprazole, omeprazole, and lansoprazole produced more rapid relief of symptoms in patients with gastric ulceration than did H_2 receptor antagonists. In those individuals with peptic ulcers refractory to long-term treatment with H_2 receptor antagonists, a number of clinical trials have demonstrated that pantoprazole, lansoprazole, and omeprazole are capable of generating effective healing.

Management of Duodenal Ulcer

A management strategy for duodenal ulcer disease.

H. pylori eradication

On determination of clinical symptomatology consistent with a putative diagnosis of peptic ulcer disease, the site and nature of the lesion should be identified. Thus, at endoscopy, the presence and site of the ulcer, as well as the presence or absence of *H. pylori*, should be determined and documented. The diagnosis of *H. pylori* can be undertaken by the use of noninvasive or invasive tests. Invasive methodology involves endoscopy with gastric mucosal biopsy and either histology culture or rapid urease testing. The rapid urease test is probably the most useful in routine practice, because in addition to being highly sensitive (85% to 95%) and specific (98%), it is easy to perform, relatively cheap, and provides a rapid result. Although the histologic demonstration of the organism has a high sensitivity (85% to 90%) and specificity (93% to 100%), its routine use is limited by its high cost.

Culture of the organism is probably the ideal diagnostic technique, but it is difficult and has a high failure rate compared to other diagnostic strategies. It is probable, however, that in the future, *H. pylori* culture may be of considerable use in checking bacterial sensitivity, particularly in individuals for whom eradication has failed as macrolide antibiotics or nitro-imidazoles are under consideration for future therapy.

The noninvasive methodologies available for the diagnosis of *H. pylori* include radiolabeled urea breath tests and enzyme-linked immunosorbent serologic assays (ELISAs). The drawbacks of the serologic studies are related to the relative lack of sensitivity, although they are easy to perform and relatively cheap. A particular problem is the fact that serologic tests are not useful in monitoring the success of eradication therapy, because IgG and IgA titers may only drop by 20% to 50% within the month of the cessation of therapy. The currently available labeled urea breath tests are the nonradioactive ^{13}C test and the radioactive ^{14}C test. Current studies suggest that both are equally specific (99%) and sensitive (90% to 98%). The ^{14}C test is less costly and has recently met with U.S. Food and Drug Administration (FDA) approval. The ^{13}C test is expensive, and the equipment is expensive and not widely available.

In the presence of peptic ulcer disease, it is important to identify the presence of *H. pylori* before the institution of therapy so that eradication of the organism can be confirmed 4 to 6 weeks after treatment. In this respect, successful eradication can be documented in duodenal ulcer patients by use of the noninvasive urea breath test. In individuals with gastric ulceration, endoscopy is necessary not only to confirm adequate healing but also to ensure that no neoplasia exists.

Under these circumstances, a biopsy sample should be used to test for *H. pylori*, preferably by means of the rapid urease test. It is important that at least two biopsy samples be evaluated (fundic and antral), because if eradication therapy has not been completely successful, the organism may be present only in small numbers and may have migrated (a consequence of acid-suppressive therapy and the alteration of its ideal pH milieu) from its original site. In those patients who exhibit relapse or recurrence of symptomatology, the presence of *H. pylori* should be meticulously assessed.

Bismuth-based antimicrobial therapy

H. pylori has been demonstrated to be sensitive to a wide variety of antimicrobial agents, including macrolides, beta lactams, ketoconazoles, tetracyclines, gentamycin, rifampicin, nitrofuran, and some quinolones. Nevertheless, the use of any of these agents alone (monotherapy) has generally proved to render suboptimal results, with eradication rates of approximately 20%. Clarithromycin, a macrolide antibiotic, is more acid stable than its counterpart, erythromycin, and is well tolerated, more effective, and has an eradication rate alone of greater than 50%. It is, however, clearly apparent that the use of more than one antibiotic has resulted in improved cure rates. The most commonly administered combinations include the classic bismuth triple therapy of bismuth, subsalicylate, or subcitrate and metronidazole in combination with amoxicillin or tetracycline (standard bismuth triple therapy). The use of this classic triple-therapy mode has limitations.

Evaluation of the two different combinations has demonstrated that triple therapy incorporating amoxicillin is significantly less effective than triple therapy that includes tetracycline, because amoxicillin is significantly less effective in eradicating *H. pylori*. A further important clinical issue is the relatively high rate of pretreatment resistance to metronidazole in some parts of the world. Patients taking less than 60% of their prescribed medication fail to achieve eradication rates greater than 70%. Alternatively, if greater than 60% of the prescribed medications is taken, eradication rates up to 95% may be expected. Because the bismuth triple-therapy regime requires the ingestion of up to 18 tablets daily, such compliance may become a serious issue. Adverse events may be predicted in between 25% and 30% of patients.

Eradication and acid-suppressive combination therapy with proton pump inhibitors

Because gastric acidity is an important component in the genesis of peptic ulcer disease, antisecretory therapy is of critical relevance in disease management. Thus, combinations of antisecretory agents with antibiotics such as clarithromycin, tetracycline, amoxicillin, and metronidazole are of considerable use. Given the fact that PPIs are more efficacious than other classes of acid-suppressing agents in the management of peptic ulcer disease as well as achieving more rapid symptom relief and ulcer healing, their combination with a variety of antibiotics has proved to be of considerable benefit. The rationale for their use is discussed in the section on *H. pylori*.

A number of studies have unequivocally demonstrated that antisecretory/antibiotic drug combinations including a PPI rather than an H_2 receptor antagonist provide better eradication of *H. pylori*. Furthermore, the combination of a PPI and one or two antibiotic agent achieves *H. pylori* eradication rates indistinguishable from those found using bismuth triple therapy. Such studies have also noted an acceleration in rapid ulcer healing, less antimicro-

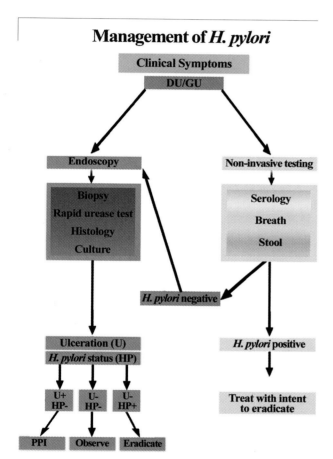

A management strategy for *H. pylori*–related acid peptic disease.

bial resistance, higher patient compliance, and fewer adverse effects compared to those identified in patients using bismuth triple therapy.

Thus, combinations of various PPIs, such as pantoprazole, lansoprazole, or omeprazole, used with clarithromycin and amoxicillin or metronidazole have all been reported to produce eradication rates and ulcer healing in excess of 90% and as high as 96%. An issue is the duration of therapy. It seems that 7 days of twice-daily combination therapy is required for effective eradication. Continued therapy with the PPI for 4 weeks is still suggested for ulcer healing, but some studies indicate that eradication is sufficient for ulcer healing, without the need for acid suppression. However, it is necessary to show a negative breath test within 1 week of therapy to enable this strategy.

Summated information from a large number of studies indicates that the optimal management strategies for either gastric or duodenal ulceration are the use of a PPI and two antibacterial agents. Under such circumstances, eradication rates of about 90% have been reported by a large number of investigators in many different countries.

In those patients for whom prior eradication therapy has been unsuccessful or in individuals who exhibit antimicrobial resistance, quadruple therapy may be contemplated. Diagnosis of clarithromycin resistance can be done by sequencing the specific region of the 23S RNA where a point mutation results in prevention of drug binding.

Diagnosis of metronidazole resistance requires *in vitro* culture. Under such circumstances, a PPI, along with a standard classical triple-therapy regime, such as colloidal bismuth subcitrate or bismuth subsalicylate, with a nitro-imidazole and either tetracycline or amoxicillin may be considered.

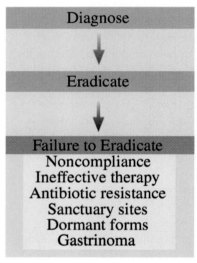

H. pylori Management Strategy

Diagnose

Eradicate

Failure to Eradicate
Noncompliance
Ineffective therapy
Antibiotic resistance
Sanctuary sites
Dormant forms
Gastrinoma

Eradication and acid-suppressive combination therapy with ranitidine and bismuth subcitrate

A newer combination of ranitidine and bismuth subcitrate with two antibiotics has also been introduced and approved for eradication. It is claimed that this form of bismuth is more soluble and more available for bactericidal action. However, significant blood levels of bismuth have been detected in some patients, and this cation is neurotoxic and nephrotoxic. Most of the data reported have not used intention-to-treat criteria, and the general impression is that eradication is less effective. Another issue is that after eradication therapy, treatment with ranitidine is continued for the routine period of 8 weeks rather than the 4 weeks for a PPI.

The treatment paradigm that is most frequently used is triple therapy with PPIs in combination with amoxicillin and clarithromycin. Usually this is a twice-daily treatment with omeprazole/lansoprazole/pantoprazole at standard dose with 1 g amoxicillin and 500 mg clarithromycin taken simultaneously, which in trials have given 90% eradication. Metronidazole may be used in substitution for either antibiotic.

Treatment failure

Although there are a number of reasons for an ulcer to recur—including failure of compliance, inadequate acid suppression, and gastrinoma—by far the most common is the failure to eradicate *H. pylori*. Thus, 70% of patients who remained *H. pylori* positive after eradication therapy were reported to have developed ulcer recurrence within 1 year, as compared to only 3% in those for whom the organism had been eradicated. Conversely, studies that have examined 1-year ulcer recurrence rates in patients in whom *H. pylori* had been successfully eradicated noted a 1.1% rate, as compared to a 67.9% rate before the introduction of eradication therapy. In this context, studies using a PPI with antibiotic regimes produced similar results, whereas monotherapy with a PPI alone is associated with *H. pylori* eradication rates of only 0% to 10%. Although it has been suggested that the failure to eradicate may actually represent reinfection, studies that have evaluated this possibility indicate that the true rate of reinfection in developed countries is probably less than 1% to 2%. The percentage may be higher in developing countries, but recurrence of *H. pylori* infection within 1 year on balance probably represents recrudescence of an original infection that was suppressed rather than eradicated and is less likely to represent a true reinfection.

Nevertheless, there does appear to be a group of patients in whom ulcers recur even after successful eradication of *H. pylori*. In such instances, once other causes of therapeutic failure (noncompliance, salicylate abuse, NSAIDs, gastrinoma) have been eliminated, maintenance antisecretory therapy should be considered. Long-term antisecretory agents should thus be reserved for individuals in whom at least two attempts at *H. pylori* eradication have failed or in those who have *H. pylori*–negative peptic disease, and possibly in individuals with complicated ulcers, particularly those prone to recurrent bleeding.

Whereas surgery had previously been the mainstay of the management of chronic peptic ulceration, and particularly its complications, the advent of H_2 receptor antagonists and, more recently, PPIs has virtually abolished elective surgery in the consideration of the management of peptic ulcer disease. Nevertheless, in a small group of patients with chronic or recurrent peptic ulcer disease, surgery may eventually become a consideration. Rarely, a patient with a chronic gastric ulcer that is unresponsive to therapy may be identified as a covert presentation of a gastric neoplasm. More usually, however, surgery becomes a consideration with the evolution of a chronic peptic ulcer into an acute complication, of which bleeding, perforation, and stenosis are the usual events. Thus, for practical purposes, apart from the issue of gastrinoma, surgery of peptic ulcer disease may be considered primarily as a strategy in the management of complications.

Gastric ulcer

Although, previously, gastric ulcer had posed a pernicious problem in terms of healing, the identification of *H. pylori* and its role in this disease process has greatly facilitated cure. Although gastric ulcer patients have overall exhibited lower levels of gastric acid secretion than healthy controls, healing is reflective of similar critical determinates, as identified in duodenal ulcer patients. In the gastric ulcer patients, it is more likely that *H. pylori* infection is present; their older age and defects in mucosal defense factors function in combination to render the disease more difficult to cure. Also, the intramural presence of acid and pepsin in

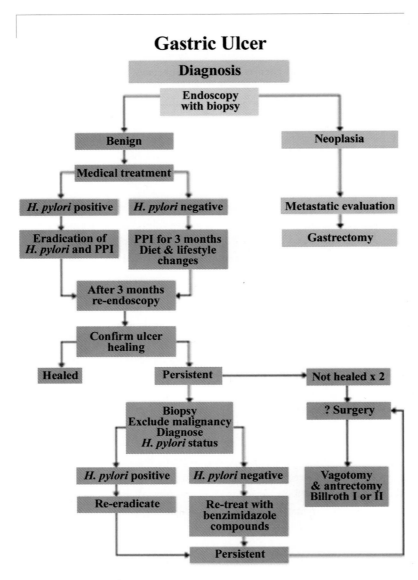

Gastric Ulcer

| Diagnosis |

Endoscopy with biopsy

Benign → Medical treatment

H. pylori positive → Eradication of H. pylori and PPI

H. pylori negative → PPI for 3 months Diet & lifestyle changes

After 3 months re-endoscopy

Confirm ulcer healing

Healed

Persistent → Not healed x 2

Biopsy Exclude malignancy Diagnose H. pylori status

H. pylori positive → Re-eradicate

H. pylori negative → Re-treat with benzimidazole compounds

? Surgery → Vagotomy & antrectomy Billroth I or II

Persistent

Neoplasia → Metastatic evaluation → Gastrectomy

A management strategy for gastric ulcer.

higher quantities than in the duodenum may play a role. In metaanalytic studies of gastric ulcer healing, the duration of treatment appeared to be the most important single determinant in predicting healing. All treatments show an increase in healing rates from 2 to 4 and from 4 to 8 weeks of treatment. Nevertheless, the degree of acid suppression is also important, because the greater suppression of 24-hour intragastric acidity produces the highest healing rates. Of relevance is the fact that suppression of 24-hour acidity appears to be more important than suppression of either nighttime or daytime acidity. Thus, maintenance of the gastric pH above 3.0 for 18 hours daily predicts healing in approximately 100% of gastric ulcers by 8 weeks, whereas a similar degree of acid suppression might be predicted to heal 100% of duodenal ulcers in 4 weeks. Clearly, such data can only be attained with concomitant eradication of *H. pylori*, if present.

At this time, there is little doubt that eradication of *H. pylori* is mandatory to ensure successful treatment of gastric and duodenal ulceration. Acid-suppression therapy alone is associated with relatively high levels of recurrence. Thus, the combination of bacterial eradication and elevation of pH appears to provide the optimal treatment not only for ensuring ulcer cure, but also for abrogating the likelihood of the development of complications such as bleeding. The therapeutic regimes available for management of uncomplicated gastric and duodenal ulceration can be evaluated under the headings of antimicrobial therapy, acid-suppressive therapy, and a combination of both entities. For practical purposes, the surgery of uncomplicated duodenal and gastric ulceration may be regarded as unwarranted except in instances of perforation, failed conservative management of bleeding, gastric outlet obstruction, and the development of neoplasia. In those patients in whom peptic ulceration may be due to a gastrinoma, surgery directed at removal of the neoplasm and/or its metastases should be considered.

Nonsteroidal anti-inflammatory drug (NSAID) mucosal ulcers

As early as 1875, reports of "dyspeptic indigestion" followed the introduction of sodium salicylate for the management of patients with dramatic disease. This class of drugs achieved widespread usage, and the further development of acetyl salicylic acid (aspirin) amplified the problem. The more recent introduction and widespread use of NSAIDs has been associated with significant morbidity and mortality given their association with gastroduodenal ulceration. Despite the fact that NSAIDs are extremely valuable and effective drugs for the treatment of musculoskeletal and arthritic disorders, they exhibit a common association with acute and chronic gastroduodenal injury. It has been calculated that the relative risk of upper gastrointestinal bleeding and ulcer perforation in individuals using nonaspirin NSAIDs increases approximately threefold and sixfold, respectively. In such situations, the patient and the physician find themselves in a dilemma, because the usefulness of treatment with NSAIDs may nevertheless outweigh the possible adverse effects of potential damage to the mucosa and the consequent ulcer-related complications. It is of interest that many patients who develop peptic ulceration on NSAID therapy are asymptomatic, and under such circumstances, both patient and physician may be unaware of the existence of any lesions until the advent of bleeding or perforation. Nevertheless, most individuals receiving NSAID therapy exhibit endoscopic evidence of erosions, of which the majority are gastric, as compared to duodenal (2 to 1 ratio). In rheumatology patients receiving NSAIDs, between 11% and 22% have ulcers, although many may be minute and only evident on rigorous endoscopic scrutiny.

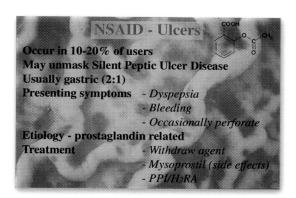

Clinical information pertinent to NSAID ulcer diagnosis and management.

Etiology

A number of putative mechanisms have been proposed to explain the relationship of NSAIDs and mucosal ulceration. The inhibition of the constitutive cox I isoform and the consequent failure to produce endogenous eicosanoids that protect the mucosa is the most widely accepted mechanism at this time. Other factors that have been implicated include associations with bile reflux and a potential direct damaging effect on the mucosa. The latter possibility is not widely accepted, and although there is substantial evidence that aspirin exerts a direct effect on the mucosa as well as inhibiting cox, it is felt that NSAIDs do not cause direct topical injury.

Of interest is the fact that depletion of circulating neutrophils in animal models has been shown to decrease the severity of NSAID-induced injury. The question of whether *H. pylori* infection plays a part in the development of NSAID ulceration has been studied in considerable detail. The current body of opinion supports a conclusion that *H. pylori* infection and NSAID use are independent and not synergistic risk factors for gastric ulceration. Thus, the prevalence of *H. pylori* infection in NSAID users and nonusers with gastric ulceration is similar, and NSAID use does not predispose to *H. pylori* infection. Evidence does exist to support the fact that NSAIDs have a potentially additive effect in promoting ulcer bleeding, possibly because of their antiplatelet effect, but there are insufficient data to support an added role for *H. pylori* in NSAID-induced ulceration. Patients at a high risk of developing NSAID ulcers require NSAID ulcer prophylaxis regardless of *H. pylori* status. It is not known whether individuals treated in the past for *H. pylori* gastric ulcers are at an increased risk for ulcers if they receive NSAIDs. It would, however, seem prudent to accept that NSAID ulcer prophylaxis is required in ulcer patients in whom *H. pylori* was successfully treated in the past if the patient requires NSAID therapy.

Risk factors for mucosal damage

The relative risk of developing mucosal damage on NSAID therapy is increased approximately fourfold. A further important factor is the duration of NSAID therapy. Paradoxically, an inverse relationship between the relative risk of complications and the duration of NSAID therapy exists. Thus, the risk of bleeding decreases by one-third when the duration of NSAID therapy is extended from 30 days to 90 days. The phenomenon of adaptation has been proposed as an explanation for this surprising observation. It is, however, evident that the risk of an NSAID-associated ulcer complication is higher in the first weeks of therapy; thus, individuals who are less susceptible to the drugs exhibit fewer problems as therapy persists. An alternative explanation is the fact that NSAID therapy may actually unmask a preexisting silent ulcer that then exhibits an acute complication early in therapy or on initiation thereof. Another explanation is that individuals who are particularly sensitive to NSAID ulcers may be progressively removed from the population taking NSAIDs by a process of elimination, and that long-term therapy essentially selects out patients not susceptible to the adverse pharmacologic effects of NSAIDs. Overall, however, the potential seriousness of this widely used drug should not be underestimated. A summation of large studies of NSAID-treated patients suggests not only an annual 2% rate of ulcer complications but also an increased ulcer mortality of three- to tenfold in individuals undergoing NSAID therapy.

Newer classes of NSAIDs are being developed that inhibit the inducible form of cox, cox II, that appear to have a lesser predilection for gastric damage and when introduced may render NSAID-related gastric ulcers obsolete.

Treatment

Because the likelihood of an NSAID-related complication is high, the consideration of ulcer prophylaxis should be regarded as an important component of therapy. An idiosyncratic sensitivity to a particular NSAID may be evaluated by altering the medication, because some drugs have been suggested to be associated with more gastroduodenal problems than others.

Ulcer prophylaxis is particularly relevant in the presence of the risk factors that have been identified for NSAID-induced ulceration. These include age older than 65 years, a past history of peptic ulceration, simultaneous use of corticosteroids, and previous problems during the administration of NSAIDs. Individuals who fall into any of the above categories should be considered for prophylactic therapy. Given the efficacy and safety profile of the PPIs, it is clear that these should be the prophylactic drugs of choice. Other less attractive alternatives, however, are offered.

The use of 200 mg of misoprostol 4 times daily for 3 months provides significant protection against gastric and duodenal ulceration in patients taking

NSAIDs. The levels of protection under such circumstances range between 75% and 90%, and the frequency of significant gastrointestinal complications is reduced by 40%. The widespread use of misoprostol, however, is somewhat limited by its tendency to cause diarrhea and abdominal pain in a significant proportion of patients. Such side effects, however, need to be weighed against the consequences of a complication of mucosal ulceration. Ranitidine therapy has also been demonstrated to be effective in healing NSAID-induced ulcers and is particularly effective if the NSAID is withdrawn.

PPIs have been demonstrated to be of superior efficacy in the management of NSAID-induced ulceration in several well-controlled clinical trials. The dose of the PPI and time of administration should be tailored to the NSAID protocol used by a particular patient for optimal prophylaxis.

The issue of whether prophylaxis should be routinely used in the management of patients taking NSAIDs raises the question of cost effectiveness. It seems likely that in the presence of one or more risk factors (advanced age, previous peptic ulceration, or concomitant steroid administration), prophylaxis is warranted given the adverse economic and clinical impact of an NSAID-induced ulcer complication.

Complications of peptic ulcer disease

The complications of acid peptic disease usually represent the sequelae of long-standing or chronic ulceration. Occasionally, such events may occur in an acute setting, but in such circumstances, the acute presentation often represents administration of a drug such as an NSAID, aspirin, or alcohol or exposure to the stress of trauma or major surgery. For the most part, bleeding and perforation are the most dramatic and the most common, with penetration and obstruction being less frequent and far less acute in their presentations.

Causes of Esophagogastroduodenal Bleeding

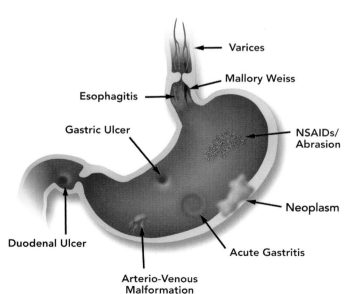

Varices

Mallory Weiss

Esophagitis

Gastric Ulcer

NSAIDs/ Abrasion

Neoplasm

Duodenal Ulcer

Acute Gastritis

Arterio-Venous Malformation

Although a wide variety of causes for bleeding are recognized, the majority can be identified at endoscopy and the specific therapeutic regime instituted.

Bleeding

Although there exists no good evidence to support the contention that bleeding ulcers are any different from nonbleeding ulcers, a different management strategy is required for this complication. Although bleeding is a relatively common complication of peptic ulcer disease, in 70% to 80% of patients, once appropriate resuscitation has been instituted, cessation is spontaneous, and no further specific intervention is required. A smaller group of such patients, however, exhibit severe persistent or recurrent bleeding, and in such instances, a mortality of between 6% and 10% may be predicted. Factors that adversely affect survival

Management of Peptic Ulcer Bleeding

Evidence of Upper GI Bleeding

Hematemesis
Collapse
Melaena
Positive Hemoccult

Resuscitate
I.V. fluids
I.V. PPI
Antibiotics

Condition stabilizes → **Elective endoscopy**

Condition unstable → **Emergency endoscopy in O.R.**

Identify Source

Ulcer (DU/GU) identified

No ulcer
- Varices
- Gastritis
- Mallory-Weiss

→ **Treatment as appropriate**

No bleeding

? Continuous bleeding

Medical therapy

Stigmata present

Bleeding uncontrollable

Endoscopic treatment: Bipolar coagulation Injection

Surgery

N/G tube PPI ICU

Control

No control

Re-endoscopy → **Re-bleeding**

A management strategy for peptic ulcer–associated bleeding.

include active bleeding or the identification of a visible vensulate at endoscopy, age older than 65 years, rebleeding in hospital, and major intercurrent medical problems, including cardiac and renal disease.

Initial strategies for the management of bleeding were mostly conservative and involved saline lavage and periulcer injection of vasoconstrictors or sclerosants. More sophisticated methodology is now available. Thus, in most endoscopy units, bipolar coagulation, laser therapy, or application of topical homeostatic agents or glue is available. The considerable success of such methodology has led to a significant decline in the need for open surgical intervention. In circumstances in which surgery may be necessary, but the patient's condition mitigates against general anesthesia and abdominal exploration, selective immobilization may be an option. Failure to specifically obliterate the appropriate arterial vessel in the stomach or duodenum, however, may result in severe sequelae, particularly in the duodenum, where mural infarction or pancreatitis may supervene.

In the event of endoscopic strategies failing to halt the bleeding, surgery should be rapidly directed at identifying the bleeding vessels that should then be under-run and over-sewn. In the past, ligation of the bleeding vessel was usually followed by a vagotomy and pyloroplasty. More recently, the recognition that adequate acid suppression and eradication of *H. pylori* will obviate recurrent bleeding has led to a diminution of the necessity to undertake surgical procedures associated with a decrease in acid secretion.

The availability and use of intravenous H_2 receptor antagonist or PPI therapy has, to a large extent, obviated the need for emergency gastrectomy and similarly decreased the incidence of recurrent bleeding from either the ulcer site or anastomotic margins.

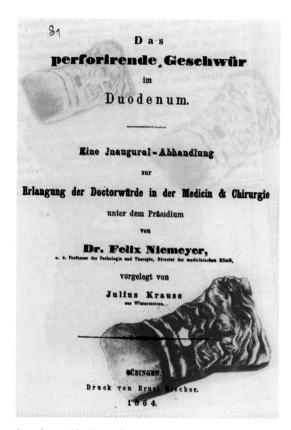

An early report by Krauss documenting perforation as a complication of acid peptic disease.

In patients whose duodenal ulcers have healed after severe hemorrhage without surgical intervention, long-term maintenance therapy with ranitidine (150 mg at night) has been reported to significantly reduce the risk of recurrent bleeding. In a similar fashion, it has been noted that the eradication of *H. pylori* infection by changing the natural history of peptic ulcer disease has been effective in the prevention of recurrent bleeding in patients who initially present with bleeding.

Thus, in one study of patients in whom *H. pylori* infection had persisted, a regime of amoxicillin plus omeprazole, which cured the *H. pylori* infection in 60% of the patients, reduced the rate of ulcer recurrence from 50.0% to 3.8% and the rate of recurrent bleeding from 33% to 0%.

Pharmacologic therapies evaluating the ability of acid suppression to prevent acute ulcer bleeding have met with limited success. On an intuitive basis, one might presume that increasing gastric luminal pH by the inhibition of acid secretion would decrease activation of pepsinogen, prevent fibrinolysis, and support the function of homeostatic mechanisms. Unfortunately, H_2 receptor antagonists produce only a relatively modest increase of intragastric pH, and, thus, studies of their usefulness have failed to document a decrease in the rate of rebleeding, surgical intervention, or mortality. Surprisingly, a study that used intravenous famotidine to maintain intragastric pH at a level above 6.0 in fasting patients with duodenal ulceration failed to decrease rebleeding rates or the need for surgery in a group of patients with bleeding peptic ulcers.

It might be that PPIs would be more efficacious, given their ability to produce a prolonged and profound inhibition of gastric acid secretion as compared to H_2 receptor antagonists. Current information using intravenous omeprazole indicated a decrease in endoscopic stigmata of rebleeding of a modest nature but no alteration in the incidence of rebleeding, surgery, or death. Nevertheless, the development of more effective intravenous PPIs with a better pharmacokinetic profile suggests that the pharmacologic management of acute peptic ulcer bleeding may be worthy of serious further consideration. Thus, the ability of intravenous pantoprazole to generate a luminal pH of greater than 6.0 within 30 minutes of administration and lasting for the duration of the infusion may be predicted to demonstrate clinical benefit.

Perforation

Although the first documented case of perforated peptic ulcer disease dates back more than 2,000 years to the western Han dynasty, the problem continues to confound physicians. In many instances, the first indication of a peptic ulcer may be the perforation itself, whereas in others, previous vague symptomatology suddenly culminates in acute perforation with peritonitis. The pathogenesis of the situation whereby an indolent or even chronic disease suddenly converts into a dramatic acute event has not been established. It is possible that this represents a locally vascular phenomenon whereby vessels supplying the base of an ulcer are acutely obliterated and a local infarction occurs. Certainly, the fact that most perforations occur on the anterior lateral border of the duodenum provided some support for the suggestion. Perforations had been previously clearly described as clinical entities by Bailey and Benjamin Travers before 1843, when Edward Crisp reported 50 cases of perforated peptic ulcer and accurately summarized the clinical aspects of the condition. Crisp expressed considerable pessimism about the outcome, stating, *"Once the perforation has occurred the case must be considered hopeless. In surgery's present state, the idea of cutting open the abdomen and closing the opening is simply too quixotic to consider."*

In 1884, Mikulicz-Radecki clearly defined the condition and provided the solution but failed to successfully treat the patient. His observations, however, were most prescient: *"Every doctor faced with a perforated ulcer of the stomach or intestine, must consider opening the abdomen, sewing up the hole, and adverting a possible or actual inflammation by careful cleansing of the abdominal cavity."*

Nevertheless, the first successful operation was undertaken on May 19, 1892, in Barman, currently a part of Wupperthal. Ludwig Heusner was summoned to the home of a 41-year-old man with a classic history of stomach ulcer, including pain and nausea for 20 years with four episodes of bleeding, who suddenly had acute peritonitis and shock. In a seemingly difficult operation, Heusner repaired the perforation, and the patient survived. This successful repair was reported by Heusner's superior, Kriege, and predated by 1 month a similar successful operation performed by Hastings Guilford in Redding, England.

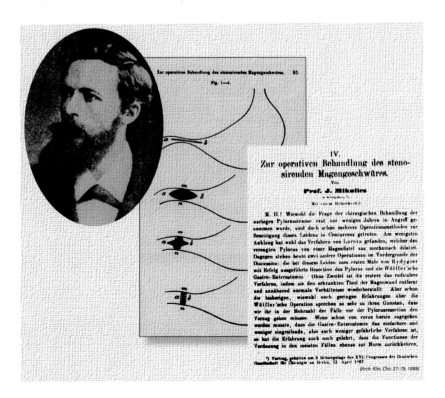

Mikulicz-Radecki had, by 1884, given considerable thought to the management of both stenosis and perforation as complications of duodenal ulcer disease.

Initial therapy for perforated duodenal ulcers involved laparotomy with omental patch repair. Occasional intrepid surgeons undertook definitive procedures such as vagotomy with pyloroplasty simultaneously, but for the most part, the need to perform surgery expeditiously and the fear of peritonitis and subphrenic abscess supported the use of patch repair alone. Modifications to decrease acid secretion included the use of highly selective vagotomy, but for the most part, surgeons were content to simply repair the perforation. Whereas early mortality rates in the pre-antibiotic era were close to 25%, most centers now report mortality rates of less than 5% to 10%, with figures as low as 3%. For the most part, mortality reflects either delay in arrival at the hospital or the presence of significant comorbid conditions consequent on age, prolonged sepsis, and cardiac or renal failure.

Despite the fact that the mortality of surgical procedures has declined exponentially, the advent of intravenous H_2 receptor antagonists and profound acid suppression by PPIs has, for the most part, precluded the need for consideration of definitive ulcer surgery. Thus, older data in the pre-PPI era suggested that after simple closure, ulcer recurrence might occur in 52% of patients, of whom 28% percent would bleed, 15% would exhibit pyloric obstruction, and 9% reperforation. Further recognition that profound suppression of acid secretion when combined with eradication of *H. pylori* virtually obviated further ulcer activity or complications has led to the growing acceptance that simple ulcer closure and appropriate medical therapy thereafter are perfectly adequate.

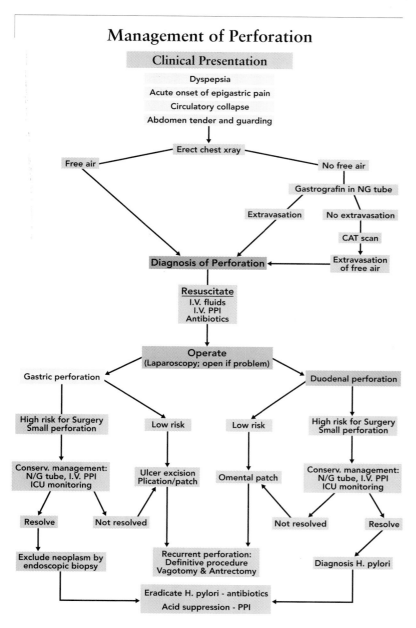

An algorithm for the management of perforation.

Interesting developments in laparoscopic surgery have led to modifications of the acute management of the perforation itself. Thus, the use of a laparoscope to identify the perforation, lavage of the abdomen, and suture or glue-in omental plugs into the defect has met with good success. A combination of

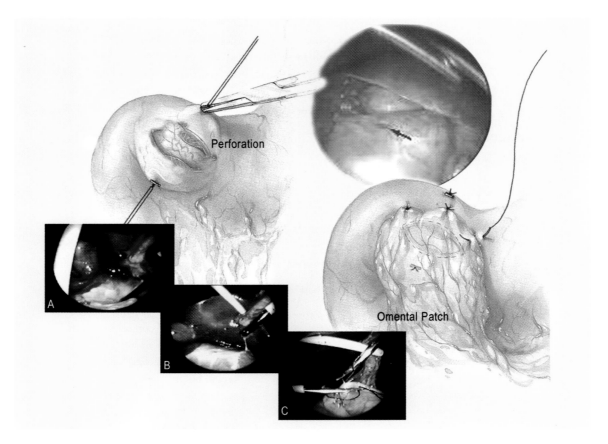

A laparoscopic view of a perforated bulbar ulcer (top right) and the series of steps for a laparoscopic approach to managing this problem (bottom). The surgical approach to the management of a perforated pyloroduodenal ulcer (background) entails lavage of the abdomen and the repair of the defect. Initially, an endoluminal endoscopic approach may be undertaken to visualize the site of the perforation (A), although this is only rarely necessary. The repair entails the mobilization of a "tongue" of omentum and its suture using interrupted silk sutures (B,C) over the perforation (Graham patch). The availability of the PPI class of drugs has rendered the need for gastric resection in the circumstance of perforation exceedingly rare.

laparoscopic and endoscopic technique whereby the laparoscopic presentation of the omentum into the duodenum is followed by the endoscopic technique of inserting the omental plug into the duodenal lumen and the suture or gluing of the omentum in place can manage even large perforations.

The management of perforated gastric ulcers has similarly undergone an evolution in much the same fashion as perforated duodenal ulcers. Before the availability of H_2 receptor antagonists and PPI therapy, the majority of perforated gastric ulcers would be managed by partial gastrectomy.

Furthermore, it was felt that gastric ulcers in the prepyloric area not only should be managed by gastrectomy, but also should include a vagotomy. More recently, with a recognition of the potency of acid-suppressive medication and the critical role of *H. pylori* in perforated gastric ulcer, placation of the perforation and omental patch have become the standard of treatment in most centers.

A formal course of PPI therapy with antibiotics to eradicate *H. pylori* has led to successful management in the vast majority of patients.

A particular consideration in the management of a perforated gastric ulcer is the need to reliably confirm the absence of neoplasia. Even if the biopsies at the repair of the acute perforation are negative, endoscopic surveillance should be undertaken at 8 weeks with four-quadrant biopsy to confirm absence of neoplasia and eradication of *H. pylori*.

Stenosis

In situations in which duodenal ulceration has either been untreated or inadequately treated over a relatively prolonged period, cicatrization may occur. Under such circumstances, the gastric outlet is narrowed, and pyloric function disturbed, with a result that gastric emptying is initially slowed and then impeded. Clinically, the patient's symptoms of dyspepsia and duodenal ulcer, such as epigastric pain relieved by food, change in character. Characteristically, a sensation of early satiety and bloating are described, followed by progression to a sensation of distention. Symptoms of reflux may also supervene as the stomach becomes filled with food and fluid, and disorder peristalsis drives food into the esophagus. The presence of undigested food in the stomach and its colonization with bacteria are associated with eructation of a classically foul-smelling nature and the patients' partners or the patients themselves may be aware of severe halitosis. The critical point is reached when gastric emptying is interfered with to the extent that projectile vomiting ensues.

In the latter stages of the disease, vomiting of a projectile nature occurs and is characterized both by the presence of undigested food eaten days before and by its foul-smelling nature. The examination of the patient usually provides evidence of weight loss, and a distended stomach with a succussion splash may be demonstrable. In most circumstances, surgery will be required to manage gastric-outlet obstruction due to progression of a chronic duodenal ulcer. It is important to determine that the underlying cause is not a prepyloric neoplasm of the scirrhous variety. Management should be initiated by passage of a large-bore nasogastric tube, with lavage of the gastric contents over a period of 3 to 4 days. Drainage should be maintained for at least 5 days, both to allow complete emptying of stomach

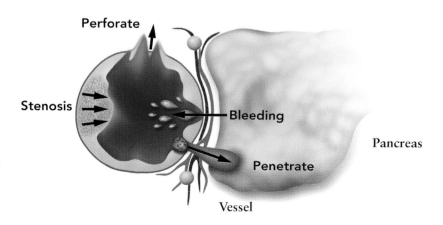

Duodenal Ulcers
Sites and Types of Complications

The complications of duodenal ulcer are to a certain extent site dependent. Perforations are usually anterolateral, penetration is posteromedial, bleeding is posteromedial, and stenosis can occur circumferentially.

and to enable it to regain tone before consideration of surgery. To facilitate surgery, the stomach should be decompressed for a reasonable length of time to decrease mucosal edema and allow the size of the organ to approach its normal proportions. The use of nonabsorbable antibiotics and antifungal agents given orally is of benefit in decreasing gastric colonization and obviating postoperative sepsis. Endoscopic balloon dilatation has been used in this situation and, in some circumstances, may be of benefit in allowing egress of gastric contents. In the vast majority of patients, restenosis occurs quite rapidly, and surgery is subsequently required. Balloon dilatation should be undertaken with caution, because perforation of the duodenal bulb under such circumstances may occur and convert a relatively benign problem into one with a serious morbidity and mortality. The surgical procedure is directed at resection of the stenotic area of the duodenum and usually involves antrectomy as a component of a partial gastrectomy. The need to resect the stenosed component of the duodenum usually prevents the construction of a Billroth I gastroduodenal anastomosis, because inadequate length may result in excessive anastomotic tension. In most circumstances, a Billroth II gastrojejunal anastomosis is constructed and particular care taken with the closure of the duodenal stump, because a leak is a catastrophic event, given both its high volume and the presence of bile, pancreatic juice, gastric acid, and pepsin. In the past, a significant proportion of the stomach, including the antrum, was removed, and a vagotomy was undertaken to ensure an adequate decrease in acid secretion to prevent the recurrence of a peptic ulcer. The widespread availability and efficacy of PPI therapy have obviated the need for vagotomy, and the degree of gastric resection should be as small as possible to resect the strictured area and facilitate a safe and patent anastomosis.

Penetration

This complication of chronic duodenal ulcer disease was relatively common in times when acid-suppressive therapy was not available and a prolonged clinical course of recurrent disease evident. Clinically, such patients present usually with a long history of untreated or inadequately treated peptic duodenal ulcer disease, classically characterized by a change in symptomatology. The customary picture of epigastric discomfort and nocturnal pain now fails to be relieved by the ingestion of food or antacids. In addition, the site of the pain shifts from the epigastrium to the back and attains a constant, boring character that is often worst at night. In most instances, the consideration of pancreatic neoplasia is raised, and even at endoscopy, the duodenal appearance may suggest a neoplasm. The constant back pain, often accentuated by food, and the failure of its relief with acid-suppressive medication usually mandate surgery. Under such circumstances, resection of the part of the duodenum containing the ulcer, with a partial gastrectomy and Billroth II anastomosis, is usually the operation of choice. Such operations may be particularly difficult given the chronic nature of the lesion, the surrounding fibrosis, and the distortion of anatomy. Particular care should be undertaken to avoid damage to the common bile duct or the head of the pancreas.

Hypergastrinemia

Background

Normal fasting gastrin levels are usually in the range of 50 pg per mL and may increase two- to threefold after a standard meal. Elevated levels of gastrin range from modest increases with H_2 receptor antagonist therapy (three- to fourfold) to levels that may be 200- to 300-fold above normal in patients with gastrinomas. For the most part, hypergastrinemia is associated with either atrophic gastritis or the use of acid-suppressive therapy, particularly the PPI class of drugs. Less common causes occur in patients with renal failure or individuals who have undergone vagotomy, especially those in whom the antrum has not been resected.

The presence of a retained excluded antrum caused by poor surgical technique is rarely evident nowadays, given the awareness of the need to resect it entirely at surgery and the virtual disappearance of gastric surgery for peptic ulcer disease. Despite its important biologic role in the stimulation of acid secretion and trophic regulation of the gastric mucosa, the effects of either acute or chronic hypergastrinemia appear to be minimal, especially if parietal cell function is inhibited (acid-suppressive drugs) or absent (diminished), as in atrophic gastritis or pernicious anemia. Indeed, prolonged, albeit modest, hypergastrinemia as evident after vagotomy has not been associated with adverse effects in numerous patients followed for as long as 30 to 40 years.

Similarly, the rigorous evaluation of patients on PPIs for up to 15 years has not revealed any significant problems. Under certain circumstances, elevated gastrin levels are associated with adverse effects that reflect the biologic actions of gastrin, particularly on gastric ECL cells. The generalized trophic effect of gastrin on mucosal stem cells may be associated with gastric mucosal thickening and occasionally polyp formation. Little evidence has emerged to support the role of elevated gastrin levels in the genesis of colonic carcinoma, and its effects are, for the most part, only relevant to the stomach. Long-standing, excessive gastrin drive culminates in ECL cell proliferation, increased histamine secretion, and, consequently, acid hypersecretion. The consequences of the former are varying degrees of ECL cell hyperplasia but rarely neoplasia. On the other hand, unregulated acid hypersecretion culminates in aggressive peptic ulcer disease and dramatic complications. The pathologic conditions associated with hypergastrinemia will be dealt with in the following section.

Common Causes of Hypergastrinemia

Atrophic gastritis

Pernicious anemia

Vagotomy

Helicobacter pylori

Duodenal/pancreatic gastrinoma

Renal failure

Proton pump inhibitors

A table of the common causes of hypergastrinemia.

Gastrinoma

The original observations of multiple, intractable, and aggressive ulcers of the duodenum and the small bowel in association with a pancreatic tumor have evolved into a well-defined pathophysiologic understanding of this entity. Previously eponymously recognized as the Zollinger-Ellison syndrome (ZES), the biologic elucidation of a gastrin-secreting neoplasm facilitated the development of rational therapy. Early reports of catastrophic multiple gastroduodenojejunal ulcerations associated with dramatic bleeding or perforation episodes have, for the most part, been supplanted by the identification of the condition in individuals whose peptic ulcer disease fails to respond to adequate acid-suppressive therapy.

Pathologically, the condition consists of one or more neuroendocrine tumors arising in either the pancreas or the duodenum that produce excessive amounts of gastrin, driving the parietal cell mass to the secretion of hydrochloric acid in quantities that overcome the mucosal barrier of the stomach, duodenum, and upper small bowel. The ensuing ulceration, which may occur in multiple sites, is aggressive, associated with bleeding and perforation as well as difficulty in maintaining healing. The duodenal or pancreatic lesions may, in rare circumstances, be part of the MEN-1 syndrome, and under such circumstances, consideration should be given to the prior surgical management of the parathyroid or pituitary problems.

The Gastrinoma Paradox

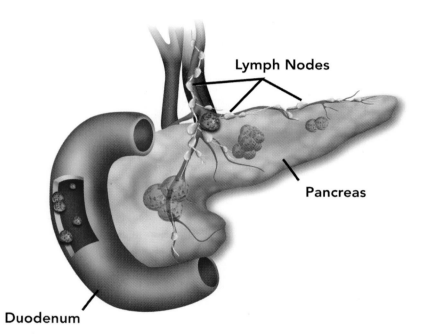

Lymph Nodes

Pancreas

Duodenum

Gastrin-producing cells are not evident in the adult pancreas, yet gastrinomas were previously considered to be predominantly pancreatic endocrine tumors. Currently, it is apparent that at least 50% of the lesions occur in the duodenum. In much the same fashion as carcinoid tumors, the majority of lesions are metastatic or multiple at diagnosis.

Although in the past diagnosis was heralded by the identification of aggressive ulceration, failure to heal, and dramatic complications, for the most part, individuals are now identified early either due to the presence of an ulcer in an atypical site (postbulbar) or the failure to heal on adequate therapy, particularly if *H. pylori* has been eradicated. Indeed, recurrent ulcer disease after demonstration of *H. pylori* eradication and appropriate compliance with PPI therapy should lead to a high index of suspicion, with early measurement of fasting gastrin levels. An important clinical clue is the presence of diarrhea in a patient with the diagnosis of peptic ulcer disease, especially if there is no evidence of intake of antacids containing magnesium or other agents known to provoke increased gut motility or secretion. Hypergastrinemia should be defined as of tumor origin by performance of a secretin-provocation test and the site of the gastrinoma then identified. The most effective topographic study is the Somatostatin Receptor Scintigram (SRS) (Octreoscan), which uses an isotopically labeled somatostatin receptor-2 subtype analogue to detect tumors and their metastases. This study has a high sensitivity and specificity (85% to 90%) for both primary and secondary lesions and is particularly effective in the detection of lymph node and hepatic metastases. Computed tomography (CT) scan and magnetic resonance imaging (MRI) are of some use and may provide further information than what is

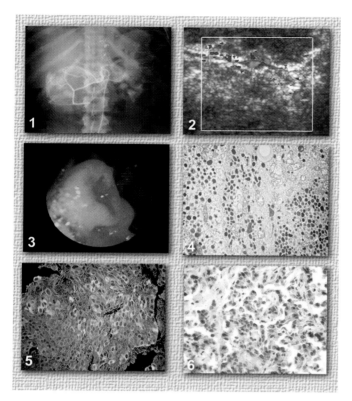

1: A gastrinoma of the head of the pancreas, demonstrated by angiography. 2: Duodenal wall gastrinoma, demonstrated by intraoperative ultrasound. 3: Duodenal wall gastrinoma at endoscopy. 4: Electron microscopy of a gastrin-secreting endocrine tumor of the pancreas. The different density and size of the granules suggest the production of more than one peptide by the lesion. 5: Immunofluorescent identification of gastrin cells. The use of immunofluorescent-labeled antibodies to a specific peptide allowed a more precise identification of the secretory granules of a particular endocrine cell. 6: An immunohistochemical photomicrograph of a gastrinoma demonstrating a high level of SST-receptor expression.

available from the SRS scan. It has proved particularly difficult to identify minute and often multiple duodenal gastrinomas. Endoscopic ultrasound has proved to be of use in this area, although often such lesions may only be detectable at surgery itself by transillumination of the duodenal wall, intraoperative ultrasound, or formal duodenotomy and palpation.

The management of gastrinomas has evolved considerably in the last decade, particularly with the advent of PPI therapy. In the past, the inability to adequately suppress acid secretion and, thus, obviate the drastic complications of aggressive peptic ulcer disease led to the widespread use of total gastrectomy to remove the target organ for gastrin. Although this therapy was reasonably successful, it did not address the underlying cause and exposed the patient to all the risks of a major operative procedure as well as the metabolic sequelae of a total gastrectomy. The early mortality of the procedure reflected technical inadequacy as well as the failure to recognize the trophic effects of gastrin and the proliferation of fundic mucosa beyond the gastroesophageal function. As a result, gastroesophageal anastomoses were often exposed to considerable acid secretion from areas of parietal cell–bearing mucosa that remained in the esophageal remnant. The subsequent anastomotic leaks and strictures marred the early results of surgery and led to the recognition that at least the lower 3 cm of the esophagus should be removed and frozen sections performed at surgery to confirm the absence of parietal cells at the margins of the anastomosis.

The introduction of H_2 receptor antagonists led to a significant diminution in the need for gastric surgery, but the high doses of H_2 receptor antagonists required to suppress acid adequately were often associated with considerable adverse effects. In addition, the tachyphylaxis associated with competitive receptor antagonism led to a diminution of efficacy and an increase of complications such as bleeding and perforation with time. The introduction of PPI therapy has, for the most part, obviated such problems, and the potency and relative lack of side effects, even at high dosage, of this class of drugs has rendered them the primary therapeutic choice in the management of gastrinomas. Those individuals whose gastrinoma is part of the MEN-1 syndrome are likely to develop gastric carcinoids within 2 to 3 years of PPI therapy. This reflects the relationship between hypergastrinemia and an as-yet uncharacterized genomic abnormality, because gastrinomas unassociated with the syndrome do not develop such lesions. Gastric carcinoid tumors should be identified and carefully monitored. If they are multiple, rapidly growing, or larger than 2 cm, consideration should be given to fundic resection to obviate the possibility of perforation, bleeding, or the development of metastases.

Somatostatin-receptor scintigraphy has proved to be of considerable value in identifying gastrinomas and their secondaries. Top: gastrinomas of the head of the pancreas and a hepatic metastasis. Bottom: gastrinoma of the head of the pancreas.

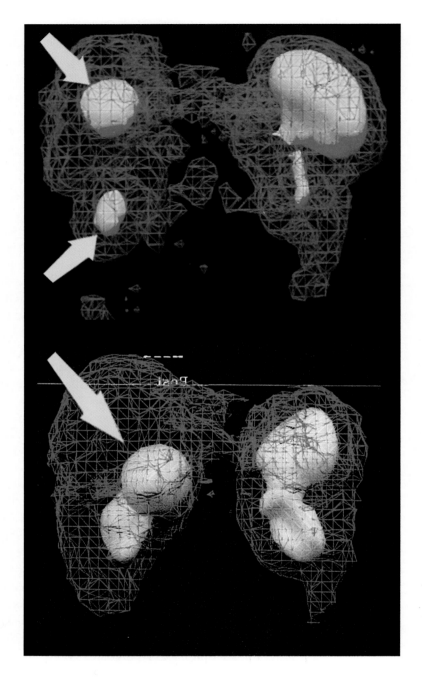

The issue of surgery for the management of gastrinoma remains a controversial question. In those rare instances when the lesion is solitary or benign, or both (less than 10% to 15%), it should be resected. Gastrinoma tumors of the pancreas appear to be of a more malignant variety and are usually multicentric and metastatic at diagnosis. The gastrinomas that arise in the duodenum, although often small, multicentric, and difficult to detect, appear to be of a more benign variety and should probably be addressed more actively. In some centers, consideration has even been given to pancreaticoduodenectomy. Such operations should be carefully evaluated against the background of the local surgical expertise, the

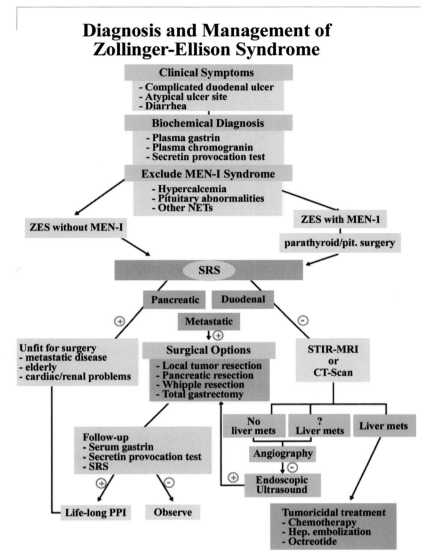

Diagnosis and Management of Zollinger-Ellison Syndrome

Clinical Symptoms
- Complicated duodenal ulcer
- Atypical ulcer site
- Diarrhea

Biochemical Diagnosis
- Plasma gastrin
- Plasma chromogranin
- Secretin provocation test

Exclude MEN-I Syndrome
- Hypercalcemia
- Pituitary abnormalities
- Other NETs

ZES without MEN-I

ZES with MEN-1
→ parathyroid/pit. surgery

SRS

Pancreatic · Duodenal

Metastatic

Unfit for surgery
- metastatic disease
- elderly
- cardiac/renal problems

Surgical Options
- Local tumor resection
- Pancreatic resection
- Whipple resection
- Total gastrectomy

STIR-MRI or CT-Scan

No liver mets · ? Liver mets · Liver mets

Angiography

Endoscopic Ultrasound

Follow-up
- Serum gastrin
- Secretin provocation test
- SRS

Life-long PPI · Observe

Tumoricidal treatment
- Chemotherapy
- Hep. embolization
- Octreotide

A management algorithm for gastrinoma.

patient's overall condition, and the question of projected life expectancy. Removal of hepatic metastases has been suggested to increase survival but should be carefully considered given the effectiveness of PPI therapy for management of the disease process and the potential risk of abdominal surgery and hepatic resection.

In gastrinoma patients who present with a major complication such as perforation or bleeding, the availability of safe intravenous PPIs, such as pantoprazole, has provided a considerable advantage in the surgical management. The ability to consistently elevate the pH of the stomach to greater than 6.0 confers a great degree of safety on anastomotic margins and minimizes the postoperative complications associated with mucosal ulceration and rebleeding. Overall, long-term maintenance therapy on PPIs appears to be the mainstay for the vast majority of gastrinoma patients, with surgical resection of tumor being a consideration only in a small proportion of highly selected individuals in institutions where special expertise for such management is available. The use of vagotomy, partial gastrectomy, and other indeterminate surgical procedures is to be abjured, because they do not decrease acid secretion adequately and confer on the patient all the risks of surgery as well as the sequelae of gastrectomy without protecting against the underlying disease process. The possibility that gastrinoma tumor growth itself may be addressed by the use of high-dosage somatostatin analogs or the introduction of high-energy isotopically labeled somatostatin analogs is under evaluation, and the preliminary results suggest that such therapy may be of some use in the future.

Idiopathic hypersecretion

Some individuals secrete high quantities of acid without elevation in serum gastrin. Their secretion is difficult to control with H_2 receptor antagonists and sometimes even with PPIs. The basis of this hypersecretion is obscure but may involve cAMP signaling in the parietal cell independent of activation of the H_2 receptor.

CHAPTER 3
GASTRIC CARCINOID

It is apparent that during proliferation of the ECL cells, a definable morphologic pattern evolves in the course of the transformation from the normal cell to the neoplastic mode. In 1988, Solcia and others delineated a system of classification for the spectrum of proliferative changes of endocrine cells of the gastric fundus. This classification is defined by histopathologic appearances ranging from hyperplasia to dysplasia to neoplasia.

Histology

The term *pseudohyperplasia* has been used to describe cell clustering unassociated with cell proliferation. The successive stages of hyperplasia are termed *simple*, *linear* or *chain-forming*, *micronodular*, and *adenomatoid*. Dysplasia is characterized by relatively atypical cells with features of enlarging or fusing micronodules, microinvasion, or newly formed stroma. When the nodules increase further in size to larger than 5 mm or invade into the submucosa, the lesion is classified as a neoplasm. This stage is divided into intramucosal and invasive forms.

The entire spectrum of endocrine cell proliferation, from hyperplasia to dysplasia and neoplasia, has been observed in MEN-1–ZES and diffuse type A chronic atrophic gastritis. Both hyperplastic and pseudohyperplastic changes occur with low frequency in the *H. pylori*–related chronic gastritis associated with ulcer disease or dyspepsia.

However, because no progression to dysplastic or neoplastic lesions has thus far been documented in these latter conditions, their role in gastric endocrine tumorigenesis appears unlikely. Carcinoid tumor is thus characterized morphologically by the criteria of size and invasion.

Biologically, however, the state of neoplasia is recognized by autonomy from the trophic effects of gastrin. A lesion that fails to regress once gastrin levels have been normalized is therefore regarded as a carcinoid tumor.

Classification of ECL Cell Proliferation

Hyperplasia	**Simple (diffuse)**
	Linear
	Micronodular
	Adenomatoid
Dysplasia (Pre-Neoplastic stage)	**Enlarging micronodule**
	Fusing micronodule
	Microinvasive lesion
	Nodule with newly formed strata
Carcinoid	
	Intramucosal carcinoid
	Invasive carcinoid

A histologic grading system for the evaluation of ECL cell proliferation. As detailed as this system is, it represents little more than pattern recognition and is unable to predict with any certainty the ultimate biologic end point of the individual aggregation of proliferating cells. In particular, histologic appearance cannot identify the critical event of gastrin autonomy. To determine the destiny of such alterations in phenotype, a molecular analysis of the cell system is required.

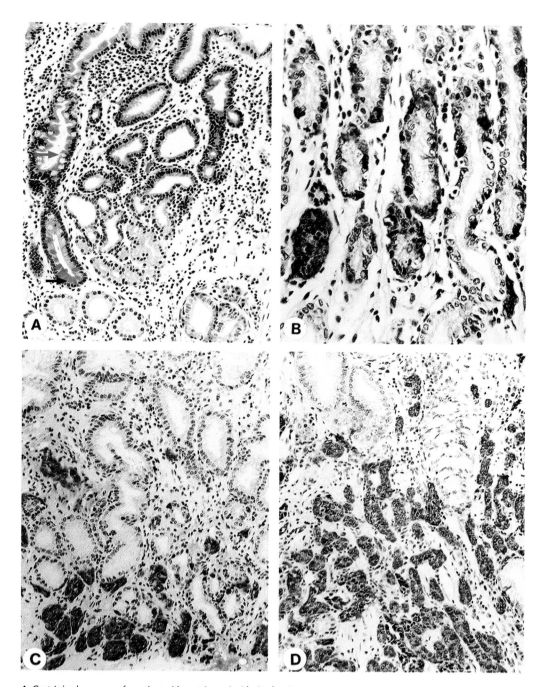

A: Gastric body mucosa of a patient with gastric carcinoidosis, showing typical features of gastric atrophy: the mucosa is thinned, parietal and chief cells are absent, and there is intestinal metaplasia (note the Paneth cells (red arrow) and goblet cells (black arrow) in the gland on the left) and a lymphoplasmacytic infiltrate (hematoxylin and eosin, ×200). **B:** Chromogranin expression in mucosa adjacent to that shown in **A.** Simple hyperplasia of ECL cells is seen in the gland on the extreme right; that in the middle of the field shows linear hyperplasia of the ECL cells (i.e., they form chains without intervening cells), whereas that on the bottom left has developed into a micronodule (immunoperoxidase, ×400). **C:** In this field, there is adenomatoid hyperplasia of the ECL cells, defined as a cluster of five or more micronodules (immunoperoxidase for chromogranin A, ×200). **D:** Intramucosal ECL cell neoplasm (immunoperoxidase for chromogranin A, ×200).

Development

In rats and *Mastomys*, it appears that a threshold value of plasma gastrin is necessary not only for ECL cell hyperplasia to occur but also for conversion to gastric carcinoid. This value reflects not only gastrin levels but also length of exposure and other factors in which female gender and, in humans and *Mastomys*, genomic events (MEN-1) are involved. In fact, in humans, the ECL cell density does not exhibit a relation to plasma gastrin levels in normogastrinemic individuals, nor does it reveal any significant differences in duodenal ulcer patients with mild hypergastrinemia. In patients on PPIs for 6 months, no significant changes in ECL cells were noted.

Furthermore, in peptic ulcer patients receiving omeprazole for more than a decade, ECL cells were not significantly affected. If plasma gastrin levels of greater than 400 pg per mL are present, significant proliferation not progressing to dysplasia has been noted. It has therefore been suggested that in patients with plasma gastrin levels greater than 400 pg per mL, gastric biopsy should be undertaken to evaluate endocrine cell status, or a decrease in the dosage of the PPIs should be considered. In patients with sustained hypergastrinemia associated with surgical vagotomy, alterations in ECL status are not significant. Although duration of exposure appears important, it has been noted that ECL cell hyperplasia may be stable with time, provided that gastrin levels do not increase significantly. With hypergastrinemia alone (e.g., sporadic ZES), ECL cell proliferation is usually limited to hyperplastic lesions of the simple or linear type. However, in patients with MEN-1–ZES or type A chronic atrophic gastritis, ECL cell lesions are usually dysplastic or overtly carcinoid in nature. Factors other than hypergastrinemia must therefore be involved in ECL cell transformation. In the MEN-1 syndrome, the loss of the tumor suppressor oncogene (menin) on chromosome 11q13 may be related.

Similarly, in atrophic gastritis, either achlorhydria or alterations in the biology of the associated mucosa, which have also been suggested to be implicated in the pathogenesis of gastric adenocarcinoma, may be involved. It has been suggested that detection of dysplastic changes or ECL cell carcinoids in a ZES patient warrant screening of both the patient and the family for a covert MEN-1 syndrome.

The hyperplastic effect of hypergastrinemia on gastric mucosal epithelial cells appears not to be restricted to the ECL cells. Foveolar cells and surface mucous cells also undergo hyperplasia in the human stomach under the influence of excessive gastrin drive, often to a considerable degree. This process may be patchy and not infrequently results in the development of endoscopically detectable polyps that are classified histologically as *foveolar hyperplasia*. Thus, to add to the confusion surrounding gastric carcinoid tumors, in patients with these lesions arising in a setting of hypergastrinemia, at least two types of mucosal polyps can be expected: those due to ECL cell proliferations and simple foveolar hyperplasias. Whether these foveolar cell hyperplasias represent an early stage on the pathway to gastric adenocarcinoma of the type that occurs with increased frequency in patients with chronic atrophic gastritis type A and pernicious anemia is not known.

In a morphometric ultrastructural investigation of sporadic ZES patients, a 168% increase in the volume density of the total oxyntic endocrine cell popula-

Distribution of Neuroendocrine Cell Types in the Fundic Mucosa

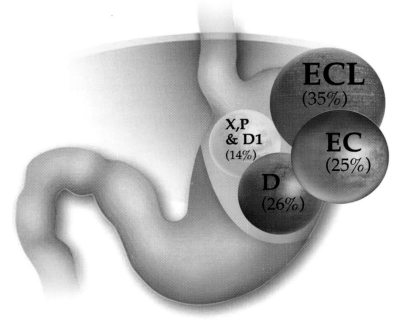

The ECL cells are the dominant fundic neuroendocrine cell type, followed by the D cells, which secrete somatostatin. The function of the other types and their biologic role have not been clearly characterized.

tion was noted. This increase was exclusively due to ECL cells, with other types showing a relatively decreased volume. However, in patients with *H. pylori*, the P and D1 cells have been reported to exhibit hyperplasia. This may reflect the metaplastic background in which endocrine cells proliferate.

The oncoprotein, BCL2, enhances cell survival by blocking programmed cell death (apoptosis) due to inhibition of mitochondrial export of cytochrome *c*. Immunohistochemical expression of BCL2 in endocrine cells of the human oxyntic mucosa has been investigated in patients with normal gastric mucosa, sporadic ZES, MEN-1–ZES, hypergastrinemic atrophic gastritis (HAG), and ECL cell carcinoids. In all patients, BCL2 immunoreactivity was exclusively located in endocrine cells located in the middle layer of the oxyntic mucosa.

The ratio of BCL2 to chromogranin A–reacting cells was low in sporadic ZES (no risk of carcinoid). It was, however, maintained in MEN-1–ZES and increased in chronic atrophic gastritis A (conditions with intermediate or high risk of carcinoid, respectively). BCL2 expression by gastric carcinoid markedly varied from one tumor to another, even in the same patient, but was low or absent in most cases. Thus, BCL2 is expressed by normal fundic endocrine cells whose intraglandular location suggests a role for the protein during migration from the neck stem zone to fully differentiated cells at the gland bottom.

Experimental model *Mastomys natalensis*

A novel rodent model available for study of the ECL cell and particularly its neoplastic transformation is the *Mastomys natalensis*. This is a sub-Saharan rodent that was initially used in the study of African plague vectors. During these studies, it was noted that a substantial percentage of the animals died of a gastric neoplasm. Initially, this lesion was identified as a gastric adenocarcinoma. It subsequently became apparent that the cell type was more compatible with a carcinoid lesion. Further investigation identified this neoplasm as a histamine-producing ECL cell tumor (ECLoma).

The tumor is histamine secreting and does not metastasize, which renders it closely comparable to the human type I gastric carcinoid tumor. If untreated, animals develop duodenal ulcers, which either bleed or perforate, resulting in demise of the tumor carrier on an acute basis. The tumor could be successfully transplanted to either subcutaneous or intraocular sites. The *Mastomys* has a genetic propensity to spontaneously develop ECLomas, with the incidence depending on the particular breeding strain. The specific genomic aberration has not been identified. The rates of tumor development vary from 20% to 70% within the lifespan of the animal. Of particular interest, however, is the observation that the use of acid-inhibitory agents in this animal result in the rapid production of hypergastrinemia, with a transformation from a normal ECL cell population to a hyperplastic state by 2 months; neoplastic lesions are evident in up to 80% of animals by 4 months. The hyperplastic ECL state is reversible at 8 weeks, but by 16 weeks, withdrawal of the gastrin stimulus fails to result in tumor regression. The use of the *Mastomys* species has therefore been of considerable use in studying gastrin-induced ECL cell proliferation and has enabled characterization of the ECL cell tumor.

Clinical considerations

Tumor classification and management

Neuroendocrine tumors of the stomach previously were felt to be responsible for approximately 0.3% of all gastric tumors and 3% to 5% of all gastrointestinal carcinoids. More recently, however, these estimates have variously risen to 11% to 41% of all gastrointestinal neuroendocrine lesions. This increase most likely represents an increase in awareness as well as an association with specific disease entities, such as atrophic gastritis.

An overall classification of such lesions (carcinoids) was developed in Munich in 1994. Essentially, it evaluates lesions on the basis of their histologic behavior and comprises four groups: (a) benign behavior: nonfunctioning, well-differentiated tumors of small size (up to 1 cm) limited to the mucosa-submucosa and without angioinvasion—usually ECL cell tumors of the fundic mucosa associated with chronic atrophic gastritis and hypergastrinemia; (b) benign or low-grade malignant behavior: nonfunctioning, well-differentiated tumors within the mucosa-submucosa of small size (larger than 1 cm and up to 2 cm) without angioinvasion or of small to intermediate size (up to 2 cm) with angioinvasion—usually ECL cell tumors of the fundic mucosa associated with chronic atrophic gastritis and hypergastrinemia, rarely MEN-1–associated or sporadic ECL cell tumors; (c) low-grade malignant behavior (low-grade neuroendocrine carcinoma): nonfunctioning, well-differentiated tumors of large size (larger than 2 cm) or extending beyond the submucosa—usually sporadic ECL cell tumors, rarely serotonin-producing tumors or others, rarely MEN-1 or chronic atrophic gastritis–associated ECL cell tumors or functioning, well-differentiated tumors of any size and extension—sporadic gastrinoma, serotonin-producing tumor (EC), or others; and

Distribution of 13,715 Carcinoid Tumors

Organ site	% of total
Gallbladder	0.2
Liver	0.3
Pancreas	0.6
Ovary	0.8
Jejunum	1.7
Duodenum	2.6
Stomach	4.1
Appendix	12.2
Rectum	13.7
Ileum	14.3
Colon, excluding Rectum	20.4
Trachea, Bronchus, Lung	24.5

Distribution of the 13,715 carcinoid tumors contained by the ERG, TNCS, and the SEER file (1950–1999) by organ site. The dominant site for carcinoid development is the gastrointestinal system. Gastric carcinoids constitute 4.1% of all carcinoid tumors.

Pathologic diagnosis of typed gastric carcinoids. **A:** Surgical resection specimen of fundic mucosa with numerous carcinoid tumor nodules (indicated by *arrows*). **B:** Gastroscopic identification of multiple carcinoid tumors in a patient with pernicious anemia. **C:** Histologic evaluation using hematoxylin and eosin staining of the fundic mucosa, with evidence of ECL neoplasia (indicated by the *arrow*). **D:** Demonstration of a microcarcinoid tumor by chromogranin A immunoreactivity (brown staining) in the fundic mucosa.

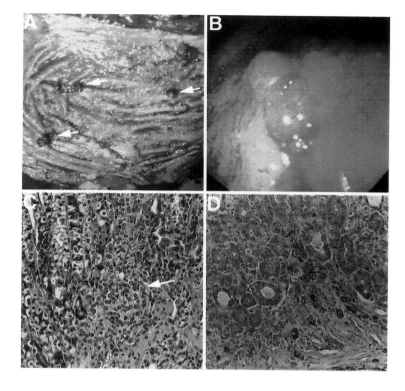

(d) malignant behavior: functioning or nonfunctioning poorly differentiated intermediate or small-cell carcinoma.

In a recent series of gastric neuroendocrine tumors, 46 of 55 tumors (83%) were well-differentiated. Only one was a G cell tumor of the antrum—the remaining 45 were well-differentiated ECL cell tumors. In reviewing the histology and pathobiology of gastric carcinoids, it is of significance to distinguish between different types of gastric carcinoids. The presence of hypergastrinemia in particular appears to connote a far more benign situation than lesions occurring under normogastrinemic conditions. Furthermore, solitary sporadic lesions are of considerably worse prognosis compared to multiple or diffuse microcarcinoid lesions. The latter occur relatively frequently in association with hypergastrinemic states, in contrast to the more rare sporadic gastric tumors.

Three patterns of gastric carcinoid (ECL cell) tumor have been proposed: (a) argyrophilic carcinoids arising in type A chronic atrophic gastritis (chronic atrophic gastritis/A), (b) argyrophilic ECL cell carcinoids in MEN-1–ZES, and (c) sporadic argyrophil carcinoids.

This classification does not include neuroendocrine carcinomas (non-ECL cell), previously known as *atypical carcinoids*. These represent an aggressive neuroendocrine neoplasm that bears greater resemblance to sporadic carcinoids than to hypergastrinemia-associated tumors. They are generally large, solitary tumors that frequently display central necrosis. Histopathologically, they feature small- to intermediate-sized poorly differentiated "protoendocrine" cells, a high mitotic index, and invasive growth. They metastasize with great frequency and progress rapidly.

Gastric Carcinoid Tumor Types

NOMENCLATURE	TUMOR CHARACTERISTICS	HISTOLOGY	HYPER-GASTRINEMIA	BIOLOGICAL BEHAVIOR
TYPE I	Generally small (<1 cm) and multiple; often nodular/polypoid	ECL cell lesion. Stages of ECL cell hyperplasia, dysplasia, and neoplasia present in adjacent mucosa	Present	Slow growth, regional or distant metastases extremely rare
TYPE II	Generally small (<1 cm) and multiple	ECL cell lesion. Stages of ECL cell hyperplasia, dysplasia, and neoplasia present in adjacent mucosa	Present	Slow growth, may metastasize more often than CAG-associated lesions
TYPE III	Solitary, often large (>1 cm)	ECL, EC, or X cells. Tumor formation w/o evidence of hyperplasia or precarcinoid dysplasia in adjacent mucosa	Absent	Relatively aggressive growth, frequent metastases to regional nodes (55%) and liver (24%)

The characteristic features of the different types of gastric carcinoid tumors.

Carcinoids arising in type A chronic atrophic gastritis (type I)

Gastric carcinoid tumors arising in the presence of type A chronic atrophic gastritis (chronic atrophic gastritis/A) constitute the most common type of gastric carcinoid (62% to 83%). Chronic atrophic gastritis/A is characterized by chronic inflammation of the oxyntic mucosa, often associated with autoimmune diseases such as pernicious anemia, and results in atrophy of the oxyntic glands and achlorhydria. Carcinoid tumors related to chronic atrophic gastritis/A are usually small, are often multicentric, and tend to behave less aggressively than sporadic gastric carcinoids.

In a series of 23 patients with gastric carcinoids, 19 of the 23 (83%) had concurrent chronic atrophic gastritis/A. Tumors in these patients were single or multiple, were associated with hypergastrinemia, and had not spread beyond the mucosa or submucosa. Solcia reported 80 cases of chronic atrophic gastritis with hypergastrinemia and found focal or diffuse endocrine cell hyperplasia in all of them. In addition, he identified 20 individuals (25%) with dysplastic (precarcinoid) lesions and 24 patients (30%) with carcinoids and concluded that dysplastic, but not hyperplastic, changes are linked to the development of multiple gastric carcinoids. Stolte studied 55 patients with gastric carcinoids, of whom 46 (83.6%) had chronic atrophic gastritis, and reported that in 27 nonoperated patients followed up by endoscopy and biopsy for an average of 3.6 years, there were no alteration in their original findings. They proposed that for patients with small (smaller than 1 cm) gastric carcinoids, expectant therapy with endoscopic follow-up may be advisable. In a series examined by Rindi, 28

A management algorithm for gastric carcinoids. Although antrectomy is a theoretically attractive surgical option, since it is based on the biologic premise that the type I and type II lesions are driven by gastrin, its application to an individual patient is flawed by the inability to determine if the proliferating ECL cells are gastrin dependent or have attained autonomy. In the latter circumstance, antral resection will not halt disease progression.

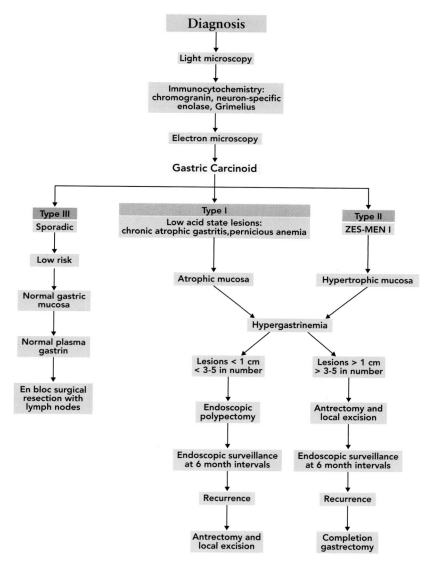

Strategy for Management of Gastric Carcinoid

of 45 (62%) patients with gastric carcinoids also had chronic atrophic gastritis/ A, and 64% of patients had multiple tumors. Of the 12 patients in whom gastrin was measured, all were hypergastrinemic. The tumors were small, with a median size of 0.7 cm, and none metastasized. Of 25 patients who were followed for an average of 6 years, 20 (80%) were alive, including 6 (24%) who did not undergo surgery. None died from causes related to their tumors. On the basis of this experience, it has been argued that expectant therapy or endoscopic removal of accessible tumors may be appropriate for gastric carcinoids associated with hypergastrinemia. This conservative form of management would reflect the relatively benign behavior of the majority of such tumors.

Others have observed that antrectomy has resulted in regression of tumors, presumably because the source of gastrin, the proposed principle promoter of

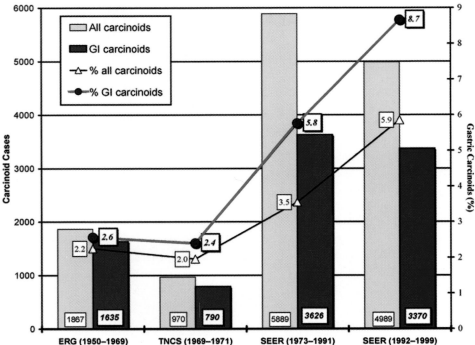

Gastric carcinoid incidence, 1950–1999. The data demonstrate that the incidence of gastric carcinoids is rising, although whether this is due to the widespread availability of endoscopy or increased awareness or whether this represents a "real" biologic phenomenon is unclear. (ERG, End Results Group; SEER, Surveillance, Epidemiology, and End Results database; TNCS, Third National Cancer Survey.)

tumor growth, has been removed. Hirschowitz et al. reported three patients with pernicious anemia, hypergastrinemia, and multicentric gastric carcinoids. After antrectomy, gastrin levels returned to normal in all three patients. Follow-up gastroscopy with biopsy 12 to 18 months postoperatively revealed foci of microcarcinoids in all three patients, but biopsies at 21 to 30 months revealed complete regression of both carcinoids and ECL cell hyperplasia. Richards and colleagues performed an antrectomy on one patient with hypergastrinemia and multiple tumors. After the operation, gastrin levels were normalized, and total regression of the tumor was reported. Eckhauser reported two cases of multicentric carcinoids, atrophic gastritis, and hypergastrinemia. One patient had tumor involving one regional lymph node, and the other had a single liver metastasis. After antrectomy (and removal of the liver nodule in the patient with hepatic metastasis), gastrin levels returned to normal in both patients. On gastroscopy with biopsy 4 to 6 months postoperatively, the patient with nodal metastasis had residual neoplasm in the stomach, and the other patient's tumor had completely regressed. Whether these lesions were ECLomas or neuroendocrine carcinomas is not clear. Caruso et al. reported one patient with atrophic gastritis and multiple gastric carcinoids. Initial management involved gastric resection with antrectomy, at which time it was noted that the largest of the tumors present was a composite carcinoid-adenocarcinoma. One month later, a complete gastrectomy was therefore undertaken, and regressive changes in the ECL cell proliferations in the gastric remnant were reported. Kern et al. described a patient with pernicious anemia, hypergastrinemia, and ECL cell hyperplasia. The patient underwent antrectomy, which resulted in resolution of his hypergastrinemia. Nine months later, the remainder of the stomach was resected, and morphometric evaluation revealed a marked reduction in the number and size of endocrine cells in the gastric mucosa. Wangberg and colleagues performed an antrectomy on a patient with atrophic gastritis, pernicious anemia, hypergastrinemia, and multiple gastric carcinoids. Although the patient's gastrin levels returned to normal, multiple fundic carcinoids developed 23 months after surgery. They proposed that antrectomy may be appropriate in the treatment of early lesions, but that large primary lesions in combination with nodular hyperplasia should be treated with total or subtotal gastrectomy. In a small number of patients, spontaneous regression of chronic atrophic gastritis/A–associated tumors has been reported.

Nevertheless, special attention is necessary for the management of patients with large (1.6- to 2.0-cm) and deeply invasive type I well-differentiated ECL tumors that tend to have a low-grade malignant behavior. This clinical profile closely matches that of the 197 chronic atrophic gastritis–associated gastric neuroendocrine tumors previously published and of the 27 similar tumors included in the series of 104 gastric carcinoids recently reported.

MEN-1–Zollinger-Ellison syndrome–associated gastric carcinoids (type II)

Individuals with MEN-1–ZES have a well-recognized propensity to develop gastric carcinoids. In a group of 48 ZES patients, Lehy et al. reported 17 with ZES and MEN-1, five of whom (29.5%) developed gastric carcinoid tumors. None of 31 patients with sporadic ZES exhibited gastric carcinoids. Despite a substantial level of hypergastrinemia, patients with sporadic ZES have very rarely been reported to develop gastric carcinoids. Hypergastrinemia is, however, associated with proliferation of ECL cells in these patients. In individuals with MEN-1, a genetic predisposition presumably exists that facilitates the development of carcinoid tumors.

More recently, Cadiot and colleagues reported the identification of loss of heterozygosity near the MEN-1 locus on chromosome 11q13 in a gastric carcinoid tumor of a MEN-1–ZES patient. They argued that this observation suggested that the MEN-1 gene was a tumor suppressor gene for fundic argyrophil tumors in ZES. Proliferating ECL cells of hypergastrinemic patients express β-fibroblast growth factor, which is known to exhibit potent mitogenic properties for a wide variety of mesoderm-derived cell types. These cells may therefore be the source of abnormally high circulating levels of the β-fibroblast growth factor–like mitogen factor that has been identified in MEN-1 patients. ECLoma-producing β-fibroblast growth factor may thus be responsible for the unusual proliferation of smooth muscle cells, presumably originating from the muscularis mucosa that is often associated with ECL cell carcinoids, particularly in areas of submucosal invasion.

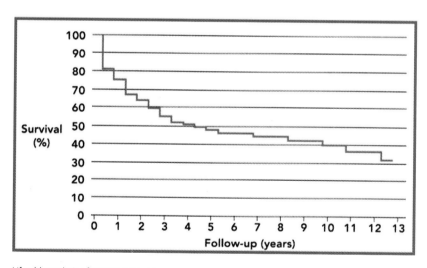

Lifetable analysis of gastric carcinoids in the SEER (1973–1991) file. The overall observed 5-year survival rate is 48.6%. This grouping may, however, reflect the outcome of a variety of different types of gastric neuroendocrine tumors. Many of the tumors were probably of the sporadic type (type III), whose prognosis is very much worse than the lesions associated with hypergastrinemia (types I and II).

Distribution of gastric carcinoid tumors by stage in the ERG (1950–1969) and the SEER (1973–1999) files. Although the percentage of localized disease increased from 45.2% through 52.9% to 67.5%, it decreased from 28.6% to 3.1% for lesions with regional metastasis and from 23.8% to 6.5% for lesions with distant metastasis. At least 50% of gastric carcinoids are nonlocalized at diagnosis. Unstaged carcinoid tumors constituted 2.4% of the ERG and 22.9% of the SEER database.

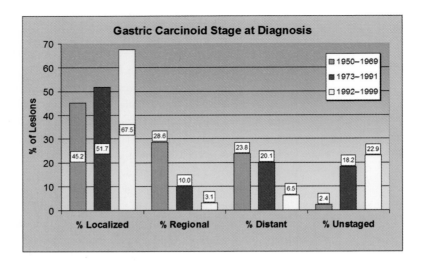

Rindi et al. described seven cases of gastric carcinoid occurring against a background of hypertrophic gastropathy. Of the seven patients, six had MEN-1–ZES. All seven of the patients displayed hypergastrinemia as well as hyperplasia and dysplasia of argyrophil cells in nontumor mucosa. The tumors in these patients were small, with a median size of 0.5 cm.

Two of the six MEN-1–ZES patients had local lymph node metastases, but none had distant metastases. None of the MEN-1–ZES patients died from tumor-related disease during a mean follow-up of 79 months. These tumors are composed predominantly of ECL cells, although some lesions contain a heterogeneous population of cell types. The behavior of gastric carcinoids associated with MEN-1–ZES appears to occupy a middle ground between that of the relatively more aggressive sporadic lesions and the more benign tumors seen in conjunction with chronic atrophic gastritis.

Sporadic argyrophil carcinoids (type III)

Sporadic argyrophil carcinoids are isolated tumors that arise against a background of normal gastric mucosa. They tend to be larger (two to three times) than the other types of gastric carcinoids and to behave more aggressively, exhibiting deep mucosal invasion. Rindi et al. reported their experience with ten sporadic tumors that ranged in size from 0.5 to 5.0 cm (median, 2.0 cm). At the time of diagnosis, six of the ten sporadic tumors had metastasized, two locally and four to the liver. In addition, eight of ten displayed lymphatic invasion. Other series have demonstrated a correlation between tumor size and metastasis for gastric carcinoids of all types. Nevertheless, minute tumors that have spread have been reported. Other factors that predict aggressive behavior by sporadic tumors include moderate cellular atypia, two or more mitoses per ten high-powered fields, angioinvasion, and deep invasion of the gastric wall. Sporadic gastric carcinoids display a fairly uniform histopathologic appearance. The cells have uniform round nuclei. Their growth pattern may be trabecular or gyriform, medullary or solid, glandular or rosette-like, or a combination of these types. The lesions are argyrophilic but not argentaffin-positive and display immunoreactivity for numerous markers, including chromogranin A, neuron-specific enolase, synaptophysin, and S-100. In addition, they may contain small numbers of serotonin, somatostatin, or even gastrin-positive cells. Ultrastructurally, the lesions appear to contain a mixture of cell types. Generally, some of the cells are identifiable as ECL cells, whereas others resemble EC or X cells. Overall, lesions of this type may be regarded as bearing greater similarity to neuroendocrine carcinomas than to carcinoids per se. Indeed, their biologic behavior is far more aggressive, with invasive growth and metastasis as predictable features in their evolution.

Complete or partial gastrectomy with local lymph node resection is recommended therapy in surgical candidates with solitary, large (larger than 1 cm), or invasive tumors. For patients with metastatic disease involving the liver, surgical resection of tumor foci may reduce symptoms and improve survival. Similarly, selective hepatic artery ligation or embolization has a beneficial effect. Chemotherapy alone has been reported to produce a 20% to 40% tumor response rate in patients with disseminated disease. Commonly used chemotherapeutic agents include streptozocin, 5-fluorouracil, cyclophosphamide, and doxorubicin. The somatostatin analog octreotide has proven effective in reducing symptoms of the carcinoid syndrome, as has leukocyte interferon in some instances.

In a series of 265 cases, Modlin reported a 52% overall 5-year survival rate for patients with gastric carcinoids of all stages, 48.6% for patients with local lesions, 39.5% for patients with regional metastases, and 10% for patients with distant metastases. This study, however, did not distinguish between different types of gastric carcinoids and therefore represents a summation of outcome information. More recent series have produced similar results for sporadic tumors. The outcome for the sporadic tumors may be regarded as poor compared to lesions that are purely of ECL cell origin or associated with hypergastrinemia, or both.

CHAPTER 4
DYSPEPSIA

Non-ulcer dyspepsia

One of the major limitations of medical practice in the management of dyspepsia is the inability to identify a mucosal lesion. To a large extent, this may actually reflect the limitations of current endoscopic technology or the macular acuity of either the endoscopist or his or her pathologist. As the discriminant index for the identification of lesions has decreased with the advent of more sophisticated technology, the group or individuals in which a diagnosis cannot be established has similarly decreased. Nevertheless, a conundrum is provided by a situation in which a patient complains vigorously of a group of symptoms that have been generically accepted by the physician as synonymous with dyspepsia if no lesion can be identified. In some circumstances, the skill of the practitioner and the attitude of the patient will allow for consideration of functional overlay. In other instances, the symptoms are not diagnostic of dyspepsia and, indeed, may wax and wane in severity as well as altering somewhat in nature as time passes.

The critical difficulty in patients of this type relates to the actual definition and meaning of the word *dyspepsia*. Although this has been broadly defined as "*pain or discomfort centered in the upper abdomen,*" this definition does not include coexisting symptoms that may occur at other sites. To override the limitations that subjective descriptions of symptomatology proffered by a patient might generate, a more cohesive definition of *functional dyspepsia* may be used. In brief, this embraces the dyspepsia complex of symptoms using three broad categories: (a) ulcer-like dyspepsia, (b) dysmotility-like dyspepsia, and (c) unspecified (nonspecific) dyspepsia. In the ulcer-like dyspepsia group, a predominant complaint should be upper abdominal pain, usually located in the epigastrium, relieved by foods and antacids, and occurring before meals or when hungry. Occasionally, this pain may awaken the patient from sleep and be associated with a timing pattern characteristic of periodicity, with remissions and relapses. It is likely that this group actually contains patients who may have acid peptic disease but in whom no overt (macroscopic) ulceration can be detected by conventional technology. In many of these patients, relief will occur with the use of H_2 receptor antagonists as well as PPIs.

In a second group—dysmotility-like dyspeptic patients—pain is not the dominant symptom, although upper abdominal discomfort is present. Usually, the discomfort is chronic and characterized by early satiety, postprandial fullness, nausea, retching, and even vomiting. Although the patient may describe a bloating sensation in the upper abdomen, no visible distension is evi-

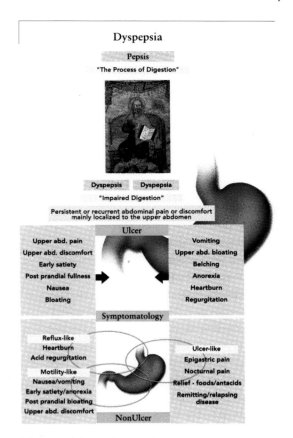

A depiction of the complex interplay between the different types of symptomatology broadly grouped together as *dyspepsia*.

dent, although it and all the above symptoms are usually aggravated by food. The symptomatology of this group of patients is not at all well understood and overall reflects the generally poor clinical understanding of motility disorders. Some of these patients, however, may not only represent abnormalities of gastric emptying but also disturbances of either gall bladder function or colonic motility.

The last group of patients, who are categorized as exhibiting unspecified or nonspecific dyspepsia, is a heterogeneous group that may include individuals with definable neurosis and demonstrable functional disorders if evaluated by a psychiatrist. Part of this group, however, may fall into the poorly understood and heterogenous syndromic collocation of *irritable bowel syndrome*. When carefully questioned, they may also allude to pain in the lower abdomen, with or without constipation, diarrhea, and mucus. It should, however, be borne in mind that the symptom repertoire of the gastrointestinal tract is relatively limited, given the fact that the neural connections are mostly of a visceral nature, rendering somatic interpretation of gastrointestinal sensation both difficult and often imprecise. Careful consideration should especially be given to patients whose complaints are not only repetitive but accurately and consistently reproducible over time. In some instances, a thorough investigation will reveal evidence of covert gall bladder disease, chronic pancreatitis, or even a carcinoid tumor of the small bowel.

A term that is almost as confusing as dyspepsia is the widely used *heartburn*. This is generally described as a symptom of "*a burning sensation under the*

A strategy for the evaluation and management of dyspepsia.

lower part of the center of the chest that rises toward or into the neck." It is frequently aggravated by consumption of food or by changes in posture, such as lying or stooping. In comparison to dyspepsia, there is considerable agreement as to the use of this term, and individuals who exhibit both heartburn and dyspepsia are considered to have symptomatic gastroesophageal reflux disease if the heartburn is the dominant complaint.

It should be recognized, however, that there are other causes of thoracic and esophageal pathology that may produce similar symptomatology, at least in the early stages of the disease. Individuals who have heartburn for at least 3 months and have no endoscopic esophagitis as well as a normal 24-hour esophageal acid exposure have been classified as suffering from *functional heartburn.* Discussions have arisen as to the precise use of the terminology *functional* whether applied to dyspepsia or heartburn.

One proposal that has no rigorous data to support its validity is that such individuals are acid sensitive, and physiologic amounts of acid in the duodenum, stomach, or esophagus generate sensations that are centrally interpreted as pain (dyspepsia or heartburn). In some such individuals, the use of acid-suppressive therapy may be of benefit.

Dyspepsia and heartburn

Approximately 25% of the general population in any Western country may have recurrent dyspepsia over a 12-month period. There appears to be no significant difference in prevalence between Europe and the United States or between men and women, although prevalence does decline significantly as age increases. Epidemiologic studies have reported that 15% of individuals suffer heartburn at least once a week, whereas 7% have heartburn daily. This number is likely to increase in pregnant women and individuals who are either overweight or whose occupation involves frequent stooping or bending. In those whose heartburn and reflux symptoms are significant enough to seek medical advice and endoscopy, 30% to 60% may exhibit evidence of esophagitis. The overall prevalence of erosive esophagitis in the general population is approximately 2%, which is 15 times less than the prevalence of reflux symptoms. Nevertheless, in individuals who are referred for endoscopic evaluation, reflux esophagitis can be documented in up to 15%. It is evident that more than 75% of patients whose symptoms may be classified as dyspepsia or heartburn never seek medical advice and self-medicate. The reasons for this are complex but include the fear of the detection of serious disease or anxiety that the physician may suggest alterations in lifestyle, prescribe medication, or initiate investigations prompting further conflict and concern.

The long-term outcome of individuals with dyspepsia whose cause cannot be identified is difficult to be certain about. Between 10% and 15% of such individuals become asymptomatic on an annual basis, and overall symptoms tend to decrease with age. Alternatively, it has been noted that in control population groups, approximately 12% to 15% on an annual basis develop symptoms of dyspepsia and heartburn for which no cause can be identified.

Despite the fact that a specific disease process in the upper gastrointestinal tract may not be definable even after serious investigation of symptoms, the disease entity per se represents a considerable socioeconomic problem. Because dyspepsia accounts for between 20% and 70% of all gastrointestinal consultation with general practitioners, a significant amount of physician time is spent evaluating the problem. Up to a third of such individuals may be referred to a gastroenterologist for further evaluation. The majority of these are treated, even if no objective evidence of mucosal ulceration is detectable. Thus the 80% receiving H_2 receptor antagonists includes 30% prescribed for heartburn and 40% for functional dyspepsia. No studies are available to determine whether the use of such medication improves the long-term outcome of the disease process.

In Sweden, in 1994, it was calculated that the costs of functional dyspepsia were greater than 55,000 U.S. dollars per 1,000 citizens. Such costs are significantly higher in the United States and will continue to increase as the cost of healthcare grows. Patients with the diagnosis of functional dyspepsia have been reported to have a two- to threefold increase in the number of days of reported sickness from their work. When studied using quality-of-life scales, they attain scores significantly lower than their cohorts.

Thus, functional dyspepsia, whether subdivided into functional heartburn or dyspepsia with motility-related disturbances, remains an area of therapeutic and diagnostic difficulty. Clearly, some of these patients have centrally mediated problems that are outside the care of the gastroenterologist, but others likely have organic pathology that has as yet not been identified. In terms of the practical management of such individuals, it is important to exclude GERD, gastroduodenal ulceration, and the presence of *H. pylori*. In the absence of any obvious pathology, a therapeutic trial of acid-suppression is warranted in those patients whose dyspepsia or heartburn falls within the ulcer-like dyspepsia classification. In individuals whose symptoms are more likely to refer to the dysmotility-like dyspepsia group, acid-suppression therapy may be combined with a prokinetic agent. If symptomatic relief is obtained in either of the two groups, it should be assumed that mucosal disease is present, and careful follow-up should be undertaken to ensure symptom relief and no recurrence of the disease process.

To ensure that *H. pylori* is not overlooked, serology should probably be repeated. In patients in whom no relief is obtained, a complex series of patient–doctor interactions is likely to occur. First, consideration should be given to ruling out the presence of any other covert disease process, particularly in the gallbladder, pancreas, or colon. Failing this, symptomatic support should be provided with counseling or the use of appropriate drugs that may decrease symptoms and allay anxiety. It is important that such individuals be carefully monitored lest their symptoms are early harbingers of some more serious medical problem.

As discussed above, specific treatment for this nonspecific disease is not available. Probably, one's reflex is to first give H_2 receptor antagonists, followed by prescription of PPIs.

Their failure is often diagnostic of non-ulcer dyspepsia (NUD). If *Helicobacter* is found, eradication is undertaken, but this has no effect on symptoms. If one takes the view that this is neurogenic in origin, then what are the gastric afferent nerve receptors that mediate the symptoms, where do they connect, and what stimulates them? Perhaps the most effective agents are PPIs. If they are given to levels at which acid is ablated, would the history of NUD change?

CHAPTER 5
INTRAVENOUS ANTI-SECRETORY THERAPY

Introduction

The concept of medication has been refined over thousands of years as physicians moved from rough herbal mixtures to crude chemicals and then to specific, albeit often impure, therapeutic agents. The subsequent development of more specific agents with defined targets led to the introduction of pharmacologic agents with distinct cellular and molecular destinations. In this respect, H_2 receptor antagonists and PPIs represent the acme of such pharmacologic developmental strategies. An essential issue, however, remains the determination of the appropriate mode of delivery of such agents, since the route of administration is critical in determining not only the rate of onset of action, but also the duration of effect. In this respect, the issue of acid suppression in situations of critical illness such as encountered in intensive care units and postoperative patients in whom oral administration may not be possible has become a matter of considerable clinical relevance. In order to consider the potential clinical implications of the use of intravenous acid suppressants, it is worthwhile to consider the evolution of the concept of systemic pharmacotherapy as an adjunct to disease management. Clearly, the utility of an agent capable of bypassing the lengthy process of intestinal absorption and targeting the cell of interest (parietal) within seconds, if not minutes, is of considerable therapeutic interest and clinical relevance. Nevertheless, issues of stability, pharmacokinetics, and safety remain considerations that need careful evaluation.

Evolution of intravenous access

In early times, most medication was administered by local ointment application or orally or rectally. In the last instance, either the condition of the patient or the vile taste of the concoction precluded oral ingestion, and elaborate clysters were developed as well as elegant enema syringes. The effect of oral medication was fraught with unpredictable absorption or even emesis, while rectal administration sometimes encountered difficulties with retention as well as noxious local effects. As a result of this parlous state of affairs, physicians of the seventeenth century considered alternative methods of delivering therapy. There is little doubt that the discovery by William Harvey of the circulation of blood represented one of the most significant events in the history of medicine. The publication of the text *De Motu Cordis* in Frankfurt in 1628 laid the basis for the consideration of intravenous medication, although almost 30 years would pass before the first substantive studies were undertaken. Nevertheless, it was soon apparent that use of the venous system as a therapeutic conduit was clearly of great medical import, and by 1664, the procedures of infusion and transfusion were considered of such magnitude that a serious dispute arose between John Daniel Major, professor of physics at Kiel, and Elshotz, the King of Prussia's physician at Berlin, as to their legitimate primacy in establishing this therapy.

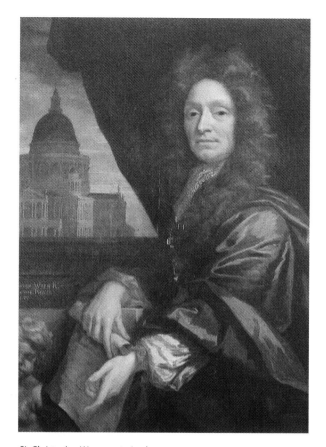

Sir Christopher Wren was trained as an astronomer and dabbled in medicine before recognizing that his future lay in architecture. One is left to ponder what a mind that conceived of St. Paul's Cathedral might have achieved if directed to medical science! He is buried under a simple unadorned black marble slab in the cathedral that he had spent 35 years building, and the plaque reads: *"Lector, si monumentum requiris, circumspice"* ("Reader, if you seek a monument, look around").

Although the acrimonious dispute was widely aired in the medical periodicals for 3 years, their respective claims were to no avail, since the primary inventor was Christopher Wren, the mathematical professor at Oxford. Michael Ettmuller, a distinguished German physician practicing in Leipzig in 1668, stated categorically that primacy was the due of Wren and that following his contributions, the technique and concepts had been improved by Clarke, physician-in-ordinary to the King of England. Thereafter, Major had begun to use it, followed shortly by Charles Fracassatus, professor at Pisa, and last of all by Elshotz and Hoffmann, Professor at Altdorf.

Although it is not well known, Wren was none other than the eminent architect Sir Christopher Wren, who built St. Paul's cathedral and the numerous other magnificent edifices that grace the cities of London and Oxford. Wren, in the words of the historian of the Royal Society, *"became the first author of the noble and anatomical experiment of injecting liquors into the veins of animals; an experiment now vulgarly known but long since exhibited at meetings at Oxford and thence carried by some Germans and published abroad. By this operation diverse creatures were immediately purged, vomited, intoxicated, killed or revived according to the liquors injected. Hence arose many new experiments and chiefly those of transfusing blood, which the Society has prosecuted in sundry instances, that will probably end in extraordinary success."*

The events that led to the investigation of accessing the blood stream were detailed by Robert Boyle, who himself was a scholar of considerable repute. Since Wren had indicated to Boyle that he thought he could easily contrive a way of conveying any liquid immediately into the blood stream, Boyle, being interested, provided a large dog, and the demonstration was carried out in the presence of some eminent physicians and other learned men.

"Wren exposed the large vein in the hind leg and applied a small brass plate, half an inch long, a quarter of an inch broad, the sides being bent inwards. This plate had four little holes in the sides near the corners through which threads could be passed, allowing it to be fastened to the vein. In the middle of the plate there was a large slit parallel to the sides and almost as long as the plate. This allowed the vein to be exposed to the lancet and kept it from starting aside. The vein was ligatured below the plate and then opened through the slit sufficient to allow of the introduction of the slender pipe of a syringe. A small quantity of a warm solution of opium in sack was injected. The effect was dramatic. No sooner had the dog's leg been untied than the opium began to show its narcotic qualities. Almost before the dog had scrambled to its feet its head began to nod, it faltered and reeled and became so stupid that wagers were offered that its life

Of particular interest was the concept embodied in the remedy referred to as *The Spirit of Human Blood* as described by no less an authority than Robert Boyle. It was an uncommon remedy, for blood was not only a commodity that was not freely available, but healthy blood was in especially short supply, *"being drawn from persons that parted with it out of custom or for prevention."* To be safe and efficacious, it was essential that the blood was obtained from healthy individuals, since that acquired from persons of dubious health was clearly unlikely to be salubrious. The blood was dried, put in a retort, and heated on a sand bath, and the material distilled in this way was the spirit (*spirit* in this context was interpreted as the volatile salt of human blood). Boyle regarded it as an alkaline material similar to that obtained by distillation of hartshorn, urine, or sal ammoniac; rather a disappointing substance compared to its name.

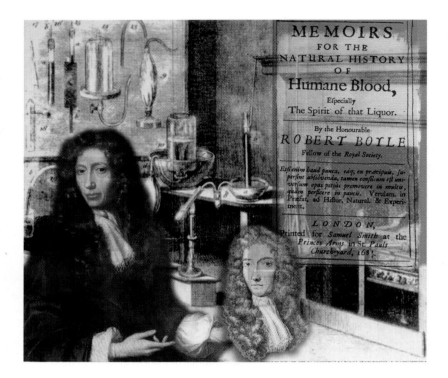

could not be saved. Boyle, however, took the dog into the garden and caused it to be whipped up and down, thereby keeping it awake and in motion, whereby it gradually came round and, being carefully tended [for a change], it not only recovered fully but grew so fat so manifestly that 'twas admired."

Thus is recorded for posterity the initiation of intravenous access! Subsequent to these studies, Wren's intellectual interest turned more toward astronomy and mathematics, and although he maintained a medical interest, he pursued physical science with considerable effect at Gresham College in London (1657) and subsequently as a professor at Oxford in 1661. While holding these posts, he not only continued to participate in medical discussions but actually illustrated Willis's classic treatise on the anatomy of the brain, published in 1664. His subsequent ventures into architecture and the magnificent contributions of his genius to that area are a subject of a separate discussion. In these early experimental years, Boyle recorded that he was informed by an "ingenious anatomist and physician" that he had obtained very good success with diuretics. Boyle therefore proposed that if it could be done without too much danger or cruelty, trial might be made on some human bodies, especially those of malefactors. This was arranged in 1657, in the house of a foreign ambassador, "a curious person" residing in London at the time.

"Infusion of crocus metallorum was injected into the veins of an unruly domestic servant who, it was recorded, deserved to be hanged. The man, as soon as the injection was given, did either really or craftily fall in'to a swoon whereby, being unwilling to prosecute so hazardous an experiment, the ambassador desisted. The only other effect was that it wrought once downward with him which yet might be occasioned by fear or anguish."

Timothy Clarke, physician-in-ordinary to King Charles the Second, recorded in the *Philosophical Transactions of the Royal Society* in 1668 that during the previous 10 years he had *"diligently labored at mixing various fluids with blood drawn from living animals and had not only caused fluids of various kinds to be infused into the living body but had also demonstrated the effects of emetics, cathartics, diuretics, cardiacs and opiates in that way."* After examining the subject of "injections" (water, beer, milk, broth, wine, and spirits of wine) in both

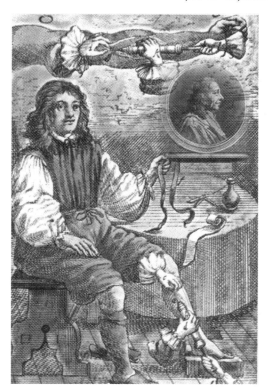

An eighteenth-century depiction of intravenous technique explored the concept of transfusion. The pioneer of the technique, Robert Lower (top right), was an original thinker whose association with Thomas Boyle and Christopher Wren at Oxford University formed a triumvirate of the greatest scientific thinkers of the generation.

animals and humans for almost 5 years, he expressed doubt as to whether the technique would ever be of benefit in the cure of disease but thought it might have potential in the study of anatomy or for the better demonstration of the nature of blood. Unfortunately, Clarke failed to document the results of his experiments—possibly because of disappointment at the poor results—and stated that he did not consider the observations sufficiently worthy to enter into controversy regarding primacy. In consequence, others recorded Clarke's experiments and subsequently claimed them as their own.

Among these, the first was John Sigismond Elshotz, who published an interesting little book entitled *Clysmatica Nova*, or the new clyster art, which described the method by which a medicine could be administered via an open blood vessel *"so that it has the same effect as if it had been taken orally."*

Richard Lower, a physician practicing in Oxford, was an early pioneer in developing the concepts and techniques of blood transfusion. Initially he used simple goose quills for uniting the blood vessels, but soon progressed to the use of silver-flanged (to facilitate a ligature) tubes connected by a piece of ox cervical artery that could be more securely fixed to the emitting and receiving blood vessels. At almost the same time in 1667, John Daniel Major, professor of physics at Kiel, published his book *Chirurgia Infusoria*, asserting angrily that the work confirmed his contributions as foremost in the new field and repudiated others who falsely claimed the credit! It is uncertain whether Major undertook any experimentation himself, and although the book resembles a compilation of the studies and opinions of others, it contains useful descriptions of the procedures as well as the earliest illustration known of an intravenous injection.

The next paper of importance was published in 1623 by a professor of anatomy at Pisa who injected into the vein of a dog some diluted *aqua fortis*. Unfortunately, the animal perished almost immediately, and on autopsy the blood in the vessels was found to be coagulated, and some of the greatest blood vessels had burst in a fashion reminiscent of those who had perished of apoplexy. An editorial in the *Philosophical Transactions of the Royal Society* referring to experimental work on intravenous injection and blood transfusion taking place on the continent explained the cultural differences in experiments as follows: *"why the curious in England make a demure in practicing this experiment upon men. The philosophers of England would have practiced it long ago if they had not been so tender in hazarding the life of men (which they take such pains to preserve and relieve) nor so scrupulous to incur the penalties of the law which in England is*

Richard Lower (1631–1691) of Cornwall and subsequently Oxford was the first to perform the successful transfusion of blood from one animal to another and repeated the procedure on one Arthur Conga in the presence of the Royal Society. Because adequate venous access was a problem, he used a primitive syringe comprising a bladder and a hollow metal tube to infuse the agent into a vein.

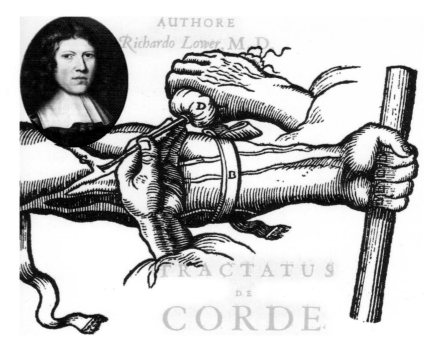

Heister described the technique and produced his own apparatus—a tube and bladder—for injecting liquors into the veins. He added a bright suggestion of his own, namely, that the morbid blood should be removed and the patient transfused with warm milk and broth in its stead.

more strict and nice in cases of this concernment than those of other nations are."

Purmann, writing on the same subject almost a decade later in 1679, provided a more balanced analysis of the subject and a more thoughtful commentary: *"That this Chirurgia Infusoria is beneficial in dangerous disease where the patient must be speedily helped, or all is lost, is very reasonable to believe; because the injected liquors speedily mix with the blood and are quickly conveyed to the heart and so through the whole body without suffering any alteration by the stomach or the several fermentative juices, but work immediately upon the diseases against which they are leveled."*

Purmann then documented some of the agents that he considered to be of particular benefit. These included *Spirit salis ammoniaci*, because it contained a volatile alkali without any oily material, *Spirit of hartshorn* and *spirit of human blood* mixed with *spirit of camphor*, since these were capable of reviving the almost extinguished natural heat and bringing the patient to a sweat, particularly if mixed with two or three drachms of clear water.

Heister in 1750 produced the best overall evaluation of the situation and commented that he believed that intravenous medication was in theory likely to be most useful in patients who could not swallow. Overall, the results were not only disappointing but even dangerous, with the therapy often worse than the disease. He noted *"almost all the patients who have been this way treated have degenerated into a stupidity, foolishness or a raving or melancholy madness or else have been taken off with a sudden death either in or not long after the operation. These lamentable and fatal consequences have brought the art of injections and transfusions into neglect at present so that being suspected and condemned by proper judges at Paris, where they most flourished, we are told they were in a little time prohibited by public edict of that Government."*

Therapeutic infusion of fluid

James Blundell, lecturer in physiology and midwifery at Guy's Hospital in 1818, had been interested for some years in the possibilities of successful blood transfusion in cases of postpartum hemorrhage. To this effect, he had undertaken numerous animal experiments and, having perfected the technique, wished to attempt a blood transfusion on a suitable human being. Fortuitously at this time, "a poor fellow named Brazier" between 30 and 40 years of age was admitted to Guy's Hospital with what was subsequently proved to be "a scirrhosity of the pylorus." Vomiting had reduced him to a helpless and hopeless appearance, and Blundell considered that transfusion alone might restore the quality of his life and enable his survival. The patient was agreeable! Three physicians, five surgeons, and several other gentlemen were present at the operation and supplied the blood. An ounce and a half was taken by syringe and immediately injected into the median vein, which had been opened by a lancet and into which a cannula had been placed and held in position by a finger. The operation began at two o'clock in the afternoon of 27 September 1818, and the procedure was repeated 10 times in the course of 30 to 40 minutes. Although no obvious change in the condition of the patient was evident during the transfusion, it was thought there were slight signs of improvement by the evening. Unfortunately, there was a dramatic deterioration in his condition the next day, and he died 56 hours after the start of the experiment. Blundell tried again without success on several occasions, but it was not until 7 December 1828 that he managed to produce a successful blood transfusion. The patient, a woman aged 25 years, was suffering from the results of a postpartum hemorrhage. Eight ounces of blood was injected during a period of 3 hours, and the patient expressed herself very strongly on the benefits of the transfusion, saying that she felt as if "life was being infused into her whole body."

During studies performed in the early 1820s, François Magendie of Paris had found on frequent occasions that the injection of warm water into the veins of a mad dog would make it quiet. Thus, in October 1823, when asked to see a man in the Hotel Dieu suffering from hydrophobia who, despite copious venesection, still had violent paroxysms and was clearly dying, Magendie elected to give an intravenous injection of water. The recovery of the patient was dramatic but, unfortunately, complications supervened, and he died 9 days later of septicemia, probably caused by the two lancets that had broken off and remained in his body after the process of blood-letting. Nevertheless, such was the reputation of Magendie in America that it prompted a dramatic medical experiment in intravenous medication in Boston. In 1824, a young physician named Hale allowed half an ounce of castor oil at a temperature of 70°F to be injected into the vein of his left arm by a friend who did not do the job very skillfully and engendered the loss of eight ounces of blood. Hale initially noted an oily taste in his mouth, which was followed by nausea and belching, trismus and dizziness, and then a major bowel evacuation. Although the experiment resulted in a month of illness, the arm in particular being swollen and inflamed, his strong constitution permitted recovery, and he was rewarded for his courage with a prize.

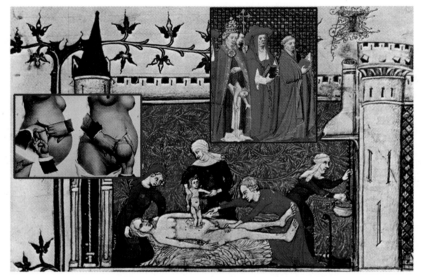

The first desperate attempts to operate on the abdomen were inspired by the desire to save the child of a dying mother. In the reign of the Roman king Numa, the cesarean operation was supported by law. Thus, the Lex Regia stated: *"Si mater pregnas mortua sit, fructus quam primum caute extrahtur"* ("If a pregnant mother dies the child [fruit] must first be removed"). The procedure was thus legally obligated to save the child in the case of death of a pregnant woman. Although it is reported that Julius Caesar was born in this manner, it is highly unlikely, since even at the time of the Gallic wars it is noted that he was writing letters to his mother. The first successful attempt at cesarean section on a living woman was reported to have been undertaken by Jacob Nufer in 1500.

In 1832, during the cholera epidemic, an Edinburgh surgeon, Thomas Latta, had been impressed by an article on the postmortem findings in that disease. It was recorded *"that there was a very great deficiency of the water and saline matter of the blood, on which deficiency the thick, black, cold state of the vital fluid depends, which evidently produces most of the distressing symptoms of that fearful complaint and is doubtless often the cause of death."* Latta attempted to replace the fluid loss by means of copious enemata of warm water with the requisite salts and by administering fluids by mouth. Finding these methods useless, and even harmful, he decided *"to throw fluid immediately into the circulation."* His first patient was an old woman on whom all the usual remedies for cholera had been tried without effect with the result that she was almost moribund and even a dangerous experimental treatment could not be deemed to harm her further. Latta inserted a tube into the median basilic vein and slowly injected 6 pints of water containing 2 or 3 drachms muriate (or chloride of soda and 2 scruples of subcarbonate of soda at a temperature of 112°F). The injection took half an hour, at the end of which time she expressed in a firm voice that she was free from all uneasiness, actually became jocular, and fancied all she needed was a little sleep. Her extremities were warm, and every feature bore the aspect of comfort and health. Delighted with the outcome, Latta departed, but soon thereafter, the vomiting and diarrhea recurred and she died 6 hours later. As a result of this sad event, Latta realized that, despite any degree of improvement, the patient should never be left, and everything held in readiness

Thomas Latta of Leith provided a classic and acutely observed description in the *Lancet* (1832) of the first resuscitative effects of intravenous saline in a case of a cholera patient who was suffering from dehydration and hypovolemic shock.

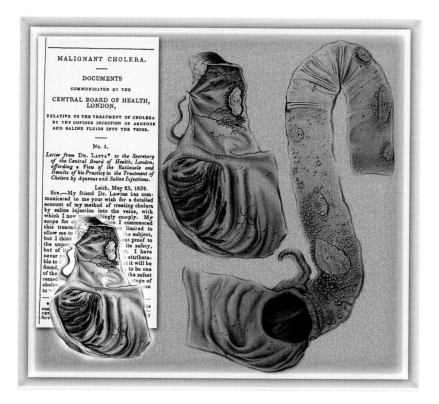

for a second or a third injection. As a result of this continuous therapy, a "very destitute woman of fifty" was given 16 and a half pints of fluid in 12 hours, and her life was saved. In yet another case, 19 pints were injected in 53 hours with a similar success, and Latta was able to present a convincing argument in favor of the early use of intravenous injections of saline in cases of cholera. Indeed, the principles of his therapy instituted in 1832 still remain in contemporary use.

Blood as intravenous therapy

The use of blood in the treatment of disease dates back to the time of primitive man. The history of this phase of human thought is very extensive and complicated, involving such apparently diverse notions as vampirism and the bloody lintel of Passover. There is a certain amount of evidence to indicate that the practice of phlebotomy itself grew directly out of magical beliefs. Blood, as far as the primitive was concerned, was the seat of life and was used in magical practices. It is a common practice of some of the tribes of Africa and the Australian aboriginals to give human blood to the sick and aged for the purpose of strengthening them.

In the seventeenth century, it was hoped that the transfusion of blood might be a useful accessory to the practice of phlebotomy. Since phlebotomy was originally used for the purpose of eliminating some supposedly noxious humor that had entered into the blood and was causing the disease, a natural extension of the idea of evacuating polluted blood was the concept of its

The earliest known form of elective surgery was the operation of circumcision. Blood loss, "although usually minimal," could be dramatic if the "mohel," or priest, was unskilled. Such catastrophes provided an early focus on the critical role of blood in life and the therapeutic power conferred by transfusion.

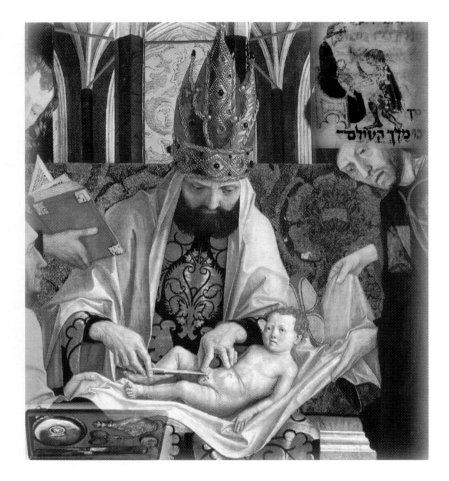

replacement with that of healthy blood, which was thought to be beneficial. Although it is not exactly clear how early this notion arose, there is evidence that early in the fifteenth century, Pope Innocent VIII was transfused and Marsilio Ficino mentioned transfusion as a possible therapeutic procedure. At the beginning of the seventeenth century, many writers suggested its use, including Andreas Libavius, who mentioned that a previous operator brought about a double fatality as a result of transfusion. In 1615, Libavius gave a full description of the technique of the operation, which involved the use of silver tubes inserted into the arteries, and in 1628, Giovanni Colle, a professor of medicine at Padua, described a similar method of transfusion. In 1653, Robert Des Bagets designed a perfusion apparatus, which differed from that originally described by Libavius by virtue of the fact that it included a pumping machine. Francesco Folli demonstrated the technique of transfusion on August 13, 1654, in the presence of Ferdinand II, and between 1657 and 1669, an English group including Christopher Wren, Boyle, and, later, Lower, performed some experiments on the transfusion of blood and the intravenous injection of drugs. In 1661, Moritz Hoffmann and also Johann Sigismund Elsholtz wrote on the subject of transfusion. Subsequent writers were Johann Daniel Major in 1667, Jean-Baptiste Denis in 1668, Paolo Manfredi in 1668, and many others both before and after. Despite widespread interest and pro-

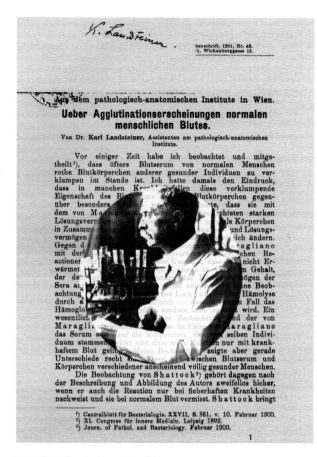

Ueber Agglutinationserscheinungen normalen menschlichen Blutes.

In 1930, Karl Landsteiner received the Nobel Prize for medicine in his discovery of the four major blood groups, which he had initially discovered in 1901. In 1927, he identified the M and N groups, and in 1940, he discovered the Rhesus (Rh) factor.

lific use, both transfusion and intravenous injection had met with such poor success that by the end of the seventeenth century, they were almost completely abandoned and preserved only as experimental procedures, although even in this respect they had fallen into disrepute. Nevertheless, the concept of transfusion remained as the last refuge of the intellectually and therapeutically destitute, such that even the venerable Malpighi was transfused in his final illness during 1694. Textbooks of surgery, such as Heister's *Large Surgery*, usually listed the methods and reviewed the literature, but injection techniques were not destined to be reemployed for therapeutic purposes until the nineteenth century, when they made their reentry not as intravenous but as hypodermic procedures. Transfusion of blood did not return until still later, after bacteriology and pathology had developed a partial appreciation of antibody formation and Landsteiner and Weiner had defined blood groups. The critical phase of the development and introduction of hypodermic injection and the development of the Pravaz syringe (Charles-Gabriel Pravaz) awaited significant advances in the purification and concentration of drugs. Indeed, while the concept of access to the venous system and the administration of systemic therapy made remarkable strides, the rate-limiting step remained the development of agents both sufficiently pure and stable to be safely administered directly into the circulation.

Intravenous medication

Despite considerable experimentation and some novel uses, textbooks of medicine before 1890 still, for the most part, referred to the saline treatment of cholera as the only example of intravenous medication. In 1890, Baccelli used quinine successfully to treat malaria, and 4 years later he used mercury to treat syphilis and carbolic acid to treat tetanus. Sodium cinnamate, under the trade name of *Hetol*, was given intravenously in 1892 to treat tuberculosis, and although even colloidal metals were injected successfully, little serious progress was made.

Indeed, in 1905, Allbutt and Rolleston's great *System of Medicine* stated: *"intravenous injection is practically only used for the introduction of large quantities of saline fluid, though ammonia has been given."* There was, however, a note in the chapter dealing with malaria of the value of quinine given intravenously, and by 1907, the intravenous use of diphtheria antitoxin had gained some degree of acceptability. The arsenic preparation atoxyl (40% arsenic) was first used intravenously in 1905 to treat trypanosomiasis, and it was advised that high doses should be administered for a long period, pushing the injections to the maximum amount that the patient could stand without headache or nausea. Salvarsan was used intravenously to treat syphilis in 1910 and, 2 years later, neo-Salvarsan was similarly administered. Thereafter, the rapid improvements of technique and device resulted in major advances in the intravenous administration of drugs. The phenolsulphonephthalein test for renal function was reported in 1910, and 3 years later paraldehyde was used to produce intravenous anesthesia. In 1921, a satisfactory sclerosing agent (a solution of quinine hydrochloride and urethane) was developed to treat varicose veins, and after years of experimentation, in 1929 the problem of identifying a suitable compound for intravenous urography was solved by the use of uroselectan. In 1930, anticoagulant therapy was initiated, and intravenous heparin was widely advocated in cases of venous thrombosis. In 1929, with the introduction of Amytal, a series of advances in the production of intravenous anesthesia were instigated. Nembutal followed in 1930, Evipan in 1933, and Pentothal in 1935. In 1936, J. S. Horsley, working at the Dorset Mental Hospital, developed the technique of narcoanalysis by discovering that administration of an intravenous barbiturate (Nembutal) before a session could dramatically amplify the conversation of his patient, facilitating a decrease in resistance and rendering emotional reactions more tolerable.

Acute control of acid secretion

Acute treatment of acid related diseases often requires a decision as to the nature of the drug to be used and the route of administration. In the vast majority of cases, oral administration of the standard formulation of available drugs is the route of choice, but in some instances, where really rapid and virtually complete inhibition of acid secretion is desired, oral dosing of the capsule or tablet forms may be less effective than required. There are then two general decisions to be made. Are liquid forms available? Can the capsule form be changed to a liquid suspension and administered as such by swallowing or via nasogastric tube? Or is the patient in a situation in which intravenous therapy is best or even mandatory?

There are no preformulated liquid forms of PPIs, but there are such forms of H_2 receptor antagonists. Hence, these are suitable in children who do not wish to swallow tablets and in those whom reasonable acid control can be achieved by H_2 receptor antagonists. However, it should not be forgotten that these drugs show tolerance, and what is apparently working early in treatment may not be adequate approximately 7 days after starting the medication. Also, withdrawal of the medication results in acid rebound.

These liquid formulations can also be administered to n.p.o. patients via a nasogastric tube, but the same considerations apply in terms of tolerance and rebound. Further, these drugs are not always effective, depending on the major stimulatory pathway that is activated.

PPIs are acid unstable, and the formulation of all of them involves gastroprotective coating. In the case of children, the formulation of omeprazole, S-omeprazole, and lansoprazole allows for opening of the capsule and suspension in orange or apple juice, whose acidity (pH ~ 3.0) keeps the enteric-coated (stable at pH <5.0) granules intact for a time long enough for the child to drink the suspension. An alternative formulation is to use high pH buffer to allow passage of the prodrug through the stomach by preventing acidification. A similar strategy has been used in n.p.o. adults, but the availability of intravenous PPI therapy should replace this approach, mainly because intravenous therapy produces faster and more reliable inhibition of acid secretion than any oral route for these drugs. The formulation currently available for pantoprazole or rabeprazole does not allow suspension, since there are not enteric-coated granules in this formulation, but pantoprazole is available in intravenous formulation—hence, modification of its tablet form is not required. A special formulation of lansoprazole for dissolution and oral administration is being developed for critical care patients and perhaps for children.

Intravenous therapy

General considerations

The presence of high volumes of an acidic solution in the stomach has long been regarded as contributing to upper GI damage in various types of patients. Here we consider those people in whom intravenous therapy is of greater benefit than oral. With the advent of cimetidine and other histamine antagonists, it became possible to control acid secretion by medical means. However, oral therapy is limited in terms of its efficacy and may not be feasible in critical care patients. Of particular clinical relevance is the patient under severe stress, such as the patient in intensive care, where stress ulcers should be avoided, and in the bleeding ulcer patient, in whom acidity of gastric contents not only would exacerbate the cause of bleeding but also would enable dissolution of the thrombus, whether naturally occurring or after a procedure such as thermocoagulation. The preoperative patient who might be at risk for aspiration pneumonia may also be a candidate for intravenous therapy. On occasion also, the Zollinger-Ellison patient requires rapid intervention to raise intragastric pH, whether gastric or duodenal ulcers or severe esophageal erosions are involved. These are summarized in the table.

Disease/Condition	Target pH/ Therapeutic Goal
GERD	**Increase pH** Reduce Volume
Bleeding/Rebleeding	**Abolish Acid Secretion** pH to 6+
Stress Ulcer Prophylaxis	**Increase** pH >4.0
Aspiration Pneumonia	**Reduce Volume** Increase pH
Zollinger-Ellison Syndrome	**Inhibit Acid** to <10mEq/Hr

A summary of some conditions in which intravenous therapy with either H_2 receptor antagonists or PPIs is to be considered.

From the table, it can be seen that there are different theoretical goals that have been suggested. The most usually invoked parameter as a therapeutic target is intragastric pH. This does not, however, necessarily reveal the pH at the gastric surface, and in the absence of a known volume of secretion, nor does it reveal the acid load in the esophagus or the antrum or the likelihood of aspiration of gastric contents. However, often the intragastric pH is the only target envisaged in antisecretory therapy in critically ill or preoperative patients. Perhaps the simplest concept is to elevate intragastric pH as high as possible—hence to approximately 6.0. As will be discussed below, this cannot be achieved with intermittent dosage of any of the drugs on the market today, whether oral or IV.

The concept that pH must be as close to neutrality as possible almost surely applies to prevention of rebleeding after coagulation therapy. The specific goal in stress ulcer prophylaxis is less obvious, but certainly an increase in pH is desirable, probably also as close to neutrality as possible. For prevention of aspiration pneumonia, not only is elevation of pH desirable, but reduction in volume is also a major goal. For patients with severe Zollinger-Ellison syndrome, it is usually thought that inhibition of acid secretion to less than 10 mEq per hour is sufficient to reduce symptoms. Perhaps the most rational end point is complete cessation of acid secretion with, therefore, minimization of volume of gastric contents. With complete inhibition of the gastric acid pump, volume of acid secretion should be reduced to zero, since the KCl gradient induced by the H,K ATPase in the secretory canaliculus of the parietal cell is the driving force for volume of secretion.

The rationale for administration of IV acid inhibitory therapy in general is based on (a) improved efficacy of the IV route and (b) inability to swallow oral medication. As will be seen below, liquid formulation of H_2 receptor antagonists is straightforward; that of PPIs is not.

H_2 receptor antagonists

The major receptor implicated in stimulation of acid secretion is the H_2 receptor on the parietal cell. However, this cell also has an activating muscarinic M_3 receptor that is not affected by H_2 receptor antagonists. The histamine responsible for stimulation of acid secretion is released by the action of gastrin on the ECL cell. The neural mediator of histamine release from this cell type is PACAP. A model of the receptors impacting the activity of the parietal cell is shown in the illustration.

The receptor antagonists are water-soluble, neutral-pH, stable compounds that can readily be formulated as solutions ready to inject. Given their stability, they can be given either as bolus or continuous infusion. The liquid formulations can also be administered orally via nasogastric tube. Both methods have been used. Cimetidine, ranitidine, nizatidine, and famotidine are all available as IV solutions, and little difference exists between these drugs in terms of acid control with IV administration. Several studies have reported that continuous infusion gives the best data in terms of control of acid secretion. Unfortunately, relatively few controlled clinical trials have been performed on the effectiveness of many of these solutions.

Resting Parietal Cell

Secreting Parietal Cell

On the left is a resting parietal cell with the acid pump, the H,K ATPase, located in cytoplasmic membrane–bound tubules. On the right, a stimulated parietal cell with the majority of the pump now located in the microvillus membrane lining the acidic space of the secretory canaliculus. The major stimulatory receptors are those for histamine and acetylcholine. Although a gastrin receptor may also be present on this cell, its role in direct stimulation of the parietal cell is obscure. A few of the known inhibitory receptors are presented on the right side of the basal membrane of the cell, the EGF, somatostatin (SST), and prostaglandin EP_3 receptor. It is important to note that the target of the H_2 receptor antagonists is only one of the activating receptors, and that the target of PPIs is only the pumps in the membrane of the active secretory canaliculus.

The major drawback in terms of continuous IV therapy with H_2 receptor antagonists is the inevitable tolerance that ensues after short-term therapy that cannot be overcome by increasing dosage of any of them. Hence, the tolerance is not due to upregulation of the receptor, and various studies have not defined the mechanism of this approximately 50% loss of efficacy. It is most likely due to upregulation of muscarinic pathways of stimulation of acid secretion. Single-bolus injections of H_2 receptor antagonists may have the drawback of short duration of action and inability to inhibit vagal pathways of stimulation of acid secretion.

In general, there has been a paucity of studies analyzing effectiveness of IV therapy with H_2 receptor antagonists. Various types of patients have been studied—those with critical care conditions and bleeding and preoperative and intensive care unit patients.

In the case of critical care patients, most studies have concluded that even intravenous infusion of H_2 receptor antagonists is not adequate to maintain pH greater than 4.0 reliably. A recent metaanalysis also concluded that, whereas these might benefit bleeding gastric ulcers, they were of little benefit in bleeding duodenal ulcers. Nevertheless, up to 75% of intensive care unit patients receive IV H_2 receptor antagonist therapy. In terms of preoperative treatment, 25% of patients receiving oral and 8% receiving IV cimetidine or ranitidine had an intragastric pH less than 2.5. Infusion is clearly superior to bolus injection. A study evaluating bolus injection of famotidine injection before cardiac surgery showed good effect and persistence for 12 hours. A detailed study on volume and acidity showed equivalence between 50- and 37.5-mg-per-hour cimetidine infusion, in which median pH was 5.3 for the former dose, and 65% of the time, gastric juice was pH greater than 4.0.

Proton pump inhibition

The advent of PPIs opened up the possibility of more reliable pH control by the intravenous route. In the case of PPI inhibition, since the target of these drugs, the H,K ATPase, is the final step of acid secretion, there is no bypass of inhibition and no tolerance of the effect. However, it is thought that PPIs require stimulation of acid secretion for efficacy. After oral administration, the half-life of PPIs is approximately 90 minutes; thus, oral administration is given with or just before meals. Further, since these compounds require an active acid pump, and not all acid pumps are active on administration, the rate of inhibition of acid secretion by IV administration may be somewhat delayed as compared to H_2 receptor antagonists. Certainly, with oral dosing, because of the separation between the time at which active pumps are present in the stomach and the dwell time of the PPI in the blood, there is improvement in inhibition of acid secretion with the days of single-dose administration, steady-state inhibition being achieved after 3 to 5 days of therapy. The mechanism of action of all the PPIs is illustrated in the figure, emphasizing the need for acid secretion for activity of these agents. Pantoprazole is used as an example.

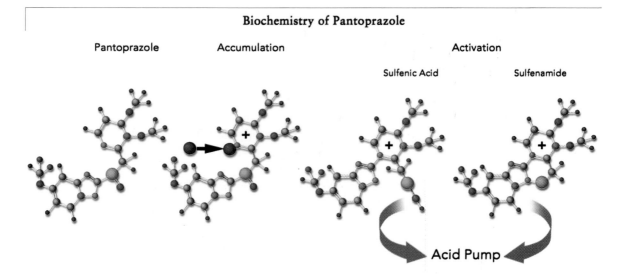

Biochemistry of Pantoprazole

Pantoprazole   Accumulation   Activation

Sulfenic Acid   Sulfenamide

Acid Pump

An illustration of the essential steps in inhibition of acid secretion by PPIs with pantoprazole as an example. The drug is administered in a gastroprotected formulation and is absorbed in the duodenum or is administered in a reconstituted IV formulation. The acidic, membrane-enclosed space of the active parietal cell's secretory canaliculus accumulates the PPI approximately 1,000-fold (pH 1.0, pK_a of drug approximately 4.0) due to protonation of the pyridine. After intramolecular transfer to the N of the benzimidazole, rearrangement of the molecule occurs to form first the cationic thiophilic sulfenic acid and then the sulfonamide, either of which reacts rapidly with cysteines on the luminal face of the pump.

The chemistry of the compounds makes it impossible in their current structure to formulate an IV solution that has sufficient shelf life, since even a solution of pH 9.0 has sufficient protons to eventually activate the drug. Since the active drug is able to react with any SH group and is positively charged, it is inactivated in the stomach or in the blood without being able to target the acid pump. Since IV omeprazole is not available in the USA and many other countries, other means of administering the compound in solution form have been devised.

Alternatives to intravenous administration

The PPIs as a class are acid-unstable drugs, an essential property to ensure targeting to the active gastric acid pump. This therefore limits their usefulness in oral therapy, where the standard enteric formulation has been dissolved to allow administration via a nasogastric tube in intensive care situations. The means of dissolving the formulation also vary. For example, omeprazole or esomeprazole is formulated in a capsule where the drug is present as enteric-coated microparticles. The enteric coating is designed to dissolve and release the PPIs at approximately pH 5.0. Hence, to use this formulation for oral administration, the capsules are opened and the granules suspended in apple or orange juice. They are then stable to gastric transit if the stomach is acidic and reasonable acid suppression may be anticipated. Other PPIs such as rabeprazole or pantoprazole are available as enteric-coated tablets, which must be dissolved at neutral pH and then administered in alkaline buffer to avoid gastric destruction. In neither case is there truly very reliable control of acid secretion by this artificial means of administering a liquid dose by nasogastric tube delivery.

Intravenous administration of proton pump inhibitors

Early in the development of omeprazole, an intravenous formulation was made available in which the drug was reconstituted in buffer immediately before bolus injection. Such an approach was first used in dogs to assess the effect of a PPI and to compare it to that of an H_2 receptor antagonist.

For example, pilot experiments in dogs used continuous pentagastrin infusion so as to mimic the effect of food stimulation and to optimize the effect of IV PPI injection. The PPI showed clear superiority in terms of duration of effect, since the release of histamine from the ECL cell by pentagastrin infusion eventually bypassed the effect of famotidine, which had disappeared from the blood.

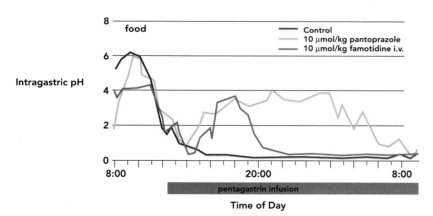

Comparison of IV Pantoprazole to H_2 Antagonist

A comparison of injection of a single dose of pantoprazole and famotidine IV on intragastric pH in dogs under continuous pentagastrin infusion. It can be seen that intragastric pH is maintained at 1.0 or below by the stimulant. Administration of famotidine results in relatively rapid elevation of intragastric pH that only lasts for approximately 4 hours, whereas the effect of pantoprazole is prolonged, to approximately at least 12 hours.

However, in humans, acid secretion is a continuous process, so that over an 8-hour period, all pumps go through a cycle of stimulation. For IV therapy, with the higher dose that can be given, it is possible that steady-state effects can be seen on acid secretion in the n.p.o. patient as would be encountered in intensive care unit settings and preoperatively, thus extending the benefit of pump inhibition to the usual IV setting.

Administration of single IV doses of omeprazole at 80 mg resulted in 80% inhibition of peak acid output at 90 minutes after dose and 60% 24 hours after dose that was about the same as that achieved by repetitive dosing for 6 days. The difference between the gradual onset of inhibition with oral dosing as compared to the first-day effect of 80 mg omeprazole injection may be attributed to the higher and longer-lasting blood levels of omeprazole achieved by this dose. Early studies on efficacy of IV omeprazole in bleeding patients showed that b.i.d. IV bolus injections of omeprazole provided markedly superior results as compared to continuous infusion of ranitidine. A study on Zollinger-Ellison patients showed also that 60 mg omeprazole administered by injection every 12 hours reduced acid secretion to 5 mEq per hour, providing at least equal efficacy to continuous IV infusion of ranitidine. After thermocoagulation to stop bleeding, the administration of an 80-mg bolus dose of omeprazole followed by an 8-mg-per-hour infusion (previously shown to elevate intragastric pH to approximately 6.0) for 3 days followed by 20 mg o.d. for 8 weeks resulted in 7% recurrence of bleeding within 30 days in the omeprazole group compared to 23% in the placebo group, with most recurrences occurring in the first 3 days of treatment. To date, there are no data on esomeprazole or lansoprazole IV in the clinical setting.

More recently, pantoprazole has been introduced in an IV formulation. It is inherently more acid stable than omeprazole, esomeprazole, or lansoprazole, and hence does not require a highly alkaline buffer for reconstitution.

As shown in the figure, a comparison of single-IV-bolus pantoprazole to IV famotidine bolus in pentagastrin-stimulated volunteers reproduced the data obtained in the dog.

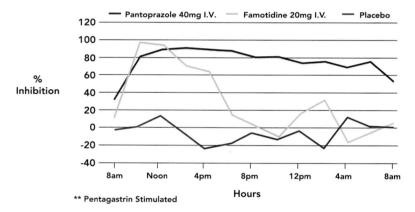

Pantoprazole 40 mg vs. Famotidine 20 mg

— Pantoprazole 40mg I.V. — Famotidine 20mg I.V. — Placebo

% Inhibition

** Pentagastrin Stimulated

Hours

A comparison of IV injection of pantoprazole to IV injection of famotidine in pentagastrin-stimulated patients showing the equally rapid onset of inhibition and the long duration of action of the PPI. Probably, current therapy indicates a bolus of 80 mg IV pantoprazole.

Early studies showed that switching to a single or b.i.d. bolus injection of pantoprazole effectively substituted for oral pantoprazole. Importantly, a controlled clinical trial compared cimetidine (bolus 300 mg and 50-mg-per-hour infusion) to various doses of IV pantoprazole administered as a bolus of 80 mg o.d., b.i.d., and t.i.d. The pantoprazole IV method resulted in as rapid an elevation to pH 4.0 or greater as did cimetidine and the t.i.d. proved superior to continuous cimetidine in pH control by the second day. Eighty mg was superior to 40 mg, indicating that 80 mg is the minimum dose to be recommended, and that t.i.d. will give better results. The tolerance to cimetidine by day 2 was clearly shown. Further, this showed the efficacy of PPIs in n.p.o. patients.

In general, therefore, IV PPIs are likely to be preferred even to infusion of H$_2$ receptor antagonists and bolus injection of H$_2$ receptor antagonists is outdated. A formulation or modification of PPI structure to allow continuous IV infusion of a neutral pH solution so as to bring gastric volume down to close to zero and to elevate pH to 6.0 is also desirable.

The superiority of acid volume control following IV as compared to oral therapy is readily observed in a comparison of individual responses to oral or intravenous therapy.

A comparison of IV bolus 80 mg pantoprazole in eight individuals (top) to 40 mg oral therapy in four individuals showing the large increase in efficacy of acid suppression with IV as compared to oral administration. Similar data are to be expected if granules of omeprazole or lansoprazole are administered by intragastric tube.

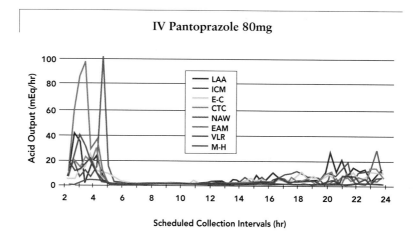

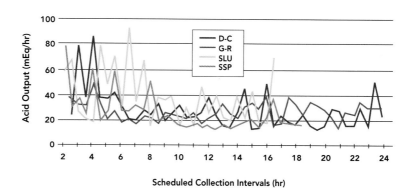

At present, therefore, in situations where rapid and effective acid control is required, IV PPI is the treatment of choice.

Clinical aspects of intravenous acid suppression

Management of upper gastrointestinal hemorrhage

Acute upper gastrointestinal hemorrhage is the most common emergency managed by gastroenterologists and, in such patients, it is usually the primary reason for presentation or referral. However, upper gastrointestinal bleeding may also be a consequence of prolonged, severe disease; in these patients, who have stress ulceration or "stress-related erosive syndrome" (SRES), management is complicated further by uncertainty as to the pathogenesis of the condition and the need to manage the underlying conditions that are, themselves, usually life-threatening.

Although upper gastrointestinal hemorrhage is a common manifestation of the stomach in distress, the stomach is not the only potential source of bleeding, and initial investigations should identify patients with specific problems, such as variceal bleeding, that will require a different approach to management. The approach to SRES is somewhat different because these patients do not generally present *de novo* with gastrointestinal hemorrhage; the principles of managing an upper gastrointestinal hemorrhage, once it has occurred, are broadly similar, regardless of whether the patient presents *de novo* or is already in an intensive care unit, but the additional challenge, for the intensive care unit patient, is to try to prevent the bleed.

Upper gastrointestinal hemorrhage and stress ulceration in critically ill patients are common events that are associated with substantial morbidity and costs to the health care system. Since many of the upper gastrointestinal tract lesions associated with these conditions are acid related, it is plausible that successful management should be based on the use of the most efficient acid-suppression medications. PPIs are the most effective medications for acid related disorders such as reflux esophagitis and peptic ulceration, but it has been surprisingly difficult to determine whether they provide similar incremental benefits in patients with more severe disease. A substantial proportion of patients with upper gastrointestinal hemorrhage have an underlying acid related lesion that will, almost invariably, be treated eventually with a PPI; however, it still remains to be established that the prompt administration of a PPI—whether orally or intravenously—will improve outcome in all patients. However, bolus IV PPI clearly provides more reliable acid inhibition than oral dosage of a PPI, however formulated. Critically ill patients may develop lesions that appear to be acid related and, although the data on the benefits of PPI therapy in this situation are sparse, PPIs are safe medications, and there is every reason to think that they will be more effective than H_2 receptor antagonists. However, there are only very limited data on which to base decisions regarding optimal therapy for upper gastrointestinal tract hemorrhage and stress ulcer prophylaxis. It will, therefore, be necessary to undertake more clinical research programs to determine the true benefit of IV as compared to oral PPI therapy, in conjunction with standard medical and endoscopic management strategies, to facilitate the development of future practice guidelines for the management of the stomach in distress.

The magnitude of the problem

Upper gastrointestinal bleeding affects more than 100 per 100,000 of the population annually, and it is most commonly attributable to peptic ulcer disease, erosive gastroduodenal disease, and variceal bleeding (see table). Bleeding ceases spontaneously in up to 80% of cases but, despite the development of new pharmacologic and endoscopic interventions, the mortality of upper gastrointestinal hemorrhage is high, ranging from approximately 10% in patients who present to a hospital with acute bleeding to more than 30% in those whose bleeding develops while they are in the hospital. Furthermore, there has been little reduction in the overall mortality over the last 4 decades, although there is some evidence that mortality rates may be less if patients are managed in a specialized gastrointestinal bleeding unit.

The majority of cases of nonvariceal upper gastrointestinal bleeding are due to peptic ulceration or gastroduodenal erosions and these are, in turn, most commonly related to underlying infection with *Helicobacter pylori*, NSAIDs, or a combination of the two. The management of upper gastrointestinal bleeding should, therefore, be based initially on minimizing the effect of these two risk factors in an attempt to prevent ulceration and hemorrhage. In the event that upper gastrointestinal hemorrhage does occur, management should then be directed at resuscitation to minimize the sequelae of blood loss, followed by

Causes of acute upper gastrointestinal hemorrhage. (Adapted from *Gut* 2002;51[Suppl IV]:iv1–iv6; *Br Med J* 1995;311:222–226; and *Gut* 1990;31:504–508.)

Causes of Acute Upper Gastrointestinal Hemorrhage	
Diagnosis	**Percentage**
Peptic ulcer	35-50
Gastroduodenal erosions	8-15
Esophagitis	5-15
Varices	5-10
Mallory-Weiss tears	15
Vascular malformations	5
Rare	5
Upper gastrointestinal malignancy	1

investigation to determine the site of hemorrhage, therapy to prevent further blood loss, and therapy to facilitate healing of the underlying lesion(s).

Physiologic stress resulting from severe illness, particularly in the setting of an intensive care unit, is associated with mucosal damage in 75% to 100% of patients. In some patients, superficial, mucosal stress erosions prevail, and there is only a low risk of hemorrhage; in other patients with stress ulceration, bleeding is much more likely, and upper gastrointestinal bleeding is the most common presentation of stress ulceration in the intensive care unit. Overt bleeding occurs in approximately 5% of patients who are clinically ill in an intensive care unit but clinically important bleeding, with hypotension, tachycardia, orthostasis, anemia, a need for transfusion, or a fall in hemoglobin of more than 20 g per L, is less prevalent, occurring in approximately 1% to 4% of critically ill intensive care unit patients. Although upper gastrointestinal bleeding may not be the direct cause of death in many patients, it is, nonetheless, associated with a high mortality rate of 9% if upper gastrointestinal bleeding was present at the time of admission, rising to approximately 50% if bleeding developed after admission.

The pathogenesis of stress ulceration and subsequent clinically important hemorrhage is multifactorial, and the management of stress ulceration in an intensive care unit setting should therefore address the underlying reasons for mucosal damage; the factors that promote progression from mucosal injury to hemorrhage; and interventions that minimize continued hemorrhage, morbidity, and mortality.

General principles

Gastroduodenal mucosal integrity is considered to be dependent on the maintenance of defense mechanisms sufficient to protect the mucosa against injurious or aggressive factors. Compromise of gastric or duodenal mucosal blood flow is associated, among other things, with increased production of nitric oxide and oxygen radicals, decreased production of prostaglandins, and reduced epithelial cell regeneration. Subsequently, the effects of mucosal ischemia can be compounded further by reperfusion injury, if blood flow increases again. These factors, combined with impairment of the protective mucus–bicarbonate barrier and back diffusion of hydrogen ions, increase the susceptibility of the mucosa to injury by luminal gastric acid and pepsin. Gastric acid and pepsin can injure the mucosa directly and impair healing, and they can also increase the risk of hemorrhage because they impair platelet aggregation and accelerate clot lysis. There are, therefore, a number of points at which therapy might be expected to prevent or minimize damage, to promote healing, or to prevent hemorrhage; however, most studies of pharmacologic interventions have concentrated on medications designed to reduce gastric acidity, and it is these medications that continue to be the mainstay of medical therapy for the stomach in distress.

Current management strategies

Gastroduodenal bleeding

The management of upper gastrointestinal bleeding encompasses initial resuscitation measures, pharmacologic therapy, endoscopic therapy, and surgery, and, although these are often considered separately, the effects of the different modalities on outcomes are interdependent.

The first step in management is a prompt clinical assessment of the patient to determine the magnitude of blood loss, the effect of this loss on health status, the cause of the bleed, and the presence of any comorbidity as a basis for determining prognosis and the most appropriate treatment. Intuitively, one would expect that a management strategy appropriate for a young, otherwise healthy, hemodynamically stable 25-year-old patient who has had a minor hematemesis following several episodes of acute, alcohol-induced vomiting would be very different from that required for a 70-year-old diabetic with ischemic heart disease who presents with frank hematemesis, maroon blood *per rectum*, and postural hypotension after a 4-week period of treatment with a conventional NSAID. Unfortunately, in practice, many patients cannot be assigned readily to low- or high-risk categories and, as economic and resource considerations assume greater importance, it is not feasible to apply intensive management strategies for all patients presenting with an upper gastrointestinal bleed. It is, therefore, necessary to develop assessment techniques that will differentiate accurately between patients who require only conservative initial management with early discharge from hospital and those who require admission for close monitoring, early investigation and therapy, and a more prolonged hospital stay.

Initial clinical assessment is important for risk stratification but, even if standardized assessment scores were not applied to determine prognosis, clinical assessment would still be an essential prelude to resuscitation, which would, itself, play a role in determining the patient's ultimate prognosis. Thus, it is very difficult to dissociate the prognostic value of a risk scoring system, such as those described by Rockall et al. and Blatchford et al., from the consequent implementation of a management strategy based on the presence of hemodynamic instability. In the final analysis, the outcome of management will depend not only on the presence of risk factors and the extent to which they are identified, but also on the subsequent management strategy and the effectiveness with which it is implemented.

After initial assessment of the patient's hemodynamic status and risk factors (such as age and comorbidities), blood tests (hemoglobin, white cell count, platelet count, urea and electrolytes, liver function tests, prothrombin time or international normalized ratio, blood group and crossmatch), and resuscitation with IV fluids and reversal, if possible, of coagulopathy should precede endoscopy. Endoscopy may be diagnostic, therapeutic, or both, but it is not a substitute for clinical assessment and resuscitation. Furthermore, the availability of endoscopy may be limited by geography or, out of hours, by economic or personnel constraints. Under these circumstances, empiric pharmacologic therapy may be considered and, if endoscopy is not available or practicable, it may be necessary to consider surgical therapy. Pharmacologic therapy includes the administration of acid suppressants (H_2 receptor antagonists or PPIs), splanchnic blood flow modulators (somatostatin, octreotide), or antifibrinolytics (tranexamic acid, epsilon aminocaproic acid). However, there are few data on the effect of empiric therapy started before endoscopy for patients with upper gastrointestinal bleeding.

The first goal of endoscopy is diagnostic; despite earlier reports that this did not affect outcome, it is important to identify patients with variceal bleeding, malignancy, and ulcers with stigmata of recent hemorrhage, since these features are prognostic. Variceal hemostasis apart, lesions with stigmata of recent or current hemorrhage may be treated endoscopically with one or more of a range of techniques, including (a) injection of adrenalin (1:10,000 in saline), sclerosants (ethanolamine, polidocanol, sodium tetradecyl sulfate, absolute ethanol), fibrin, or glue; (b) application of heat (heater probe, multipolar coagulation, laser or argon plasma coagulation); and (c) the application of mechanical clip or loop. If hemostasis is documented at endoscopy, pharmacologic therapy is then initiated with the options of repeat endoscopy if bleeding recurs, followed by surgery if hemostasis cannot be achieved.

In the longer term, therapy should be directed at the underlying cause for the gastrointestinal bleeding; standard ulcer healing therapy is appropriate with eradication of *H. pylori* infection if this is present. For patients who had received NSAIDs before presentation, discontinuation of NSAIDs, a change of NSAID medication, prophylactic therapy (with a PPI or misoprostol), and *H. pylori* eradication may also be considered. Rarer causes, such as a Dieulafoy lesion and vascular lesions, may also require more chronic therapy.

"Stress" ulceration

The management of stress ulceration is, in large part, prophylactic. Once clinically significant SRES supervenes, the major complication is upper gastrointestinal hemorrhage, and the management principles for patients with stress ulcer–related hemorrhage are similar to those for patients who present *de novo*, with upper gastrointestinal hemorrhage, albeit the former are already at greater risk because of their severe comorbidities.

Thus, the management of stress ulceration is based on aggressive medical therapy of the underlying condition in a critically ill patient to achieve optimal tissue oxygenation and fluid and electrolyte repletion with antimicrobial therapy for documented or presumed sepsis. Although mucosal ischemia is considered to play a role in the pathogenesis of SRES, luminal acid plays a dominant role, either by damaging the mucosa directly or by contributing to a fall in intraepithelial pH. Prophylactic therapy to prevent or minimize the risk of stress ulceration is therefore based on reduction of luminal acidity or on protection of the mucosa from the injurious effects of acid and acid-dependent peptic activity. The major prophylactic treatment options are antacids or sucralfate, administered nasogastrically, and H_2 receptor antagonists or PPIs, administered intravenously. The major concern that has arisen, particularly with the use of intravenous acid suppressants, is that an increase in gastric pH favors bacterial colonization of the stomach and that subsequent aspiration of gastric contents will therefore increase the risk of pneumonia and mortality compared with sucralfate. This fear appears to be without foundation, and mucosal protective agents are generally considered to be without effect.

Evidence for individual management strategies

Gastroduodenal bleeding

Pharmacologic therapy

Somatostatin, at high doses, reduces gastric acid secretion and splanchnic blood pressure while increasing duodenal bicarbonate secretion; however, although it is used widely in variceal hemorrhage, the evidence for its use in nonvariceal hemorrhage is limited. A metaanalysis by Imperiale of 14 trials in 1,829 patients (12 trials, somatostatin; 2 trials, octreotide) reported a relative risk (RR) of 0.53 compared with H_2 receptor antagonists for rebleeding, with a somewhat higher RR of 0.73 in "investigator-blinded" studies. However, most of the studies included were of low quality, and the analysis did not control for confounders such as the prior use of endoscopic therapy.

Tranexamic acid, an inhibitor of fibrinolysis, was subject to a metaanalysis by Henry et al., including six trials in 1,267 patients but, although tranexamic acid produced a significant reduction in rebleeding and surgery compared with placebo, there was no difference in the mortality rate. Furthermore, the trials reviewed were conducted before the use of endoscopic therapy became routine.

On the basis of these metaanalyses, neither somatostatin nor antifibrinolytic agents can be recommended for the routine management of upper gastrointestinal hemorrhage. There has been no single study demonstrating that H_2 receptor antagonists provide significant benefit in the management of upper gastrointestinal hemorrhage, although a large metaanalysis of 27 randomized, controlled trials of ranitidine (3 trials) or cimetidine (24 trials) in 2,670 patients reported that H_2 receptor antagonists produced a 10% decrease in rebleeding ($p > .05$), a 20% decrease in surgery ($p < .05$), and a 30% decrease in mortality ($p = .02$). However, a more recent metaanalysis by Levine et al. reported that intravenous H_2 receptor antagonists were of no benefit in bleeding duodenal ulcer and, although they produced a significant reduction in risk of rebleeding, surgery, and death in bleeding gastric ulcer (7.2%, 6.7%, and 3.2%, respectively), the effect was small. These authors concluded that, because PPIs have a greater inhibitory effect on gastric acid secretion than H_2 receptor antagonists, they may be more effective in ulcer bleeding; however, this expected benefit has been surprisingly difficult to document.

The first, large double-blind, controlled trial of a PPI was conducted by Daneshmend in 1,147 patients with nonvariceal upper gastrointestinal hemorrhage who were randomized to placebo or omeprazole given intravenously (200 mg) for 24 hours, then orally (40 mg b.i.d.) for 3 days; this study did not show any significant benefits with respect to hemorrhage, transfusion requirements, or surgery. The design of this and subsequent studies, such as that by Khuroo et al., has been criticized because there was no endoscopic intervention before pharmacologic therapy, although the latter study, in which 220 patients with a bleeding ulcer were randomized to placebo or oral omeprazole, did report that omeprazole produced a significant reduction in hemorrhage and transfusion requirements with a trend to a decreasing mortality. A number of current studies, generally using higher-dose, continuous-intravenous infusions of omeprazole, have shown greater benefit than the original study reported by Daneshmend et al., and the potential benefit of PPI therapy is supported by a recent metaanalysis by Zed et al. This metaanalysis, including 9 trials in 1,829 patients, reported that PPIs produced a 50% reduction in the relative odds of rebleeding (OR, 0.50; 95% CI, 0.33 to 0.77; $p = .002$), a 53% reduction in the relative odds of surgery (OR, 0.47; 95% CI, 0.29 to 0.77; $p = .003$), and a nonsignificant 8% decrease in the odds of death (OR, 0.92; 95% CI, 0.46 to 1.83, $p = .81$). They concluded that PPIs are superior to H_2 receptor antagonists and placebo in preventing rebleeding and surgery, although they do not appear to reduce mortality. Perhaps the amount of blood lost in the mortality group is too large and too much damage has occurred before medical intervention.

Endoscopic

Endoscopic therapy encompasses direct control of bleeding, by injection therapy, application of heat and mechanical hemostatic methods, alone or in combination. A metaanalysis, including 30 randomized controlled trials by Cook et al., reported significant reductions in rebleeding (OR, 0.38; 95% CI, 0.32 to 0.45), surgery (OR, 0.36; 95% CI, 0.28 to 0.45), and mortality (OR, 0.55; 95% CI, 0.40 to 0.76) when all patients and all treatment modalities were considered; these findings were confirmed in high-risk patients, with an actively bleeding vessel or a nonbleeding visible vessel with comparable reductions in rebleeding (OR, 0.23; 95% CI, 0.15 to 0.27), surgery (OR, 0.26; 95% CI, 0.17 to 0.32), and mortality (OR, 0.62: 95% CI, 0.38 to 0.98). Comparison of the different treatment modalities—injection therapy, thermal contact therapy, and laser therapy—showed that they all produced similar outcomes with respect to rebleeding, surgery, and mortality. A more recent review of endoscopic therapy by Church et al. concluded that adrenaline (1:10,000) is an effective agent and that the addition of sclerosants increases the risk of adverse events without any concomitant benefit. However, the results of two large trials by Kubba and Rutgeerts suggest that adrenaline, combined with a thrombogenic agent (thrombin or fibrin glue), may confer additional benefit by stimulating the formation of a stable blood clot. Alternatively, Hiele has suggested that there may also be merit in combining injection with a thermal technique, although the same group reported that this was shown to be significant in only one study, which used a bipolar "gold probe" in combination with adrenaline injection. As Hiele noted, there is no convincing evidence that endoscopic mechanical techniques are superior to current injection or thermal methods, or that the combination of injection and mechanical techniques confers any advantage compared with either modality alone.

The role of repeat endoscopy for patients who have recurrent bleeding after successful endoscopic hemostatic therapy remains somewhat controversial. Lau et al. randomized 100 patients with recurrent peptic ulcer bleeding to immediate endoscopic retreatment or surgery, and they concluded that endoscopic retreatment reduces the need for surgery without increasing the risk of death and is associated with fewer complications than surgery. However, the decision to undertake repeat endoscopy or proceed to surgery remains a matter of clinical judgment based, in part at least, on the initial endoscopic findings (including the extent and accessibility of the initial lesion) and on the risks of surgery in the individual patient.

"Stress" Ulceration

As documented by Tryba and Cook, antacids have been shown, in placebo-controlled trials, to reduce the frequency of stress ulcer–related gastrointestinal tract hemorrhage. A metaanalysis by Shuman in 1987 of data from 16 trials reported that there was no significant difference in the rates of overt bleeding between antacids (3.3%) and cimetidine (2.7%; $p = .69$). Furthermore, both agents produced lower rates of overt blood loss than placebo (15%; $p < .001$). A more recent metaanalysis by Cook in 1991 of data from 42 eligible trials reported that antacids (OR, 0.40; 95% CI, 0.20 to 0.79) and H_2 receptor antagonists (OR, 0.29; 95% CI, 0.17 to 0.45) decreased the incidence of overt bleeding, and that H_2 receptor antagonists were more effective than antacids (OR, 0.56; 95% CI, 0.33 to 0.97), although there was no difference in mortality between treated and untreated patients.

In a randomized, controlled study comparing sucralfate with antacids plus H_2 receptor antagonists, the authors reported no difference in bleeding between the treatment groups, but they did report a lower incidence of pneumonia in those who received sucralfate (9.1%) compared with combination therapy (23.2%) and a lower mortality rate (23.6% vs. 46.4%, respectively). In a subsequent metaanalysis undertaken in 1996, Cook et al. reported that sucralfate and H_2 receptor antagonists were both associated with decreased rates of overt bleeding compared with placebo, and they also reported that sucralfate was associated with a decreased risk of pneumonia and mortality. In contrast, a subsequent formal, randomized, multicenter, double-blind, controlled trial in 1,200 ICU patients undertaken by the same group showed that ranitidine (50 mg IV every 8 hours) reduced the risk of clinically important bleeding (1.7%) compared with sucralfate (1 g via nasogastric tube every 6 hours; 3.8%; $p < .02$), whereas there were no significant differences between the groups with respect to the incidence of ventilator-associated pneumonia (respectively, 19.1% vs. 16.2%; $p = .19$) or mortality.

If the benefit of H_2 receptor antagonists is due to reduction in gastric acidity, PPIs would be expected to produce a greater decrease in stress ulcer–related complications. As both Netzer and Merki independently reported, this may be in part because PPIs are, *ab initio*, more effective than H_2 receptor antagonists at increasing gastric pH and, in part, because tolerance to intravenous H_2 receptor antagonists develops in all patients within 72 hours of starting therapy.

Unfortunately, there are very few data on the efficacy of PPI therapy for stress ulcer prophylaxis. In two trials conducted by Phillips and Lasky, there was no indication of clinically significant bleeding in patients receiving a suspension of omeprazole granules. Similarly, Levy et al., in another trial, noted that clinically significant bleeding occurred in 31% of patients receiving intravenous ranitidine and in 6% of patients receiving omeprazole suspension (p <.05). However, there are limitations to these trials, including small sample sizes, the lack of a comparison group, an open-label trial design, and different definitions of clinically important bleeding from those used in previous trials. Thus, for the present, there are no convincing data to support the prophylactic use of PPIs, orally or intravenously, to prevent the development of stress ulceration in critically ill patients. Nevertheless, if the physician considers gastric acidity to be a risk factor, then PPIs are the medication of choice.

Management reality

The variability of practice in the management of upper gastrointestinal hemorrhage and stress ulceration may be, in part, a reflection of regional differences in disease prevalence and severity, but is probably as much due to variations in individual clinicians' assessment and application of published evidence. It has been suggested that improved outcomes in specialist units are attributable to the development and implementation of clear protocols and guidelines as much as technical resources and prowess, and there is therefore a clear need for practice guidelines in both of these areas.

Gastroduodenal bleeding

The most recent guidelines were developed by the British Society of Gastroenterology (BSG) Endoscopy Committee and are founded on an evidence-based review of the literature. These guidelines share, with other writings on the subject, an approach rooted in the basic principles of managing any potentially seri-

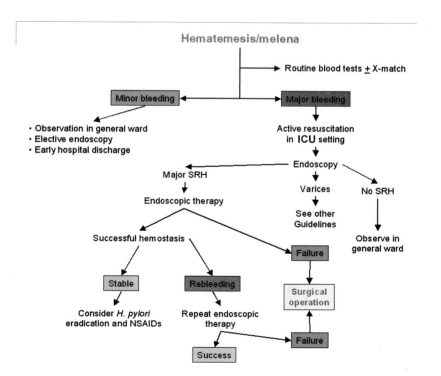

Algorithm for the management of acute gastrointestinal hemorrhage proposed by the British Society of Gastroenterology Endoscopy Committee. (ICU, intensive care unit; NSAIDs, nonsteroidal antiinflammatory drugs; SRH, stigmata of recent hemorrhage.) (Adapted from *Gut* 2002;51[Suppl IV]: iv1–iv6.) (Courtesy of D. Armstrong.)

Rockall Score for Rebleeding and Death

Variable	Score			
	0	1	2	3
Age (years)	< 60	60-79	> 80	-
Shock	No shock	Tachycardia	Hypotension	-
Systolic BP	> 100	> 100	< 100	
Pulse	< 100	> 100	> 100	
Comorbidity	Nil major	Nil major	Cardiac failure Ischemic heart disease Any major co-morbidity	Renal failure Liver failure Disseminated malignancy
Diagnosis	MW tear No lesion No stigmata	All other diagnoses	Upper GI malignancy	-
Major recent stigmata	None Dark spot	-	Blood in UGI Adherent clot Visible vessel Spurting vessel	-

Rockall score for risk of rebleeding and death in patients presenting with an upper gastrointestinal bleed. (MW, Mallory-Weiss.) (Adapted from Gut 1996;38:316–321.) (Courtesy of D. Armstrong.)

ous condition; namely, initial assessment of the patient's condition, resuscitation as needed in an appropriate environment, investigation to determine the cause of the condition, directed therapy, and appropriate monitoring as the patient recovers. The initial recommendations, based on consensus, identify the need for a medical or surgical gastroenterology specialist involvement aided by 24-hour support from medical and nursing staff and the availability of a high-dependency unit. There was also consensus that blood transfusion and endoscopy facilities should be available 24 hours a day, 7 days a week, and that each institution should follow an agreed-on management protocol with standardized documentation of all interventions. The algorithm for the management of upper gastrointestinal bleeding shown here identifies patients with hematemesis or melena who are then assessed for bleeding severity. The guidelines describe the Rockall score (see table) as a means to stratify patients into low- (≤2) or high- (>8) risk groups. However, the Rockall score is based, in part, on endoscopic findings, and, because risk stratification may be needed—particularly out of hours—to determine which patients should undergo emergency endoscopy, an approach such as the Blatchford score (see next table) may be preferable for initial screening, based on the patient's clinical status and blood tests. Early assessment and resuscitation are based on prompt blood tests (hemoglobin, white cell and platelet count, prothrombin time or international normalized ratio, urea, creatinine, electrolytes, liver function tests, blood group, and crossmatch) and appropriate intravenous access and hemodynamic monitoring to permit necessary replacement of blood and other fluids. These measures are essential to ensure that the patient has been resuscitated as fully as possible before endoscopy is undertaken by an experienced endoscopist able to perform therapeutic procedures.

Blatchford score showing features, which, if all are present, indicate patients at low risk of requiring intervention for upper gastrointestinal bleeding. (Adapted from *Lancet* 2000;356:1318–1321.)

Blatchford Score for Gastrointestinal Bleeding

Feature	Value
Blood urea	< 6.5 mmol/L
Hemoglobin: *men*	> 130 g/L
women	> 120 g/L
Systolic blood pressure	> 110 mm Hg
Pulse	< 100 beats/min

The aims of endoscopy are (a) to identify the cause of bleeding, (b) to assess the risk of rebleeding and mortality, and (c) to perform a therapeutic hemostatic procedure in patients with major stigmata of recent hemorrhage. As noted by Cook, endoscopic therapy reduces the rebleeding as well as decreases the need for surgery and mortality, but it remains less clear which hemostatic technique is most effective. Injection of 1:10,000 adrenaline solution is probably the least expensive technique, and there is no evidence that a second injection with a sclerosant solution provides any additional benefit. Techniques based on the application of heat (heater probe, multipolar coagulation, argon plasma coagulation) are also effective, with outcomes comparable to injection hemostasis, and there is some evidence that a combination of injection and thermal hemostasis may be better for patients with active arterial bleeding. Mechanical hemostasis with, for example, clips, may be effective, but there are few comparative data.

The guidelines recommended medical therapy with high-dose intravenous omeprazole (80 mg bolus, followed by an infusion of 8 mg per hour for 72 hours) after endoscopic hemostasis in patients presenting with major ulcer bleeding, noting that there were no convincing data to support the use of H_2 receptor antagonists in this setting. Based on the available evidence, neither somatostatin nor antifibrinolytic drugs (tranexamic acid) were recommended for routine use. Routine, "second-look" endoscopy was not recommended, but repeat endoscopy was considered reasonable in the event of a suboptimal initial therapeutic attempt and in the event of rebleeding; uncontrolled hemorrhage and rebleeding were considered to require urgent surgery, in collaboration with an experienced surgeon who had been involved in the patient's care from the outset. The guidelines also addressed the roles of *H. pylori* eradication and NSAID discontinuation in patients who had had an ulcer bleed, as well as the need for endoscopic follow-up in patients with gastric ulceration. The BSG guidelines form a basis for managing patients with upper gastrointestinal hemorrhage but, as the authors indicated in their introduction, the specific elements of the guidelines need to be incorporated into institution-specific protocols to allow full implementation, but the role of long-term ulcer prophylaxis was not reviewed.

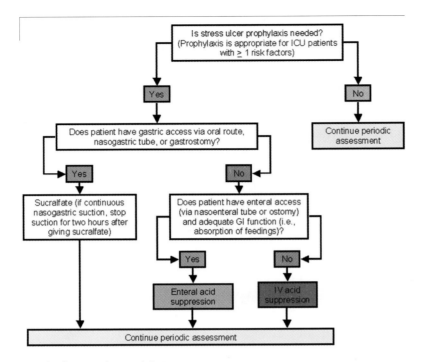

Algorithm for stress ulcer prophylaxis in adult patients proposed by the American Society of Health-System Pharmacists. (Adapted from *Am J Health-Syst Pharm* 1999;56:347–379.)

Stress ulceration

The most detailed guidelines regarding stress ulcer prophylaxis are those developed by the American Society of Health-System Pharmacists (ASHP). This publication provides an extensive review of the pathogenesis of stress ulceration and an evidence-based review of the literature as a basis for the guidelines. The administration of stress ulcer prophylaxis is based on an assessment of the patient's risk and is recommended if an intensive care unit patient has a coagulopathy, requires mechanical ventilation for more than 48 hours, has a history of gastrointestinal ulceration or bleeding within the previous 12 months, or has at least two of the following risk factors: sepsis, intensive care unit stay of more than 1 week, occult bleeding lasting 6 days or more, and use of high-dose corticosteroids (see table below). Other, more specific, indications

Risk factors for upper gastrointestinal bleeding in critically ill patients. (Adapted from *N Engl J Med* 1994;330:397–381.)

Risk Factors for Upper Gastrointestinal Bleeding in Critical ill Patients

Risk Factor	Risk Ratio (multivariate)	*p*-value
Respiratory failure	15.6	< 0.001
Coagulopathy	4.3	< 0.001
Hypotension	3.7	0.08
Sepsis	2.0	0.17
Hepatic failure	1.6	0.27
Renal failure	1.6	0.26
Glucocorticoids	1.5	0.29
Enteral feeding	1.0	0.99

for stress ulcer prophylaxis are also listed in these guidelines; prophylaxis is not recommended for adult patients in non–intensive care unit settings with fewer than two risk factors for clinically important bleeding.

However, although there is clear delineation of the patients who require stress ulcer prophylaxis, there is less clarity concerning the choice of prophylactic agent or agents. Indeed, after reviewing the literature, the guidelines state that the choice between antacids, H$_2$ receptor antagonists, and sucralfate should be made on an institution-specific basis, taking into account concerns regarding administration (e.g., functioning gastrointestinal tract), adverse-effect profile, and total costs. The guidelines noted that there were insufficient data to allow any recommendation on the use of misoprostol or PPIs or novel therapies, such as free-radical scavengers. However, the guidelines were issued before any IV PPI had been in use in the United States.

The algorithm presented in the guidelines (shown above) was accompanied by the caveat that institution-specific guidelines should be developed on the basis of economic modeling. One the one hand, as the ASHP guidelines noted, if H$_2$ receptor antagonists and sucralfate are assumed to have equal efficacy, sucralfate is the most cost-effective agent, although an H$_2$ receptor antagonist (ranitidine) can be considered, either enterally or parenterally, if sucralfate cannot be given due to lack of oral or enteral access. On the other hand, if ranitidine is assumed to be more effective than sucralfate without increasing the risk of pneumonia, it would be the drug of choice and would also result in a cost saving, although less than that achieved with sucralfate.

Thus, for this complex and difficult condition, recommendations as to optimal practice are constrained by a lack of evidence and, although there is some agreement on who should receive prophylaxis, the nature and duration of the prophylaxis remain controversial.

SUGGESTED READING

Armstrong D. The stomach in distress: a critical appraisal of management with reference to proton pump inhibitors. *J Clin Gastroenterol* 2003 (*in press*).

Blatchford O, Murray WR, Blatchford M. A risk score to predict need for treatment of upper gastrointestinal haemorrhage. *Lancet* 2000;356:1318–1321.

Brunner GH, Thiesemann C. The potential clinical role of intravenous omeprazole. *Digestion* 1992;51(Suppl 1):17–20.

Church NI, Palmer KR. Injection therapy for endoscopic hemostasis. *Bailliere's Clin Gastroenterol* 2000;14:427–441.

Collins R, Langman MJS. Treatment with histamine H_2 antagonists in acute upper gastrointestinal hemorrhage: implications of randomized trials. *N Engl J Med* 1985;313:660–666.

Cook DJ, Guyatt GH, Salena BJ, et al. Endoscopic therapy for acute non-variceal upper gastrointestinal haemorrhage: a meta-analysis. *Gastroenterology* 1992;102:139–148.

Cook DJ, Witt LG, Cook RJ, et al. Stress ulcer prophylaxis in the critically ill: a meta-analysis. *Am J Med* 1991;91:519–527.

Daneshmend TK, Hawkey CJ, Langman MJS, et al. Omeprazole versus placebo for acute upper gastrointestinal bleeding: a randomized, double-blind, controlled trial. *Br Med J* 1992;304:143–147.

Driks MR, Craven DE, Celli BR, et al. Nosocomial pneumonia in intubated patients given sucralfate as compared with antacids or histamine type 2 blockers: The role of gastric colonization. *N Engl J Med* 1987;317:1376–1382.

Durrant JM, Strunin L. Comparative trial of the effect of ranitidine and cimetidine on gastric secretion in fasting patients at induction of anaesthesia. *Can Anaesth Soc J* 1982;29(5):446–451.

Freston J, Chiu YL, Pan WJ, et al. Effects on 24-hour intragastric pH: a comparison of lansoprazole administered nasogastrically in apple juice and pantoprazole administered intravenously. *Am J Gastroenterol* 2001;96(7)2058–2065.

Henry DA, O'Connell DL. Effect of fibrinolytic inhibitors on mortality from upper gastrointestinal hemorrhage. *Br Med J* 1989;298:1142–1146.

Hiele M, Rutgeerts P. Combination therapies for the endoscopic treatment of gastrointestinal bleeding. *Bailliere's Clin Gastroenterol* 2000;14:459–466.

Hogan DL, McQuaid KR, Koss MA, et al. Gastric acid suppression is greater during intravenous ranitidine infusion versus bolus injections of famotidine. *Aliment Pharmacol Ther* 1993;7(5):537–541.

Imperiale TF, Birgisson S. Somatostatin or octreotide compared with H_2 antagonists and placebo in the management of acute non-variceal upper gastrointestinal hemorrhage: a meta-analysis. *Ann Intern Med* 1997;127:1062–1071.

Jansen JB, Lundborg P, Baak LC, et al. Effect of single and repeated intravenous doses of omeprazole on pentagastrin stimulated gastric acid secretion and pharmacokinetics in man. *Gut* 1988;29(1):75–80.

Karlstadt RG, Hedrich DA, Asbel-Sethi NR, et al. Acid-suppression profile of two continuously infused intravenous doses of cimetidine. *Clin Ther* 1993;15(1):97–106.

Khuroo MS, Yattoo GN, Javid G, et al. A comparison of omeprazole and placebo for bleeding peptic ulcer. *N Engl J Med* 1997;336:1054–1058.

Kubba AK, Murphy W, Palmer KR. Endoscopic injection for bleeding peptic ulcer: a comparison of adrenaline with adrenaline plus human thrombin. *Gastroenterology* 1996;111:623–628.

Lasky MR, Metzler MH, Phillips JO. A prospective study of omeprazole suspension to prevent clinically significant gastrointestinal bleeding from stress ulcers in mechanically ventilated trauma patients. *J Trauma* 1998;44:527–533.

Lau JYW, Sung JJY, Lam Y, et al. Endoscopic retreatment compared with surgery in patients with recurrent bleeding after initial endoscopic control of bleeding ulcers. *N Engl J Med* 1999;340:751–756.

Lau JY, Sung JJ, Lee KK, et al. Effect of intravenous omeprazole on recurrent bleeding after endoscopic treatment of bleeding peptic ulcers. *N Engl J Med* 2000;343(5):358–359.

Levine JE, Leontiadis GI, Sharma VK, et al. Meta-analysis: the efficacy of intravenous H2-receptor antagonists in bleeding peptic ulcer. *Aliment Pharmacol Ther* 2002;16(6):1137–1142.

Levy MJ, Seelig CB, Robinson NJ, et al: Comparison of omeprazole and ranitidine for stress ulcer prophylaxis. *Dig Dis Sci* 1997;42:1255–1259.

Merki HS, Wilder-Smith CH. Do continuous omeprazole and ranitidine retain their effect with prolonged dosing? *Gastroenterology* 1994;106:60–64.

Metz DC, Forsmark C, Lew EA, et al. Replacement of oral proton pump inhibitors with intravenous pantoprazole to effectively control gastric acid hypersecretion in patients with Zollinger-Ellison syndrome. *Am J Gastroenterol* 2000;96(12):3274–3280.

More DG, Raper RF, Munro IA, et al. Randomized, prospective trial of cimetidine and ranitidine for control of intragastric pH in the critically ill. *Surgery* 1985;97(2):215–224.

Morris J, Karlstadt R, Blatcher D, et al. Field intermittent intravenous pantoprazole rapidly achieves and maintains gastric pH ≥4.0 compared with continuous infusion H2 receptor antagonist in intensive care unit (ICU) patients [abstract 117]. *Crit Care Med* 2003;31(Suppl):A34.

Netzer P, Gaia C, Sandoz M, et al: Effect of repeated injection and continuous infusion of omeprazole and ranitidine on intragastric pH over 72 hours. *Am J Gastroenterol* 1999;94:351–357.

Phillips JO, Metzler MH, Palmieri TL, et al. A prospective study of simplified omeprazole suspension for the prophylaxis of stress-related mucosal damage. *Crit Care Med* 1996;24:1793–1800.

Pisegna, JR, Lew EA, Martin P, et al. Inhibition of pentagastrin-induced gastric acid secretion by intravenous pantoprazole: a dose response study. *Am J Gastroenterol* 1999;94:2874–2880.

Postius S, Brauer U, Kromer W. The novel proton pump inhibitor pantoprazole elevates intragastric pH for a prolonged period when administered under conditions of stimulated gastric acid secretion in the gastric fistula dog. *Life Sci* 1991;49:1047–1052.

Rockall TA, Logan RFA, Devlin HB, et al. Incidence of and mortality from acute upper gastrointestinal haemorrhage in the United Kingdom. *Br Med J* 1995;311:222–226.

Rutgeerts P, Rauws E, Wara P, et al. Randomised trial of single and repeated fibrin glue compared with injection of polidocanol in treatment of bleeding peptic ulcer. *Lancet* 1997;350:692–696.

Shuman RB, Schuster DP, Zuckerman GR. Prophylactic therapy for stress ulcer bleeding: a reappraisal. *Ann Intern Med* 1987;106:562–567.

Tryba M, Cook D. Current guidelines on stress ulcer prophylaxis. *Drugs* 1997;54:581–596.

Vinayek R, Frucht H, London JF, et al. Intravenous omeprazole in patients with Zollinger-Ellison syndrome undergoing surgery. *Gastroenterology* 1990;99(1):10–16.

Wagner BK, Amory DW, Majcher CM, et al. Effects of intravenous famotidine on gastric acid secretion in patients undergoing cardiac surgery. *Ann Pharmacother* 1995;29(4):349–353.

Zed PJ, Loewen PS, Slavik RS, et al. Meta-analysis of proton pump inhibitors in treatment of bleeding peptic ulcers. *Ann Pharmacother* 2001;35:1528–1534.

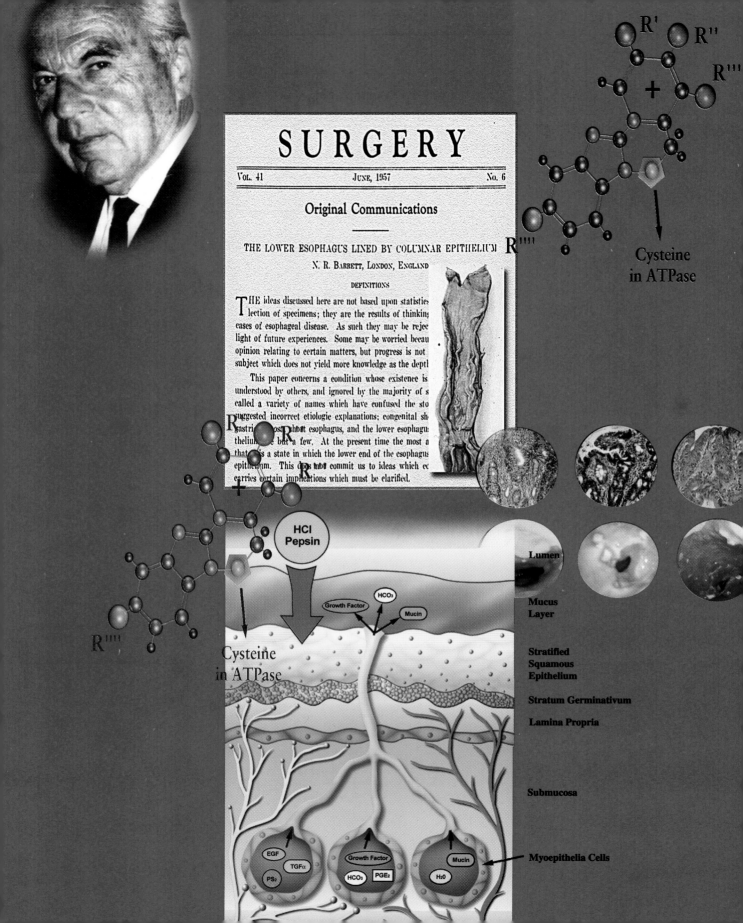

SURGERY

Vol. 41   June, 1957   No. 6

Original Communications

THE LOWER ESOPHAGUS LINED BY COLUMNAR EPITHELIUM

N. R. BARRETT, LONDON, ENGLAND

DEFINITIONS

THE ideas discussed here are not based upon statistics
lection of specimens; they are the results of thinking
cases of esophageal disease. As such they may be reje
light of future experiences. Some may be worried becau
opinion relating to certain matters, but progress is not
subject which does not yield more knowledge as the dept

This paper concerns a condition whose existence is
understood by others, and ignored by the majority of s
called a variety of names which have confused the sto
suggested incorrect etiologic explanations; congenital sh
gastric mucosa about esophagus, and the lower esophagus
thelium are but a few. At the present time the most a
that this is a state in which the lower end of the esophagus
epithelium. This does not commit us to ideas which e
carries certain implications which must be clarified.

R'   **R''**

R'''

R''''

Cysteine
in ATPase

R''''

Cysteine
in ATPase

HCl
Pepsin

Growth Factor HCO_3 Mucin

Lumen

Mucus
Layer

Stratified
Squamous
Epithelium

Stratum Germinativum

Lamina Propria

Submucosa

Myoepithelia Cells

EGF   TGFα PS_2

Growth Factor HCO_3 PGE_2

Mucin H_2O

GASTRO-ESOPHAGEAL REFLUX DISEASE

CHAPTER 1
EVOLUTION OF THE DISEASE AND ITS MANAGEMENT

Introduction

The apparent late recognition of esophagitis as a widespread disease has given cause for much discussion. Surprise has been expressed at the relative lack of reference to it before the mid-nineteenth century, and even thereafter it was noted to be quite rare. Numerous factors reflect the apparent obscurity of the disease until recently. These include the lack of a clear understanding of the anatomy and physiology of the organ, confusion regarding differentiation between its symptomatology and that of the stomach, and, lastly, the lack of opportunity and technology to adequately study it. Of particular importance in terms of the latter aspect of the problem was the advent at the beginning of the twentieth century of rigid endoscopy and the introduction of first bismuth and then barium upper gastrointestinal radiologic studies. The subsequent evolution of fiberoptic endoscopy in the 1960s provided major access to the esophageal lumen, as did the introduction of manometry and pH probe devices to the elucidation of the function of the lower esophageal sphincter (LES). The delineation of the secretion of acid and the ability to document its relationship to acid peptic disease, as well as the recognition of the concept of reflux as a related but separate disease process, facilitated the ability of physicians to focus on the esophagogastric junction as an area of considerable medical relevance.

The prolonged anatomic course of the esophagus caused confusion in the attribution of symptoms. Thus, upper area complaints were often considered to be of oral or throat origin and pathology in the mediastinal course erroneously attributed to the heart. Similarly, at the lower end, the symptoms, as well as their relationship to ingested food, often led to the conclusion that the problem was of gastric origin. Furthermore, the path of the esophagus deep within the posterior mediastinum rendered its study difficult, and speculation rather

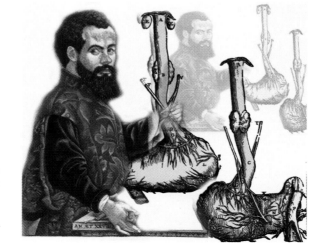

The peripatetic Flemish anatomist Andreas Vesalius (1513–1564) (left), with the aid of the Basel printer J. Oporinus (Herbst) (1507–1568), in 1543 produced an exquisite anatomic folio in which the relationship of the stomach and esophagus was delineated. The dissections were undertaken in Padua and the drawings produced by Stephen van Calcar, a pupil of Titian. Although Vesalius captured the intimate association of the vagus nerves with the upper digestive tract and demonstrated clearly what would later become known as the angle of His, he failed to comment on the functional nature of the LES.

On May 16, 1957, at the Broadmoor hotel, Dr. John Tilden Howard (right), the president of the American Gastrointestinal Endoscopy Society, eschewed his privilege to deliver the presidential address. He elected to yield the floor to Basil Hirschowitz, who presented the first studies of the fiberoptic endoscope (bottom). The subsequent evolution of fiberoptic endoscopy led to the elucidation of esophageal disease, which Tilden himself had previously declared *terra incognita* (no man's land).

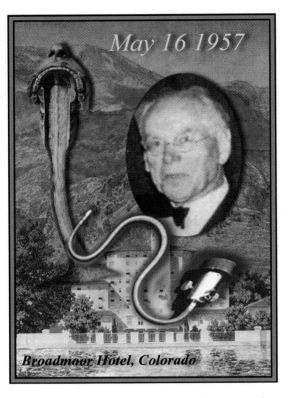

May 16 1957

Broadmoor Hotel, Colorado

than evaluation confounded a clear elucidation of its pathology and delayed the evolution of its rational therapy. Indeed, well into the twentieth century, the upper third was regarded as the province of the otolaryngologist, whereas the lower component was considered a part of the stomach. Few physicians laid claim to the middle third, because most cardiothoracic surgeons directed their attention to the more dynamic structures of the heart and lungs. Indeed, as early as 1946, John Tilden Howard, the secretary of the American Society of Gastrointestinal Endoscopy, had been vocal in pointing out to gastroenterologists the need to examine the esophagus. By the 1950s, the advent of therapeutic strategies for esophageal disease rendered it apparent that the esophagus was no longer *terra incognita*, or no man's land.

Ye meri or ysopaghus

Although seemingly a straightforward topic, the consideration of the esophagus and its disease has proved to be a subject of considerable vexation to physicians. The esophagus has long languished as an organ not highly regarded by any group and little understood by either laypersons or physicians. Some wits even referred to it as the *humble organ*, because so little attention had been devoted to it. To some extent, this reflected its course through three different anatomical territories—the neck, mediastinum, and abdomen—and the reluctance of the medical specialists of each group to claim the organ as their own. Even its name is poorly understood, and much conjecture exists regarding the origin of the term. Although the name is considered to have originally derived from an old Homeric term for the gullet, the meaning became transmuted to reflect a combination of swallowing and food, thus becoming interpreted as "*a tube that conveys food.*" Aristotle claimed that the name derived from its narrowness and length, and some etymologists have even linked the origin of the word to an osier twig, because the old Greek term could also be translated as an "*eater of osiers.*" Whether this reflected the early usage of such flexible branches in the treatment of esophageal obstructions is not recorded. Although the earliest English use of the term is recorded in 1398 in a manuscript in the Bodleian collection that refers to "*Ysophagus, that is the wey of*

mete and drinke," by 1541, Guydon stated, "*the Meri otherwise called Ysophagus is ye way of the mete & this Meri commeth out of the throte and thyrleth
the mydryfe unto ye bely or stomacke.*"

The etymology of symptomatology

The history of the subject of esophagitis is mired in the confusion regarding
the terminology used to describe its symptomatology, as well as by a failure to
appreciate the organ as a separate entity from the stomach or the mouth. Thus
dyspepsy, or, as it is more latterly referred to, *dyspepsia,* was in 1656 referred
to by Blount as *dyspesie* and in 1661 by Lovell as an "*imbecility of the stomach, which is a vice of the concocting faculty and is called apepsy, bradys-
pepsy, or dispepsy and diaphthora.*" The recognition that it might be caused
by both acid and bile appears to reside in the 1829 notation of Southey, who
in *Epistle* in *Anniversary* noted the sensations evoked "*by bile, opinions, and
dyspepsy sour!*" The relationship between the mind, stress, and acid disorders
may have been first noted by Lowell, who in the 1848 *Fable for Critics* opined
that an individual had been "*brought to death's door of a mental dyspepsy.*"
Similarly, the subject of heartburn, which was initially regarded as a heated
and embittered state of mind that is felt but not openly expressed, was
described by Shakespeare in *Richard III* as "*A long continued grudge and
hearte brennynge betwene the Quenes kinred and the kinges blood.*" An
awareness of this problem dates back to 1591, when Percivall described "*a
sharpnes, sowernes of stomack, hartburning.*" Thereafter, Swan, in 1635,
expressed the opinion that "*Lettice cooleth a hot stomach called heart-burning.*"
As early as 1607, Topsell noted the potential severity of the disease, commenting on the "*the hearts of them that die of the heart-burning disease.*" Of note
was the fact that in 1747, Wesley identified that heart burning was "*a sharp
gnawing pain at the orifice of the Stomach.*"

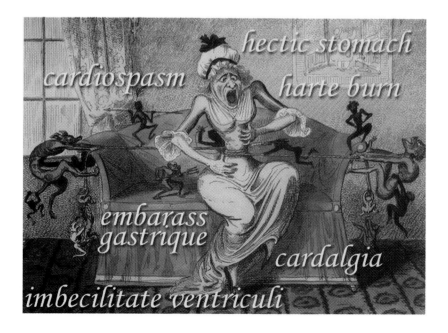

An eighteenth-century British cartoon
accurately attests to the wide public
awareness and familiarity with the
"*Demon of Dyspepsia.*" Confusion as
to the source of visceral pain led to the
evolution of a nomenclature that confused the origin of the symptoms with
the stomach, the heart, or even the
brain. Many believed all chest symptoms emanated from the heart, and
reflux symptoms were referred to as
cardiodynia or *cardalgia*! Indeed, two
centuries later, the basis of esophageal
pain is as little understood now as it
was then!

Nevertheless, the esophagus claimed early medical attention, given the propensity of foreign bodies to obstruct it and the rapid onset of symptoms once ingress of fluids or liquids into the stomach was impaired. Furthermore, there was the disturbing sensation in the chest that caused intense discomfort and was associated with the eating of certain kinds of food. Given the location of the pain and the concept of cardiac dominance in medicine, it was assumed that the origin of the discomfort was the heart and not the esophagus; hence, *cardalgia* and *cardialgy* were terms first used to describe the uneasy burning sensation in the lower part of the chest. The cause was believed to be indicative of putrefactive fermentation in the stomach. This confusion was further amplified by anatomic nomenclature that referred to the upper portion of the stomach as the *cardia*. An additional term, *cardiodynia*, was also used in the nosology of Cullen and was a part of a complex classification that sought to characterize a wide variety of "pain," thereby further defining the origin of a particular disease. Since the time of Harvey and the description of the circulation of the blood, the ebb and flow of bodily fluids through valves and orifices had been acceptably described as examples of flux and reflux. It was therefore well accepted that food might reflux out of the gastric storage vat, and the descriptive term used to describe the consequences of reflux thus alluded not only to the burning sensation, *heartburn*, but its sequela, namely, *cardiospasm*. As early as 1597, Gerard, in his *Herbal*, noted that "*a small stonecrop is good for hart-burne*," whereas Buchan, in 1790, could state with assurance, "*I have frequently known the heart-burn to be cured by chewing green tea.*" A more contemporary comment by Beale, in 1880, stated, "*chalk or magnesia is taken for the relief of heartburn.*"

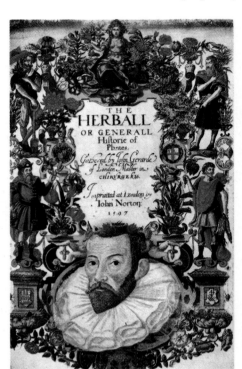

The frontispiece of the *General Herbal* written by John Gerard (1545–1612) (bottom), a master surgeon of London, in 1597. This encyclopedic tabulation of the known therapeutic strategies of the time included a number of putative remedies for the treatment of the vexatious question of "*Ye dreaded lurgy of Harte Burne*"!

Esophagitis

The first description of the disease by Galen was accurate, although somewhat incomplete. Nevertheless, he duly noted that, although difficulties with swallowing may be due to tumors or paralysis, the esophagus, when inflamed, interfered with swallowing by itself acting as a hindrance due to the associated excruciating pain. In 1884, Morell Mackenzie defined esophagitis as an "*acute idiopathic inflammation of the mucous membranes of the esophagus giving rise to extreme odynophagia and often to aphagia.*" It was this Anglicized description that was used to qualify the disease known as *esophagitis*, which had first properly been described by John Peter Frank in 1792.

Although similar observations had been made previously in 1722 by Boehm, who described an acute pain "*which reached down even to the stomach and which was accompanied by hiccup and a constant flow of serum from the mouth,*" he had not defined the condition as accurately. Honkoop published a thesis on inflammation of the gullet in 1774, and in 1785, Bleuland, a physician himself, was struck down with the disease and carefully recorded the details of his

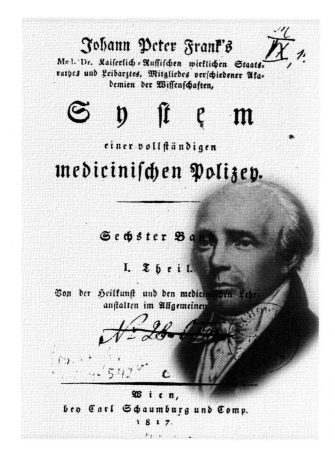

Johann Peter Frank's

Med. Dr. Kaiserlich-Russischen wirklichen Staats-
rathes und Leibarztes, Mitgliedes verschiedener Aka-
demien der Wissenschaften,

System

einer vollständigen

medicinischen Polizey.

Sechster Band

I. Theil.

Von der Heilkunst und den medicinischen Lehr-
anstalten im Allgemeinen.

Wien,
bey Carl Schaumburg und Comp.
1817.

John Peter Frank (1745–1821) was born in Rotalben in the Palatinate of Germany and studied medicine at several German and French universities, receiving an M.D. at Heidelberg before becoming a Professor of Surgery at Pavia, Vienna, and Moscow. Frank is best known for his publication of a *System of a Complete Medical Policy*, in which he described a comprehensive system of medical care combining preventative and curative medical services. His intellectual capacity to appreciate disease was wide ranging. In this respect, he was the first to accurately describe and define the condition now known as *esophagitis*.

illness. The first reports of the condition of esophagitis in children originated with Billard, who, in 1828, published a statement regarding the ailments of newborns. In 1829, Mondière wrote a thesis describing his own severe personal experiences with esophagitis and in addition collected much of the extant material on the subject. His laborious compilation represents more industry than discrimination, but the thesis provides a good overview of early nineteenth-century thoughts on the esophagus. Indeed, it is from the work of Mondière that much of the literature sources of esophageal diseases were drawn for the next century. These included Velpeau's *The Esophagus–A Dictionary in Four Volumes*, Follin's essay "Considerations of Esophageal Disease," and Copland's *Dictionary*. In 1835, Graves of Dublin made some observations on the disease but, thereafter, confined his attentions to the thyroid, achieving eponymous recognition for his contributions to the subject. In 1878, Knott, in Dublin, published *The Pathology of the Esophagus* and included in it the cases of esophagitis described by Roche, Bourguet, Broussais, and Paletta, as well as some original illustrations of diseases of the organ. The topic of the esophagus was further illuminated by communications from Hamburger, Padova, Laboulbène, and a number of other distinguished physicians of the time, but little novel was added to the understanding of the subject.

Although Mackenzie regarded the condition to be of unknown etiology (1884), he carefully defined the chief symptom as excruciating burning or tearing pain—*odynophagia*—induced by any attempt to swallow or any movement of the laryngeal muscles. He also noted that such patients developed considerable thirst but were unable to achieve relief by drinking, because the pain was so severe. In adults, he reported that there was a constant expectoration of frothy saliva, and although patients might not always have a fever, they often became delirious. Mackenzie believed the lesion to represent a diffuse catarrhal inflammation of the mucosa of the upper end of the gullet and felt the diagnosis was based on the history of extreme pain and the absence of pharyngeal inflammation on examination!

Although the description by Mackenzie of esophagitis is very different from that now recognized to represent the contemporary understanding of the disease, his is the first lucid attempt to define the subject. His text *Diseases of the Throat and Nose* contains a fascinating and detailed analysis, as well as classification of esophagitis, but sometimes fails to accurately distinguish between disease of the lower and upper end of the gullet. In the twentieth century, the term *esophagitis* has become referable almost solely to an entity involving the lower part of the gullet. Nevertheless, Mackenzie recognized that the inflammatory conditions of the upper part of the gullet were

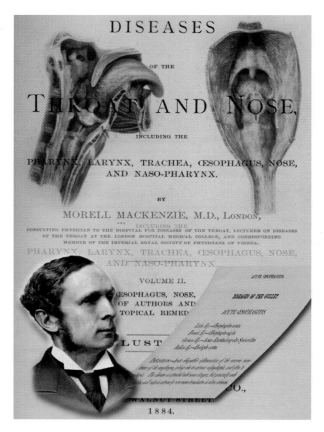

DISEASES

OF THE

THROAT AND NOSE,

INCLUDING THE

PHARYNX, LARYNX, TRACHEA, ŒSOPHAGUS, NOSE,
AND NASO-PHARYNX.

BY

MORELL MACKENZIE, M.D., LONDON,

CONSULTING PHYSICIAN TO THE HOSPITAL FOR DISEASES OF THE THROAT, LECTURER ON DISEASES
OF THE THROAT AT THE LONDON HOSPITAL MEDICAL COLLEGE, AND CORRESPONDING
MEMBER OF THE IMPERIAL ROYAL SOCIETY OF PHYSICIANS OF VIENNA.

VOLUME II.

1884.

Sir Morell Mackenzie (1837–1892) was regarded as the leading ear, nose, and throat surgeon of London at the end of the nineteenth century. His definitive text on the subject included substantial information on the esophagus and an erudite chapter on the subject of acute esophagitis and its treatment. Unfortunately, his medical contributions were somewhat overshadowed by his role in the debacle that led to the tragic demise of the German Emperor (Frederick III of Prussia) from laryngeal cancer.

Most therapy of the nineteenth century was permeated by the belief that disease reflected some noxious property present in the blood. Venesection as a means of therapy was widely accepted and vied with the use of leeches for primacy in efficacy. In France, the use of leeches to remove blood from ill persons was so prevalent that demand exceeded supply to the extent that leeches became a huge import commodity during the early part of the nineteenth century. Such was the presumed widespread benefit of leech therapy that even esophagitis was deemed amenable to leech application.

specific and included diphtheria, thrush, tuberculosis, syphilis, actinomycosis, and corrosive damage. Some of the associated nonspecific conditions (myalgia, general hyperesthesia) alluded to by Mackenzie are no longer recognized, but as late as 1900, all inflammatory conditions affecting the gullet were still regarded as varieties of esophagitis. Of particular interest were the treatments proposed in the management of this vexatious condition. It was considered mandatory that the organ be maintained in a state of absolute rest. Thus, feeding was undertaken by nutrient enemata and morphia administered by hypodermic injection to facilitate resolution of inflammation and abolish pain. Poultices were applied along the upper part of the spine, or, if the pain was particularly severe, anodyne embrocations, such as oleate of morphia or belladonna lineaments, were rubbed into the back. Mondière, following the French practice of the time, believed in venesection and cupping as well as leech applications (12 to 30 at a time).

Counterirritation by the application of mustard poultices or moxas was also widely recommended. By 1884, however, Mackenzie was able to declare that bleeding or even the local abstraction of blood was of little value, and that he himself had found counterirritation to be of no effect. He favored derivatives and especially recommended the use of extremely hot

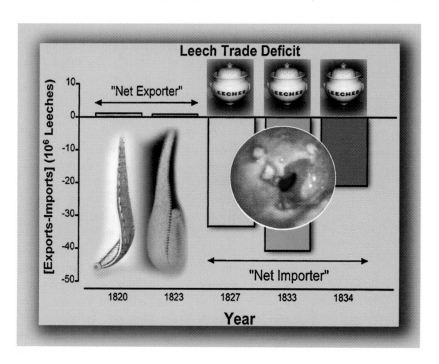

pediluvia. Bleuland used blisters *loco dolenti* between the shoulders with success, and Pagenstecher reported the use of hydrochloride of ammonia to great advantage. This agent had long been a favorite of German and Dutch physicians and was used as a remedy for many different kinds of diseases. Mackenzie was adamant that the passage of bougies was dangerous and should never be attempted, because it was likely to cause rupture of the esophagus. Once convalescence commenced, the patient could be changed from a liquid to a solid diet gradually, and if pain returned, immediate return to a liquid diet should once again be undertaken.

Despite the attention to the gullet provided by Mackenzie, esophagitis per se was not commonly recognized, and little was known about it. In 1906, Wilder Tileston carefully defined at least 12 different types of ulceration, which included carcinoma, corrosive, foreign bodies, acute infectious diseases, decubitus, aneurysms, catarrhal inflammations, those associated with diverticulum, tuberculosis, syphilis, varicose, and ulcers due to thrush. Tileston was particularly drawn to the disease that he referred to as *peptic ulcer of the esophagus*, which he claimed exactly simulated the behavior and appearance of chronic gastric ulcer. He noted that, although a rare entity, it had initially been described by Albers in 1839 and thereafter sporadically noted by pathologists. No less an authority than C. Rokitansky (1804–1878) had concurred that peptic ulcer of the lower esophagus was a real and definable entity and represented the aftermath of gastric juice in the gullet. Nevertheless, when Tileston reviewed the literature, as far as 1906, there had only been 44 clear-cut examples of the condition published. The ulcers described were usually single and often associated with chronic peptic ulcer in the stomach or the duodenum. They were large, penetrating lesions sometimes 6

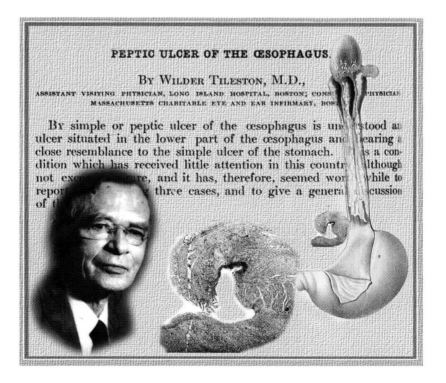

In 1906, Wilder Tileston, while a pathologist at Harvard, was able to identify at least 12 potential types of esophageal ulcerations. In particular, he noted a disease that simulated the behavior and appearance of chronic gastric ulcer, which he referred to as *"peptic ulcer of the esophagus."* His seminal manuscript of 1906 reported forty-four cases of this rare and novel disease entity. His precise description of the condition accurately noted the typical "overhanging edge" of the healing mucosa (center).

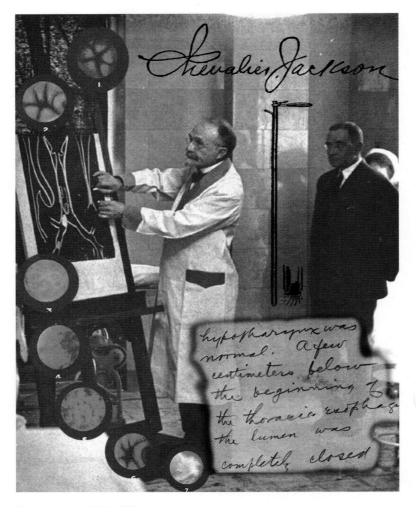

to 8 cm in length that lay *"above the cardiac sphincter"* and, although often longitudinal, might also encircle the entire gullet.

The patients were elderly, and many had no symptoms referable to the esophagus until their admission to the hospital. Death usually occurred from perforation into a large vessel, the pericardium, the mediastinum, or the pleural cavity, although some died of pneumonia. Of interest was the fact that few exhibited symptoms of esophageal obstruction. Tileston further reported that the histology of such ulcers was identical to that of chronic gastric ulcer, and that the adjacent mucosa was gastric in type. He assumed it to be "ectopic," because it lined the lower part of the gut in the mediastinum.

The understanding of ulceration of the esophagus and esophagitis itself became further obfuscated with the advent of radiology and esophagoscopy at the turn of the nineteenth century. The use of these diagnostic tools enabled the identification of a variety of esophageal lesions, particularly ulcers and inflammation at the lower end of the gullet not previously apparent to clinicians. Thus, by the 1920s, it was apparent that pathologists, clinicians, and endoscopists, although assuming that they were describing the same entity when they referred to peptic ulcer of the esophagus or esophagitis, were each unclear as to the exact nature of the disease process. In 1929, Chevalier Jackson, a virtuoso esophagoscopist, reported 88 cases in 4,000 consecutive endoscopies, whereas Stewart and Hartfall in the same year claimed that they were able to identify only one example of esophagitis in 10,000 consecutive autopsies.

The subsequent reports of Lyall (1937), Chamberlin (1939), and Dick and Hurst (1942) provided further insight into the nature and occurrence of these lower esophageal lesions. The further substantial contributions by Paul Allison and Johnstone of Leeds (1943, 1946, and 1948) left little doubt that the authors were confident in their ability to recognize and diagnose "peptic ulcer of the esophagus" or "esophagitis."

Chevalier Jackson (1865–1958), an ear, nose, and throat surgeon of Philadelphia, made important contributions to the subject of endoscopy and the esophagus. Jackson was erudite, artistic, sophisticated, and a brilliant surgeon to boot, and by 1930, his perspicacity enabled him to consider the concept of gastric juice as one of the causes of inflammation of the lower esophagus (text). In this respect, he was able to provide strong support for the proposal put forward by Winkelstein in 1934 that peptic esophagitis was a disease entity worthy of serious consideration.

The Beatitude of Barrett

Norman Barrett believed that the early descriptions of ulcer by Tileston, Stewart, and Lyall differed significantly from those identified by clinicians such as Allison. He felt that the former were rare and of little clinical significance, whereas the latter were common and important entities. He further proposed that this confusion had arisen because the pathology of the former had been tacked on to the symptomatology of the latter. Indeed, it was Barrett's opinion that the condition described in 1948 by Allison actually represented *reflux esophagitis*, and that this was the best name for the lesion.

The assessment of the situation at the lower end of the esophagus by Allison was prescient. He was of the opinion that chronic esophageal ulcers could develop into lesions similar to gastric ulcers and noted that the features of esophageal ulcers that complicate reflux esophagitis are that they are situated in the esophagus and represent digestion of the squamous epithelium. Allison opined that these lesions arose in areas of general acute inflammation and manifested initially as erosions that could either heal or persist, depending on the amount of gastric juice that had access to the gullet. Such areas remained as superficial defects for a considerable period in the majority of individuals, but eventually, when the site had become significantly scarred, they burrowed through the muscularis. It was Barrett's proposal that the stricture of the esophagus generated by this chronic inflammation had been mistakenly regarded as the esophagus, whereas it was, in fact, a patch of stomach partially enveloped by peritoneum that had been drawn up by scar tissue into the mediastinum. Barrett therefore concluded that it was this stomach that was the site of the chronic gastric ulcer, and that the ulcers that had been described in the lower gullet were in truth gastric and not esophageal, and that they were located below the stricture.

To defend his novel and somewhat provocative assertion, he asked two questions: First, what is the esophagus? And second, what is meant by *heterotopia* of the gastric mucosa in relation to the esophagus? Barrett regarded the esophagus as that part of the alimentary canal extending from the pharynx to the stomach, lined by squamous epithelium. As regards heterotopia and ectopia, he believed the terms to be interchangeable and to refer to small islets of gastric epithelium found in the esophagus and surrounded on all sides by normal squamous epithelium. He proposed that the alternative scenario in which gastric mucosa, in direct continuity with the rest of the stomach, extended up into mediastinum in one sheet was due to a congenital and pathologic condition that was denoted by the term *short esophagus*. His views on the relationship of islets of gastric epithelium to chronic peptic ulcer of the esophagus were novel. In his opinion, such ulcers arose in the esophagus in islets of ectopic gastric mucosa themselves or as a consequence

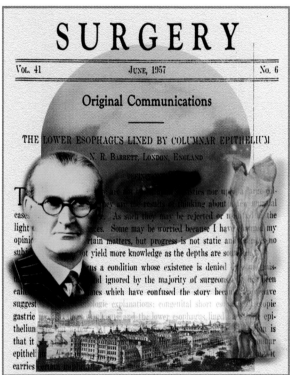

Norman (Pasty) Barrett (1903–1979), originally of Adelaide, Australia, studied in London and as a consultant surgeon at St. Thomas Hospital (bottom) developed novel concepts relating to the subject of peptic esophagitis and the consideration of a putative condition that he referred to as a "short esophagus." His reflections on the subject of ectopic gastric mucosa (1957) subsequently spawned a gastroenterologic obsession that led to the development of an entirely novel disease entity. Well known for his eccentricity, sailing skills, and idiosyncratic persona, Barrett, if alive today, would certainly regard the pursuit of this illusory biologic phenomenon of the "short esophagus" as the medical equivalent of Lewis Carroll's *The Hunting of the Snark*.

of the secretion of acid into the gullet by such islets. The history of these ectopic islets of gastric mucosa in the esophagus is actually quite intriguing. Although first described by F. A. Schmidt in 1805, the observation was overlooked until Schridde, in 1904, reported that microscopic ectopic islets were present in 70% of all gullets and always situated in the postcricoid region. Taylor of Leeds, in 1927, in examining 900 cases, had identified in six, at the top of the gullet, areas large enough to be visible to the naked eye. Terracol, in 1938, reported similar lesions at the top of the gullet, whereas Rector and Connerly (1941) identified in infants 56 examples at the upper end and seven somewhat lower down. Barrett did not believe that these isolated islets secreted acid, or if they did, the volume was of such paucity that it could not cause ulcers. Indeed, he claimed, *"nor were there any reports of ulcers associated with such islets."* His interpretation of the papers by Tileston, Stewart, and Lyall was that the massive ulceration described by them was in an area of stomach that extended beyond the crura of the diaphragm, and that the ulcers were in actual fact chronic gastric ulcers occurring in a pouch of "mediastinal stomach." In contradistinction, Lyall and his colleagues had

A cross section of a normal esophagus (center), surrounded by endoscopic and histologic views of Barrett's esophagitis. Endoscopic grades I (top left) and II (bottom right) are shown with the corresponding histologic views of type I (top right) and dysplasia of the esophagus (bottom left). Given the anatomy of the esophagus and the nonlinearity of the metaplastic mucosa, the biopsy sampling remains the critical issue.

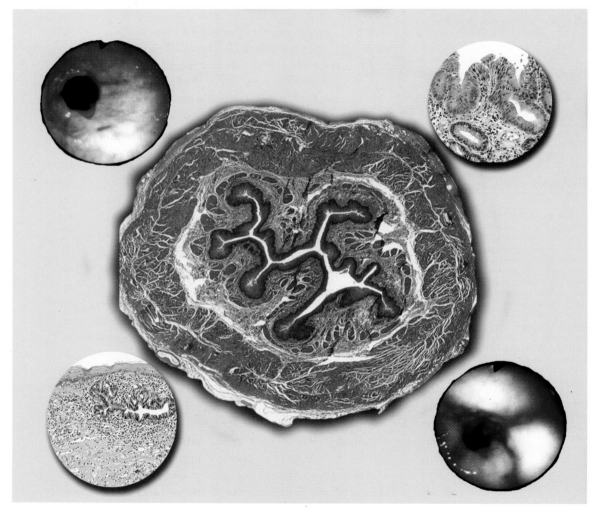

regarded the ulcers to be in the esophagus and had called the columnar mucosa with which they were associated *heterotopic*.

The final conclusion that Barrett arrived at in his provocative but seminal comments on esophagitis was that the word had now become a blunderbuss term and was being used to cover many different pathologic lesions. He believed that its use should always be qualified by the descriptive adjective *reflux esophagitis*, and that this condition was common and could produce ulceration of the esophagus and stricture formation. He further believed that this particular lesion was separate from the condition regarded by pathologists as peptic ulcer of the esophagus, which he felt to be an example of a congenital short esophagus. In the latter, there was neither evidence of general inflammation nor stricture formation, but a part of the stomach extended up into the mediastinum and even into the neck, and it was in this type of stomach that a typical chronic gastric ulcer could form.

Asher Winkelstein

Although there is much debate over who first noted reflux esophagitis and what its precise etiology might be, the contributions of Winkelstein require consideration. At the eighty-fifth annual session of the American Medical Association, held in Cleveland on June 13, 1934, Winkelstein of Mt. Sinai Hospital, New York, presented to the Section of Gastroenterology and Proctology a paper entitled "Peptic Esophagitis—A New Clinical Entity." He noted that, although the causes of esophagitis were generally regarded as irritative

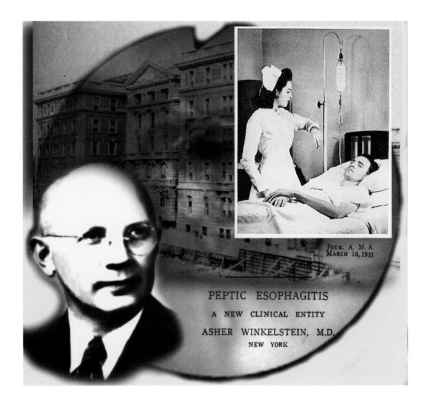

Asher Winkelstein (1893–1972) (bottom left), as the Chief of Gastroenterology at Mount Sinai Hospital in New York, deserves credit for the initial description of peptic esophagitis (right). Possessed of a brilliant mind unfettered by dogma, he also was the first to propose the milk drip for the treatment of peptic ulcer disease (top right), advocate the use of surgical vagotomy years before its introduction by Lester Dragstedt (1893–1975), and note the relevance of nocturnal acid secretion.

(alcohol, tobacco), specific (syphilis, tuberculosis), or secondary to complications of cardiospasm, diverticuli, or neoplasm, he believed that there existed a different and separate entity. *"Recently I have observed some patients with a type of esophagitis that does not seem to fit into this classification. The features of these cases are so distinctive as to impress one with the probability that they form a separate clinical entity."*

In the discussion of this pivotal presentation, the doyen of American esophageal disease, the venerable Chevalier Jackson of Philadelphia, rose to comment, stating:

I am in hearty accord . . . chronic esophagitis is a common disease due to a variety of causes not all of which are known or, at least proved. . . . The cause of this kind of esophagitis is similar to the causes of gastric ulcer. . . . I think that the word "peptic" is justified by the fact that all of these ulcers in the esophagus, stomach and duodenum are within the area of the gastric juice, and for parallel reasons this form of esophagitis, which is also within the area flooded by the gastric juice. I think it is quite properly called peptic.

In 1935, in the March 16 issue of the *Journal of the American Medical Association*, Winkelstein further noted, *"one cannot avoid the suspicion that the disease in these five cases is possibly a peptic esophagitis i.e. an esophagitis resulting from the irritant action on the mucosa of free hydrochloric acid and pepsin."* Indeed, it was the culmination of Winkelstein's proposal and Allison's later concept of a chronic reflux of gastric contents that finally assured the place of the term *reflux esophagitis* in the literature. The subsequent arguments as to whether anatomic and mechanical factors, such as a hiatus hernia, were responsible engendered much discussion. In 1968, E. D. Palmer, in a powerful paper, cast considerable doubt on the relationship between hiatus hernia and esophagitis. It is of interest to note that he had a short time previously similarly disparaged the proposed relationship between the spiral bacteria noted in gastric biopsies and washings and peptic ulcer disease! In a 22-year prospective study, he reported that many patients with hernias had neither reflux symptoms nor esophagitis, and that many other patients had esophagitis in the absence of a hiatus hernia. At this stage, the role of the LES became an area of critical relevance in establishing the primary mechanism of reflux disease.

Hiatus hernia

Although diaphragmatic hernia was first described by Ambrose Paré as far back as 1580, historically, the hiatus hernia had hardly been described before the X-ray era and reflected the classic autopsy technique of that time, in which the esophagus was cut just above the diaphragm and taken out with the heart and the lungs, losing all its connections with its abdominal segment and with the stomach. In 1884, Postempski reported the successful repair of a diaphragmatic hernia by a transthoracic approach, and within a year, six further cases had been reported in his clinic.

Bernstein, in reviewing the subject of hiatus hernia in 1947, noted some of the causes for the relatively low numbers of diagnoses of the condition.

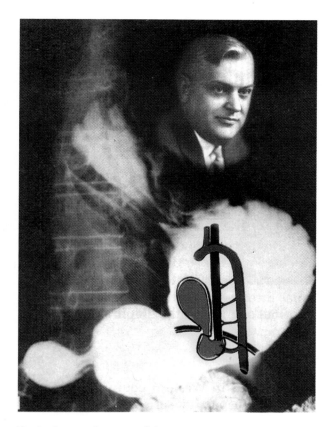

The development of contrast radiology in the first decade of the twentieth century, 70 years before endoscopic identification of esophagitis enabled radiologists such as Russell Carmen (1875–1926) (top right) of the Mayo Clinic to identify the presence of a hiatus hernia. The putative relationship between such herniation and reflux-induced mucosal disease escaped consideration for decades until the contributions (1943–1956) of the surgeons, Norman Barrett (1903–1979) of London and Philip Allison (1904–1974) of Leeds. The relationship of this radiologic observation to clinical symptomatology became a matter of considerable dispute, as surgeons sought to address a much-venerated target that had long been a part of their idealized therapeutic domain, namely, the repair of a hernia. The center inset diagrams Barrett's original concept of the paraesophageal hernia (right).

At autopsy, with all muscles relaxed and the intra-abdominal pressure diminished, this condition may easily be overlooked, and only scattered reports of a few cases were therefore known in the literature of the pre-radiological era. The conventional technique of X-ray examination of the stomach with the patient in upright posture usually also fails to visualize these hernias. Examination in recumbent or even Trendelenburg position with application of manual pressure toward the upper abdomen is necessary to produce and demonstrate the condition under the fluoroscope. It is usual for these hernias to disappear as soon as the patient is brought back into upright posture or the increased abdominal pressure is released.

The rarity of the condition may best be considered by the work of H. Eppinger, who, in 1911, summarized the literature on diaphragmatic hernia and reported that of 635 cases of herniation through various portions of the diaphragm, only 11 involved the esophageal hiatus. In 1923, Richards could review 23 observations. By 1925, 30 cases had been seen at the Mayo Clinic. It was, therefore, only when such a specially adapted technique of examination was introduced by Akerlund in 1926 that the relatively frequent occurrence of this condition was generally recognized. Akerlund thereafter reported 30 more cases and proposed a classification of hiatus hernia that for many years was regarded as definitive. From then on, the number soon became legion. Knothe observed 300 cases at the Charite Hospital in Berlin, representing 8% of all patients subjected to gastrointestinal roentgen examination. In 1930, Ritvo, a Boston radiologist, published a series of 60 cases, all in adults, and, in commenting on the differential diagnosis, cited cardioesophageal relaxation as a distinct pathologic process. Although Ritvo reported epigastric pain, heartburn, nausea, vomiting, and regurgitation as clinical correlates of "esophageal orifice hernia," he failed to postulate gastroesophageal reflux as the cause of these symptoms. Harrington subsequently reported 680 cases of diaphragmatic hernia seen at the Mayo Clinic. From 1930–1946, 984 articles on diaphragmatic hernia were quoted in the *Quarterly Cumulative Index Medicus*. Bernstein himself noted that in the 2 years before his publication, he had identified 38 cases of diaphragmatic hernia in 994 gastric examinations—3.8%. From all these publications, containing reports of numerous cases each, and from his experience, he stated, "*hernia of the esophageal hiatus is a very common condition indeed.*" He concluded that, on the average, the incidence in relation to the number of patients examined varies from 2% to 5%.

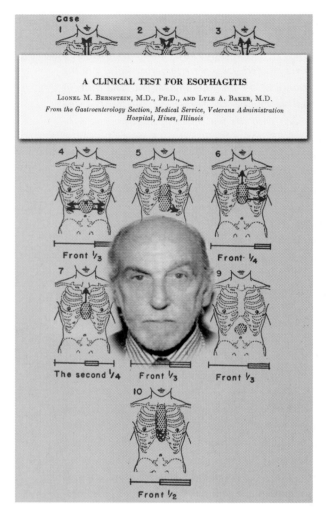

In 1961, Bernstein (center) and Baker published their acid-based test, which attempted to identify patients with esophagitis by reproducing the symptoms of heartburn. As such, this test (acid or saline infusion) allowed for the determination of whether chest or back pain (background) was due to acid in the esophagus and was indicative of GERD. It is of interest that, 4 decades later, R. Fass, by using the "enantiomeric" concept of abrogating acid secretion, was able to describe an equally effective diagnostic-therapeutic test for identifying the nature of chest pain (acid suppression test).

The early writings of Harrington and Kirklin, Hedbloom, and others in the twentieth century concentrated on anatomic problems, and for practical purposes, surgical intervention was concerned principally with returning the stomach to the abdomen. In 1935, Winkelstein first called attention to peptic esophagitis secondary to reflux and, thereafter, a number of physicians, particularly Bernstein, in 1947, commented on the clinical relevance of this consideration. It became well recognized that hiatal hernia was a common condition, and Harrington reported that over half of the patients undergoing laparotomy for other conditions could be shown to have an asymptomatic hiatal hernia. It was thus accepted that only when reflux esophagitis was present did hiatal hernias become symptomatic. In 1949, Kramer and Ingelfinger, using "modern" technology, revived the early work of Kronecker and Meltzer that had documented the physiology of the swallowing mechanism. The subsequent studies of the acidity of the lower esophageal contents by Bernstein and Baker and others made it possible to accurately determine the necessity for surgical correction and also enabled an objective evaluation of the completeness of the surgical repair. The further expansion of the gastroesophageal horizon of disease was proposed in 1962, when J. H. Kennedy implicated reflux symptoms in the production of pulmonary symptomatology, and in 1968, Cherry and Margulies suggested that laryngeal abnormalities might be secondary to gastroesophageal reflux. By 1990, Sontag had demonstrated that more than 80% of asthmatics exhibited reflux, and the disease of GERD had assumed almost epidemic proportions. Indeed, epidemiologic studies indicated that up to one-third of the people in developed countries, such as the United Kingdom and the United States, suffered from the disorder.

The evolution of surgical strategies

During the first half of the twentieth century, surgeons were somewhat mechanistically inclined and were thus especially excited by the concept that an organ that protruded through a muscle, possessed a sac, and was called a *hernia* could indeed be treated like a hernia. Thus, if the patient was deemed capable of sustaining a major operation that consisted of an anatomic repositioning of the stomach, then such was the resolution of the problem. If the

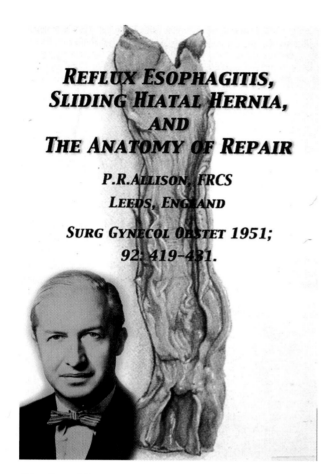

REFLUX ESOPHAGITIS, SLIDING HIATAL HERNIA, AND THE ANATOMY OF REPAIR

P. R. ALLISON, FRCS

LEEDS, ENGLAND

SURG GYNECOL OBSTET 1951; 92: 419–431.

Philip Allison of Leeds, England, was among the first to consider that the entity of reflux esophagitis could be managed surgically by appropriate repair of a sliding hiatus hernia. Despite meticulous surgical technique, analysis of the outcome demonstrated that a hernia repair alone was inadequate in securing long-term relief from reflux esophagitis.

operation were deemed risky, the alternative of ablating the phrenic nerve or snipping the hiatal rim to release the supposedly "throttled" stomach was considered acceptable. As usual, there existed some discussion as to how large the hernia should be to qualify for fixing and, of course, whether the repair should be done through the chest or abdomen. Surgeons who had failed to comprehend the significance of gastroesophageal reflux and were uncertain of the precise relationship of hiatus hernia to esophagitis responded by proposing a wide variety of operations destined to restore anatomic "purity" to the region. Thus, the subject of hiatal hernia was relegated to chapters dealing with inguinal, scrotal, and other celomic "ruptures."

By 1950, there was no doubt that hiatus hernia had to be corrected surgically by placing the abdominal segment of the esophagus, the cardia, and the fundus into the abdomen below the diaphragm. In the 1940s, Pettersson had tried to correct the hiatus hernia by paralyzing the left hemidiaphragm, which he accomplished by crushing the phrenic nerve. This idea had been proposed earlier by Harrington and Manseck. However, the results were unpredictable, and the method was therefore abandoned.

The demise of this doctrine of anatomic preoccupation was ushered in by publication of Allison's classic article in 1948, in which he proposed that the symptoms of an ordinary sliding hiatal hernia derived from acid damage inflicted on the lower esophagus secondary to reflux. To remedy this situation, Allison described a procedure whereby he united the two halves of the right crus and reattached the splayed-out phrenoesophageal membrane to the undersurface of the diaphragm. This operation was accepted as the logical treatment of hiatus hernia, and it was believed that the anatomic repair would also correct the pathophysiology. Unfortunately, this technique failed to prevent gastroesophageal reflux and often even aggravated the situation. Indeed, in 1973, Allison himself reviewed 421 of his own cases, operated between 1950 and 1970, and reported a recurrence of the hernia, gastroesophageal reflux, or both in 49% of sliding hiatus hernia repairs. This experience was shared by numerous surgeons of the time, including Sweet, Husfeldt, Pettersson, Wanke, Rehbein, and others. As a result, in 1955, Boerema proposed the anterior gastropexy, that is, the fixation of the lesser curvature of the stomach to the anterior abdominal wall, as the sole necessary procedure in the surgical repair of hiatus hernia.

Unfortunately, it now seems apparent that the latter component of the technique probably distracted and opened the dysfunctional sphincter even more. Because reposition of the hernia alone proved valueless in preventing gastroesophageal reflux, new techniques were developed to reestablish or accentuate the angle of His, thus forming an antireflux valve. Duhamel was among the first to use such a technique and, in January 1953, published his first eight cases of reconstruction of the angle of His with six excellent and two good results. Thereafter, Bettex proposed a broader back-to-back suturing of the fundus to the lower esophagus and achieved better long-term results.

Although Allison's operation represented a novel idea, and he was among the first to embrace the notion of the relationship to hernia and reflux, the procedure failed to endure, and enthusiasm for the "reflux thesis" might have waned considerably had it not been for the more or less simultaneous and independent achievements in the Kantonsspital, Basel, and the Frenchay Hospital in Bristol by Rudolf Nissen and Ronald Belsey, respectively.

Nissen and fundoplication

The first rational surgical therapy for the condition now ubiquitously referred to by the "generic" acronym of *GERD* can be attributed to Rudolf Nissen and the technique of fundoplication. In his original account of the procedure, Nissen, who was at that time chairman of the department of surgery at the Bürgerspital, Switzerland, treated two patients with chronic reflux disease. He termed the operation a *gastroplication*. In the original description of the open fundoplication, two broad folds were wrapped around the esophagus and fixed anterior to the esophagus using four to five sutures. In the course of this operation, major exposure of the esophagogastric junction was required and an incision of the lesser omentum undertaken, leading to the transection of numerous branches of the vagal nerve, particularly the right trunk. This inadvertent denervation was responsible postoperatively for considerable gastric motility–related morbid symptomatology. As a result, the original fundoplication was modified by Nissen and his colleagues, as well as by others, to preserve the vagal branches. The "anterior wall technique" (Rosetti-Hell total fundoplication) uses the anterior wall of the gastric fundus to create the total wrap, thus obviating the extensive mobilization and division of the short gastric vessels. A further modification of the original fundoplication procedure, the "short floppy cuff," introduced in 1977 by Donahue and Bombeck, significantly reduced concomitant side effects such as dysphagia and gas bloat symptoms. This technical modification proposed a complete mobilization of the fundus and gastroesophageal junction, a short wrap length (2.0 to 2.5 cm), and preservation of the vagal nerves. In addition to the initial total fundoplication procedures used, a partial fundoplication may be performed whereby partial fundal wraps are placed either anterior or posterior to the gastroesophageal junction. A variety of similar procedures has been described and includes a posterior crurally fixed partial fundoplication (Toupet) or an anterior 180-degree fundoplication (Dor). Watson's operation comprises a full mobilization of the lower esophagus and gastroesophageal junction, crural repair, fixation of the esophagus to the crura, and anterior 180-degree Dor-type fundoplica-

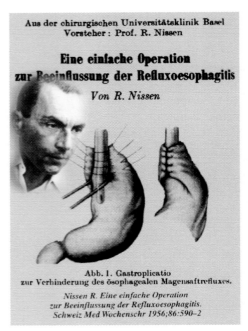

Aus der chirurgischen Universitätsklinik Basel
Vorsteher : Prof. R. Nissen

Eine einfache Operation zur Beeinflussung der Refluxoesophagitis

Von R. Nissen

Abb. 1. Gastroplicatio
zur Verhinderung des ösophagealen Magensaftrefluxes.

Nissen R. Eine einfache Operation zur Beeinflussung der Refluxoesophagitis. Schweiz Med Wochenschr 1956;86:590–2

Rudolf Nissen, a peripatetic surgeon of Berlin, Istanbul, Boston, Brooklyn, and Basel, is best remembered for establishing fundoplication as the "definitive" surgical procedure for the management of GERD. Few recall that he operated on Albert Einstein.

The evolution of antireflux surgery. The Nissen fundoplication (top), a complete 360-degree wrap of the gastric fundus posteriorly around the esophagus; the 240-degree to 270-degree partial wrap of the Toupet fundoplication (right); and the Hill procedure (bottom) all represent surgical attempts to bolster the sphincter. The latter included the fixation of the LES in the abdomen and created an angulation in the lower esophagus to prevent reflux. The Collis gastroplasty (left) was developed to generate a tension-free fundoplication in the setting of a shortened esophagus.

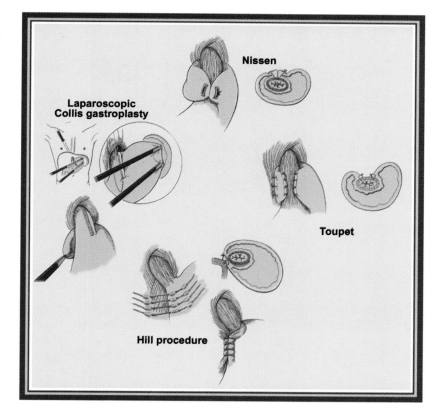

tion (the Belsey Mark IV consists of an anterior 270-degree partial fundoplication, fixed to the undersurface of the diaphragm and performed through the left chest—more on this later). In general, it was felt (by surgeons) that such procedures had a good outcome and were associated with fewer side effects such as dysphagia and gas bloat. In particular, it was apparent that the partial fundoplications were most useful in patients with evidence of significant esophageal hypomotility. Overall, however, the wide variety of procedures, their high morbidity, and the absence of rigorous evaluation of the outcome have generated a sense of suboptimal enthusiasm for their use.

Belsey of Bristol

Although it may appear that the discovery by Nissen of the beneficial effect of fundoplication was a serendipitous observation, it nevertheless remains a fact that in undertaking surgery that folded the stomach over an esophagogastric anastomosis to protect it from leaking, he inadvertently also protected the esophagus from the predictable acid reflux associated with resection of the LES. On the contrary, the surgical strategy adopted by Belsey reflected the culmination of many years of observations in the Frenchay endoscopy unit and subsequent careful correlation of these findings with the symptomatology of the patient. Using a rigid 50-cm esophagoscope and examining the sedated but awake patient in the sitting position, Belsey concluded that competency at the cardia depended on its lying well below the diaphragm. Thus, when the gastro-

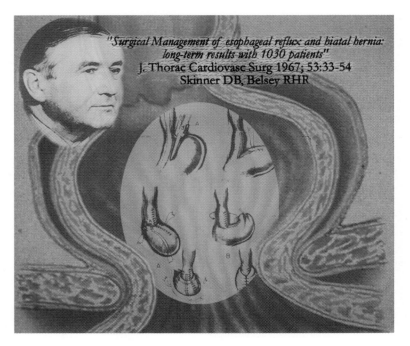

"Surgical Management of esophageal reflux and hiatal hernia:
long-term results with 1030 patients"
J. Thorac Cardiovasc Surg 1967; 53:33-54
Skinner DB, Belsey RHR

Ronald Belsey (top left) of Bristol, England, was not only a surgeon of considerable technical virtuosity, but possessed of an independent and inquiring mind. His thoughtful evaluation, over a period of years, of the nature of the disease of the lower esophageal sphincter led to his development of a series of procedures (Belsey Mark I-IV) designed to surgically obviate the problem of reflux. The results of these data, an analysis of 1,030 patients over a decade, were published in 1967 (top) and for years were widely regarded as the definitive contribution to the field. A number of American surgeons (Skinner, Baue, Ellis) who trained with him at the Frenchay Hospital in Bristol played an important role in disseminating Belsey's concepts of fundoplication to the North American surgical community.

esophageal junction was dislocated from its usual relationship with the right crus, the cardia gaped and gastric contents could be detected as rising into the esophagus with deep inspiration.

Belsey described this situation as "*a patulous cardia*" and proposed that the operative goal should be to fix the gastroesophageal junction 2 or 3 cm below the diaphragm. A series of different surgical strategies was thereafter undertaken in an attempt to maximize the efficacy of this procedure. The Mark I operation was essentially the Allison approach, whereas the Mark II and III procedures represented various degrees of fundoplication. These culminated in the crescentic overlay of stomach in the Mark IV procedure, which was achieved by trial and error as a means of obtaining tissue more substantial than the naked esophagus into which the anchoring sutures could be passed. Of interest is the fact that Belsey's criteria of a good operation included the ability to teach the procedure to others and achieve durable relief from reflux while preserving the other esophageal functions (i.e., agreeable swallowing, venting of gas, protection of the airway, and maintenance of the capacity to vomit). The Mark III operation, with three rows of plicating sutures, failed both tests, because it was difficult to teach, and because the valve was more competent than acceptable. During the early trial period (1949 to 1955) with the Mark I, II, and III operations, unsatisfactory results were identified in approximately one-third of the patients; there were also seven postoperative deaths. In contrast, 85% of the 632 patients operated on between 1955 and 1962 had a good or excellent result. Belsey delayed formal publication of the Mark IV repair procedure for patients with the isolated condition of *patulous cardia* for 6 years before considering it to be of sufficient durability to publish the results and a full 12 years before the publication of the long-term cumulative results with Skinner. Indeed, the most salient lesson of this classic report was the remarkable restraint exhibited by Belsey in deferring publication until more than 2 decades had passed and more than 1,000 patients had been treated. Pearson, in a recent presidential address to the American Association of Thoracic Surgery, quoted Belsey as saying "*The battlefields of surgery are strewn with the remains of promising new operations which perished in the follow-up clinic.*" The lessons of the publication remain as valid now as they were almost 50 years ago when gastroesophageal reflux was firmly established as a correctible affliction if the appropriate patient was selected and an experienced surgeon identified. Of particular interest is the recognition that these results were obtained based on astute observations made decades before the availability of cineradiography, manometry, pH studies, and flexible endoscopy.

Surgery redivivus— laparoscopy

The introduction of laparoscopic antireflux surgery in 1991 by Geagea, a Lebanese surgeon practicing in Canada, and Dallemagne in Belgium had a profound impact on the management strategy for patients with GERD. In much the same fashion as had followed the introduction of laparoscopic cholecystectomy, the novel procedure was widely embraced by surgeons anxious to use technical skills to resolve the vexatious problem of GERD. As a result of the perceived advantages of the procedure, surgeons began to undertake laparoscopic fundoplication, often without adequate training and unaware of the appropriate indications. Although the advantages of minimally invasive surgery were evident, initial enthusiasm resulted in failure to initiate prospective randomized trials to critically evaluate the relative merits of the open procedure or long-term PPI usage. Nevertheless, early results seemed to confirm all the advantages of the minimally invasive approach (once the learning curve had been negotiated), with early outcomes not significantly different from those reported for the open procedure.

In general, the laparoscopic approach follows the same principles as the open Nissen fundoplication. A particular advantage is the excellent visibility of the gastroesophageal junction at operation and the relatively atraumatic nature of the procedure as compared to a major upper abdominal incision. A short (1 to 2 cm) wrap is advocated to avoid postoperative dysphagia. Other modifications that have been proposed include either division of the short gastric vessels to establish a tension-free fundoplication using a mobile posterior portion of the fundus or, alternatively, nondivision with the use of a more anterior portion of the fundus.

Pediatric issues

Gastroesophageal reflux and peptic esophagitis were referred to in the medical literature as early as the eighteenth century by J. P. Frank, and the first case of esophagitis in a child was published in Paris in 1829 by Billard. By 1931, the British otolaryngologists Findlay and Kelly had described nine children with partial intrathoracic stomach, shortening of the esophagus, and stenosis just above the cardia in a paper entitled *Congenital Shortening of the Esophagus and the Thoracic Stomach Resulting Therefrom.* But the role of gastroesophageal reflux was overlooked and cause and effect inverted, as may be judged by review of the title. Subsequently, between 1941 and 1943, Allison demonstrated that this type of esophageal stricture was not a congenital abnormality but was secondary to esophagitis induced by reflux of gastric contents. In 1947 and 1950, Neuhauser and Berenberg in Boston described esophageal chalasia or cardioesophageal relaxation as a cause of vomiting in infants. Shortly after that, Duhamel, Sauvegrain, and Masse, in Paris, tried to synthesize all that was then known and for the first time considered hiatus hernia, esophageal relaxation or chalasia, gastroesophageal reflux, peptic esophagitis, short esophagus, and peptic esophageal stricture as different forms and grades

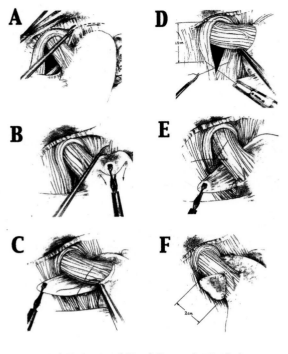

Surgical Treatment of Hiatal Hernias by Fundoplication and Gastropexy (Nissen Repair)

S. KRUPP, M.D., M. ROSSETTI, M.D.

From the Department of Surgery, University of Basel, Basel, Switzerland

Ann. Surg. 1966; 164:297-304.

Innumerable modifications of the original gastric fundoplication procedure proposed by Nissen have emerged. Whether the variety of permutations and commutations of the techniques proposed represent advances or attest to the fact that no procedure of this kind is adequate remains a source of considerable disagreement among both surgeons and gastroenterologists. The Rosetti modification depicted (**A–F**) achieved widespread popularity among pediatric surgeons. Whether young infants or children warrant surgery as opposed to acid-suppressive medication remains a subject of controversy.

of the same affliction. As early as 1962, in the United States, Ravitch expressed a similar opinion in regard to the plurality of the disease process.

At approximately the same time, a general feeling emerged that the entity of hiatus hernia represented a gradation of a single disease process, and that minor forms could develop into major forms or in infants even disappear by the age of 1 to 2 years, as reported by Carré. Those physicians who were involved in pediatric care were of the opinion that all forms of hiatus hernia could lead to peptic esophagitis and even considered that this was more frequent with the minor forms than the major hernias. The fact that, without treatment, 20% of patients with hiatus hernia culminated in peptic stenosis was in the pediatric population a major incentive to propose surgical intervention. Thus, by the early 1950s, it was well accepted that the malformation of the lower esophagus and cardia, which we called hiatus hernia, led to gastroesophageal reflux and, in 20% of cases, to esophageal stenosis. Thus, pediatric surgeons were satisfied with the description of the pathologic entity and with its role in the pathogenesis of gastroesophageal reflux, peptic esophagitis, and peptic stenosis of the esophagus. Furthermore, it seemed that surgical correction of this malformation had a sound scientific rationale.

In the early 1960s, the American literature contained relatively few papers on hiatus hernia in children and in both the first edition (1962) and the second edition (1969) of *Pediatric Surgery*, the chapter on hiatus hernia was written by an Englishman, David Waterston. In contrast, the European pediatric literature commented in detail on what was considered to be a well-recognized disorder of children. Nevertheless, most North American pediatricians and surgeons claimed the condition to be rare and a European phenomenon. They opined that few such children were seen in America, stating, *"we never see such cases in America, probably because we feed our infants differently and allow them to lay on their bellies."*

In the late 1960s, however, a change became apparent in the United States as Judson Randolph initiated an era of operative intervention for pediatric hiatus hernia. Oddly, Randolph worked in Washington, D.C., only a few miles away from the great medical centers in Baltimore and Philadelphia, where hiatus hernia had been previously claimed to be nonexistent! By the 1970s, papers on gastroesophageal reflux and hiatus hernia began to appear all over the United States, and in 1979, Randolph, in the third edition of Benson's *Pediatric Surgery*, and, in 1980, Holder and Ashcraft in their own textbook on *Pediatric Surgery*, affirmed the validity of reflux-preventive operations in the New World. Thus, fundoplication, according to Nissen's and Belsey's Mark IV operation, became widely accepted as the best method of treatment in the pediatric age group. This state of mind persisted until the late 1980s, when the recognition that adequate acid suppression initially by the histamine receptor–antagonist class of drugs was as, if not more, effective as surgery. The subsequent introduction of the PPI class of drugs, particularly in a suspension that could be easily ingested by young children, allowed therapy to move toward a pharmacologic strategy in the majority of patients.

Current status

Peptic ulcer of the esophagus was first reported by Albert in 1839 and its histology described in 1879 by Quinke. However, by 1906, Tileston could report a mere 44 patients. The disease was regarded as so rare and obscure that in 1926, von Hacker and Lothiesieu could only collect 91 cases, although few were verified by autopsy. In 1929, Friedenwald and his colleagues reported 13 cases, and their experimental results in animals documented that esophageal ulcer healed rapidly if hydrochloric acid was withheld from the lesion. Stewart noted one esophageal ulcer in 10,000 autopsies in 1929, and in the same year, Sir Arthur F. Hurst, the doyen of British gastroenterology, could only document 11 patients. In Philadelphia, Chevalier Jackson, in 1929, in reviewing 4,000 consecutive esophagoscopies, identified 88 cases (21 active and 67 healed). The alteration in incidence and recognition of this disease process in the remainder of the century was remarkable and is worthy of consideration.

In recent years, there has been an increased awareness among both patients and physicians of the increasing prevalence of GERD. It has been estimated that as much as 20% of the population of the United States experiences symptoms associated with the disease. Of interest is the observation that the incidence of diagnosis appears to be increasing in a linear fashion in countries that are generally regarded as of the first world, whereas in less developed areas, the disease is still relatively rare. Indeed, in the early part of the twentieth century, the disease was virtually unknown, and as late as 1930, the literature contained information on fewer than 100 patients. Current information suggests that the disease has reached almost epidemic proportions in some areas and has raised the specter of a similar increase in the identification of Barrett's esophagus. This increase in diagnosis and awareness has been associated with recent changes in the availability of effective pharmacologic and surgical treatments for the condition and an increasing knowledge of some of the basic mechanisms underlying gastroesophageal reflux.

The prevalence of GERD varies considerably from country to country and reflects not only the level to which subjective symptomatology is investigated but also the psyche of the population and its physicians. Overall, it may range from less than 1% in Senegal to almost 23% in the United Kingdom. Gastroesophageal reflux is now the most common upper gastrointestinal disorder in the Western world. Thus, 7% to 10% of the adult population may report daily heartburn, whereas up to 30% to 40% of patients complain of symptoms compatible with the disease on a monthly basis. The spectrum of complaints ranges from only occasional heartburn to a far more severe course. This may include increasing degrees of esophageal injury with associated progressive sphincter

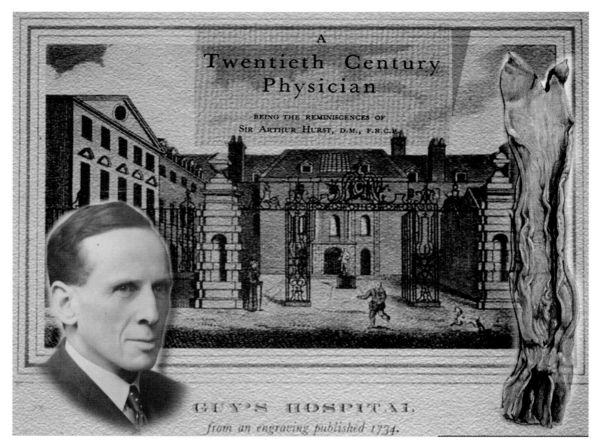

A

Twentieth Century
Physician

BEING THE REMINISCENCES OF
SIR ARTHUR HURST, D.M., F.R.C.P.

GUY'S HOSPITAL.
from an engraving published 1734.

Sir Arthur Hurst (1879–1944) (bottom left) was born in Bradford, England. The great physicist Henrich Rudolf Hertz was his father's cousin. In 1908, Hurst (the name change reflected British sensitivities to Germanic origins) published a detailed account of the movement of the stomach, intestine, and colon, having been influenced by the pioneer X-ray studies of W. B. Cannon. After being appointed to the staff of Guy's Hospital at the age of 27 years, he established himself as a general physician with a special interest in gastroenterology. Hurst was particularly interested in ulcer disease, achalasia, and constipation and wrote definitively on these and diverse gastrointestinal subjects. In 1936, Hurst established the Gastroenterologic Club (subsequently the British Society of Gastroenterology) and at its first meeting, in 1937, was elected president.

dysfunction, culminating in the development of Barrett's metaplasia and even adenocarcinoma. This disease currently represents one of the fastest growing categories of cancer in the United States, with a threefold increase during the period from 1983 to 1987, as compared to the rates from 1973 to 1977. Although up to 40% of adults complain of heartburn, only 2% of this group show erosive esophagitis to an extent that warrants pharmacologic therapeutic intervention. Complications have been variously reported to develop in up to 21.6% of such patients. These may include either ulcer (2% to 7%), hemorrhage (less than 2%), stricture (4% to 20%), or Barrett's esophagus (10% to 15%). Symptomatic GERD is a chronic disease requiring long-term management in most patients. Although the treatment initially exhibited a bias toward surgical management, it has become pharmacologically orientated during the past 2 decades. The introduction of two classes of gastric acid–inhibitory agents—the H_2 receptor antagonists and PPIs—resulted in a massive amplification of the usefulness of medical therapy. Two pivotal issues have required consideration in management. The first is the recognition that relapse continues to be a significant event in the pharmacologic management of such patients. More than 80% of the patients relapse within 6 months after the cessation of therapy. Long-term drug therapy is usually necessary. The second is the recent availability of minimally invasive surgery and the suggestion that the nature and consequences of surgical intervention now require reevaluation. The enthusiasm for laparoscopically undertaken antireflux procedures has mounted exponentially

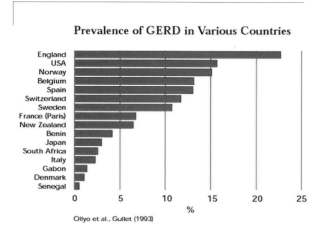

Prevalence of GERD in Various Countries

Ollyo et al., Gullet (1993)

The increased prevalence of GERD appears to be reflected in the economic and social developments of countries. The basis for this incidence is unclear.

since the initial experience reported by Dallemagne in 1991. It is a widely held belief among surgeons that a laparoscopic procedure combines the potential of excellent long-term results with low morbidity/mortality and significant cost-effective advantages. Whether such claims can be substantiated in the long-term remains to be resolved.

The recognition in the first part of the twentieth century that mucosal damage was caused by acid ("no acid—no ulcer"), and that this acid could be decreased by luminal neutralization, resulted in application of antacid preparations, bland diets, and milk infusion as therapeutic options. The subsequent categorizing of the H_2 receptor antagonists and the development of agents specifically capable of blocking this receptor revolutionized the management of acid related diseases and virtually abrogated surgery as a therapeutic option for peptic ulcer except in cases of emergency. However, the relatively large relapse rates for GERD even on high-dose H_2 receptor antagonist therapy still engendered considerable enthusiasm for surgical intervention in the management of reflux disease. The more recent identification of the specific molecular mechanism of acid secretion—the proton pump (H,K ATPase)—resulted in the development of a new class of therapeutic agents, the PPI class of drugs. These are significantly more effective in the treatment of GERD, given their improved efficacy as acid-secretory inhibitors. Generalized concepts of loss of sphincter tone, inability to clear the lower esophagus of refluxed acid peptic material, and the insidious effects of a variety of ill-defined noxious agents are all tenable etiologic factors in these diseases. Nevertheless, the principle of decreasing gastric acid secretion and increasing the pH in the lower esophagus has been clearly demonstrated to be therapeutically effective. Arguments regarding which compound, which dosage, and which schedule of administration should be used appear to be reasonably specious at this time, based on the obvious recognition that the longer the period for which the pH is elevated, the greater the degree of symptom relief and healing. Similarly, the higher the level of pH achieved, the better the results. This observation reflects the well-defined enzyme kinetics and pH optima for pepsin,

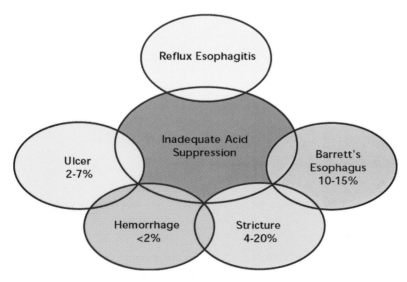

Complications of GERD

Reflux Esophagitis

Inadequate Acid Suppression

Ulcer 2-7%

Barrett's Esophagus 10-15%

Hemorrhage <2%

Stricture 4-20%

The concept of GERD progressing into a series of potential complications is linked to the uncontrolled reflux of acid and pepsin into the lower esophagus.

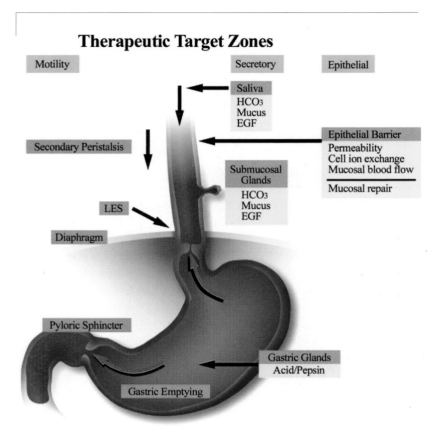

Therapeutic Target Zones

Motility

Secondary Peristalsis

LES

Diaphragm

Pyloric Sphincter

Gastric Emptying

Secretory

Saliva
HCO3
Mucus
EGF

Submucosal Glands
HCO3
Mucus
EGF

Gastric Glands
Acid/Pepsin

Epithelial

Epithelial Barrier
Permeability
Cell ion exchange
Mucosal blood flow

Mucosal repair

The possible sites of therapeutic intervention in GERD are related to the areas of pathophysiology involved in the genesis of the disease process. The most likely candidate target is the modulation of transient LES relaxation.

which probably plays a major catalytic role in the genesis of mucosal damage and, in addition, obviates optimal healing.

Using such criteria, the PPI class of drugs today are clearly the primary therapeutic agents. A secondary pharmacologic option that may well be of considerable clinical relevance once appropriate agents are developed is the use of motility-directed or prokinetic substances to facilitate clearance of acid-peptic material from the lower esophagus. Similarly, the introduction of agents to increase the LES tone, thus further inhibiting the ability of gastric contents to regularly enter the lower esophageal area, would confer an obvious advantage. The current failure to identify a specific agent capable of targeting the LES has, to date, hindered the widespread clinical use of this type of strategy.

Unfortunately, although drugs can be delivered via existing anatomic routes, the surgical option required a significant degree of trauma to obtain its quotient. For this reason, the introduction of laparoscopic surgery has engendered extraordinary enthusiasm based on the swelling chorus of acclamation relating to its minimally invasive nature. A further significant consideration is that surgery in a definable fashion increases (albeit unpredictably) LES pressure, thus ameliorating reflux. Such surgery appears to have advantages as regards reduced hospital stay and faster return to activity, thus supporting a notion that it is cost-effective. Additionally, both surgeons and patients purport to express a high degree of satisfaction with this procedure.

Etiology

The esophagus, stomach, and duodenum should be a one-way system for the transit of food into the rest of the gastrointestinal tract. The stomach functions both as a reservoir and as a pump. Gastric peristalsis results in an increase in pressure whereby the valve constituted by the pylorus opens at a lower pressure than the LES. The gastric pacemaker initiates pressure waves directed toward the pyloric valve, further ensuring that food mixed with acid and pepsin exits from the gastric pump/reservoir in an aboral fashion. The reflux of gastric contents into the esophagus is an abnormal situation and generally has been accepted as reflective of failure of the esophageal component of the system. It is, however, worthy of consideration that the failure of the pylorus to relax appropriately or the gastric peristaltic wave to be coordinated with the function of both sphincters may also play a part in the genesis of the reflux scenario. Under such circumstances, the LES, which normally opens intermittently to permit food to enter the stomach, exhibits an inability to remain closed as gastric pressure increases to force food toward the pylorus, through it, and into the duodenum. In mechanical terms, therefore, reflux simply represents leakage of the proximal (LES) valve system of a one-way cycling pump (the stomach). As a result of failure of either motility coordination or valve competency, or both, noxious agents are delivered into the lower esophagus for varying lengths of time.

The ability of the esophagus to withstand the presence of barrier-breaking agents, such as acid, pepsin, and occasionally bile, is generally maintained by the stratified squamous epithelial barrier. In addition, protection is afforded by the secretion of glands in the lower third, as well as the presence of esophageal "stripping" waves, whereby refluxate is readily and efficiently cleared from the esophagus back into the stomach. Under circumstances in which a number of different factors may function suboptimally (decreased pressure of the LES, decreased clearance of lower esophageal contents, decrease in the barrier function), inflammatory sequelae are initiated in the lower esophagus. Because the stratified squamous epithelium of the lower esophagus does not have either the tight junctions or the apical barrier properties of the gastric mucosa, damage to it results in inflammation that may be difficult to heal. Indeed, metaanalysis data indicate that the pH of the lower esophagus needs to be significantly greater than that in the duodenum to ensure healing.

Repeated episodes of inflammation with incomplete healing presumably reflect an ongoing pathologic process that culminates in both the loss of esophageal glands and the development of scar tissue. A further progression of the ongoing healing/damage cycle is the alteration in the phenotype of the mucosa toward a columnar epithelium predominance and, ultimately, intestinal metaplasia. Presumably, the interface between the squamous epithelium of the esophagus and the columnar of the stomach represents a junctional zone with a degree of instability and even susceptibility to damage. Once injury has failed to heal or been initiated on a number of occasions, the area presumably becomes more vulnerable, and esophagitis remains in place, with constant susceptibility to further reflux and damage. Under such circumstances, the chronic nature and relapsing course of GERD are understandable.

The clinical problem is best characterized by the loss of an efficient reflux barrier, which results in a retrograde passage of gastric contents in the esophagus. Although the mean basal pressure of the LES is significantly lower in patients with GERD, especially in those with severe esophagitis, there is signif-

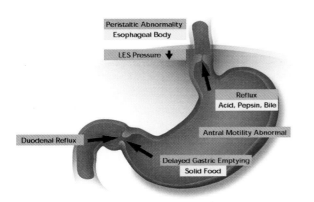

Reflux Etiology

Peristaltic Abnormality
Esophageal Body

LES Pressure ↓

Reflux
Acid, Pepsin, Bile

Duodenal Reflux

Antral Motility Abnormal

Delayed Gastric Emptying
Solid Food

Current concepts in the etiology of GERD. Irrespective of the wide variety of abnormalities that have been proposed as the genesis of GERD, the common denominators are dysfunction of the LES and damage of the esophageal mucosa. It is likely that the fundamental abnormality may lie within the pacemaker system of the stomach. Thus, aberrant electrophysiologic function results in gastric contraction and incoordinated closure of the pyloric valve and opening of the LES.

icant overlap between normal and GERD patients. Whether this is a *post hoc* phenomenon or reflects the primary etiology of the disease has not been adequately established. Nevertheless, it seems apparent that transient LES relaxation not associated with swallowing may be responsible for GERD in some patients with mild to moderate disease. The spectrum of alterations in LES pressure, however, is wide. Thus, in some circumstances, basal LES pressure may be normal but the number of transient inappropriate LES relaxations abnormally high. Alternatively, in some individuals, a persistent but as-yet uncharacterized defect of LES control is associated with permanent low resting-sphincter pressure and almost constant reflux. It is unknown at present what regulates the transient spontaneous relaxation of the LES, but it is apparent that in up to 80% of GERD patients, reflux episodes are associated with transient LES relaxation. The modulation of LES function has been determined to include at least vagal pathways, hormones such as gastrin and cholecystokinin, nitric oxide, and a number of other regulators, including VIP, ACh, and serotonin.

Botulinum toxin has been demonstrated to result in profound LES relaxation and proposed to be of some putative efficacy in the management of achalasia. Although its current application by endoscopic injection is somewhat impractical, it may provide a viable avenue for further exploration of the function of the smooth muscle system at the gastroesophageal junction. Presumably, the delineation of the function of the gastric pacemaker and its efferent regulatory mechanism will be needed to further define the regulation of the pumping action of the stomach and its associated valves.

Once reflux has occurred, the degree of mucosal damage reflects a number of variables: first, the ability of the esophagus to clear the reflux material; second, the precise nature of the refluxate; and last, the degree of mucosal resistance. It is clearly apparent that there exists a direct correlation between the exposure of the esophagus to acid and the severity of GERD. Thus, individuals with severe disease suffer from longer reflux periods and demonstrate more frequent reflux episodes. Moreover, their esophageal pH remains below 4.0 for significantly longer periods than in those patients with milder forms of the disease.

The stomach itself is an important variable in determining GERD. Indeed, it has even been proposed that the entire disease process may be a consequence of disordered gastric motility. Abnormalities in antral motor motility either due to disordered pacemaker cycling or in-coordinate peristalsis may result in gastric contents being inappropriately moved in a retrograde fashion towards the oral valve (LES). Under such circumstances, alterations in the rate of gastric emptying, duodenogastric reflux, and the volume of gastric contents as determined by the degree of gastric accommodation and distention may be critical variables in the establishment and maintenance of GERD. In many individuals, delayed gastric emptying is demonstrable, and, in fact, the gastric emptying rate can be related to the degree of esophageal damage.

Of further importance is the fact that patients with GERD who are resistant to medical therapy have been demonstrated to display delayed gastric emptying of solids more often than those who respond well to treatment. Thus, it becomes more apparent that the mechanical issues relating to reflux may be the primary determinant of the disease process, whereas the inflammatory responses simply reflect the sequelae of the refluxate itself. Under such circumstances, treatment directed toward the diminution of damage to the lower esophagus should be recognized as addressing the aftermath of the problem rather than dealing with the problem itself. In this respect, the motor function of the corpus fundus region of the stomach is little understood. This area, which is directly adjacent to the LES, is primarily responsible for the regulation of intragastric pressure whereby the physiologic function of accommodation is used to increase the gastric capacitance without a concomitant increase in pressure. Although a complex interrelationship between the smooth muscle fibers of the LES and the gastric wall of this region has been anatomically defined, little knowledge is available regarding the physiologic interface between the lower esophagus and the gastric fundus as a functional unit. A loss of regulatory interaction between the gastric fundus and the lower esophageal area, which involves alteration in the function of the LES, therefore, might easily be a critical component of the initiating pathogenesis of this disease process. It has been demonstrated that in patients with GERD, fundic distention results in an LES pressure response when compared to healthy controls. Under such circumstances, it might be predicted that delayed gastric emptying of either liquids or solids would facilitate gastroesophageal reflux.

In summary, esophagitis should be regarded as a mucosal inflammatory disease secondary to mechanical events that infringe on the function of the LES. The high relapse and recurrence rate of GERD may be predicted based on the fact that the majority of current therapy is directed at dealing with the consequences of the pathology (inflammation) and its healing rather than the primary etiology, which is an as-yet inadequately characterized mechanical or electrical phenomenon, probably of gastric origin. Under such circumstances, it may be predicted that once a certain degree of damage has been inflicted on the lower esophageal mucosa, acid-suppressive therapy is only able to ameliorate symptomatology and maintain or stabilize the damage and scar already present. In this respect, medical therapy, although successful in facilitating healing, can do little more than maintain a steady state while the motor abnormalities of the stomach, pyloric valve, and LES persist.

CHAPTER 2
BIOLOGY

**The esophageal
epithelium**

The junctions between the squamous epithelial cells lining the esophagus are quite different from the junctions between epithelial cells in other regions of the gastrointestinal tract, where tight junctions link the luminal ends of columnar epithelial cells by a functional "belt" comprising specialized membrane and intracellular proteins such as occludin and Zoo-1. Such tight junctions can be classified based on the number of strands into "tight" and "leaky" tight junctions. The gastric epithelium has "tight" tight junctions with as many as 15 adhesive strands of protein. At best, the tight junctions visualized in the first layer of the esophageal epithelium contain two or so strands and must be extremely leaky. In the stratified squamous epithelium of the esophagus, adjacent epithelial cells are joined more loosely by desmosomes (gap junctions) connected by intracellular intermediate filaments. The barrier function of the cells lining the esophagus is therefore normally dependent not on tight junctions but on the multiplicity of cell layers comprising the stratified epi-

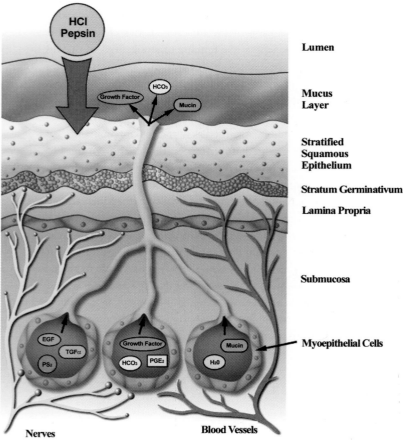

The Esophageal Gland System

HCl Pepsin

Growth Factor

HCO₃

Mucin

EGF

TGFα

PS₂

Growth Factor

HCO₃

PGE₂

Mucin

H₂O

Lumen

Mucus Layer

Stratified Squamous Epithelium

Stratum Germinativum

Lamina Propria

Submucosa

Myoepithelial Cells

Nerves

Blood Vessels

The lower end of the esophagus has a limited supply of glands. These are of importance as a component of the defense mechanism to reflux and may be of relevance in healing. Although the relative contributions of the various defense mechanisms to reflux are not certain, it is evident that a complex system is in place to protect the lower esophagus from damage. Probably of more relevance are the biologic mechanisms whereby healing occurs. There is, however, little information available on the mechanistic regulation of this process.

thelium and the intercellular spaces between these cell layers. The esophagus may be considered as analogous to "wet skin" and in this respect even behave in a similar fashion when damaged.

In GERD, the spaces between squamous epithelial cells enlarge, thereby perhaps allowing luminal contents more access to the submucosa. Whether enlargement of the intercellular space is the primary event or secondary to cell shrinkage is not entirely clear and remains to be determined.

Esophageal anatomy and physiology

The esophagus is normally a collapsed empty tube. During swallowing, transient phrenic ampulla form as a consequence of physiologic herniation associated with longitudinal muscle contraction during peristalsis. The process of esophageal emptying slows significantly with formation of the phrenic ampulla from the approximately 3-cm-per-second characteristic of peristalsis to approximately 1 cm per second. The ampulla appears to form as a result of longitudinal shortening of the esophagus, thus forming a closed chamber bound above by the distal esophagus and below by crural diaphragm. Because the LES moves approximately 2 cm with each swallow, an important part of its anatomic stabilization is the elastic recoil provided by the phrenoesophageal ligament. Emptying of the ampulla occurs in conjunction with relengthening of the esophagus. These mechanistic descriptions have anatomic implications.

There appears to be a sequential activation of esophageal longitudinal muscle with progression of the peristaltic contraction. It is possible that each longitudinal section is subsequently reelongated by contraction of the adjacent distal segment. The distal end of the esophagus is anchored to the diaphragm by the phrenoesophageal (PE) membrane, formed by the fused endothoracic and endoabdominal fascia. The PE membrane has elastic properties and inserts circumferentially into the esophageal musculature close to the squamocolumnar junction, normally residing within the esophageal hiatus. Thus, the PE ligament is stretched with each swallow, and its elastic recoil is responsible for pulling the squamocolumnar junction back to its normal position after shortening. This repetitive stress subjects the PE ligament to substantial wear and tear, making it a plausible target of age-related degeneration.

Gastroesophageal junction

The gastroesophageal junction is a complex sphincter composed of both a diaphragmatic element and the smooth muscle LES. This anatomically and physiologically complex organ is vulnerable to dysfunction by several mechanisms. Mechanically, the gastroesophageal junction must protect against reflux in both static and dynamic conditions. Failure to adequately prevent reflux is associated with both the initiation of GERD and relapse and chronicity of the disease.

A prerequisite for the development of GERD is movement of acid and pepsin from the stomach into the esophagus. Under normal circumstances, gastroesophageal reflux is prevented by a competent gastroesophageal junction.

This antireflux barrier is an anatomically complex zone whose func-

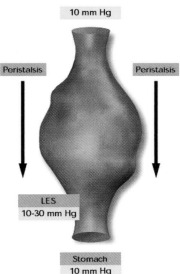

Gastroesophageal Junction Pressure Zone

10 mm Hg

Peristalsis

Peristalsis

LES
10-30 mm Hg

Stomach
10 mm Hg

The lower 5 to 7 cm of the esophagus function as a dynamic peristaltic mechanism or ampulla serving both to empty swallowed material into the stomach and to dispose of gastric refluxate. The mm Hg values indicate that, in general, the LES pressure is higher than that in the gastric fundus and, hence, reflux only occurs during transient LES relaxation or if there is sphincter dysfunction. It is possible that incoordinate gastric pacemaker function may result in inappropriate pyloric valve closure with the result that the gastric peristaltic pressure exceeds LES pressure and reflux occurs, but no proof of this hypothesis exists.

tional integrity has been variably attributed to intrinsic LES pressure, extrinsic compression of the LES by the crural diaphragm, intraabdominal location of the LES, integrity of the PE ligament, and maintenance of the angle of entry of esophagus into the stomach (His).

It is most probable that competence of this barrier is attributable to more than one of these factors, and incompetence becomes increasingly severe as more mechanisms are compromised.

However, evidence for functional integrity is most compelling in the cases of the LES and the crural diaphragm.

The lower esophageal sphincter

Over the last 3 decades, considerable attention has focused on those factors that are normally responsible for maintaining the LES contraction yet allowing for transient relaxation during a swallow. It is known from animal models that electrical stimulation of the LES leads to relaxation. Early research on the control of sphincter tone led to the cholinergic hypothesis, in which it was felt that the tone of the LES was controlled by cholinergic nerves. However, not all of the experimental evidence fits neatly. For example, in humans, vagotomy does not in general reduce this tone. Also, in the 1970s, gastrin was demonstrated to be a modulator, but because none of the classical neurotransmitters or peptide hormones then identified accounted for all LES tone, an inherent myogenic tone was also proposed as a component of the system.

Most recently, studies have shown that at least 50% of the neurons innervating the LES possess nitric oxide synthase, thus implicating nitric oxide as a possible mediator in relaxation of the LES. In an animal model, the LES can be induced to contract or relax when exposed to arachidonic acid and its metabolites. Because arachidonic acid is produced by the action of phospholipase A_2 and is a precursor of prostaglandins and leukotrienes, these proinflammatory substances may also be implicated in LES pathology.

The LES is a 3- to 4-cm–long segment of tonically contracted smooth muscle at the distal end of the esophagus. Resting tone varies between 10 and 30 mm Hg in normal individuals and is least in the postcibal period and greatest at night. Intraabdominal pressure, gastric distention, peptides, hormones, various foods, and many drugs affect this pressure. LES tonic contraction itself is a property of both the surrounding muscle and the extrinsic innervation. Anatomically, the proximal margin of the LES is effectively approximately 1.5 cm above the Z line, which is in close proximity to the PE ligament. In contrast, the distal margin is approximately 2 cm distal to the Z line, bounded inferiorly by the angle of His. The resultant is a segment whose distal portion herniates through the hiatus as a consequence of esophageal shortening, with the formation of the phrenic ampulla.

The crural diaphragm encircling the LES serves a sphincteric function. The diaphragm appears to augment the LES during transient periods of increased intraabdominal pressure (e.g., inspiration, coughing). Electrical and mechanical inhibition of the crural diaphragm has been demonstrated during transient LES relaxations. The concept of the intrinsic pressure zone augmented by an extrinsic system has enabled consideration of a dual mechanism known as the *two-sphincter hypothesis of gastroesophageal junction competence.*

CHAPTER 3
PHYSIOLOGY AND FUNCTIONAL STUDIES

Esophageal function testing

Motility

The detection of reflux and abnormal motility, as well as of disturbances in gastric emptying, is easily accomplished using fluoroscopy. Although fluoroscopy displays patterns of transit secondary to motor events with excellent resolution, manometry is usually required to define the underlying patterns that may be radiologically revealed. Imaging is useful in demonstrating obstruction and even reflux but is not particularly effective in identifying "underpowered" peristalsis, which is best delineated using manometric techniques. The identification of reflux events on fluoroscopy can be misleading in the short period of such an examination and require esophageal pH monitoring and even manometric studies to fully define and confirm the clinical relevance of such events.

Intraluminal pressures in the esophagus may be measured by either water-perfused manometric assemblies connected to external pressure transfusers or recording assemblies using intraluminal transfusers. The latter technique does not require water perfusion, which is an advantage but is expensive, fragile, and costly to repair. The perfused manometric assemblies are therefore most widely used, given their relatively low cost, easy maintenance, and reliable function. They consist of an extrusion with multiple fine channels, each of which opens sideways at the esophageal lumen at different levels, thus enabling recordings of pressure simultaneously at multiple levels. Using a low-compliance manometric pump, each hole and its associated channel transmits pressure to an external transducer, enabling a pressure profile of the sphincteric zone and the area of interest to be developed. Because the LES has a maximal pressure zone that is only a few millimeters, positioning is of critical importance, especially given the fact that the LES moves approximately 10 cm each time a swallow occurs. The pull-through technique was previously used to precisely identify the pressure zones but is uncomfortable for the patient and involves repeated manipulation of the manometric assembly. For the most part, swallow-induced esophageal peristalsis is used to define the site of the LES and measure its function. A perfused sleeve of 6 cm in length provides reliable monitoring of both basal and swallow-induced changes of sphincteric pressure, because this length is adequate to accommodate the predictable movement of the LES relative to the manometric assembly. Primary peristalsis can be evaluated using 5-mL water boluses and provides informa-

Normal Esophageal Peristalsis in Response to Water Swallows*

Esophageal peristalsis is a complex electromyometric series of descending sequenced contractions culminating in a terminal sphincter (LES) relaxation. The progression of the waves over time demonstrates the progression of the descending esophageal peristaltic wave following a swallow of water. The LES (red) relaxes intermittently to allow passage of the bolus into the stomach.

tion that enables the termination of appropriate esophageal clearing. A peak threshold pressure of 33 mm Hg per mL is reached in the distal esophagus for reliable fluid transport by primary peristalsis. Esophageal transport of solids depends in a large part on secondary peristalsis, because the primary peristaltic wave moves too rapidly to propel solids in the esophageal body, thus passing over them and moving them only a small part of the esophageal length. Secondary peristalsis is the event that follows the primary peristaltic wave and initiates a powerful, initially static contraction that occurs directly around the boluses. Abnormalities in primary and secondary peristalsis need to be defined in patients with GERD, particularly in those for whom a surgical remedy may be sought.

The best methodology for evaluating secondary peristalsis is to abruptly insufflate 10 mL of air into the midesophageal body via the wide-core lumen of a manometric extrusion system. The motor response of the esophagus to this distention can then be evaluated.

The measurement of LES relaxation is of particular importance, not only in the early diagnosis of achalasia and the assessment of dysphagia after antireflux surgery but also to determine the appropriateness of LES contraction and relaxation. Water swallow–induced LES relaxation has a duration of 4.1 (3.0 to 5.4 range) seconds, with a mean nadir pressure of relaxation of 1.0 (0.2 range) mm Hg. Some conditions, such as achalasia or diffuse esophageal spasm, can be easily defined, but in some instances, only a *nonspecific motor defect* is evident. This somewhat vague term embraces individuals with "underpowered" peristalsis and results in the failure of development of an adequate propulsive force to clear the esophagus.

The identification of a manometric abnormality is important in helping define the cause of GERD or the failure of acid-suppressive medication to provide adequate relief and healing. In addition, it provides information necessary to confirm the need for a prokinetic agent. Under circumstances in which defined motor abnormality is evident, the use of surgery should be carefully considered, because wrap procedures performed under such circumstances may not function adequately. In individuals who meet the criteria for elective surgery based on demonstration of abnormal LES function, manometric evaluation is useful as a quantitative tool to evaluate efficacy of the surgery or alternatively define causes for its failure.

Esophageal pH monitoring

Esophageal pH monitoring is an important adjunct to clinical assessment and endoscopy in the diagnosis of GERD. Methods of esophageal pH monitoring have advanced substantially in the last decade. Better and more versatile recording equipment has been developed and is now widely marketed. Computers and purpose-designed software have extended the scope of interpretation of the recordings and made this process more time dependent.

In contrast to endoscopy or the Bernstein test, ambulatory esophageal pH monitoring records spontaneous reflux events and measures directly the degree of esophageal acid exposure, fundamental factors in the pathogenesis of this disease. Not surprising, therefore, is the regard by many that this is the gold standard for the diagnosis of reflux disease. However, as in any medical test, it is not without limitations. There are both methodologic and inappropriate approaches to analysis and interpretations of the results.

Equipment

The major components are the pH electrode, data recorder, and software. There are three main types of pH electrodes: glass, monocrystalline antimony, and ion-selective field effect transistor (ISFET) electrodes. The first two are the most widely used. Glass electrodes are distinguished by having a linear response over a pH range from 1.0 to 12.0 and are relatively drift free, particularly when used with an internal reference in the form of a combination electrode. They are also the most durable of electrodes (can be chemically sterilized) and have a service life of approximately 100 studies. Their main disadvantages are their expense, fragility, and relative bulkiness. The result is that they are often difficult to pass and require extra care with handling. Indeed, nasal passage, particularly with combination electrodes, can often be difficult and uncomfortable. Antimony electrodes are cheaper than their glass counterparts, are smaller in size, and are more resistant to mechanical shock. The caveats are that they are less sensitive than glass electrodes and exhibit nonlinear responses even over the physiologic pH range from 1.0 to 7.0. In addition, they exhibit some drift and temperature sensitivity. They also have a limited lifespan because of corrosion and oxidation and are not chemically resistant, making them easily damaged by glutaraldehyde. Nevertheless, studies directly comparing glass and antimony electrodes demonstrate both the accuracy of the latter and similar results in clinical studies. A reference electrode is a prerequisite for accurate results. Both intraluminal and external (skin) references are used, the former providing the more accurate recordings (skin-enteric potential differences introduce errors up to 0.6 pH units). The pH signal is digitized and stored in a portable data storage device or data recorder, which may have up to four channels. For clinical purposes, a single channel (recording pH in the distal esophagus) is usually sufficient. Most data recorders sample the pH signal at eight samples per minute (0.13 Hz), which provides sufficient information for the calculation of mean or median values. However, accurate determination of individual pH fluctuations or reflux episodes requires a sample rate of at least 1 Hz (one sample per minute). Software should be able to display both a numeric summary and a time course of esophageal pH onto which can be added indicators for specific periods (e.g., supine, postprandial, and symptom events). Most programs can calculate reflux indices, circadian plots, and frequency curves.

Technique

It is not unusual for pH monitoring to be performed without the patient taking any antireflux therapy.

Before the study, H_2 receptor antagonists and prokinetics should be stopped for 24 to 72 hours. pH monitoring, however, is flexible enough to assess the efficacy of antireflux treatment on esophageal physiology. Before beginning a study, the electrode should be calibrated in a neutral and acid buffer (pH less than 2.0) and again at the end to check for electrode drift. Glass electrodes

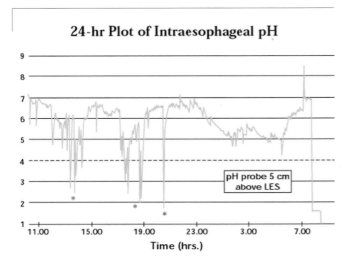

24-hr Plot of Intraesophageal pH

pH probe 5 cm above LES

Time (hrs.)

There is a clear relationship between esophageal mucosal damage, the hydrogen ion concentration, and the acid dwell time in the esophagus. Episodic reflux events are documented by a sudden drop in esophageal pH (*).

should not exceed 0.2 pH units in drift. Antimony electrodes require special buffers, because they can be irreversibly damaged by many of the standard buffers. For standard pH monitoring, the electrode is positioned 5 cm above the proximal margin of the LES. Variation from this position can significantly influence the recorded value for esophageal acid exposure; the closer to the LES, the greater the level of acid exposure. Location of the electrode relative to the LES is best done by reference to manometric definition of LES position. Less adequate alternatives include using both the step up in pH that occurs as the electrode is withdrawn from the stomach and endoscopic measurements. Patients are encouraged to continue normal physical activity as much as possible, with the exclusion of acidic foods and drinks and antacids. Maintenance of an accurate diary is essential, with the recording of minimum information (meals, snacks, sleep). Traditionally, ambulatory pH monitoring is performed over a 24-hour period.

Analysis

There are two major considerations in the analysis of pH recordings: measurement of the amount of reflux and the relationship between the patient's symptoms and reflux. Interestingly, these two issues are not necessarily related and rather appear often to be complementary aspects of the analysis and interpretation of pH recordings. Traditionally, reflux is thought to occur when esophageal pH falls below 4.0. This threshold is clinically relevant, because heartburn occurs at a pH of less than 4.0, and peptic activity diminishes rapidly above this level. Interestingly, it is common for buffering of gastric contents early in the postprandial period to lead to reflux of gastric contents with a pH of above 4.0. In addition, falls in pH that do not reach a pH of 4.0 can also be symptomatic, and in some circumstances (e.g., gastric resection), it may be appropriate to set the threshold above pH 4.0 or 5.0. The end of the reflux period is defined as the point at which esophageal pH rises above 4.0 (or 5.0); it is recommended that a minimum time (18 seconds) should elapse before a new reflux period is scored. Reflux events occurring at a pH of less than 4.0 are not currently identifiable but do not have an adverse impact on the clinical importance of pH monitoring. Shifts in esophageal pH to greater than 7.0 (alkaline pH events) have been interpreted as reflux of alkaline duodenal contents. However, more recent analysis has suggested that these may be as a result of swallowed saliva. Inclusion of such events in the final analysis is, therefore, potentially inappropriate. The duration of pH below 4.0, usually expressed as a percentage of the recording time, is the variable most often used in the analysis of esophageal pH recordings. It is a measure of the degree of esophageal exposure to acid and correlates with the severity of esophagitis. The overall 24-hour esophageal acid exposure, however, appears to be the best single determinant to discriminate between normal subjects and patients with esophagitis.

The upper level for normal for total duration of esophageal acid exposure ranges between 5% and 7%. Reasonable intrasubject reproducibility (75% to 86%) has been recorded in patients with esophagitis. However, actual values may differ by as much as threefold. Unfortunately, reproducibility is lowest in endoscopy-negative patients or those with atypical symptoms, as well as in studies shorter than 24 hours. Although much emphasis has been placed on the measurement of esophageal acid exposure to classify patients as either normal or having reflux disease, this approach has its limitations. Levels of exposure to acid do not indicate whether the symptoms are related to reflux. This suggests the necessity, therefore, of a symptom analysis. Minor increases in the level of exposure above normal should be interpreted with caution. Assessment of the relationship between reflux and the patient's symptoms has proven to be a significantly greater challenge than quantification of acid exposure. The problem lies in the potential independent relationship of these two variables. Despite the many attempts to express the relationship objectively (symptom specificity index, symptom sensitivity index, symptom associated probability, and binomial symptom index), an ideal approach has yet to be devised.

Applications

Esophageal pH monitoring is not essential in all patients with suspected GERD. Endoscopy is the investigation of first choice, because it is the most sensitive means of diagnosing reflux esophagitis and assessing its severity, which then is the major factor influencing initial therapy. Esophageal pH monitoring is most applicable in those patients with troublesome symptoms but without endoscopic signs of esophagitis in whom a trial therapy has failed, in patients with atypical symptoms that cannot be clearly related to reflux, and in patients considered for antireflux surgery. It is also useful in assessing the adequacy of acid suppression in patients who fail to respond to what would appear to be adequate levels of acid-suppressant therapy. In summation,

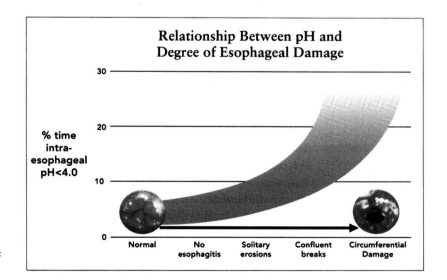

The longer the period the esophagus is exposed to a pH less than 4.0, the greater both the likelihood and extent of damage.

esophageal pH monitoring is an important adjunct to clinical assessment and endoscopy in the diagnosis of reflux disease. Although it is the gold standard for the measurement of esophageal exposure to acid and assessment of relationships of symptoms to reflux, the weaknesses in both these functions should be understood when applying this test for the diagnosis of reflux disease.

Pathophysiology

It is well recognized that, whereas the etiology of GERD is due to impaired function of the LES, the pathologic effects of this are mostly or entirely mediated by acid and pepsin reflux.

The esophageal epithelium appears more susceptible to acid damage than either the gastric or duodenal epithelium, and the explanation for this is found in the structural and secretory properties of the squamous lining of the esophagus adjacent to the stomach.

Malfunction of the LES results in acid reflux into the esophagus. Reflux is mostly episodic, so that the esophagus is not often presented with a continuous acid load.

Prediction of esophageal disease related to reflux takes into account the pH of the refluxate and the duration of reflux. Expulsion of the refluxate back into the stomach shortens the time of exposure. The volume of reflux is also an important parameter for estimation of the acid load on the esophageal epithelium. It is the magnitude of this acid load that determines the presence or absence of pathology or symptoms. Intraesophageal pH monitoring provides an approximate measure of the acid load to the lower esophagus.

The human esophageal epithelium is a multilayered, stratified squamous epithelium. Afferent nerves are present, reaching into the superficial layers of the mucosa. With incompetence of the LES, acid reflux results, with pain and damage to the epithelium depending on the pH of the refluxate.

Rather than being protected by a continuous tight junction, this epithelium has largely regional cell-to-cell contact via desmosomes, but, being multilayered, provides a winding path for proton diffusion into the epithelium. It is nevertheless significantly more acid sensitive than the gastric epithelium, which is provided with "tight" tight junctions.

The threshold of acidity for damage and pain may be different. A higher acidity is likely needed for damage to the epithelial cells, compared to the acidity required for stimulation of the pain fibers. This is probably because the epithelial cells have acid-recovery mechanisms (such as Na^+/H^+ or anion exchange), which are mostly absent in the pain fibers. It is also likely that the pain fibers have acid-sensing ion channels (ASICs). Here, protons displace Ca^{2+} from the channel, resulting in activation and pain fiber discharge. Depending on the location of the pain fibers and access thereto of H^+, different individuals will have different sensitivities to luminal acidity. The therapeutic aims of acid control may vary, being elevation of mean diurnal pH for healing of erosions or prevention of acidic excursions for symptom relief, or both. The acid load presented to the esophagus is likely to be the major determinant of heartburn or erosion. Reflux is mainly episodic, so that the esophagus is not often presented with a continuous acid load. Expulsion of the refluxate back into the stomach shortens the time of exposure.

The volume of reflux is also an important parameter for estimation of the acid load on the esophageal epithelium. Finally, the pH of the gastric contents that are refluxed into the esophagus also determines the possible damage. Intraesophageal pH monitoring provides an approximate measure of the acid load to the lower esophagus in terms of the pH of refluxate and dwell time of the acid solution and is probably the most useful semiquantitative measure of the degree of exposure of the esophageal epithelium.

The human esophageal proximal epithelium is a multilayered, stratified squamous epithelium. Afferent nerves are present reaching into the superficial layers of the epithelium. With incompetence of the lower esophageal sphincter (LES), acid reflux results with consequently the possibility of pain and damage to the epithelium depending on the pH of the refluxate. Rather than being protected by a continuous tight junction, this epithelium has largely regional cell-to-cell contact via desmosomes. There is some evidence for the presence of tight junctions in the first layer of the epithelium, but the very few strands seen on EM freeze fracture show that these at best are "leaky" tight junctions. This epithelium, being multilayered, provides a winding path for proton diffusion into the deeper layers of the epithelium. It is significantly more acid sensitive than the gastric epithelium that is provided with "tight" tight junctions.

The threshold of acidity for damage and pain may be different. A higher acidity is likely needed for damage to the epithelial cells compared to the acidity required for stimulation of the pain fibers. This is probably because the epithelial cells have acid recovery mechanisms (such as Na^+/H^+ or anion exchange) mostly absent in the pain fibers. Dependent on the location of the pain fibers and access thereto of H^+, individuals will have different sensitivities to luminal acidity. The therapeutic aims of acid control may vary, being elevation of mean diurnal pH for healing of erosions or prevention of acidic excursions for symptom relief or both.

Given the absence of continuous tight junctions or only leaky tight junctions, the lower esophageal epithelium is an inviting target for acid back diffusion. Mucus is an aqueous gel and is unlikely to provide a significant barrier to acid. In water, protons can move faster than other cations due to their ability to jump from water molecule to water molecule, and there are continuous chains of water in aqueous gels.

Resistance to acid may therefore depend more on the ability of the esophageal epithelium to neutralize an acid load than on restriction of entry of acid between the cells. Neutralization of acid occurs at the surface, due to net HCO_3^- secretion, and also in the paracellular pathway, since the epithelial cells can produce buffer or absorb H^+. However, once damage has occurred, this paracellular pathway is shorter or more open and the lesion consequently more sensitive to acid than the normal epithelium. The measured average net flux of bicarbonate is approximately 78 mmol/30 minutes/10 cm in the human esophagus. It appears to be subject to regulation by muscarinic receptors, responding to the vagal stimulation of acid secretion by the stomach. It is possible to approximate the pH of unbuffered refluxate that can be neutralized by esophageal surface secretion. If buffering is present, such as that due to amino acids or weak acids such as citrate, the acid load will be greater in the buffering range of gastric contents and reflect not only pH.

With reflux of unbuffered gastric contents at a pH of 4.0, there is a load of acid equivalent to 100 nmol/mL. If 10 ml of gastric contents at that pH is refluxed each minute for 30 minutes and spreads over a length of 10 cm, 30 mmol of acid is presented to this length of the esophagus in that 30-minute time span. This is within the average neutralizing ability of the secreted HCO_3^-. Reflux at pH 4.0 should therefore be largely neutralized at or close to the esophageal surface. This calculation may explain the results of a metaanalysis of the ideal pH elevation for the most rapid healing of esophageal lesions as discussed below.

At pH of 3.0, there is tenfold more acid, and 300 mmol of acid is presented to the lower esophagus with 10 mL refluxing each minute. This is beyond the capacity of net HCO_3^- secretion to neutralize the HCl. Acidification of intercellular spaces is likely, which may result in pain in some individuals. Epithelial cell pH may remain within viable limits given adequate Na^+/H^+ or Cl^-/HCO_3^- exchange.

At pH 2.0, the limits of the HCO_3^- response are greatly exceeded and the intercellular spaces will acidify even more and to a deeper level. At this stage, the ability of the epithelial cells to maintain constant intracellular pH may be overcome due to the higher acid load, with resultant erosion. As the more superficial cells are eroded, pepsin may also back diffuse, adding proteolytic insult to acid injury. These calculations, although fraught with assumptions, do predict that elevation to a mean diurnal pH of >4.0 will optimize healing of erosions of the lower esophagus. Gastric contents contain pepsin in addition to acid. Proteolytic activity of pepsin requires a pH <3.0, and there is probably adequate neutralization of intercellular pH if the refluxate does not fall much below 3.0. At a refluxate of pH 2.0, because the esophageal surface cannot neutralize this acid load, peptic activity may begin to contribute to esophageal damage. Peptic activity is less likely to contribute directly to pain.

The central hypothesis regarding the pathogenesis of esophagitis is dependent on the extent of esophageal injury, which itself is a reflection of the mucosal acidification time. Overall motility disorder as a basis for esophagitis can therefore be considered as due to either a markedly increased propensity to incur reflux events (LES abnormality) or a markedly impaired acid clearance (peristaltic dysfunction).

The dominant abnormality leading to the development of esophagitis and GERD can vary from patient to patient and may even evolve with time as scarring and damage progress.

At this time there are three theories that consider gastroesophageal junction incompetence or variations thereof as the critical issue in the genesis of GERD: (a) excessive transient LES relaxations (TLESRs), (b) a hypotensive LES without any accompanying anatomic abnormality, or (c) an anatomic disruption of the junction by hiatal hernia. It has been proposed that the dominant mechanism may vary as a function of disease severity or possibly even be a determinant. Thus, LES may predominate in mild disease, whereas mechanisms associated with a hiatal hernia or weak sphincter may be more prevalent in individuals with more severe disease.

It seems likely that TLESRs account for the majority of reflux events in normal individuals and in patients with normal LES pressure at the time of reflux. Transient lower esophageal relaxations probably represent a physiologic

Reflux in the Presence of a Hiatus Hernia

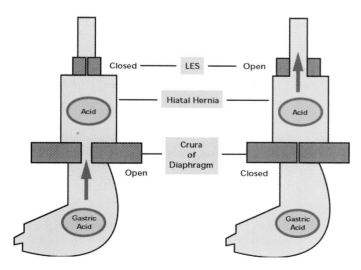

In the presence of a hiatus hernia, the diaphragmatic crura play a role in producing an "acid space" above the diaphragm and increasing the likelihood of reflux. Hiatus hernia was initially thought to be "the" cause of GERD. Subsequent revisionist consideration declared it to be nothing more than a correlatable epiphenomenon. More recent evidence has been advanced to support its role in the genesis of GERD.

response to gastric distention by food or gas and are the primary mechanisms responsible for gastric gas venting. Acid reflux (at the same time) would therefore appear to be an associated phenomenon. Investigations suggest that the functional LES consists of integrated motor responses involving not only LES relaxation but also crural diaphragmatic inhibition and contraction of the costal diaphragm. They appear to occur without an associated pharyngeal contraction, are unaccompanied by esophageal peristalsis, and persist for longer periods (longer than 10 seconds) than do swallow-induced LES relaxations. However, not all LESs are accompanied by reflux.

GERD may take place during episodes of diminished LES pressure associated with either stress reflux or free reflux. Stress reflux (which is an unusual mechanism of reflux) appears to occur when a hypotensive LES is transiently overcome by an abrupt increase in intraabdominal pressure and the LES is overcome. Observations of the antireflux mechanism during stress maneuvers, such as leg raising and abdominal compression, suggest a pinching effect of crural contraction (the second sphincter) that augments the antireflux barrier. Vulnerability to reflux under abrupt increases in intraabdominal pressure (e.g., bending, coughing) depends on both the susceptibility of the LES and the diaphragmatic sphincter to dramatic pressure change.

Patients with hiatal hernia exhibit progressive disruption of the diaphragmatic sphincter that is proportional to the extent of axial herniation. Although neither hiatal hernia nor hypotensive LES alone results in severe gastroesophageal junction incompetence, the effects of the two on this complex are probably synergistic.

Free reflux, on the other hand, is characterized by a fall in the intraesophageal pH without an identifiable change in either intragastric or LES pressure.

Instances of free reflux only occur when the resting LES pressure is within 0 to 4 mm Hg of intragastric pressure. Nevertheless, it is likely that a substantial number of individuals with mild or moderate GERD are susceptible to stress reflux when their LES pressure has been temporarily diminished by specific foods (chocolate, onion, coffee), drugs, or personal habits.

A number of discrete observations have provided evidence to suggest that hiatal hernias may play a significant pathogenetic role in up to 50% of instances of GERD. It would appear that hiatal hernias constitute only an aberration from normal anatomy, based on the concept of the well-documented physiologic herniation observed during swallowing. It has been proposed that the PE membrane, which is stretched during each peristaltic contraction, gradually loses its elasticity with the passage of years. As the PE membrane weakens, the extent of herniation during swallowing gradually increases, with the resultant sequelae. Under such circumstances, it is plausible that large hernias may impair the normal process of esophageal emptying, thereby prolonging the clearance time of acid and increasing the mucosal acidification exposure time of the esophagus, particularly in the supine position. Therefore, hiatal hernias, although not an initiating factor in GERD, may be considered as providing a significant contribution to the chronicity of the disease. A critical issue, however, is the need to think in more precise terms in regard to the identification of the hiatus hernia itself. Thus, axial length, both at rest and during distention, needs to be evaluated as well as the competence of the diaphragmatic hiatus.

The pathogenesis of GERD probably does not lend itself to reductionist thinking. Integration of both anatomic and physiologic studies of the gastroesophageal junction suggests the multifactorial nature of the anatomic disruption of the diaphragmatic hiatus, the physiologic dysfunction of the LES, and the resulting diseases—esophagitis and GERD. However, it is clear that GERD is due to abnormal acid reflux.

CHAPTER 4
MANAGEMENT

Lower esophageal sphincter function in gastroesophageal reflux disease

When placed in the esophagus, more than 90% of acid is cleared into the stomach by a rapid peristalsis, but the other 10% is cleared more slowly by saliva and other host defenses. Most diseases of the esophagus, including GERD, do not cause a loss of peristalsis but do reduce the amplitude of the contractions of the fast peristaltic phase. A hiatus hernia may thus interfere with normal peristaltic waves and, therefore, prevent complete acid clearance, because acid can become trapped in the hiatal pouch. Experimentally, cisapride, a 5-HT$_4$ agonist, has effects not only on the sphincter but also on increasing salivary volume, which have been proposed to be of benefit in facilitating the esophageal clearance of acid.

GERD may be due to an extremely hypotensive sphincter, and this was the rationale for the use of metoclopramide in the past. But it is now appreciated that this abnormality is rare and that most GERD is probably due to spontaneous but excessively prolonged (30 to 60 seconds) relaxation of the LES. The issue of transient LES relaxation (TLESR) and its role in GERD is an exciting area of pathophysiology and potentially important therapeutic development.

Current evidence indicates that TLESRs are mediated primarily via vagal pathways and that, although the basal rate for TLESRs is relatively low, gastric distention appears to be a major stimulus in initiating their occurrence. Presumably, pressure signals are transduced via mechanoreceptors in the proximal stomach (gastric cardia) that relay to the vagal sensory nucleus in the brainstem by way of vagal afferent pathways. Of particular interest is the consistent and complex nature of TLESRs, which suggests that they occur in a programmed manner, probably controlled by a pattern generator in the vagal nuclei. The currently accepted explanation as to the function of the system is that when afferent signals from the proximal stomach reach a given intensity, they excite the discharge of a pattern generator, thereby triggering LES relaxation and other complex elements (perhaps antral motility and pyloric tone) of this motility response. It is evident that the motor arm of this response resides in the vagus nerve and that it almost certainly shares common elements with swallow-induced LES relaxation. Clearly, however, so complex a system requires numerous parallel and interfaced circuits, of which few are at present defined. It is apparent, however, that pharyngeal stimulation and cholecystokinin influence TLESRs and that sleep, anesthesia, and the supine position are inhibited by them.

The stimulus for prolonged relaxations may be excessive distention of the fundus, for example, by large meals, and perhaps aberrant signals from the pharynx. Chronic reflux patients may have numerous episodes of these prolonged relaxations, even up to 12 per hour. It is also apparent that transient LES incompetence is more common with age. In this respect, the role of hiatus hernia, which had been out of vogue, has once again enjoyed an etiologic renaissance as a component of the causation of GERD. Thus, the age-related increase in prevalence of hiatal hernias, which are capable of interfering with normal gastric mechanoreception in the fundus, may lead to delayed gastric emptying of solids and over-distention of the stomach. The debate concerning the association of a hiatus hernia and gastroesophageal reflux disease has gone back and forth for many decades. However, current beliefs are that a hiatus hernia is indeed contributory to GERD, and sophisticated analyses examining the effect of a hiatus hernia on the mechanics of gastroesophageal reflux and sphincter tone support this view.

The wide variety of surgical options available to improve the tone of an incompetent sphincter, both laparoscopic and open, suggests that none is perfect. Even different surgeons performing what they believe to be the same operation may not agree on the precise details, so it is often difficult to compare surgical results between centers and between individuals. Generally, the more the surgeon does, the more likely is the patient to be cured of reflux but also to develop dysphagia and the disabling symptoms of an inability to belch. Clearly, an experienced surgeon is the most important determinant of surgical success, and because of the potential problems of the surgery, a careful preoperative assessment of peristaltic function by a motility study is mandatory. The identification of individuals with poor motor function who will not do well with surgery is critical to avoid iatrogenically induced accentuation of the GERD. It is also necessary to make a positive diagnosis of GERD before surgery; either by endoscopy or 24-hour pH measurement. A trial of a PPI is a useful predictor of likely surgical success—if the patient's symptoms are markedly improved by this drug, then they will probably also be helped by surgery.

Therapeutic targets

The lower esophageal sphincter

Although considerable attention has been directed to acid-pepsin refluxate in the genesis of GERD, it is the LES that remains one of the critical variables in the disease process. Unfortunately, current knowledge of sphincter physiology is limited, and in the case of the lower esophagus, this is particularly apparent. In most situations, the diagnosis of GERD is undertaken on a clinical basis, although endoscopy is used if alarm symptoms are present or a particular patient demands endoscopic confirmation of the diagnosis before institutional therapy. For the most part, however, study of the LES itself and the esophageal peristalsis is usually reserved for patients who fail acid-suppressive therapy, exhibit obvious symptoms consistent with motility problems, or are being contemplated for surgery. Documentation of the function of the LES and the motility status of the esophagus are important in the management of such individuals.

The LES in GERD appears to malfunction either by exerting a pressure zone, which is too low to prevent reflux from the stomach, or, alternatively, by producing transient episodes of relaxation that are either too frequent or prolonged. In the 1950s, surgical techniques were developed to wrap a mobilized portion of gastric fundus around the LES (Nissen, Belsey) in an attempt to increase LES pressure and obviate reflux. Innumerable modifications of this

The Principles of Fundoplication (Wrap)

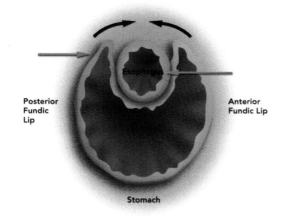

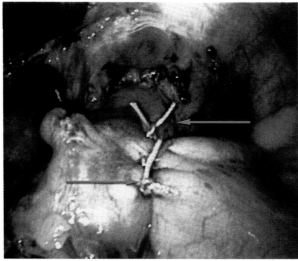

The principle of the wrap technique is diagrammatically depicted above. Below is a laparoscopic view of the completed wrap. In the photograph, the diaphragm is superior, and the mobilized esophagus emerges through the hiatus for a distance (*arrow*) of 2 to 3 cm before being obscured by the mobilized stomach that is wrapped over it and sutured in place (*arrow*). The principle of the procedure is to wrap the LES within a "doughnut" comprised of gastric fundic mucosa. The wrap is then maintained by the insertion of a number of sutures that fix the stomach both to itself and to the underlying esophagus.

procedure failed to provide a reliable high-pressure barrier zone to reflux, and the morbidity of the operation as an open procedure was substantial (12% to 18% complications). Furthermore, the inability to precisely calibrate the increase in lower esophageal pressure generated by the wrap led to failures due to either excessive wrapping or inadequate pressure increase. The subsequent development of prokinetic agents, such as metoclopramide, designed to pharmacologically ameliorate motility disturbances associated with GERD met with limited success. This reflected the relative nonselectivity of the agent and a high incidence of adverse effects. It is, however, apparent that in certain circumstances the mechanical defects associated with GERD, which are principally located in the area of esophageal peristalsis, and particularly LES pressure, need to be addressed.

Fundoplication

In circumstances in which the patient is young, requires maintenance acid-suppression therapy, is fit for surgery, and desires an operation, manometric testing should be undertaken to confirm the absence of esophageal peristaltic abnormalities and define the function of the LES. If all the criteria for surgery are met, the most appropriate operation at this time appears to be a Nissen fundoplication undertaken by laparoscopic technique. In brief, this consists of the introduction of a number of ports into the upper abdomen whereby dissection and mobilization of the fundus of the stomach and the esophagus can be undertaken. A gastric wrap is performed, having mobilized the lower 4 to 5 cm of the esophagus and moved the stomach behind it before suturing it anteriorly in front of the esophagus through the residual portion of the gastric fundus, which has been mobilized but not moved behind the esophagus. Critical areas involve the need to avoid damage to the stomach and esophagus as well as to the vagus nerves.

The diameter of the esophagus embraced by the wrap is determined by insertion of a large bougie through the gastroesophageal junction from the mouth. Results using this technique have been reported as successful in up to 85% of patients with a morbidity level varying between 10% and 15%. The precise details of surgery and its advantages and disadvantages have been dealt with in the surgical section. Under some circumstances, however, both physicians and patients would prefer to avoid surgery, and in such cases, the use of prokinetic drugs in addition to antisecretory agents should be strongly considered.

The most common antireflux procedure is the Nissen fundoplication. The procedure can be performed through the abdomen or the chest either open or through a laparoscope. Nissen described the procedure as a 360-degree fundoplication around the lower esophagus for a distance of 4 to 5 cm. Although this provided good control of reflux, it was associated with a number of side effects, which have encouraged modifications of the procedure. These include taking care to use only the gastric fundus to envelop the esophagus in performing the fundoplication, sizing the fundoplication with a 60-French bougie, and limiting the length of the fundoplication to 1 to 2 cm. The elements necessary for the performance of a transabdominal fundoplication are common to both the laparoscopic and the open procedure. The surgical steps are illustrated in the pictures. 1: Crural dissection and identification and preservation of both vagi and the anterior hepatic branch. 2: Circumferential dissection of the esophagus. 3: Crural closure. 4: Fundic mobilization by division of short gastric vessels. 5: Traction of the fundus behind the esophagus. 6: Creation of a short, loose fundoplication by enveloping the anterior and posterior walls of the fundus around the lower esophagus over a 60-French bougie in the esophagus. 7: Suture to each other and anterior wall of stomach. 8: Completed wrap.

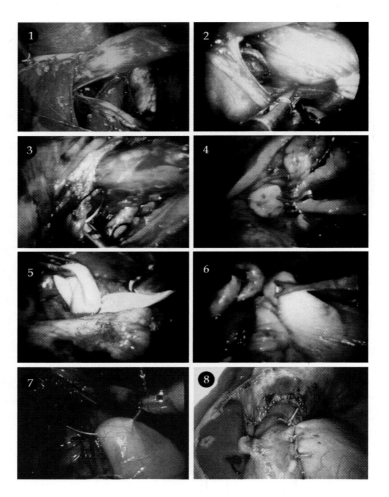

Prokinetic agents

Given the fact that acid appears to be a major inciting event in esophagitis, initial attention was directed at neutralization or suppression of acid secretion. The issue of decreasing reflux by addressing sphincter function, esophageal clearance of acid, or gastric emptying has led to an interest in identifying pharmacotherapeutic targets and agents that have a motor rather than a secretory function. Although most successful therapies have decreased acid secretion and volume with H_2 receptor antagonists and especially PPIs, the use of either mucosal protectants, such as sucralfate, or prokinetic agents, such as cisapride, has had minimal effect on the treatment of GERD except in occasional patients. Thus, in spite of serious consideration that GERD is a motility disorder, such promotility drugs as bethanechol, metoclopramide, and cisapride have had marginal efficacy in treating GERD patients except in patients with nonerosive disease or dyspepsia with associated delayed gastric emptying. Although a variety of mechanisms were proposed whereby such agents purportedly increased LES pressure and improved acid clearance, in retrospect, it is probable that they did little more than improve gastric emptying. Of particular relevance to current concepts of GERD etiology, it is apparent that none of these putative promotility agents had any effect on the major motor mechanism underlying reflux episodes, TLESRs.

Because TLESRs appear to be a key mechanism underlying most episodes of gastroesophageal reflux, the ability to regulate them pharmacologically is paramount to the success of therapy. It is now evident that TLESRs account for virtually all reflux episodes in healthy subjects and most (55% to 80%) reflux episodes in GERD patients. Although such patients usually exhibit no esophagitis (NERD) or only mild erosions, they collectively account for as much as 80% of all patients with reflux disease. Furthermore, it is apparent that individuals with severe esophagitis not only reflux via TLESRs but also have frequent reflux episodes during periods of prolonged absent basal LES pressure.

Prokinetic agents are those that are intended to restore, normalize, and facilitate motility in the gastrointestinal tract. The development of this group of pharmacologic agents is historically traceable to the appreciation of the role of dopaminergic receptors in gut smooth muscle. The recognition of their presence stimulated an investigation of agents that would even neutralize or antagonize the inhibitory effects of dopamine on gut motility. The first agent of this class was metoclopramide, which was useful in that it improved gastric emptying, accelerated transit through the small bowel, and provided for the first time an agent capable of modulating gut motility. Unfortunately, metoclopramide crosses the blood–brain barrier, resulting in CNS antidopaminergic effects, and up to 20% of individuals suffered from experimental side effects of varying degrees of intensity. Further problems related to the generation of hyperprolactinemia include breast enlargement, nipple tenderness, galactorrhea, and menstrual irregularities. To a certain extent, these disadvantages were overcome by the development of domperidone, which, although it had minimal experimental side effects, still caused hyperprolactinemia and its related symptomatology. Its effect on enhancing motility of the esophagus, stomach, and small bowel was useful, but its primary therapeutic usefulness was its antiemetic properties at the chemoreceptor trigger site.

The subsequent development of cisapride, an agonist of the serotonin receptor 5-HT$_4$, was a significant improvement over both previous agents. This prokinetic agent facilitates the release of ACh from postganglionic cholinergic fibers within the myenteric plexus. The overall result of this biochemical effect has been to improve propulsive motor activity of the esophagus, stomach, small bowel, and large bowel. In addition to its motor effects, cisapride has been documented to enhance salivary secretion by stimulation of the esophagosalivary reflex, with the result that increased saliva flow as well as the protective agent within it (bicarbonate, glycoconjugate, EGF, and PGE$_2$) are delivered in larger quantities to the LES area and are postulated to accentuate healing. Cisapride is a substituted piperidinyl benzamide, which is chemically related to metoclopramide but did not exhibit the major CNS effects. Nevertheless, somnolence and fatigue have been reported as well as some experimental effects.

The particular problem with cisapride has been its relative nonselectivity in terms of a target of smooth muscle function. In some individuals, serious diarrhea and abdominal pain have proved to be major drawbacks in its use. Nevertheless, cisapride has been demonstrated to significantly increase lower esophageal pressure as well as to promote gastric emptying. Given its positive effects on promoting esophageal peristalsis, the sum of these pharmacologic events has been to produce a prokinetic agent of therapeutic benefit in patients with GERD. Indeed, in individuals in whom acid suppression may not adequately obviate relapse, the use of cisapride as an adjuvant agent has been met with some reasonable success.

A number of studies have demonstrated that cisapride alone is more effective than placebo in symptom relief and healing in patients with heartburn of the esophagitis grade 0 to 3 range. Similarly, it has been reported that episodes of gastroesophageal reflux are decreased in patients taking cisapride, and that in individuals using acid suppression in combination with cisapride, efficacy of symptom relief and healing are greater than when acid suppression alone is used. The widespread distribution of the 5-HT$_4$ receptor has resulted in very serious side effects, particularly in children. This drug has thus been withdrawn from the market. Perhaps, also, the selectivity of this agonist is less than that required, and the side effects are due to actions on other receptors.

Tweaking transient lower esophageal sphincter relaxations

In the 1990s, the ability to manipulate TLESRs pharmacologically became possible with the identification of several agents that substantially diminished this phenomenon. Although the magnitude of TLESR reduction required to achieve a clinically significant reduction in reflux symptoms has not been precisely defined, it has been suggested that a reduction of at least 50% is necessary to assure clinical efficacy. To date, a wide variety of agents, including CCK$_1$ antagonists, anticholinergic agents, nitric oxide synthase inhibitors, morphine, and γ-aminobutyric acid β (GABA$_\beta$) agonists have been studied in humans.

Anticholinergic agents

After the observation in healthy volunteers that intravenous atropine reduced the rate of TLESRs by nearly 60%, a study in GERD patients produced similar findings. Current evidence suggests a central site of action, because selective peripheral anticholinergic agents, which do not cross the blood–brain barrier, fail to inhibit TLESRs. It is, however, unlikely that anticholinergic agents will be clinically effective because of their deleterious effects on supine acid clearance and worrisome side-effect profile.

Cholecystokinin

Given the well-accepted data reporting the presence of a variety of CCK receptor subtypes on neurons and the LES muscle and the demonstration that meals and/or gastric distention stimulate the release of CCK, it was predictable that the peptide would influence TLESRs. Furthermore, because animal studies showed that CCK infusion increased the rate of TLESRs triggered by gastric distention, the augmentation of TLESRs by food intake and gastric distention provided a logical potential treatment target. Thus, devazepide, a CCK$_1$ but not a CCK$_2$ antagonist, was demonstrated to be effective in decreasing gastric distention–induced TLESRs. Because devazepide was not effective when administered into the CNS, it seemed likely that CCK was acting either via the proximal stomach or on the afferent nerves. Subsequent human studies demonstrated that the CCK_1 antagonist loxiglumide inhibited the rate of TLESRs induced by meals and gastric distention by approximately 40%, further suggesting a potential therapeutic opportunity. Unfortunately, an orally effective CCK_1 antagonist is not yet available, and the feasibility of TLESR management using intravenous preparations seems low.

Nitric oxide

The role of nitric oxide in sphincter function remains an exciting area of debate, and, indeed, nitric oxide is the major postganglionic inhibitory neurotransmitter to the LES, and nitrergic neurons are present in the dorsal motor nucleus of the vagus. Its potential role in the modulation of LES pressure was confirmed by a series of animal studies that reported not only that the nitric oxide synthase inhibitor L-MNME inhibited the rate of TLESRs but also that the effect could be reversed by L-arginine. Of further interest were human volunteer studies that reported that L-NMMA inhibited TLESRs induced by gastric distention by more than 75%. Although the reduction in meal-induced TLESRs was only 25%, the potential of such compounds is indisputable. Unfortunately, no orally effective nitric oxide inhibitor is currently available, and the inhibition of nitric oxide is associated with widespread alterations in gastrointestinal motility and substantial changes in the cardiovascular, urinary, and respiratory systems.

Morphine

Because opioid nerves have been demonstrated in the myenteric plexus of the LES in humans, and morphine has been noted to inhibit LES relaxation caused by swallowing and balloon distention, a possible therapeutic role has been proposed. Thus, the demonstration that intravenous morphine given to GERD patients inhibited TLESRs by 50% while also decreasing the number of reflux episodes further supported the contention that a therapeutic role might exist. Because the effect of morphine is blocked completely by naloxone, it is likely that its activity is mediated through opioid receptors located in the CNS. The likelihood of a central effect is further substantiated by the fact that the peripherally active opioid—loperamide—does not effect TLESRs. At this time, the unacceptable side effects of the agent, including addiction and constipation, seriously preclude its consideration as a viable therapeutic strategy.

$GABA_B$ agonists

$GABA_B$ is one of the major inhibitory neurotransmitters of the CNS, and $GABA_B$ receptors are present at numerous sites within the CNS and peripheral nervous system. Baclofen, the prototype agent, acts through inhibition of transmitter release from muscle spindle afferents and is currently used clinically for the treatment of muscle spasticity but has been demonstrated to be a powerful inhibitor of TLESRs. Although the precise mechanism of its action has not been defined, animal studies suggest that baclofen exerts its effect by modulating the trigger sensitivity of gastric mechanoreceptor and the central pathway between vagal afferents and efferents.

In both healthy subjects and those with GERD, single oral doses (40 mg) of baclofen have been demonstrated to decrease the rate of TLESRs by more than 50%, with a concomitant 60% decrease in the rate of reflux episodes. Thus, in a field (sphincter function regulation) where there are few reasonable candidates, GABA$_B$ agonists currently appear to be the most promising new class of agents for controlling the rate of TLESRs. A subsequent encouraging preliminary study in healthy subjects and reflux patients found that oral baclofen (40 mg twice a day) decreased acid and nonacid reflux and symptoms associated with these refluxates. Of note is the fact that, compared with other available agents, baclofen is available as an oral agent and does not exhibit adverse effects on basal LES pressure or acid clearance. Unfortunately, side effects are common and include drowsiness, nausea, and the lowering of the threshold for seizures. Thus, although baclofen appears promising in principle, it is evident that novel agents with more precisely defined molecular targets are necessary before widespread clinical use is possible.

Gastric acidity

Gastric juice is harmful to esophageal squamous mucosa. In general, the secretion of acid, pepsin, and bile as measured by classic secretory studies using nasogastric tubes is no different in patients with or without GERD, suggesting that hypersecretion is not the cause of the disease. Indeed, most experimental models suggest that it is not acid alone that is injurious. The damage is due to the presence of other contents of the refluxate, including at least pepsin, bile, ingested material, and lysolecithin.

Although acid may have direct effects on the esophageal mucosa, including widening intercellular spaces and altering the esophageal potential difference, its main function may be to facilitate the damage initiated by pepsin and bile as well as activating pepsinogen to pepsin. Although acid may not be the only cause of the damage in GERD, acid suppression is a very effective treatment. In the evaluation of data acquired by metaanalysis, it is apparent that the greater the acid suppression, the better the healing of esophagitis and the more rapidly the symptoms are relieved. It is interesting that certain regulatory agencies have failed to accept this concept and still require head-to-head clinical studies between individual acid-suppression medications to prove efficacy. In general, the most effective acid suppression is achieved with PPIs, and there are currently several of these available, including pantoprazole, lansoprazole, and omeprazole. The latter agent was the initial pump inhibitor, shown to be far more effective than H$_2$ receptor antagonists in the healing of GERD, but subsequently, many compounds of the PPI class of drugs have been shown to exhibit equivalent superiority.

More recently, esomeprazole, an (S)-isomer of omeprazole, has been developed. It is the first PPI to be developed as an optical isomer and appears to

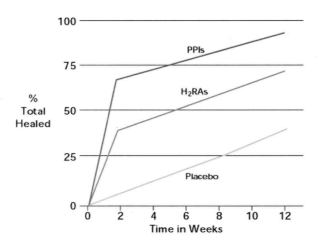

Esophagitis Healing by Drug Class

The proton pump inhibitor class of drugs is significantly more effective than H$_2$ receptor antagonists in healing esophagitis. This reflects their ability to provide a far greater sustained level of acid suppression.

have an improved pharmacokinetic profile that confers increased systemic exposure and less interindividual variability compared with omeprazole. It is proposed that this produces more effective suppression of gastric acid production compared with other PPIs. Of note are the observations that esomeprazole is well tolerated, with a spectrum and incidence of adverse events similar to those associated with omeprazole. Several large, double-blind, randomized trials have noted higher rates of endoscopically confirmed healing of erosive esophagitis and resolution of heartburn in patients with GERD receiving 8 weeks of esomeprazole, 40 mg o.d., compared with those receiving omeprazole, 20 mg o.d., or lansoprazole, 30 mg o.d. Similarly, esomeprazole, 10, 20, or 40 mg o.d., was significantly more effective than placebo in two 6-month, randomized, double-blind trials in the maintenance of healed erosive esophagitis. In a separate 6-month, randomized, double-blind trial, esomeprazole, 20 mg o.d., was more effective than lansoprazole, 15 mg, in the maintenance of healed erosive esophagitis, and healing of esophagitis was also effectively maintained by esomeprazole, 40 mg o.d., in a 12-month noncomparative trial. Esomeprazole, 20 or 40 mg o.d., effectively relieved heartburn in patients with GERD without esophagitis in two 4-week, placebo-controlled trials. Similarly, studies in endoscopy-negative patients, or in both esophagitis- and endoscopy-negative patients, have demonstrated good efficacy for esomeprazole, with high levels of symptom control achieved in the first 7 days of therapy. The greatest advantage for esomeprazole appears to be its improved healing rates in the more severe grades of esophagitis as compared to omeprazole, although recent studies suggest that there is no appreciable difference between it and pantoprazole, and that on a milligram-for-milligram basis, all PPIs appear to be equivalent.

There is little difference in the 1-month healing rates between any of these agents. Lansoprazole at a dose of 30 mg daily is claimed to be more effective than omeprazole, 20 mg daily, for symptom relief, perhaps just reflecting the higher dose or superior bioavailability of lansoprazole. There is also some person-to-person variability in the secretory response to omeprazole and, to a lesser degree, to lansoprazole. Pantoprazole appears to have the most advantageous pharmacokinetic profile and is negligible in its effects on the hepatic P450 cytochrome system. This latter factor may be of relevance in the context that the vast majority of older patients take other medications as well as PPIs.

Despite the efficacy of these medications, at least 10% of all patients continue to have symptoms after 2 months of PPI therapy. This reflects the fact that many patients present for treatment at a point well into the evolution of the disease process and exhibit an esophagus that is either scarred or so damaged that the healing process cannot maintain mucosal integrity in the presence of anything other than the presence of the most limited amounts of acid or pepsin. This further emphasizes the need not only to tailor treatment for GERD to the individual patient but also to ensure early institution of therapy with PPIs rather than observation of repeated recurrence of symptomatology and accentuation of damage during a trial of inadequate acid inhibitory therapy.

Gastroesophageal reflux disease and esophageal pH

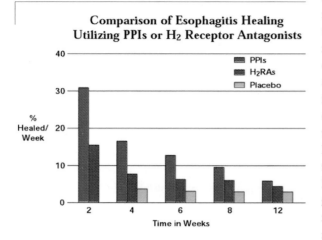

Comparison of Esophagitis Healing Utilizing PPIs or H₂ Receptor Antagonists

The percentage of patients with esophagitis that heal over time is dependent on the class of agent used for acid suppression.

There is a clear predictive relationship between intragastric pH and intra-esophageal pH, as both correlate with the healing of esophagitis. The greater the severity of the esophagitis, the greater the requirement for acid suppression. The conventional pH threshold for aggressive versus nonaggressive reflux is regarded as a pH of 4.0, and this has been supported by pH measurements in patients with defined severities of GERD. Overall, it is apparent that the severity of mucosal injury in GERD is dependent on the pH of the reflux material and its dwell time in the esophagus. In this respect, 24-hour esophageal pH monitoring has proved to be the most effective measurement of gastroesophageal reflux, because it records both the pH of the reflux and the duration of the exposure. It is evident that the daily duration of time for which the intragastric pH is elevated to 4.0 or higher correlates closely with the healing of erosive reflux esophagitis. Nevertheless, esophageal pH monitoring studies reveal in some patients the presence of GERD despite normal or near normal acidic exposure values.

This paradox probably reflects alterations in reflux patterns that vary from day to day as well as variations in pH between different regions of the esophagus. Esophageal pH rises as the distance from the LES increases, and in addition, pH appears to be lower at the peaks of the esophageal folds, which are exposed to acid as opposed to the tufts, where there is a greater degree of protection afforded by bicarbonate and mucus. This variation in esophageal pH is presumably responsible for the linear distribution of erosive esophagitis evident at endoscopy in some patients. Overall, it does not appear that patients with GERD are acid hypersecretors. Nevertheless, repeated measurements of 24-hour intragastric acidity in individual patients reveal considerable variations.

In some patients, abnormal duodenal gastric reflux may make gastric juice especially aggressive to esophageal mucosa. In this respect, delayed gastric emptying may contribute significantly to pathologic gastroesophageal reflux. Similarly, abnormally frequent transient LES relaxation, as well as inappropriate esophageal clearance and the presence of a hiatal hernia, may contribute to the development of GERD. Twenty-four-hour esophageal pH monitoring in endoscopically negative or mild reflux disease has shown that most acid exposure occurs during the day in the postprandial state. Furthermore, several esophageal-monitoring studies have demonstrated that individuals with Barrett's esophagus exhibit high levels of esophageal exposure to gastric reflux. Nevertheless, rigorous data supporting that Barrett's esophagus is linearly related to the level of acid reflux are not available.

The key role of acids in the development of GERD is best exemplified in patients with gastrinoma disease, in which peptic esophagitis is directly related to the level of acid suppression achievable. It is likely that the marginal efficacy of H₂ receptor antagonists in the management of GERD is related to their failure to control esophageal acid exposure. Other factors involved in the development of GERD that are pH related include the ability of the esophagus to clear acid and to deal

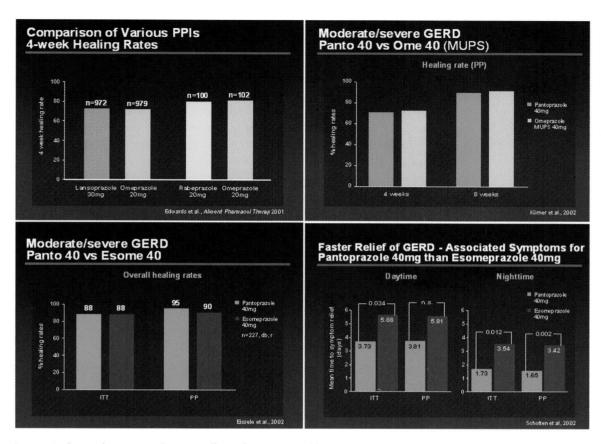

A composite data set demonstrating the varying efficacy of proton pump inhibitors on esophageal disease. Similar 4-week healing rates have been determined for this drug class (top left). In addition, pantoprazole, 40 mg, is as effective as omeprazole, 40 mg, in the treatment of moderate to severe GERD (top right) and has similar overall healing rates (bottom left). Pantoprazole, however, demonstrates faster relief than omeprazole for the treatment of the symptoms of GERD (bottom right).

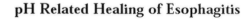

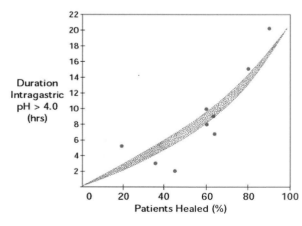

The more sustained the duration of pH above 4.0, the greater the percentage of esophagitis healing.

with activated pepsinogen. In up to 50% of patients with GERD, it has been demonstrated that the higher the acid concentration in the refluxate, the longer it requires for clearance. The reasons for the diminished rate of clearance are at this time unclear but may represent either abnormally low swallowing rates or ineffective primary or secondary peristalsis. Although salivary bicarbonate is of importance in determining esophageal acid clearance, little information is available on salivary gland function in GERD patients. The pH necessary to activate pepsinogen is an important variable in the sensitivity of the esophageal epithelium through acid peptic insult. The higher the pH, the further outside the optimum pH profile for pepsinogen activation and, hence, the less the likelihood of damage. A similar pathogenesis is probably involved in damage caused by bile acids, but this usually reflects a smaller subgroup of patients who have had previous gastric surgery or exhibit major motility disorders.

Given the fact that the degree of esophageal acid exposure correlates almost linearly with the severity of esophagitis, the primary aim of acid-suppression therapy is to raise the pH of the refluxate. In this respect, H_2 receptor antagonists are not effective in anything other than the mildest of GERD situations due to their inability to maintain a pH greater than 4.0 for a sustained period. A number of metaanalytic studies have indicated that a threshold of pH 4.0 appears to be the critical determinant for ensuring esophageal healing. Thus, the longer the esophageal acid exposure to a pH greater than 4.0, the more likely it is that healing will occur. The rapid relapse of esophagitis on withdrawal of acid-suppressive therapy indicates that the duration of therapy is of critical relevance in determining complete healing. In this respect, agents such as the PPI class of drugs are clearly superior, given their ability to not only provide a higher degree of acid suppression but also to maintain pH levels elevated both during the daytime and the nighttime, regardless of stimulation by meals. It may well be that the efficacy of the prokinetic agents is to a certain extent provided by their effect on acid clearance. Relatively poor responses to prokinetic agents suggest that abnormally delayed gastric emptying may be a relatively minor factor in the pathogenesis of GERD. Because they do not result in a major decrease in the frequency of reflux episodes, it seems likely that, at this time, the suppression of gastric acid secretion will remain the primary means of GERD therapy.

Helicobacter pylori

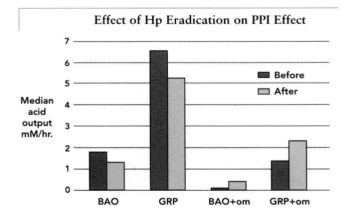

Effect of Hp Eradication on PPI Effect

Median acid output mM/hr.

Before
After

BAO GRP BAO+om GRP+om

Eradication of *H. pylori* alters the acid-secretory response of the stomach to GRP (gastrin releasing peptide) stimulation and omeprazole inhibition. The precise mechanism by which the effects of *H. pylori* on acid secretion occur have not been defined. They include both a direct effect of the organism on parietal cells and effects on the neuroendocrine cells responsible for the regulation of acid secretion. The generation of NH_3 by the organism in acid is able to have a significant neutralizing effect, particularly when acid secretion is severely inhibited by PPIs. Recent prospective trials suggest that *H. pylori* eradication does not affect the outcome of PPI therapy.

It is interesting to note that the increase in the reported prevalence of GERD has coincided over the last 50 years or so with a natural decline in *H. pylori* infection in the West. This has led to some speculation that the two may be causally related and that *H. pylori* may have been of some symbiotic benefit to humans. One possible mechanism by which *H. pylori* may influence GERD is through engendering an alteration in acid secretion.

Although *H. pylori* increases acid secretion in patients with duodenal ulcer disease, it may be responsible for decreasing acid secretion in those individuals infected early in life who develop gastritis of the gastric corpus. Several lines of evidence support this view. Thus, in Japan, the gastric cancer and *H. pylori* incidence rates have fallen dramatically over the last 20 years, and there has been an associated increase in gastric acid secretion in the population, as well as an increasing recognition of GERD. It has been reported that the eradication of *H. pylori* in a series of people with duodenal ulcer disease led to some of them developing GERD for the first time. Although this finding remains controversial, it raises interesting questions and cannot be ignored. The issue of whether harboring *H. pylori* in the stomach is associated with an unexpected beneficial effect of the bacterium by the protection afforded from GERD may be quixotic but requires examination.

Another observation of relevance is that lower doses of antisecretory medications appear effective in the management of GERD when *H. pylori* is present. The generation of NH_3 by *H. pylori* is likely able to neutralize a significant portion of nighttime acid secretion when this is already inhibited by PPIs. This would explain the observation that eradication of the organism decreases intragastric pH, particularly at night. Currently, the consensus appears to be that eradication of the pathogen has little effect on the incidence of GERD in the infected population. The potential benefit to the individual of retaining his or her *H. pylori* to lower the PPI dose when treating GERD is offset by the reports suggesting that the development of gastric atrophy, a preneoplastic change, is accelerated by the presence of *H. pylori* in patients taking omeprazole. This controversial finding initially provoked considerable skepticism but has more recently acquired further support in studies that addressed the same question. Given the considerable support for the use of maintenance PPI treatment in the management of GERD, this issue is of critical relevance and requires definitive resolution. At this time, the safest approach is eradication of *H. pylori*–positive GERD in patients taking PPIs on a chronic basis.

Determination of gastroesophageal reflux disease and management

In general practice, dyspepsia occurs in approximately half of the population, and even patients who have reflux symptoms often also have ulcer-like symptoms. The endoscopic evaluation of esophagitis remains an area of both controversy and difficulty. There is no completely satisfactory classification, and many schemes vie for widespread acceptance. Even within individual classifications, agreement between the classifiers is not uniform. Although agreement between observers is good for severe changes of esophagitis—stricture and erosions—there is often extremely poor agreement between observers for minor changes. Because the prevalence of endoscopy-negative reflux disease far outweighs those

A number of different classification systems have been developed to enable objective endoscopic quantification of the severity of the disease process. Although the LA classification system is probably the most widely used, the MUSE system shown here has proved particularly effective in facilitating assessment of esophagitis.

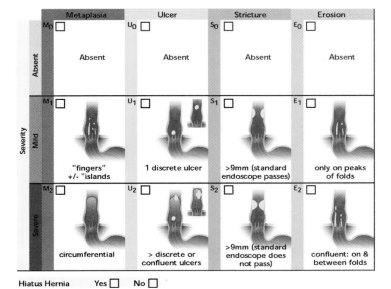

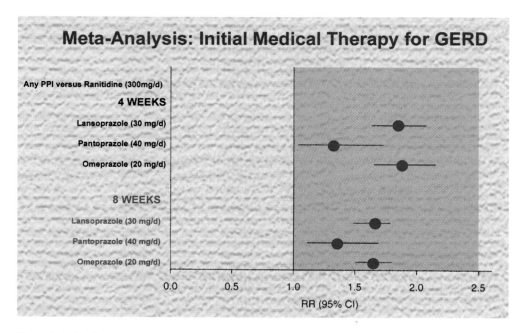

Metaanalysis of healing rate ratios (RR) and 95% confidence intervals (CI) for proton pump inhibitors compared with ranitidine at 8 weeks. The rate ratios were estimated by dividing the average healing rates for the treatments being compared with the estimates of omeprazole or ranitidine. (Adapted from Caro JJ, Salas M, Ward A. Healing and relapse rates in gastroesophageal reflux disease. *Clin Ther* 2001;23:998–1017.)

who have positive endoscopic findings, the precise role of endoscopy in diagnosis needs serious consideration. Given its expense, invasiveness, and relative insensitivity as a diagnostic tool, initial enthusiasm has been replaced by a healthy degree of skepticism. A once-in-a-lifetime endoscopy, toward the beginning of treatment rather than later, is probably a useful maneuver, if only to rule out other unexpected lesions. However, repeat endoscopy in a patient with uncomplicated GERD is probably not indicated unless Barrett's esophagus has been identified and verified. In such individuals, cost-effectiveness analyses have suggested that surveillance should be performed every 5 years, although given the current reduction in endoscopy costs in the United States, the financial equation may change in favor of more frequent evaluation.

Medical strategies

A number of algorithms have been developed for the management of erosive esophagitis. These tend to be somewhat different from country to country or between different health systems. Once the diagnosis of GERD has been established, an attempt at lifestyle modification, with or without antacids, mucosal protectant agents, or alginic acid, is usually undertaken as an initial step. If unsuccessful, an acid-inhibitory agent is then introduced into the therapeutic regimen. In patients with mild disease (grade 1 to 2), an H_2 receptor antagonist is often used. If this fails (failure to relieve symptoms or relapse on cessation of therapy), a PPI is usually used. Because a significant number of patients fail to heal with the H_2 receptor antagonist therapy or, alternatively, relapse, PPIs have increasingly been rightly considered as a first line of therapy. Within broad parameters, the general algorithm used includes initial evaluation by endoscopic examination with biopsy, followed by 24-hour pH monitoring and measurement of LES pressure, followed by an 8-week course of a PPI. If symptom relief and healing do not occur under these circumstances, a second course of PPI ther-

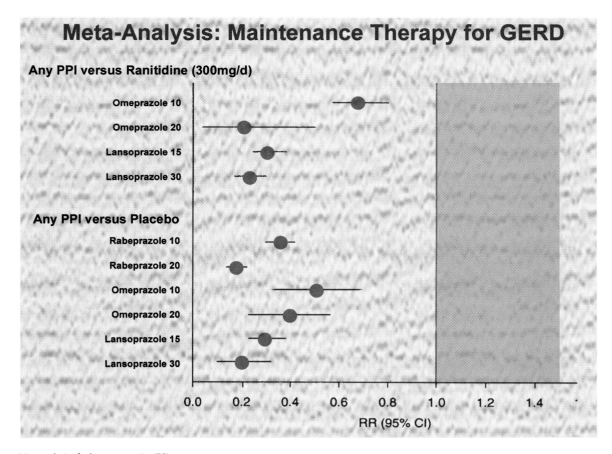

Meta-Analysis: Maintenance Therapy for GERD

Metaanalysis of relapse rate ratios (RR) and 95% confidence intervals (CI) for proton pump inhibitors compared with ranitidine or placebo after 6 months. (Adapted from Caro JJ, Salas M, Ward A. Healing and relapse rates in gastroesophageal reflux disease. *Clin Ther* 2001;23:998–1017.)

apy is usually undertaken (often at a higher or divided dosage). Depending on the age of the patient, severity of symptomatology, and the physician's level of concern, a number of relapses may lead either to the introduction of a prokinetic agent or, alternatively, to the consideration of surgery. For the most part, the latter option now entails laparoscopic surgery. In those individuals who at initial diagnosis exhibit evidence of a complication of GERD, the use of short-term medical therapy before surgical intervention is usual. Using this general management strategy or reasonable variations thereof, it appears that between 85% and 95% of all patients can be adequately managed medically, and some 5% to 15% of patients either exhibit complications or are nonamenable to long-term acid-inhibitory therapy and thus require consideration for surgery.

In a review of 31 randomized studies performed between 1986 and 1995, initial medical therapy over 8 to 12 weeks resulted in an overall healing rate with PPIs of 87.1% (n = 1,725 patients), H_2 receptor antagonists of 57.2% (n = 2,262), prokinetic agents of 66.0% (n = 209), and placebo of 23.7% (n = 719). The prokinetic data are probably too small to enable reasonable comparison. In a further evaluation of 36 studies undertaken between 1989 and 1995, the relapse rate for H_2 receptor antagonists was 77.3%, compared to an overall relapse rate of 26% for the PPI group of drugs. When analyzed individually on an agent-specific basis, the relapse rate after short-term treatment was 39.2% for omeprazole, 22.3% for lansoprazole, and 17.5% for pantoprazole.

In regard to the long-term outcome after maintenance therapy with omeprazole or lansoprazole, a remission rate of 79% to 90% can be achieved over a 12-month period. The issue of adverse events using medical therapy was evaluated in 16,816 patients, comprising nine studies performed between 1989 and 1995. The majority of these events were minor and rarely required cessation of the therapy. They included headache, diarrhea, abdominal pain, skin rash, and drowsiness. When summated, treatment-related incidents occurred in the H_2 receptor antagonist group in approximately 23%, whereas use of the PPI class of agent was associated with reportable events in approximately 18%. This difference was not statistically significant. Individually adverse effects were reported with pantoprazole in 13.0%, lansoprazole in 18.0%, and omeprazole in 22.3% of patients. These are no different from placebo events.

Surgical and endoscopic strategies

Endoscopic antireflux therapies

There has been widespread enthusiasm to find less invasive strategies for dealing with reflux than surgery and to decrease life-long exposure to acid-suppressive medications. As a consequence, luminally delivered physical antireflux therapies are being explored to obviate some of the limitations or disadvantages of medical therapy or conventional laparoscopic antireflux surgery. This has led to the introduction of a variety of procedures that are minimally invasive; intended to be undertaken as a same-day, outpatient procedure; and suitable for retreatment, reversal, or both, although absolving patients from the necessity of daily medication. Over the last decade, a diverse spectrum of such candidate therapies has emerged. Unfortunately, most focus on the relatively simplistic notion of augmenting or bolstering the LES. Furthermore, few techniques have been subjected to rigorous scrutiny or evaluated in prospective randomized studies; hence, the data on their efficacy are less than assured. An additional problem with most of these novel strategies is that patients with less severe levels of esophagitis have been treated; hence, results may be optimistically unrealistic. The notion that the therapy is luminally delivered has led to a false perception that it may, therefore, be deemed safe; such is clearly not the case.

Radiofrequency energy delivery

The principle of this technique is based on the concept that heat-induced damage will lead to some degree of scarring of the LES and, hence, decrease reflux. It has been demonstrated that the procedure decreases the rate of transient LES relaxation in both dogs and humans. The radiofrequency energy [Stretta procedure (Curon Medical Inc., Sunnyvale, California, USA)] is delivered via a specially designed catheter passed orally that has three retractable needle electrodes mounted radially around a balloon. A radiofrequency energy generator monitors both the tissue temperature and impedance during treatment and, in this fashion, controls the amount of energy delivered via each electrode. The current treatment protocols are designed to produce up to 80 predominantly submucosal lesions in the distal esophagus, LES, and gastric cardia. The assessment data of the technique are not uniform. Thus, a recent multicenter study in 47 patients demonstrated symptomatic improvement with

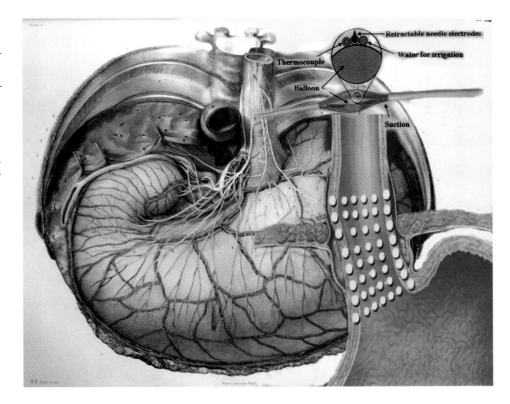

The Stretta device is a balloon-tipped three- or four-needle catheter that delivers radio-frequency energy to the smooth muscle in the area of the gastro-esophageal junction. The subsequent heat-induced damage engenders local fibrosis, which may be of benefit in decreasing reflux. Definitive studies to substantiate this hypothesis are as yet lacking, although the concept remains both intriguing and attractive.

a significant reduction in 24-hour acid exposure (10.2% to 6.4%) at 6 months, with a symptomatic response being sustained up to 12 months of follow-up. A randomized sham procedure controlled trial has produced somewhat less optimistic results.

Endoscopic suturing

Endoscopic suturing requires an overtube and a sewing capsule that is attached to the end of a standard gastroscope. The mechanisms of action of endoscopic suturing are not clear but potentially include an increase in basal lower esophageal pressure and a theoretic increase in LES length. It has been reported that suturing results in a modest decrease in the number of transient LES relaxations 6 months after endoscopic suturing, although this had no impact on the rate of postprandial reflux events or on acid exposure. It has

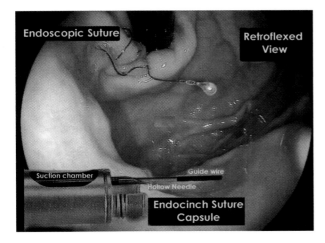

The EndoCinch device is a suturing system that allows endoscopists to create plications in the mucosa of the LES area. The technique requires considerable technical expertise and is therefore significantly operator dependent in its outcome. Some studies have reported significant improvement in symptoms and enabled a decrease or elimination of dependence on acid-suppressive medication.

been proposed that the creation of a series of plications at the gastroesophageal junction might potentially alter the angle of His; however, this speculation remains to be proven. An issue of considerable concern remains regarding the durability of the stitches over time.

The technique involves insertion of a stitch through tissue captured in the suction chamber of the sewing capsule. The needle is then reloaded externally, and another stitch is placed adjacent to the first. Sutures are placed just distal to the gastroesophageal junction. Because the procedure requires considerable manual dexterity and is relatively difficult to perform, the outcome is likely to be considerably operator dependent.

In general, there is a lack of systematic information on the best number of sutures and whether these should be placed vertically or circumferentially. A U.S. multicenter study that involved 64 patients followed for 6 months without a placebo group reported an improvement in symptoms and a modest decrease in the rate of reflux episodes and esophageal acid exposure, regardless of whether patients had a linear or circumferential plication.

Luminal-Technical Antireflux Therapies
Injection techniques
Bovine dermal collagen
Polytetrafluoroethylene (Polytef)
Polymethylmethacrylate (PMMA)
Hydrogel (Gatekeeper)
Ethinyl-vinyl-alcohol (EVA, Enteryx)
Sodium morrhuate
Suturing
Bard EndoCinch
Wilson-Cook Flexible Endoscopic Suturing Device
Thermal methods
Nd:YAG laser
Radiofrequency energy (Stretta)
Plication and valvuloplasty
NDO Surgical Plicator

Endoscopic injection techniques

The development of this technique was based on early experiences with the use of injection techniques. As a result of a perceived putative efficacy, attention was directed to the identification of inert, biocompatible substances that might safely function as "bulking agents" at the LES. An early report in 2001 by Feretis described a technique of endoscopic submucosal injection of polymethylmethacrylate microspheres suspended in gelatin into the LES of ten patients. At 7 months' follow-up, there was a significant fall in 24-hour acid exposure (24.5% to 7.2%) that was, in addition, supported by a comparable improvement in symptom scores.

The Gatekeeper (Medtronic, Minneapolis, USA) uses prostheses that are placed submucosally at the gastroesophageal junction using an endoscopic technique. Each cylindrical prosthesis measures only 1.5 mm by 15.0 mm when inserted in its dehydrated state but, subsequent to hydration, swells to 6 mm in diameter. Because between three and six of these prostheses are inserted, there is substantial alteration (indentation) of the lumen in the sphincter region. It is proposed that this results in an augmentation of both the consistency and force of closure of the sphincter, thereby decreasing reflux. Preliminary uncontrolled data from 40 patients indicate a reasonable symptom response, although the impact on decreasing esophageal acid exposure was not as convincing.

Enteryx (Boston Scientific Corporation, Natick, Massachusetts, USA) is a radio-opaque liquid ethinyl vinyl acetate (EVA) that is injected into the lower esophageal muscle endoscopically. On contact with the tissue, the EVA polymerizes and forms a spongy cushion that becomes trapped in the sphincter region. The procedure requires that several injections be made under fluoroscopic control to create a circular cushion that theoretically might function in a fashion designed to increase the consistency and force of sphincter closure. In actuality, animal studies demonstrate that EVA injection has only a minor impact on the measures of sphincter function evaluated. Thus, no effect on basal pressure or length was demonstrable, although an increase in gastric yield pressure was recorded. Similarly, preliminary uncontrolled data on 127 patients suggest a modest symptomatic benefit and concomitant decrease in acid exposure.

Overall, there remains considerably more enthusiasm than data regarding these novel techniques for obviating reflux, and at this time, it is not possible to determine or to identify those that will gain an established place in routine management. Certainly, the past experience with open surgical techniques leads to the conclusion that mechanical methodology for bolstering sphincter function may ultimately prove disappointing. Thus, conjecture in regard to the development of a full-thickness plicator, and the introduction of a nipple valve–forming procedure valvuloplasty, although intriguing, may ultimately suffer the same fate as the continent ileostomy valve of 3 decades ago.

Surgery

The majority of surgeons concur that clearly defined requirements for an antireflux procedure have to be fulfilled before consideration of a patient for surgery. These include (a) pathologic esophageal acid exposure on 24-hour pH monitoring, (b) significantly decreased LES pressure, (c) normal parameters of esophageal contractility, and (d) normal esophageal length. In the published literature, surgical intervention is for the most part regarded as a laparoscopic Nissen fundoplication (LNF), although other procedures, including the Toupet, have been used with considerable success. The difficulty with the evaluation of surgical techniques is that few of the studies have been performed in a prospective randomized fashion and even fewer have been evaluated by blinded observers. Similarly, although most patients undertaking medical therapy at centers are included in cumulative reports, few surgeons rush to press to report their failures or to amplify in the public domain the complications of surgical intervention. This difference is further reflected in that, before the introduction of a new therapeutic agent, not only are levels of evaluation (phases I, II, III) required but, in addition, federal approval is necessary. In contrast, the introduction and acceptance of a novel surgical procedure is usually a result of informal generalized approval by peers.

Thus, surgical data may err quite significantly on the side of optimistic evaluation. In evaluating all published series that embraced the management of antireflux surgery over the last 5 years, it was apparent that there had been a substantial shift to the use of laparoscopic antireflux procedures. Although follow-up is somewhat limited, it is apparent from these reports that between 85% and 95% of all patients can be predicted to improve after surgery, irrespective of the technique used. The complications for laparoscopic surgery appear to be approximately half of those reported for open surgery, although this may reflect the fact that only experts are undertaking laparoscopic antireflux surgery, whereas open antireflux surgery is still regarded as the province of almost all general surgeons. The mortality for laparoscopic surgery was 0.4%, whereas that reported for open surgery was 0.5% (review of 11 nonrandomized studies from 1991 to 1994 comprising 1,237 patients). This significant difference may again reflect selection bias of patients and the comparison of expert surgeons functioning under extremely rigorous conditions, as compared to summated information from many different levels of hospitals.

It is worth noting that in a comparison of randomized versus nonrandomized studies of antireflux surgery, the symptomatic improvement remains the same, whereas the complications reported for individual patients of the randomized group were higher. Nevertheless, few of these complications were of any major significance, and no deaths were reported. The postoperative problems most often reported include dysphagia, gas bloat, and flatulence. Those individuals who fail to benefit from antireflux surgery may, under certain circumstances, return for further surgical intervention. Although accurate data are difficult to collect in this group, it is evident that the reoperative (for the most part by open procedure) complication rates in such patients are significantly higher and the mortality substantially increased. Thus, surgical therapy carries an initial morbidity and mortality, and reoperative surgical intervention substantially amplifies this problem. This should be contrasted with failure of medical therapy, which is not associated with such grave consequences.

A recent prospective randomized trial by Spechler of medical and surgical antireflux treatments in 247 patients with complicated GERD to evaluate the

Laparoscopic Antireflux Surgery

Author	Year	No.	Improve (%)	Complications Intra op	Complications Post op	Mortality
Cuschieri A	1993	116	91	14.0	1.3	0
Gooszen HG	1993	62	73	8.0	?	0
Geogan T	1994	59	100	minimum		0
Jamieson GG	1994	155	99	1.9	1.9	0.6
Hallerback B	1994	60	90	6.7	0	0
Hinder R	1994	198	97	3.5	2.5	0.5
Pitcher DE	1994	70	100	8.6	4.3	0
Anvari M	1995	168	100	1.2	2.4	0
Cadiere GB	1995	162	98	2.5	1.8	0
Coster DD	1995	52	90	11.5	5.8	0
Dallemagne B	1995	368	90	4.0		0
McKeman JB	1995	283	100	3.5		0
Patti MG	1995	68	98	2.9	1.5	0
Watson DI	1995	230	98	3.0	2.6	0.4
Bell RCW	1996	102	excellent	3.9	2.9	0
DePaula AL	1996	110	94	2.7	2.7	0
Galloway GQ	1996	207	96	4.0		0
Samas G	1996	79	92	2.5	2.5	0
Paluzzi MW	1997	99	96	3.9		0
Collet D	1997	123	91	4.9	4.9	0.8
Ritter DW	1997	78	86			
Fingerhut A	1997	133	96	4.5	10.5	0
Laine S	1997	55	100	9.0		0
Alexander HC	1997	54	98	13.0		
Cordiere GB	1997	224	84	2.2	1.8	
Kiviluoto T	1998	200	98	5.0		0
Frantzides CT	1998	362	96	7.0		
Landrenean RJ	1998	150	94	1.3	3.3	0
Dallemagne B	1998	622	92	2.3		0
Lefebvre JC	1998	100	93	4.0	1.0	0
Rothenberg S	1998	220	excellent	2.6	7.3	0
Leggett PL	1998	138	excellent	10.9	1.5	0
Althar R	1999	100	100	2.0		0
Dick AC	1999	50	excellent	8.0		0
Zaninotto G	2000	621	92	2.9	7.3	0
Kiil J	2001	100	91	3	2.0	0
Allal H	2001	142	excellent	0.5	2.0	0
Finley CR	2001	557	excellent	0.4	1.3	0.2
Ray S	2002	310	97	0	3.2	0
Pimpalwar A	2002	54	83	5.6	16.7	0
Pessaux P	2002	1470	94	2.1	2.9	0.1
Granderath FA	2003	668	89	0.6	7.6	0

A summation of published data on the results of laparoscopic antireflux surgery (1/1/2003, I.M. Modlin).

A summation of the reported complications of laparoscopic antireflux surgery (1/1/2003, I.M. Modlin).

Complications of Laparoscopic Antireflux Surgery

SURGICAL	Range (%)	Mean (%)
Esophageal or gastric perforation	0 - 5.1	1.24
Hepatic lesion	0 - 1.0	0.6
Splenic lesion	0 - 6.9	1.66
Splenectomy	0 - 1.7	0.54
Inadvertent vagotomy	0 - 6.3	0.6
Wound infection	0 - 4.4	1.34
Incisional hernia	0 - 1.9	0.37
Intraperitoneal, mediastinal abscess	0 - 1.9	0.41
Herniation into chest	0 - 1.0	0.23
Severe stricture	0 - 1.0	0.2
Post-operative bleeding	0 - 3.4	0.6
Non Surgical	1.2-11.4	4.3

n = 3,874 patients (26 studies)

long-term outcome of medical and surgical therapies provided some interesting insights. The mean (median) duration of follow-up was 10.6 years (7.3 years) for medical patients and 9.1 years (6.3 years) for surgical patients. Two hundred thirty-nine (97%) of the original 247 study patients were identified (79 were confirmed dead). Among the 160 survivors (157 men and three women; mean age, 67 ± 12 years), 129 (91 in the medical treatment group and 38 in the surgical treatment group) participated in the follow-up. Eighty-three (92%) of 90 medical patients and 23 (62%) of 37 surgical patients reported that they used antireflux medications regularly (p <.001). During a 1-week period after discontinuation of medication, mean (SD) GRACI symptom scores were significantly lower in the surgical treatment group [82.6 (17.5) versus 96.7 (21.4) in the medical treatment group; p = .003]. It is of considerable relevance that no significant differences between the groups were found in grade of esophagitis, frequency of treatment of esophageal stricture and subsequent antireflux operations, Medical Outcomes Short Form-36 standardized physical and mental component scale scores, and overall satisfaction with antireflux therapy. Survival during a period of 140 months was decreased significantly in the surgical treatment group (relative risk of death in the medical group, 1.57; 95% confidence interval, 1.01–2.46; p = .047), largely because of excess deaths from heart disease. Patients with Barrett's esophagus at baseline developed esophageal adenocarcinomas at an annual rate of 0.40%, whereas these cancers developed in patients without Barrett's esophagus at an annual rate of only 0.07%. There was no significant difference between groups in incidence of esophageal cancer. Spechler and his colleagues concluded that antireflux surgery should not be advised with the expectation that patients with GERD will no longer need to take antisecretory medications or that the procedure will prevent esophageal cancer among those with GERD and Barrett's esophagus.

Pros and cons of surgery

There remains some controversy as to the use and efficacy of surgery, given the fact that GERD is an essentially benign disease for which safe and effective medical therapy is available. Proponents of surgery argue against life-long drug therapy, whereas opponents perseverate about substantial morbidity, learning curve issues, unpredictable outcome, and even mortality. The precise role of surgery should be considered within the "known" parameters of the causes of GERD. Thus, the most important aspect of the pathophysiology of GERD is the competency of the antireflux barrier and the factors that contribute to its integrity. These include the LES pressure, the occurrence of transient LES relaxations, and the presence or absence of a hiatal hernia. In addition, an LES pressure of less than 6 mm Hg, LES length less than 2 cm, and intraabdominal length less than 1 cm are usually associated with GERD. The relationship with hiatus hernia reflects the role of the crural diaphragm, which contributes substantially to the integrity of the LES. In individuals with a hiatal hernia, the spatial relationship of the crural diaphragm and the LES is altered, and as a result, sphincter competence is diminished. Other factors, such as transient LES relaxation at the time of a reflux episode, poor esophageal clearance, and delayed gastric emptying may play a variable role in contributing to the severity of GERD in certain individuals. Those who advocate surgical relief of GERD maintain that antireflux surgery is the only available therapy that reliably increases LES pressure and LES length, decreases the frequency of TLESRs, and corrects the hiatal hernia. Furthermore, there exist several studies that purport to demonstrate that antireflux surgery may improve esophageal motility and speed gastric emptying. The crux of the problem is that, overall, individuals with GERD have a poor quality of life, and that after laparoscopic fundoplication, the quality of life improves and becomes comparable to that of healthy individuals. Indeed, patients with severe gastroesophageal reflux have an extremely low quality of life, as assessed by the Medical Outcomes Short Form-36, equivalent to a control population with congestive heart failure, and several studies demonstrate that these scores consistently increase to that of a control population of healthy volunteers after antireflux surgery.

In further support of the surgical argument, there are numerous studies that demonstrate the efficacy of antireflux surgery. A report by Peters of 100 patients with positive 24-hour pH studies and "typical" symptoms of GERD who underwent antireflux surgery reported relief of the primary symptom of GERD in 96% followed for a mean of 21 months. Thus, 71 were asymptomatic, three had gastrointestinal symptoms requiring medical therapy, and two were worsened by the procedure. Clinically significant complications occurred in only four patients, and dysphagia was present in only two patients 1 year after surgery. This study, however, represents the apogee of surgical reports in that it documents patients who are the ideal candidates for antireflux surgery undertaken by highly skilled and experienced surgeons and is thus representative of the best results possible.

An issue not addressed by this study, however, is the question of the longevity of the surgery. In fact, there is a paucity of studies on the long-term durability of laparoscopic antireflux surgery, and only a few have examined patient status at 5 years of follow-up. Hinder, in 2001, reported a series that provided data at a mean of 6.4 years after surgery on 171 of 291 patients who had undergone an LNF. Overall, 96.5% of patients were satisfied with the result of the procedure, although many patients were experiencing symptoms. Thus, 14% remained on continuous PPI therapy; 6% had chest pain, heartburn, and regurgitation; 20% had abdominal bloating; 12% had diarrhea; and 27% had dysphagia, with 7% requiring esophageal dilation. In addition, to evaluate their status, 21% required either endoscopy or a barium swallow, or both, postoperatively. The majority of patients on PPIs was, surprisingly, using the drug to relieve abdominal discomfort and was reported as free of heartburn. In this respect, the 1998 report of de Beaux noted in a study of 312 patients that many of the so-called postfundoplication sequelae clearly predated the surgical repair. Thus, in their report, although antireflux surgery was noted to decrease the symptoms of heartburn, epigastric pain, regurgitation, bloating, dysphagia, odynophagia, nausea, vomiting, diet restriction, nocturnal coughing, and wheezing, it was also associated with a significant increase in inability to belch, diarrhea, and passage of flatus. In a monumental series of more than 10,000 patients assembled from the surgical literature by Carlson and Frantzides in 2001, they concluded that the overall success rate, as defined by Visick I or II grades, was greater than 90%. The average follow-up period for published series, however, was shorter than 2 years.

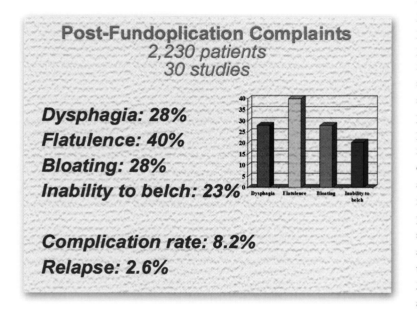

Postfundoplication complaints after a total fundoplication. The ranges for each of these parameters are as follows: dysphagia, 0% to 71%; flatulence, 30% to 60%; bloating, 1% to 38%; and inability to belch, 4% to 80%. The ranges for the complication and relapse rates were 1.9% to 26.0% and 0% to 8.6%, respectively. (Adapted from Lundell L. Anti-reflux surgery in the laparoscopic era. *Baillieres Best Pract Res Clin Gastroenterol* 2000;14:793-810.)

Antireflux surgery has been performed for more than 50 years to relieve symptoms of GERD yet, despite the development of better medical therapy for GERD, the number of adult antireflux procedures performed in the United States more than doubled from 11,000 per year in 1985 to 25,000 in 1997. Not surprisingly, this amplification of the use of the technique was coincident with the introduction of laparoscopic surgery. It would not be unreasonable, however, to note that, despite a huge increase in surgery, the population-level frequency of adverse events after antireflux procedures and its relationship to surgical experience has not been well studied.

In 2002, Flum reported the nationwide frequency of major adverse outcomes in antireflux surgery using two parallel retrospective, population-based cohort studies based on the Washington State discharge and the United States Health Care Utilization Project (HCUP) database. The frequencies of case fatality, splenectomy, and esophageal injury were measured, as well as the relationship of adverse outcomes to the cumulative number of procedures performed by a given surgeon in case order. Overall, an estimated 86,411 patients underwent antireflux surgery between 1992 and 1997, with associated splenectomy in 2.3%, esophageal laceration in 1.1%, and in-hospital death in 0.8%. Of particular note was the observation that adverse events were significantly more likely when procedures at case order less than or equal to 15 (median) were compared with those at case order greater than 15. Flum noted that as the case order increased by 1, the risk of death decreased by 1.7% ($p = .001$), and the risk of splenectomy and injury repair decreased by 1.6% ($p = .001$). Conversely, if the adverse event were examined based on inexperience at a case order of less than 15, the odds of splenectomy were 2.7 times, esophageal laceration repair 2.3 times, and death 5.6 times greater than the odds of adverse outcomes for procedures performed at later case orders. These data confirmed previous suggestions that, although morbidity and mortality associated with antireflux surgery performed in the 1990s was quite low, it was substantially higher than suggested by individual case series mostly published by experienced surgeons in centers of excellence. The observation that surgical experience with the procedure was linked to better outcomes provided no dramatic revelation but formally confirmed a widespread belief.

In terms of decision making, the final argument might be considered to lie within the comparison of the two modes of therapy, namely, surgical and medical. Indeed, the most impressive studies in favor of antireflux surgery are those that compare the two modalities. Thus, Allgood and Bachman, in 2000, published a systematic review of six randomized trials and three cohort studies published between 1966 and 1999 and reported improved objective outcomes in five of six randomized trials and in two of three cohort studies after surgical therapy compared with medical treatment. Similarly improved subjective outcomes, including symptoms and patient satisfaction, were more common among surgical patients in all but one study that assessed them. To date, the two largest published studies are Spechler's VA Cooperative Study and Lundell's Nordic study, both of which showed marked superiority of surgical therapy. The former study enrolled patients with complicated GERD in the mid-1980s and demonstrated that surgical therapy was markedly superior to the, albeit limited, medical therapy of the era, namely, H_2 receptor antagonists and metoclopramide. The Lundell study involved 310 patients with erosive esophagitis, of which 155 patients were randomized to continuous PPI (omeprazole) therapy, and 155 were randomized to open antireflux surgery. At 3 and 5 years of follow-up, there were more treatment failures in patients who were randomized to omeprazole treatment. Furthermore, although the study protocol permitted dose adjustment in patients allocated to omeprazole therapy to either 40 or 60 mg daily in case of symptom recurrence, the failure rates still remained in favor of surgery (although not statistically significant), even if the adjustment was considered. Nevertheless, quality-of-life assessment revealed values within normal ranges in both therapy arms during the 5 years.

A further issue that has been used to support the position of surgery has been the notional consideration that antireflux surgery should decrease health care use. A retrospective matched cohort study of Tennessee Medicaid patients compared the costs of medical and surgical treatment for GERD in 1996. The study compared 135 patients who had fundoplication with 250 randomly selected patients from a group of more than 7,000 who were treated medically.

Surgically treated patients used more GERD-related outpatient resources in the 3 months before operation, particularly physician visits and diagnostic testing, whereas the mean number of inpatient days for the fundoplication procedure was 3.2. Overall, surgical treatment led to a 64% reduction in GERD medication use, with no increase in the use of other medical services in the following year. Thus, successful antireflux surgery may be claimed to correct the underlying pathophysiology, improve symptoms, normalize quality-of-life scores, reduce health care use, and produce outcome results that are as good as, if not better than, medical therapy in large comparative trials.

Despite the powerful case that is made by advocates of surgical therapy, there are two significant reasons that have led to powerful opposition to antireflux surgery. The first and dominant one is that more than a decade of medical therapy has led to the widespread acceptance that it is extremely safe, very effective, and well tolerated. The second and most compelling argument put forward by the surgical opposition is that surgical therapy can be associated with serious, albeit rare, complications and even death. Thus, even the most optimistic published surgical series describe some dramatic complications, and even the Peters report, with its 96% improvement rates in the primary symptom of the patients, noted that 2% were worse as a result of the surgery. Although long-term results suggest a satisfaction rate of 96%, as many as 14% of patients require medication postsurgery, and many patients have some gastrointestinal symptoms. Furthermore, much of the surgical data is optimized, because most long-term follow-up data are from a few highly specialized centers. Thus, Carlson and Frantzides demonstrated that the majority of data available for review have a follow-up of less than 2 years. Their analysis of more than 10,000 patients revealed a perioperative complication rate of approximately 5.0%, with a mortality rate of 0.08%. Of particular relevance was the observation that the need for reoperation ranged from 2% to 6% and was actually increasing toward the end of the 1990s. A most significant report by Vakil in 2001 documented the experiences of a community-based group and reported a 57.0% satisfaction rate, a 67.0% rate of development of new postoperative symptoms, and a 6.7% reoperation rate at 1 year. Such data are particularly worrisome, because they may in actuality represent the real options for most American patients who are not able to attend centers of excellence where surgeons with substantial experience are available. Given the overall safety, ease of delivery, and efficacy of PPI therapy, a surgical complication rate greater than 0% may justifiably be considered unacceptable. It is worthy of note that at the turn of the century (2000), Hogan and Shaker, gastroenterologists possessed of considerable esophageal experience and judgment, noted with serious concern, "*an esophagus disabled by an inappropriate or dysfunctional fundoplication wrap is a terrible price to pay for control of acid reflux.*"

Arguments have been made that the two large, randomized series showing "superior" results with antireflux surgery may also be interpreted as being in favor of medical therapy. Thus, in the Lundell Nordic study that randomized 310 patients with erosive esophagitis to omeprazole therapy or to open antireflux surgery, at 3 and 5 years of follow-up, surgical therapy was far superior to omeprazole, 20 mg daily. This difference disappeared, however, when patients were allowed to increase the dose of the omeprazole in accordance with what is perceived to be the standard of care. Furthermore, there were no significant differences in costs or quality-of-life measures. Similarly, the initial report on the Spechler VA Cooperative study that showed marked superiority of surgical therapy over medical therapy was altered on subsequent review. Thus, follow-up for at least 10 years on the 247 patients in this trial revealed that no significant differences could be identified between the groups in the grade of esophagitis, frequency of treatment of esophageal stricture and subsequent antireflux operations, Medical Outcomes Short Form-36 standardized physical and mental component scale scores, and overall satisfaction with antireflux therapy. Of particular interest was the observation that more than 60% of the surgically treated patients required medical therapy. A notable observation was the fact that death from heart disease significantly decreased survival in the surgical group compared with the medical treatment group. Of further relevance was the fact that although nearly half of the patients in this study had Barrett's esophagus at the time of enrollment, there was no significant difference between groups in incidence of esophageal cancer after 10 to 13 years.

Although it is commonly believed that patients having laparoscopic surgery have comparable success rates at lower costs, with lower morbidity and mortality compared with the open procedure, there are at least two studies that refute this position. Sipponnen reported that in Finland over a 10-year period (1986–1997), of the 5,502 antireflux operations performed, 43 fatal complications occurred. Furthermore, the serious complication rate was twice as high with laparoscopic fundoplication compared with open fundoplication. In addition to this disconcerting report was the Dutch experience detailed by Bais, which documented the termination of the only multicenter randomized trial to compare laparoscopic with open Nissen fundoplication because of the high incidence of complications (mostly dysphagia in the laparoscopic group). Although this study was resoundingly criticized by surgeons who have claimed that the trialists were inexperienced in laparoscopic fundoplication, the antisurgery group has been vocal in maintaining that this is precisely the issue and that the results of surgery are clearly not as good in less experienced hands.

A further issue held against surgery is that, historically, antireflux surgery has been recommended for patients with refractory or complicated disease, and in this group, the results are not as good. Thus, it is well accepted that individuals with Barrett's esophagus generally have the poorest surgical success rates, which may range from 40% to 92%. Furthermore, some studies have reported that reoperation is more likely in patients with Barrett's esophagus (6% to 8%) compared with controls (approximately 2%). The consideration that surgical therapy may decrease the development of dysplasia and esophageal cancer is based largely on the fact that cancer rates in such studies were lower than expected; this claim has not been supported by any rigorous data. Indeed, counterargument studies by both Sampliner and Richter demonstrated comparable data for patients in surveillance programs on PPI therapy. The overall opinion among most is that surgery for Barrett's esophagus should not be considered based on any expectation that antireflux surgery will decrease the risk of the development of esophageal cancer.

The question of considering surgery for stricture management has produced some interesting debate. Although it has long been accepted that GERD can culminate in esophageal stricture by causing chronic fibrosis and scarring in response to prolonged esophageal acid exposure, more recently, it has been suggested that NSAIDs play a role in stricture formation. It is of note that medical therapy with PPIs markedly improves dysphagia and lessens dilation requirements in 94% of patients, although it is evident that successful antireflux surgery also decreases the need for further dilation. Nevertheless, experience suggests that stricture patients generally have poorer surgical success rates than do uncomplicated patients (70% compared to 91%). Thus, although there are no ideal comparative studies, it is generally accepted that therapy with a PPI and intermittent dilation is as good as or better than surgical therapy.

In summary, it seems that, given the safety of PPI therapy, even the small risk of surgery is not justifiable in patients with uncomplicated GERD that has responded to medical therapy. Furthermore, complicated GERD, which in the past was almost an automatic indication for antireflux surgery, may need to be more carefully considered in patients who are comfortable and well managed with medical therapy.

Symptoms and healing

It has been established that elevation of the pH in the esophagus leads to healing of esophagitis and that this healing is almost linearly related to the level of pH reached and the duration of the elevated pH. The relationship to symptomatology is an additional feature that requires clarification. Numerous clinical studies have defined the relative efficacy of the various treatment choices by comparison of rates of healing at specific but arbitrary time intervals. In these studies, the results of healing did not reflect a true rate but rather represented a proportion of those healed as compared to those treated at any given time. The two medications that might both heal esophagitis completely achieve the same healing proportion of 100%, although one medication might heal in 4 weeks and the other takes 12 weeks or longer. Thus, the true rate or speed at which healing occurs is considerably different. It is evident that the

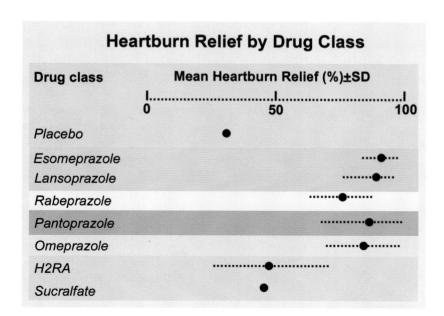

A metaanalysis of the rate of symptom relief in esophagitis compared to the class of drug used for therapy.

greater the severity of the esophagitis, the less effective are H_2 receptor antagonists. Metaanalytic studies of acid-suppression data support the statement that healing of erosive GERD and the healing proportions are directly related to the degree and duration of acid suppression. Nevertheless, to the patient, the proportions of individuals who are healed are less important than the speed at which healing takes place. The healing rate may be determined by the slope of a healing time curve and can be assessed as the percentage of erosive esophagitis healed per unit of time. By comparison of such information, the speed of healing and the speed of symptom relief may be deduced, thus providing information relevant to both patient and physician. Overall, the PPIs provide the highest healing proportion ($83.6\% \pm 11.4\%$) irrespective of drug dose and duration of therapy. Other drug classes, especially sucralfate, showed inconsistent healing. The H_2 receptor antagonists provided an overall healing proportion of $51.9\% \pm 17.1\%$. There appeared to be little therapeutic gain obtained with using higher dosages of H_2 receptor antagonists, even if the higher dose levels were given for as long as 12 weeks. Indeed, in comparison with PPIs, H_2 receptor antagonists' healing rates were still significantly lower than those observed with PPIs even after shorter (6 weeks) duration. Nevertheless, it was evident that the efficacy of H_2 receptor antagonists can be improved up to a point; however, this requires four-times-daily dosing, significant compliance, and substantial increases in costs. In this respect, the great efficacy and once-daily dosage of the PPI therapy appeared more satisfactory.

With regard to speed of healing, it is apparent that PPIs heal at a rate approximately twice as fast as H_2 receptor antagonists at all time points, and the largest gain in efficacy is evident early in the treatment period. As the duration of therapy becomes prolonged, the larger proportion of esophagitis patients are healed, and the speed of healing decreases, because there are fewer patients left to be healed. Nevertheless, even at this component of the time sequence, PPIs maintain a significant advantage. It is estimated that PPI patients healed at an average rate of $11.7\% \pm 0.5\%$ per week, which is almost twice as fast as H_2 receptor antagonists, which heal at $5.9\% \pm 0.2\%$ per week, and is four times faster than placebo healing rates of $2.9\% \pm 0.2\%$ per week. It is likely that the more prolonged and greater degree of acid suppression established by PPIs is responsible for the greatest speed of healing.

Of importance is the observation that H_2 receptor antagonists are less effective than PPIs in the management of grade II disease than has been previously proposed. Thus, the concept of H_2 receptor antagonists being more useful in lower-grade levels of esophagitis remains unsubstantiated. Also of note is the fact that in the patients studied with peptic strictures, the necessity for repeat dilatation and reports of greater relief of dysphagia further support the use of PPIs as compared to H_2 receptor antagonists, even at the higher grades of esophagitis. Thus, in terms of acute healing of esophagitis, therapeutic targeting of a greater and more sustained pH elevation is clearly achieved by the PPI class of drugs and is clearly more effective than H_2 receptor antagonists. Because in a substantial proportion of patients, especially those with erosive esophagitis, recurrence is common, the issue of maintenance therapy is of considerable relevance. In this respect, a number of studies using different PPIs have demonstrated that maintenance of esophagitis healing is consistently superior when compared to H_2 receptor antagonists.

From the patients' point of view, however, the issue of symptom relief may, in the short term, be more critical than the issue of healing. In this respect, studies of PPI-treated patients demonstrate a significantly greater overall proportion of patients free of heartburn at the end of the study and nearly twice as many as noted with individuals receiving H_2 receptor antagonists. It is apparent that the speed of healing and the rate of symptom relief are closely correlated. Thus, in PPI-treated patients, the speed of heartburn relief was 30.7% ± 7.5% patients per week, becoming asymptomatic by week 2. This was approximately twice as fast as identified in patients treated with H_2 receptor antagonists. The rate of symptom relief declined for both classes of drugs with longer duration of treatment, as the increments of patients who were still symptomatic became smaller. Thus, by week 2, 58% ± 16.9% of PPI-treated patients were heartburn free, and 63.4% ± 6% of such patients were healed. It is thus apparent that healing rates correlate almost directly with symptom relief. Analysis of symptom-relief studies using linear regression analysis has demonstrated that PPIs provide the fastest overall rate of symptom relief (11.5% ± 0.8% per week), which is almost twice as fast as that detected with H_2 receptor antagonists. Of relevance, however, is the fact that the slopes of symptom relief time curves are comparable to the slopes of the healing time curves for both PPIs and H_2 receptor antagonists. This would suggest that symptom relief and healing occur in parallel. In studies that use scoring systems to grade symptoms, it was evident that more complete heartburn relief occurred with PPIs as compared to H_2 receptor antagonists. Thus, at the termination of such studies, more than 50% of the patients who had received H_2 receptor antagonists persisted with mild to moderate heartburn even after 8 weeks of treatment, whereas after 4 weeks, only 18.4% of patients still had residual mild to moderate heartburn if treated with PPIs. The PPI class of drugs, therefore, appears not only to provide patients with more complete heartburn relief but also to facilitate its occurrence in a more rapid fashion.

Atypical gastroesophageal reflux disease manifestations

Despite the fact that the majority of patients with GERD present with heartburn and its constellation of related symptoms, an ever-increasing percentage exhibits an atypical symptom complex. The initial group that was recognized was those with atypical or noncardiac chest pain. A second group of ever-increasing prevalence is composed of individuals, often children, who exhibit asthma-like symptoms. A third group comprises individuals with a diversity of ear, nose, and throat (ENT) complaints, of which laryngitis may be the most common and often misinterpreted presenting complaint.

Noncardiac chest pain

It has been estimated that between 20% and 30% of individuals undergoing coronary angiography for chest pain have normal studies. This group of individuals has been designated as suffering from chest pain of noncardiac origin. In 40% to 45% of this group, acid reflux has been identified, and episodes of chest pain can be correlated with reflux episodes. In some circumstances, albeit rarely, both coronary artery disease and reflux may occur in the same individual and require both Holter and pHmetry monitoring for identification.

Conditions Associated with GERD

Disease	Putative Mechanism
Hiatal Hernia	LES function disorganized
Obesity	Increased Intra-abdominal pressure
Laryngitis, hoarseness	Acid reflux material; vagal reflex
Chronic obstructive pulmonary disease	Aspiration of reflux contents; smoking delays gastric emptying; decreased LES pressure
Coronary artery disease	Treatment with nitrates and calcium antagonists, which decrease the LES pressure; detection bias with chest pain evaluation
Diabetes	Delayed gastric emptying (autonomic neuropathy)
Duodenal ulcer	Detection bias of upper gastrointestinal endoscopy
Pregnancy	Increased intra-abdominal pressure; decreased LES tone by estrogens
Rheumatoid arthritis	Treatment with NSAIDs resulting in erosive esophagitis and stricture; possibly also impaired peristalsis
Degenerative joint disease	NSAIDs
Sicca syndrome	Impaired salivation; diminished clearance of reflux contents; secretion of epidermal growth factor diminished
Systemic sclerosis, CRST syndrome	Impaired peristalsis and decreased clearance of reflux material
Mental retardation	Unknown neural regulation of LES impaired or incoorinate peristalsis and decreased clearance of reflux
Achalasia (post-myotomy)	Myotomy or dilation; disruption of LES barrier to reflux
Zollinger-Ellison syndrome	Increased acid output; increased LE acid load

A variety of conditions have been associated with GERD. In not all of the circumstances is the nature of the relationship clear.

In the past, the acid infusion or Bernstein test was used to confirm the diagnosis, but for the most part, this has proven to be relatively insensitive and has been superseded by the use of esophageal pH monitoring. Once the diagnosis has been confirmed, treatment with PPIs has been shown to be effective in up to 85% of patients. In some centers, individuals have undergone fundoplication, with comparable resolution of symptomatology.

Asthma

Although the association between asthma and a distended stomach was first remarked on more than 100 years ago by Sir William Osler, it is only recently that the relationship between GERD and asthma has become well-defined. Asthmatics have an increased frequency of GERD, with a prevalence that varies between 34% and 89%. Because as many as 20% of adults may experience intermittent bronchospasm, the potential benefits of identifying a subgroup of patients whose disease is initiated by GERD is of considerable clinical relevance.

It is likely that at least two mechanisms are operative in the interface between GERD and asthma. The most commonly accepted cause is microaspiration of gastric contents. Alternatively, it has been suggested that a vagally mediated reflex exists whereby acid reflux into the lower esophagus initiates bronchoconstriction via a shared autonomic innervation between the esophagus and the bronchi based on their common embryonic origin. Support for the latter proposal is based on two lines of evidence. First, acid infusion of the esophagus in asthmatic children results in increased airway resistance, which can be reversed with antacids. Second, the infusion of antacids into the distal esophagus of asthmatic children during sleep induces bronchoconstriction, suggesting the presence of a protective mechanism.

The possible relationship between acid reflux and GERD can be established by the use of a barium esophagogram, upper gastrointestinal endoscopy, and esophageal manometry. By far the most useful, however, is pH monitoring, because increased acid reflux can be identified in more than 50% of asthmatics and may occur in 70% to 80%. In approximately 50% of wheezing episodes, no relationship to reflux can be established, indicating that many other factors are involved in the genesis of asthma even if acid reflux is involved.

The best management of asthma-related GERD involves aggressive acid suppression with PPIs, which not only significantly reduce the asthmatic episodes but also considerably improve pulmonary function in almost 80% of patients. In those individuals who underwent a fundoplication procedure, as many as 75% were cured or improved significantly.

Ear, nose, and throat

This recently recognized association is now understood to be common. Patients may present with hoarseness, chronic cough, throat clearing, chronic laryngitis, globus, vocal cord granulomas, laryngeal or tracheal stenosis, and even carcinoma of the larynx. Only 40% of such individuals may exhibit the typical signs and symptoms of GERD itself. Indeed, in some circumstances, ear, nose, and throat complaints may be the sole manifestation of GERD. Thus, 10% of persistent coughers, 5% to 10% of patients with hoarseness, 25% to 50% of individuals with a globus sensation, and a small number of patients with laryngeal neoplasia exhibit GERD as a primary etiologic factor. The relationship is based on at least four possible mechanisms. First, the presence of a vagally mediated reflex in which acid in the lower esophagus mediates a response that involves chronic repetitive throat clearing and coughing that culminates in laryngeal symptoms and finally lesions. The second involves the deposition of refluxate by aspiration directly onto the laryngeal structures themselves, with ensuing inflammation and damage. A further factor that has been defined is the identification of lower levels of upper esophageal sphincter (UES) pressure in patients with reflux into the pharynx. Third, it is evident that in individuals with esophagopharyngeal reflux, UES pressure decreases significantly at night, potentially leaving the pharynx unprotected from nocturnal esophageal reflux. Fourth, it has been noted that in up to 60% of individuals with persistent ENT symptoms, esophageal motility disorders were evident, with almost 80% exhibiting abnormal acid clearance from the lower esophagus.

Once the ENT diagnosis has been established, the existence of GERD needs to be validated. Prolonged esophageal pH monitoring with a dual pH probe system (one in the hypopharynx or just below the UES and a second probe at the LES) is the most sensitive and specific method for diagnosing GERD-related ENT disease. Proximal pH monitoring is difficult, however, because the probes may dry out or, in the large space, reflux may actually be missed. If the diagnosis is satisfactorily established, long-term administration of PPIs has proven to be the most efficacious method of treating ENT symptoms. Under unusual circumstances, consideration may be given to antireflux surgery.

Economics

One of the most vexatious questions faced by society in dealing with a chronic disease of relatively inexplicable etiology is the issue of cost. Because heartburn affects 7% of the U.S. population daily, and 10% to 15% of Americans have heartburn at least once per week and 36% monthly, the magnitude of the problem is not inconsequential. GERD is thus a common problem, and most patients with erosive GERD require long-term treatment, without which relapse is common. Because the cost of ongoing medical care for GERD is substantial, and patients with symptomatic GERD have impaired quality of life, treatment strategies for GERD should aim to improve patient outcome at a reasonable cost. In addition, because of the chronic nature of GERD, there is not only significant impairment in quality of life and substantial aggregate lifetime treatment costs but also the issue of the overall cost to society. It is therefore mandatory that clinicians choose not only an effective therapy for GERD but one that is also cost conscious and appropriate for the individual patient. In this respect, the use of cost-effectiveness analyses to help determine the most cost-effective therapy for GERD has provided clinicians with the utility of applying the results of these economic analyses to practice settings. The application of cost-effectiveness methodology has facilitated the integration of costs and patient outcomes, thereby providing the clinician with information that allows a choice of the most cost-effective therapy in a variety of clinical circumstances. In this respect, the overview analysis of the subject provided by O'Connor and colleagues provides the best basis for understanding the complexity and importance of an issue that has become of fundamental relevance to all clinicians.

The published studies demonstrate that PPIs are the most cost-effective initial and maintenance medical therapy for GERD under most circumstances. However, variations in drug acquisition costs, such as may occur in managed-care practice settings, have in some circumstances led to H_2 receptor antagonists being preferred. In the long-term management of GERD, laparoscopic surgery is effective, but its high initial cost makes it less cost effective than PPIs in the early treatment years. Also, recent data suggest that the long-term morbidity is higher than previously suspected.

Acute-phase gastroesophageal reflux disease treatment

In 1994, Hillman compared phase I therapy (combined with antacids) to ranitidine, 150 mg twice daily, and omeprazole, 20 mg each day, in patients with persistent GERD for at least 3 years and grade II or worse esophagitis. To account for the complexities of managing these patients in clinical practice, the authors addressed both empirical and nonempirical approaches to treating GERD. In the empirical approach, patients were treated without prior endoscopy or 24-hour esophageal pH testing. In the nonempirical approach, both of these procedures were performed to confirm GERD, and treatment was offered only to those in whom GERD was confirmed. Recurrences were treated with a second course of therapy; patients relapsing on ranitidine, 150 mg twice daily, neither received a higher dose of ranitidine nor crossed over to treatment with omeprazole. In the nonempirical arm, patients with heartburn symptoms but negative 24-hour pH testing and a negative upper endoscopy did not receive any treatment. The analysis was restricted to a 7-month period—4 to 8 weeks of initial treatment and 6 months of follow-up. The study found that, irrespective of whether an empirical or diagnostic approach was taken initially, omeprazole, 20 mg each day, had the lowest cost (approximately $4,900) and the lowest number of symptomatic months (0.2). Omeprazole was the dominant therapy, because it had the lowest cost and the best outcome. Ranitidine cost more than omeprazole but less than antacids and was second in effectiveness, yielding 2.2 symptomatic months out of the 7 months of follow-up.

In 1995, Zagari used a decision-analysis model for the treatment of patients with erosive GERD over a 1-year time horizon. Three initial strategies were compared: (a) lansoprazole, 30 mg each day; (b) cimetidine, 800 mg twice daily; and (c) ranitidine, 300 mg twice daily. The H_2 receptor antagonists were further subdivided into generic versus brand formulations. Patients whose esophagitis healed on lansoprazole, 30 mg each day, received maintenance therapy with 15 mg each day of lansoprazole for the rest of the year. Those who did not respond within 2 months received 30 mg of lansoprazole each day for an additional 2 months. Patients who failed to respond to the prolonged therapy with 30 mg each day, or who experienced a relapse while taking the higher dose, were reevaluated with endoscopy to rule out more serious conditions such as esophageal strictures and Barrett's esophagus. Patients responding to the high-dose H_2 receptor antagonist specified above were maintained on ranitidine, 150 mg twice daily, or cimetidine, 400 mg twice daily. If erosive GERD recurred during the year, they again received high-dose H_2 receptor antagonists, whereas those who had a second recurrence were given lansoprazole, 30 mg each day.

Most of the input data for the model were derived from published literature, whereas drug costs were average at prevailing wholesale prices. The authors performed two analyses: The first was a cost analysis to determine the least costly initial strategy for the treatment of erosive GERD, and the second was a cost-effectiveness analysis examining the incremental cost per treatment failure avoided with PPIs versus H_2 receptor antagonists. Results over the 1-year period showed that the costs of treatment with PPIs and generic H_2 receptor antagonists were $1,192 and $1,152, respectively. Branded H_2 receptor antagonists were the most expensive, at $1,495. However, the H_2 receptor antagonists were considerably less effective than pump inhibitors. For example, healing rates at the end of 1 year were 80% for patients who received PPIs as initial treatment versus 15% for patients who received H_2 receptor antagonists. The incremental cost-effectiveness ratio of PPIs as compared to receptor antagonists indicated that PPIs cost $36 to avert one additional treatment failure. A weakness of this study is the fact that the time horizon was limited to 1 year, which is a short time horizon considering that erosive GERD is a chronic condition.

Bloom, in 1995, gathered economic data in a single, blind, randomized controlled trial comparing omeprazole, 20 mg each day, to ranitidine, 150 mg each day, plus metoclopramide, 10 mg four times daily, in 184 patients with erosive esophagitis. Esophagitis was verified by endoscopy before entry into the trial. Healing was confirmed by endoscopy at the end of 4 weeks and, if necessary, at the end of 8 weeks of treatment. Patients kept a daily symptom diary and also recorded the numbers and types of medical services used outside those required by the protocol and direct nonmedical costs, such as meals outside the home, parking fees, and patient and spouse time lost from work because of the illness. Cost for services rendered as part of the trial were derived from mean payments from two large private insurers in the United States. Drug costs were obtained from a survey of actual consumer payments at the time of dispensing. The perspective of the study was that of the payer (insurer). At 8 weeks, 81.5% of the omeprazole group had healed versus 45.7% of the ranitidine/metoclopramide group. Omeprazole patients had 19.6 symptom-free days versus 13.5 symptom-free days in the combination therapy group—a 31% difference. Mean gastroenterology-related costs were $154.52 in the omeprazole group versus $145.91 in the ranitidine/metoclopramide group. The average cost per patient healed was $189.60 in the omeprazole group versus $319.28 in the ranitidine/metoclopramide group. Finally, the incremental cost per extra symptom-free day associated with the use of omeprazole compared to ranitidine/metoclopramide was $1.41.

Maintenance treatment of gastroesophageal reflux disease

Medical therapy comparison

Harris, in 1997, compared three maintenance treatment strategies (lansoprazole, 15 mg each day; ranitidine, 150 mg twice daily; and ranitidine, 300 mg twice daily) in patients with erosive esophagitis after initial healing. The perspective adopted was that of the health care system, which included all health-related costs but excluded indirect costs, such as time lost from work. The model followed a hypothetical cohort of patients for 1 year. Patients who had a recurrence on maintenance ranitidine were treated with lansoprazole, 15 mg per day, whereas further recurrences were treated by increasing the dose of lansoprazole to 30 mg per day and, finally, 45 mg per day. The model assumed that no patients would recur on lansoprazole, 45 mg per day, and recurrence rates on lansoprazole were derived from a single randomized controlled trial whose outcome variable was endoscopic recurrence of esophagitis. However, the authors appropriately noted that symptomatic recurrences, rather than endoscopic recurrences, are more often measured in everyday clinical practice. Endoscopic recurrences were therefore transformed into symptomatic recurrences using an expert panel, which "estimated" that 81% of endoscopic recurrences would also be symptomatic. Nonpharmacologic cost inputs for the model were derived from Medicare resource-based relative-value scale for physician fees, whereas input values for drug costs varied from average wholesale price, representing fee-for-service setting costs at the upper end to managed care costs at the lower end.

The results of the study were reported under two practice scenarios: (a) the average wholesale price of drugs and (b) managed-care cost of drugs. The study concluded that, in most situations, high-dose H_2 receptor antagonists are more costly and less effective than lansoprazole. The authors did not measure quality of life in reflux patients but used sensitivity analysis to assess the impact of decreased quality of life on the absolute and relative cost effectiveness of each of the treatment strategies. Under managed-care costs, a quality-of-life decrement of only 1.4% was associated with PPIs being the preferred treatment option, whereas under government drug procurement costs, an 18.2% decrement in quality of life was needed before PPIs became more cost-effective.

Intermittent versus continuous therapy

Stalhammar (1993) constructed a model comparing two strategies in patients with reflux esophagitis. All patients began the model in remission and either received or did not receive maintenance omeprazole therapy. In the maintenance-therapy group, patients were given omeprazole, 20 mg each day, and relapses were treated with 40 mg each day. In the intermittent strategy, no maintenance therapy was given initially, but relapses were treated with 20 mg each day. Patients who were not healed after 8 weeks received 40 mg each day. Patients could transition from a healed to a nonhealed state on a monthly basis and were followed over a 1-year time horizon. Data from the model were obtained from a metaanalysis of clinical trials comparing omeprazole and ranitidine, and all cost data were derived from Sweden. The input values for 28 capsules of omeprazole, 20 mg; 60 tabs of ranitidine, 150 mg; and a physician office visit were USD $84.00, USD $51.54, and USD $83.60, respectively. The clinical outcome measure in the model was the number of healthy (symptom-free) days. A 5% annual discount rate was applied to both costs and benefits. The model was analyzed both with and without allowance for indirect costs. Results of the model indicate that continuous maintenance therapy yielded 353 healthy days (maximum, 365). Intermittent therapy yielded only 290 healthy days—63 fewer healthy days. When direct costs only were considered, the maintenance therapy cost USD $1,063, and the intermittent therapy cost USD $762. Therefore, the incremental cost-effectiveness ratio of continuous compared with intermittent maintenance therapy was USD $4.77 per additional healthy day. When indirect costs were included, the incremental cost-effectiveness ratio fell to USD $1.90 per additional healthy day. Because Swedish drug costs are lower than in the United States, the model has limited application to practice in the United States. Nonetheless, it supports the cost effectiveness of common clinical practice using continuous rather than intermittent maintenance for erosive reflux esophagitis.

Surgical versus medical therapy

In the treatment of chronic GERD, laparoscopic fundoplication is (probably) as effective as and is less costly than open surgery and has a lower morbidity rate and almost no mortality. Surgery is associated with a substantial initial cost, accruing benefits over the ensuing years with minimal additional costs, making fundoplication an attractive long-term treatment option for some patient subsets.

One of the most comprehensive models comparing long-term medical and surgical therapy for reflux esophagitis was provided by Heudebert in 1997. This paper analyzed the example of a hypothetical middle-aged male with moderate to severe reflux esophagitis. In the model, patients were initially assigned to either LNF or omeprazole and followed for 5 years. Data and probabilities for the maintenance omeprazole treatment were chosen from the 1994 report by Klinkenberg-Knol. Maintenance treatment began with omeprazole, 20 mg each day for most patients, and those who relapsed on 20 mg each day were increased to 40 mg each day for 90 days and, if relapse again occurred at that dose, were increased to 60 mg each day. Patients relapsing on 60 mg each day crossed over to LNF. Costs for medications, office visits, and procedures were derived from reimbursements from Blue Cross/Blue Shield of Alabama. Direct medical costs associated with the evaluation of reflux esophagitis, such as upper endoscopy and 24-hour pH testing, were included. However, indirect costs, such as time lost from work, were not included, because the model's perspective was that of a third-party payer. Because at the time of the study there were no long-term data on the effectiveness of LNF, the authors assumed equal efficacy between open and laparoscopic procedures over a 5-year period. Patients who had a symptomatic recurrence after LNF had the choice of either repeat fundoplication via open approach or medical treatment. The authors assumed that 25% of patients with recurrent symptoms would choose repeat surgery.

Over the 5-year period of the model, LNF generated 4.334 quality-adjusted life years (QALYs), whereas omeprazole generated 4.332 QALYs—a difference of 18 hours. However, the costs were significantly different, with surgery costing USD $9,426, compared to USD $6,043 for omeprazole—a 36% savings. Therefore, the average cost-effectiveness ratio of omeprazole was USD $1,398 per QALY versus $2,186 per QALY for laparoscopic surgery. The incremental benefit in effectiveness of LNF was 0.002 QALYs, at an additional cost of USD $3,383. Therefore, the incremental cost-effectiveness ratio of laparoscopic fundoplication compared to omeprazole therapy was USD $3,383/.002, which is $1.6 million per QALY. The longer the hypothetical patients were followed in the model, the more cost-effective laparoscopic surgery became relative to medical therapy, because the high initial surgery costs were gradually offset over time by lower relapse rates and, thus, lower subsequent costs. However, at 10 years of follow-up, even though the cost of laparoscopic fundoplication and omeprazole were approximately equal, the marginal cost-effectiveness of laparoscopic fundoplication over omeprazole remained high, at USD $300,000 per QALY.

In sensitivity analysis, decreasing the cost of LNF to USD $4,100 from a baseline of USD $7,500 made both strategies cost the same. Increasing the cost of omeprazole to USD $120 per month (baseline = USD $70) also made both strategies comparable in cost. There are some important points to be made concerning the assumptions of this model. First, the authors assumed that all patients were symptom-free after surgery. This also assumes no long-term adverse consequences of surgery, such as gas bloat syndrome or dysphagia. Recent data challenge these assumptions. Any possible decrement in quality of life related to such symptoms is important, because even a small disutility of 0.01 units after surgery has a significant impact on the effectiveness of the surgical strategy. Also, the model is biased toward laparoscopic fundoplication, because the authors did not attempt to model a decline in the cost of omeprazole once its patent expires. In addition, the morbidity, mortality, and efficacy estimates for LNF are derived from tertiary care centers, where skill level is high, whereas community hospital standards may differ.

Nevertheless, this study uses a clinically reasonable algorithm and accounts for a decrement in the quality of life for symptomatic GERD. Of all the available studies, it provides the practitioner with the best, albeit imperfect, assessment of the relative costs and consequences of medical and surgical maintenance therapy for erosive GERD.

Viljakka, in a 1997 Finnish study, compared the lifetime costs of surgical versus medical treatment for severe gastroesophageal reflux. Surgical costs

Table of the base cost effectiveness in USD of different PPI management in GERD. (Adapted from Dean BB, Siddique RM, Yamashita BD, et al. Cost-effectiveness of proton pump inhibitors for maintenance therapy of erosive reflux esophagitis. *Am J Health Syst Pharm* 2001;58:1339–1346.)

Financial Costs - Proton Pump Inhibitors

Management Strategy	Average Cost per Patient ($)	Incremental Cost ($)	Effectiveness (% Symptomatic Recurrences Prevented)	Average Cost-Effectiveness Ratio ($/Symptom Recurrence Prevented)
Rabeprazole	1,414	.....	86	1,637
Lansoprazole	1,671	257	68	2,439
Omeprazole	1,599	185	81	1,968

were derived for both open and LNF and included costs for postoperative complications, such as wound infection and pneumonia. The authors also calculated sick leave and the financial losses due to fatal outcomes. Surgical costs were calculated as the average of costs from three referral centers in Finland. Antireflux surgery was priced at USD $2,609 for laparoscopic fundoplication and USD $2,370 for open fundoplication. Comparative medication costs over 1 year were USD $1,262 for omeprazole, 20 mg each day; USD $537 for ranitidine, 150 mg each day; and USD $1,073 for ranitidine, 300 mg each day. All costs were discounted at 6% per year, and the model was run over the average life expectancy of men and women separately, beginning at various ages, from 20 to 69 years. The cost of ranitidine, 150 mg each day, varied from USD $5,428 in patients aged 65 to 69 years to USD $8,961 in women aged 20 to 24 years. Similarly, the lifetime cost of omeprazole, 20 mg each day, varied from USD $12,758 for women aged 65 to 69 years to a high of USD $20,402 for women aged 20 to 24 years. The total cost for fundoplication, including the operation, time lost from work, and the calculated economic losses from a surgical death, ranged from USD $5,239 to USD $5,872. The authors conclude that treatment with ranitidine, 150 mg each day, was cheaper than surgery in women older than 60 to 64 years and in men older than 55 to 59 years. Lifelong omeprazole therapy at 20 mg each day was never cheaper than surgery. A limitation, from the perspective of practice in the United States, is that the cost of antireflux surgery is considerably lower in Finland than in the United States.

Van den Boom in the Netherlands, in 1996, developed a complex cost-effectiveness model comparing medical and surgical treatment in patients with severe or refractory GERD. The study compared long-term maintenance medical versus surgical therapy in patients with healed reflux esophagitis. Based on a metaanalysis of several studies, they determined that two out of three patients would remain in remission on maintenance therapy with omeprazole, 20 mg each day. Of those relapsing, 80% went into clinical remission on omeprazole, 40 mg each day. However, patients unresponsive to omeprazole, 40 mg each day, were considered resistant to medical maintenance therapy and did not have any additional treatment. The model assigned an effectiveness of 90.5% to Nissen fundoplication. The assigned values for procedural and surgical costs were reimbursements as proxies of true costs. For example, the total costs for surgery, including preoperative endoscopy, manometry pH testing, and follow-up outpatient visits, was USD $6,988—considerably less than comparable costs in the United States. Costs in the medically treated group included both initial and ongoing medication costs, costs of assessing a relapse with endoscopy, and an increased dose of medication. However, the costs for the surgical group were limited to the initial costs of preoperative assessment and surgery itself. The costs were discounted at 6% per year. Analysis of the model found that at 18 months, the cost of omeprazole was the same as that of laparoscopy, whereas open fundoplication cost the same as omeprazole therapy after 4 years.

A more recent study by Romagnuolo addressed the direct medical costs and utilities of laparoscopic fundoplication and long-term treatment with a PPI (omeprazole) for erosive reflux esophagitis using a Markov model calculation. Assuming probabilities over a 5-year time horizon for transitions from one disease state to another, the authors estimated utilities (quality of life and, thus, QALYs) and accumulated direct medical costs (in Canadian dollars) for the medical and surgical treatment options. The base case used was a 45-year-old man with erosive reflux esophagitis refractory to H_2 receptor antagonists who underwent either an LNF fundoplication or long-term treatment with PPIs. For surgical treatment, a number of major assumptions for the base case were made. Thus, the likelihood of performing LNF was 94.2% and conversion to open surgery was assumed to be 5.8%. Costs of LNF surgery were CAD $3,520, including a 1.2-day hospital stay, and CAD $8,069 for open fundoplication, including a 7-day stay. Laparotomy for surgical complications was set at 1.5%. The operative mortality of LNF was assumed to be 0.2% and that of laparotomy 1.4%. The annual rate of failure of fundoplication—that

A simplified analysis of the potential costs involved in GERD management (c. 1998). Although numerous models have been proposed to examine this question, there appears to be no definitive resolution to the question of which particular modality of treatment is most cost effective. Because the costs of surgical therapy and medication vary in different countries, a variety of assumptions are part of all models that have been proposed to assess this question. Furthermore, the cost of the various acid-suppressive medications is constantly decreasing, and some agents are soon due to come off patent. In essence, if one assumes that surgery and medication are equally effective, the fact that medication has few or no cost-related adverse effects suggests that it may be the preferred treatment option. Similarly, because medication has no mortality-related events and no morbidity, costly interventions associated with such clinical scenarios are avoided. The diagonal lines above each operation represent the potential increase in cost generated by a complication. Although laparoscopic procedures are claimed to be more cost effective, their cost is underestimated, because some hospital costs are transferred to home services and often are not included in calculations. In an evolving economic environment, it is likely that the introduction of novel agents will result in the fall of costs with the passage of time.

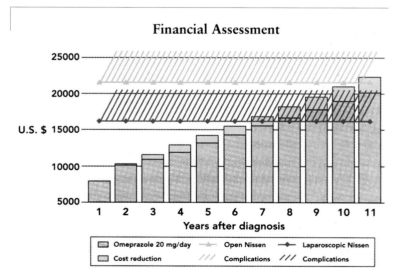

is, recurrence of reflux symptoms requiring the use of medical treatment—was estimated at 1.1%, and it was estimated that one-third of such patients (0.4%) would choose to have repeat surgery. The only long-term complication of fundoplication considered was dysphagia needing dilatation in 1.2%. On medical treatment, rates of healing and recurrence of reflux during treatment were derived from the Klinkenberg-Knol long-term study (1994). In this compassionate-use study of omeprazole, the cumulative healing rate with 40 mg daily was 64% after 1, 82% after 2, 95% after 3, and 99% after 4 months. The current Canadian drug costs were CAD 137.30 for 1 month with a daily dose of 40 mg. Relapse rates during long-term treatment with omeprazole, 20 mg, were taken from the same publication. Treatment of relapse (and subsequent maintenance) was accomplished by increasing the daily PPI dose by 20 mg, with a maximal dose of 60 mg. One-fifth of the patients on 60 mg received fundoplication—that is, 0.6% after 1 year. It appears that there was no dose reduction after healing of relapses, and it is unclear from the description of the methods whether the progress of healing was determined by repeated endoscopies. For calculations of utilities (quality of life), the 5-year total duration of the model was reduced by the time spent at less-than-perfect health, and QALYs were estimated. For instance, regular intake of medication was attributed a utility of 0.99, reflux symptoms 0.935, the 2 postoperative weeks after surgery 0.5, and death 0. For sensitivity analysis, all these values were varied within reasonable ranges. Finally, a Monte Carlo simulation was performed in which all individual input values were randomly varied within these ranges. Cost and utility values were discounted at 3% per annum. Using these base case assumptions, utilities of surgical and medical treatments were very similar, with 4.334 and 4.350 QALYs, respectively. This means that over the period of 5 years, medical treatment "saved" 0.35% of "perfect" time, or approximately 5.5 days. On the other hand, the costs amounted to CAD 3,520 for surgical and CAD 5,465 for medical treatment. This corresponds to an incremental cost of CAD 129,665 per QALY gained. Because in surgical treatment most expenses occur at the beginning, whereas in medical treatment the expenses accumulate nearly linearly over the entire 5-year period, surgical treatment is more expensive at the onset. Equal costs were reached after 3.1 years. The most important contribution to total cost of surgery is, of course, the initial intervention, whereas the expenses of medical treatment are determined mainly by drug costs. For the 5-year time horizon assumed for this calculation, LNF would have to cost at least CAD 5,296 to render it less cost-effective than medical treatment. Conversely, the monthly cost of 20-mg omeprazole would have to be $38.60 at most. However, surgery would become less expensive after 5 years in both instances. Also, increasing the failure rate of surgery up to 10% (instead of 1.1%) would raise the 5-year costs of surgical treatment to CAD 4,030 only, but this would be associated with a dramatic loss of utilities for surgery. Although the authors concluded that LNF was a cost-effective alternative to long-term maintenance therapy with PPIs, the data are clearly subject to critique, given the optimized assumptions made on behalf of the surgical component of the model.

CHAPTER 5
BARRETT'S

Malignant transformation of the esophageal epithelium

As with neoplasia elsewhere, the transformation from normal to a malignant mucosa occurs through a series of morphologic changes accompanied by specific molecular genetic events. The histologic changes in the squamous mucosa exposed to gastroesophageal reflux include an increase in the height of the rete pegs and an increase in the number of cycling epithelial cells. Whether the latter phenomenon is a direct effect of exposure of the gastric contents to the esophageal squamous epithelium or whether it is indirect is not known. Similarly, whether direct damage, including erosions, is necessarily the stimulus for transformation from squamous to columnar epithelium, as in Barrett's esophagus, is not clear. Currently, it is thought that the development of a Barrett's-type mucosa containing gastric, small intestinal, or colonic-type cells often together in the same metaplastic esophageal gland is due to an altered process of differentiation from the pluripotent epithelial stem cells. The presence of abundant growth factors in the esophageal gland system suggests that a process analogous to that described for the UACL system may be implicated in the local repair process. As in many other cancers, p53 mutations and aneuploidy are common in esophageal dysplasia and cancer, and alterations of other molecules, such as cyclins and *rab* proteins, have been described. The precise relevance of such diverse molecular events to the pathobiology of the system is at this stage unclear. Indeed, the sequence of genetic events occurring in esophageal cancer is not as well established as in the colon, although the potential use of these markers for screening purposes and possibly prognostic information is an area of considerable clinical and scientific interest.

SURGERY

VOL. 41   JUNE, 1957   No. 6

Original Communications

THE LOWER ESOPHAGUS LINED BY COLUMNAR EPITHELIUM
N. R. BARRETT, LONDON, ENGLAND

DEFINITIONS

THE ideas discussed here are n[...] statistics nor upon a large collection of specimens; they [...] thinking about a few unusual cases of esophageal disease. [...] rejected or modified in the light of future experiences. [...]ecause I have changed my opinion relating to certain [...]ot static and there is no subject which does not yiel[...] pths are sounded.

This paper concerns [...] is denied by some, misunderstood by others, and [...] surgeons. It has been called a variety of names[...]tory because they have suggested incorrect etiolog[...] short esophagus, ectopic gastric mucosa, short esoph[...]agus lined by gastric epithelium are but a few. At [...]st accurate description is that it is a state in which the [...]hagus is lined by columnar epithelium. This does not com[...]hich could be wrong, but it carries certain implications which [...]rified.

Although Norman Barrett initially proposed that the columnar-lined lower end of the esophagus was stomach, he subsequently revised his view, recognizing that the structure was esophagus that now possessed a columnar lining.

Barrett's esophagus

History

Norman Barrett, in 1950, published a report in the *British Journal of Surgery* in which he defined the esophagus as *"that part of the foregut, distal to the cricopharyngeal sphincter, which is lined by squamous epithelium."* He went on in this article to describe a number of patients who had ulcerations in a tubular, intrathoracic organ that appeared to be the esophagus except that its distal portion was lined extensively by a gastric type of columnar epithelium. Because the esophagus was by definition a squamous-lined structure, Barrett believed that the columnar-lined organ was a tubular segment of stomach generated by traction induced by a congenitally short (squamous-lined) esophagus and tethered within the chest. In this report, Barrett did not identify intestinal features (goblet cells) in the columnar lining of the tubular organ, nor did he raise the question of intestinal metaplasia. This issue was first noted in 1951 by Bosher and Taylor, who commented on the appearance of heterotopic gastric mucosa in the esophagus with ulceration and stricture formation. They noted that "*the gastric mucosa was composed of glands which contained goblet cells but not parietal cells.*"

A year later, Basil Morson, together with Belcher, commented on the relationship of adenocarcinoma of the esophagus and ectopic gastric mucosa. They noted that in an individual with adenocarcinoma, the esophageal mucosa exhibited "*atrophic changes with changes towards an intes-*

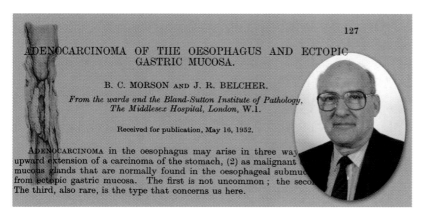

In 1952, in the *British Journal of Cancer*, Morson (right) and Belcher noted that a 56-year-old male patient with adenocarcinoma of the esophageal mucosa exhibited "*atrophic changes with changes towards an intestinal type containing many goblet cells.*" They postulated that the cancer might have arisen from a "congenital abnormality" of the esophagus associated with ectopic gastric mucosa.

tinal type containing many goblet cells." In 1953, Allison and Johnstone proposed that Barrett had misidentified the columnar-lined intrathoracic structure as stomach and that, in reality, it was the esophagus lined with gastric mucous membrane. They noted that, in contrast to the stomach, the structure lacked a peritoneal covering, often harbored islands of squamous epithelium, and possessed some mucosal glands and a muscularis propria characteristic of the esophagus. Thus, 7 years after his original report, Barrett reversed himself and concurred that the columnar-lined organ that he had previously believed to be the stomach was, in fact, the esophagus and suggested that the condition now be called "*lower esophagus lined by columnar epithelium.*" Despite this *volte-face*, the condition to this time remains known as *Barrett's esophagus* and continues to evoke as much confusion as when initially described.

In the first decade of its recognition, most believed that the esophageal columnar lining was congenital in origin but noted a common association with hiatal hernia and severe reflux esophagitis. It remained until 1959 for Moersch and his colleagues to propose that the columnar epithelium was not congenital in origin but acquired as a sequela of reflux esophagitis. Hayward, in 1961, commented on the vulnerability of the squamous epithelium at the site where it joined the gastric epithelium. He felt that it would be liable to digestion at this junctional zone and proposed "*a buffer zone of junctional epithelium which does not secrete acid or pepsin but is resistant to them and has to be interposed.*" For the subsequent 2 decades, the histology of the columnar-lined epithelium remained a controversial issue. Various investigators described an esophagus lined by junctional epithelium, some noted the presence of acid and an acid-secreting fundic type of epithelium, and others described an intestinal type of epithelium with goblet cells. In 1976, Paull clarified the situation in patients with Barrett's esophagus by obtaining biopsy specimens at specified levels throughout the esophagus using manometric guidance.

Using this technique, the distal esophagus was noted to possess a combination of one to three types of columnar epithelia: (a) a junctional type of epithelium, (b) a gastric fundic type of epithelium, and (c) a distinctive type of intestinal metaplasia that was termed *specialized columnar epithelium*. The former two epithelial types were noted to be indistinguishable from the columnar epithelium normally identified in the stomach. However, the specialized intestinal metaplasia with its prominent goblet cells could readily be distinguished from normal mucosa. In addition, the three epithelial types were noted to occupy different zones in the esophagus, with a specialized intestinal metaplasia adjacent to squamous epithelium in the most proximal segment of the columnar lining. The junctional-type epithelium was noted to be present in the most distal esophageal segment, and the gastric fundic–type epithelium was directly adjacent to the columnar mucosa of the stomach, which it joined.

The Histological Evolution of Barrett's Esophagus

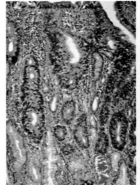
Mild dysplasia

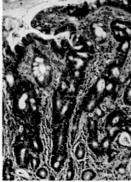
Severe dysplasia

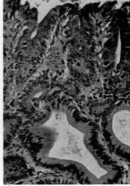
Carcinoma

Continued damage to the lower esophagus over a varying period results in transformation of the cell type and may culminate in neoplasia.

By the 1970s, it was firmly established that the columnar-lined esophagus was often associated with severe GERD. There was controversy as to whether normal esophagus could be lined by columnar epithelium.

Because the association of large hiatal hernias with extensive esophageal inflammation often obscured the endoscopic landmarks of the junction between the esophagus and the stomach, false-positive diagnoses of Barrett's esophagus abounded.

This became a source of considerable concern with the widespread recognition of the relationship between adenocarcinoma and Barrett's esophagus. In the latter instances, the columnar epithelium surrounding the tumor invariably contained specialized intestinal metaplasia that often exhibited dysplasia. The recognition that specialized intestinal metaplasia was the epithelial type that predisposed to dysplasia and cancer development generated a major interest in the biology of this lesion and its early identification.

Current status

The last decade has led to disagreement as to the diagnosis and management of Barrett's esophagus, particularly as it relates to the possible evolution of malignant disease. To a large extent, the issue has been fueled by the extraordinary rise in incidence of adenocarcinoma of the esophagogastric junction and the gastric cardia in particular.

The critical questions that have arisen have not as yet been adequately resolved. Thus, the precise definition of Barrett's esophagus by the identification of the extent of esophageal columnar lining has not been confirmed. Furthermore, problems in defining Barrett's esophagus by the presence of intestinal metaplasia require certainty as regards biopsy sampling sites and histologic identification.

Finally, there exists a considerable degree of confusion with regard to the relationship between the extent of the esophageal columnar lining, specialized intestinal metaplasia, and GERD.

It is apparent, however, that the greater the length or extent of the esophageal columnar lining of the esophagus, the greater the frequency of the finding of intestinal metaplasia. Indeed, the frequency of specialized intestinal metaplasia at the squamocolumnar junction may be said to vary linearly with the extent of columnar epithelium lining the esophagus.

Given the degree of confusion that exists regarding the term *Barrett's esophagus*, an alternative classification that does not rely on arbitrary and imprecise endoscopic measurements has been proposed by Spechler. Thus, when columnar epithelium is detected in the esophagus, regardless of its extent, the condition should be called *columnar-lined esophagus*, as originally proposed by Barrett. Once biopsy samples have been obtained from this esophageal columnar lining, the use of histologic criteria can then be used to classify the condition as either *columnar-lined esophagus with specialized intestinal metaplasia* or *columnar-lined esophagus without specialized intestinal metaplasia*.

This proposal provides considerable improvement in clarity for both physicians and pathologists with regard to the entity under consideration in a particular patient.

Although both conditions may be associated with GERD, the association is variable and appears to be related to the extent of the columnar lining. Thus, individuals with long segments of esophageal columnar lining often exhibit both severe GERD and specialized intestinal metaplasia. Signs and symptoms of GERD, however, may be absent in patients with short segments of columnar lining in the distal esophagus, even when biopsy specimens reveal specialized intestinal metaplasia.

Thus, endoscopic surveillance for adenocarcinoma may be recommended in individuals who have columnar-lined esophagus with intestinal metaplasia, irrespective of the extent, whereas columnar-lined esophagus without specialized intestinal metaplasia does not require endoscopic surveillance.

In the situation in which the distal esophagus appears normal and specialized intestinal metaplasia is identified at the squamocolumnar junction, which does not extend appreciably above the anatomic junction of the esophagus and the stomach, the condition should be called *specialized intestinal metaplasia at the esophagogastric junction*. It has not been established whether this condition is related to GERD, nor is it evident that the risk of cancer applies to patients with this condition.

Complications of Barrett's Esophagus

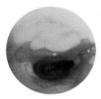 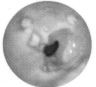

| Barrett Esophagus | Barrett with stricture | Barrett with carcinoma |

The histologic changes in the lining of the lower esophagus are associated with topographic alterations of considerable biologic and clinical importance.

Barrett's esophagus had been identified primarily in patients with the signs and symptoms of GERD and in whom endoscopic examination revealed a long segment of columnar epithelium extending well up into the esophagus. Biopsy specimens taken from the columnar lining usually reveal an unusual form of intestinal metaplasia called *specialized intestinal metaplasia*, and the intestinal lining is invariably evident in the columnar epithelium surrounding Barrett's adenocarcinomas. As a result of such observations, Barrett's esophagus with specialized intestinal metaplasia became recognized as a major risk factor for adenocarcinoma at the gastroesophageal junction. The similar recognition that adenocarcinoma of the gastroesophageal junction was increasing at a dramatic rate in the United States and western Europe led to the development of a high level of interest in the pathology, early identification, and treatment of the condition. Of note is the observation that individuals who undergo esophagectomy for adenocarcinoma at the gastroesophageal junction often do not exhibit endoscopically apparent Barrett's esophagus but more often have short inconspicuous segments of specialized intestinal metaplasia only evident at histologic examination of the specimen. This observation accords well with reports that in 18% of elective endoscopy patients with no evidence of Barrett's esophagus (columnar-lined epithelium less than 3 cm of the distal esophagus), biopsies of the Z line (squamocolumnar junction) revealed specialized intestinal metaplasia. It is evident from this and other similar studies that short inconspicuous segments of specialized intestinal metaplasia can be frequently found at the Z line in predominantly Caucasian populations.

The precise relevance of the metaplasia, however, is not certain. In particular, the question of whether columnar metaplasia develops as a sequela of GERD has not been resolved. Thus, different studies have variously reported (a) an association with GERD symptoms, (b) no association with GERD, (c) no association with endoscopic esophagitis, and (d) an occasional association with histologic esophagitis. Given these inconsistent observations, the traditional concept that intestinal metaplasia develops as a consequence of GERD requires further scrutiny. Similarly, the cancer risk for individuals with short segments of intestinal metaplasia is unknown. Indeed, given the relatively high prevalence rates reported for intestinal metaplasia at the Z line and the infrequency of cancers at this location (irrespective of the rise in incidence), it seems likely that the risk associated with the short segments of specialized intestinal metaplasia is quite small.

Nevertheless, the concerns with regard to neoplasia in relation to GERD and Barrett's esophagus remain a source of concern. In 1990, Cameron and colleagues showed that for every case of Barrett's esophagus in a patient with esophageal cancer, many more are unrecognized.

Clinical Relevance of Barrett's Esophagus

Classification	Association with GERD	Association with Adenocarcinoma	Endoscopic Surveillance Recommended
Columnar-lined esophagus with specialized intestinal metaplasia	Variable	Yes	Yes
Columnar-lined esophagus without specialized intestinal metaplasia	Variable	Unlikely	Probably not
Specialized intestinal metaplasia at the esophagogastric junction	Unclear	Probable	Unclear

A reevaluation of the approach to Barrett's esophagus has been proposed by S. Spechler and R. Goyal. Intestinal metaplasia may represent the critical variable of most pathologic significance. Unfortunately, the histologic recognition of the entity does not necessarily enable accurate prediction of its biologic behavior.

Similarly, in at least five separate studies, it has been demonstrated that of all individuals undergoing endoscopy, up to one in five individuals will have specialized intestinal metaplasia at the gastroesophageal junction, whether or not abnormalities are evident at the time of endoscopy.

Despite the screening recommendations for Barrett's esophagus mentioned above, a recent study in the United Kingdom has suggested that the yield of a Barrett's surveillance program may be too low to justify economically.

Interesting issues have been raised with regard to the relationship between *H. pylori* and GERD and in particular between these two disease entities and the possible relationship to adenocarcinoma at the gastroesophageal junction. Similarly, claims that acid-inhibitory therapy may be implicated in the genesis of gastroesophageal junction intestinal metaplasia and neoplasia are not supported by data. At this time, any such pathogenic linkage is speculative, and rigorous studies are required before such relationships can be substantiated.

At present, given the advances in endoscopic detection and a better understanding of metaplasia, the definition and pathogenesis of Barrett's esophagus seem less clear than previously envisaged. Thus, the definition of Barrett's solely by the presence of specialized intestinal metaplasia, regardless of its extent, may serve to significantly overestimate the disease process (by this definition, one in every five endoscoped patients has Barrett's esophagus). It is probably more realistic to restate the observation in terms of the identification of a condition known as *columnar epithelium–lined esophagus with specialized intestinal metaplasia*. On identification of such an entity, a specific focus can then be developed to identify cellular or molecular markers consistent with the development of dysplastic and neoplastic transformation. The wide use of the term *Barrett's esophagus* and its associated emotive and artificially numinous connotations of GERD and neoplasia should be avoided lest it engender overly emotional therapeutic responses.

If the principal issue is to impact the incidence of adenocarcinoma of the esophagus, which is currently the most rapidly increasing cancer in the United States, and amplify therapeutic gain, a different strategy is required.

Thus, better tests to identify at-risk patients than the use of endoscopy in patients with known Barrett's esophagus are needed. In particular, the identification of molecular markers of cell transformation in the esophagus is mandatory to facilitate the identification of individuals whose metaplasia is of pathologic significance.

Barrett's esophagus and adenocarcinoma

Diagnosis and evaluation

The consideration of both the presence and the management of Barrett's esophagus is usually accompanied by clinical excitement and characterized by views that are often both emotional and passionate. To a large extent, this reflects the fact that the therapeutic strategies for its management are as ill defined as the endoscopic criteria used for its diagnosis and measurement of extent. Of particular concern is the fact that the criteria currently in use for the most part do not reflect a systematic evaluation of either their clinical relevance or use.

A major issue has been the ability to identify the disease and characterize its type and extent. The development of magnification endoscopy has facilitated the detailed assessment of the topography of the surface of metaplastic esophageal mucosa, especially when combined with dye spraying. A recent report by Endo has clearly demonstrated that the visible topography using these techniques provides information with regard to both histologic features and mucin phenotypes. A further important issue relates to the need to define the length of the Barrett's esophagus. In this respect, it has proven difficult to provide a consistent endoscopic diagnosis of short-segment lesions, which are variably defined as up to 3 cm of endoscopically visible columnar metaplasia. Because as many as 12% of patients presenting for endoscopy have short-segment metaplasia, the identification of the precise nature and length of the abnormality is important. To assure accuracy of such a diagnosis, it is therefore vital that there be accurate localization of the anatomic gastroesophageal junction. Unfortunately, even the best endoscopic criteria used to the define this junction cannot always enable identification of a precise, reproducibly determined location. As a result of this quandary, it is advisable that the endoscopic diagnosis of short segments of columnar metaplasia include histologic criteria that confirm that the columnar mucosa are truly of esophageal (as opposed to gastric) origin and that specialized intestinal metaplasia is evident. To reliably establish this information, chromoendoscopy and special histopathologic approaches, such as cytokeratin analysis or DNA analysis, are required.

Short-segment Barrett's esophagus

There is considerable controversy regarding the precise clinical relevance of short-segment Barrett's esophagus. In essence, the issues that arise when this diagnosis is established are as follows: First, do patients with short-segment Barrett's esophagus represent a subset of patients with "traditional" Barrett's esophagus? Second, does this constitute a cancer risk? Third, how should they be managed? It seems apparent that individuals with short-segment Barrett's esophagus are generally male Caucasians who, overall, have less severe esophageal acid exposure when compared to "traditional" Barrett's patients. Current data suggest that the prevalence of short-segment Barrett's esophagus is age dependent, and that its extent does not change over time, similar to what occurs in patients with long-segment disease. In this respect, therefore, it seems that short-segment Barrett's esophagus is a distinct subset rather than a group with a long segment in evolution. As regards the precise cancer risk that such individuals are exposed to, there exist no adequate long-term prospective data to provide a reliable answer. Nevertheless, it is clear that cancer does arise in short segments, although it is far from certain whether the length of the Barrett's epithelium directly influences cancer risk. Factors that further compound the understanding of this issue include the fact that some studies that have reported an association between length and cancer have often excluded patients with short segments, and, indeed, the prevalence of high-grade dysplasia in short segments is not only low, but regression of the dysplasia has also been recorded in some circumstances.

Given the degree of uncertainty in this area, it is not surprising that agreement on management strategies for short-segment Barrett's has been a vexatious subject. To a large extent, this reflects a serious lack of understanding of the biology of the disease process, with the result that clinical practice in different centers is often widely divergent. Of particular relevance in this respect is the unresolved question of whether suspected short segments should be routinely biopsied. Unfortunately, few rigorous data exist to allow for definitive recommendations, although they are seriously needed, because the economic consequences of managing short-segment Barrett's esophagus effectively are substantial, given its prevalence.

The esophageal adenocarcinoma issue

The recognition that there is an increase in the incidence of esophageal adenocarcinoma in many countries has led to widespread speculation not only as to the cause but also as to the relationship to Barrett's esophagus. It is indubitable that there is a real increase in the condition, but it is possible that this has been overestimated, and, indeed, Foreman has recently examined this issue in considerable detail. Such a likelihood reflects both changes in cancer coding practices and a greater awareness that adenocarcinoma at the gastroesophageal junction could be the result of distal esophageal adenocarcinoma rather than cancer arising from the extreme upper extent of the gastric mucosa. Of direct relevance to the observation of an increase in adenocarcinoma is whether the strategies for the surveillance of Barrett's esophagus should be influenced by data on adenocarcinoma conversion rates. In addition, the somewhat different incidences in different countries, such as the United States and the United Kingdom, need to be further explored. Nevertheless, these data are vital, because they form the basis for determining the level of risk for adenocarcinoma development and thereby are critical determinants in guiding management strategy. A U.S. study has demonstrated differing epidemiologic patterns of esophageal adenocarcinoma and adenocarcinoma of the cardia. Thus, data gathered in the United States by El-Seraq regarding the different patterns of change in the overall age-adjusted incidence of esophageal junction adenocarcinoma provide important information with regard to this topic. When expressed as incidence per 100,000 of the population (95% confidence limits), the incidence of esophageal adenocarcinoma between 1987 and 1991 rose from 1.8 (1.7–1.9) to 2.5 (2.3–2.6) in the period from 1992 to 1996, whereas adenocarcinoma of the gastroesophageal junction in the same period was 3.3 (3.2–3.4) and 3.1 (3.0–3.3), respectively. The decreasing rate of gastric cardia cancer seen in the United States, however, is inconsistent with the increase in gastroesophageal adenocarcinoma reported in 2002 for the Netherlands by Wijnhoven. It is probable that, given the complexities of mucosal biology of the junctional zone in the area of the gastroesophageal junction, at least two types of cancers may occur in this region, and only one is related to esophageal columnar metaplasia. The resolution of this conundrum requires the development of a more sophisticated molecular analysis of the involved cell systems.

Mucosal markers for adenocarcinoma

Given the obvious shortcomings of dysplasia as a biomarker for the malignant potential of Barrett's epithelium, investigators have sought to identify alternative biomarkers (see table). The current strategy of screening and then

Malignancy Biomarkers in Barrett's Esophagus
Cell proliferation markers - Ki67
Ornithine decarboxylase
Carcinoembryonic antigen mucus abnormalities
Flow cytometry
Aneuploidy
Abnormal cellular proliferation
Chromosomal abnormalities (allelic imbalance in 3q, 4q, 5q, 6q, 9p, 10q, 12p, 12q, 17p, l8q)
Oncogenes
c-Ha-ras
c-erb-B
Tumor-suppressor genes (p53)
Growth regulatory factors
Epidermal growth factor
Epidermal growth factor receptor
Transforming growth factor-α

surveying patients over time for the presence of dysplasia in mucosal biopsies suffers from major limitations of cost, sensitivity, and practicality. Because dysplasia occurs focally, multiple biopsies must be performed and examined histologically to ensure that there has been adequate mucosal sampling, because routine white-light endoscopy cannot recognize areas of dysplasia. An option for improving the current situation is to devise special endoscopy techniques that reveal dysplastic areas to target biopsies. Techniques with the potential to do this include high-resolution endoscopy with dye spraying, fluorescence imaging and spectroscopy, Raman spectroscopy, optical coherence tomography, light-scattering spectroscopy, chromoendoscopy, confocal fluorescence endoscopy, and immunofluorescence endoscopy.

A further issue is the need to seek specific molecular clues that will allow identification of cells that appear capable of attaining neoplastic status. Candidate markers include abnormalities of the p53 and p16 genes, ploidy status, markers of cell proliferation, cox-II and villin expression, telomerase activity, and the loss of the Y chromosome. In particular, attention has focused on the p53 tumor-suppressor gene located on the short arm of chromosome 17 (allele 17p). Expression of mutated p53 protein and deletion of a 17p allele have been reported for a number of human malignancies, including cancers of the lung, breast, and colon. In these tumors, carcinogenesis appears to involve mutation of one p53 gene, with deletion of the 17p allele that harbors a normal p53 gene (loss of heterozygosity). It is of particular interest that allelic deletions of 17p have been found in the majority of cancers in Barrett's esophagus. Furthermore, enhanced expression of p53 protein by the metaplastic epithelium adjacent to the cancers has been found in one-half to two-thirds of cases. In patients with no apparent adenocarcinoma, immunohistochemical staining for p53 has been shown to correlate with the histologic finding of dysplasia, and p53 abnormalities can be found occasionally in metaplastic mucosa with no histologic signs of dysplasia. A recent report by Cawley described the finding of antibodies to p53 in the serum of 11 of 33 patients with esophageal carcinoma and in three of 36 patients with benign Barrett's esophagus.

DNA abnormalities in Barrett's esophagus can be recognized by flow cytometry, a technique in which cell nuclei prepared from tissue specimens are treated with a fluorescent dye that binds to DNA. The treated nuclei are passed through a flow cytometer wherein the DNA-bound dye is excited by laser irradiation, and an estimate of DNA content is obtained by measuring the intensity of fluorescent light emitted. Flow cytometry can identify aneuploid cell populations and can provide information on the proportion of diploid cells (cells in the G_0/G phase of the cell cycle that contain two copies of each chromosome) and tetraploid cells (cells in the G_2/M phase that contain four copies of each chromosome) in the sampled tissue.

In a prospective study, Reid reported flow-cytometric abnormalities (aneuploidy or increased G_2/tetraploid populations) in biopsy specimens of Barrett's mucosa obtained during the initial endoscopic evaluation for 13 of 62 patients. During a mean follow-up period of 34 months, 9 of the 13 patients with flow-cytometric abnormalities on initial evaluation developed high-grade dysplasia, adenocarcinoma, or both. In contrast, none of the 49 patients without flow-cytometric abnormalities developed high-grade dysplasia or cancer. During the apparent progression from dysplasia to adenocarcinoma, flow cytometry frequently showed multiple aneuploid populations of cells. No patient in this series progressed to invasive cancer without first exhibiting high-grade dysplasia, however.

The studies mentioned above suggest that flow-cytometric and p53 abnormalities may be earlier and more specific markers for cancer development than the histologic finding of dysplasia. Nevertheless, these markers do not yet provide sufficient additional information to justify their routine application in clinical practice. Indeed, none of the biomarkers listed in the table provides such information. Despite the problems, at this time, the finding of dysplasia remains the most appropriate biomarker for the clinical evaluation of patients with Barrett's esophagus.

Adenocarcinoma risk management

There exist few rigorous data to enable a definitive strategy to be enunciated. Indeed, the area represents a quagmire for the clinician confronted with the anxiety of the patient who has been apprised of a recognized (albeit numerically uncertain) risk of developing esophageal adenocarcinoma. The physician is between Scylla and Charybdis as he grapples with medico-legal issues, patient expectations that risk be minimized, and the concerns of health care providers who insist that only proven "cost-effective" risk-minimization strategies be used. Dent has elegantly summarized the situation in commenting that risk management is supported variously with protagonists, each of whom is armed with enthusiasm and blind faith, because there are remarkably few authoritative clinical data. Thus, current approaches are mainly justified by *"perceived biological plausibility, studies in animal models, anecdotes from clinical practice and surrogate outcomes in clinical studies that are usually seriously underpowered."*

Overall, the approach to risk minimization may be considered to fall into two main categories: first, measures that reduce the risk of development of esophageal adenocarcinoma and, second, those that may be directed to the early diagnosis of esophageal adenocarcinoma. It is clearly evident that early diagnosis by surveillance is definitely beneficial, as survival is vastly superior in patients whose adenocarcinoma has been detected by surveillance. Although this is encouraging for an individual in whom Barrett's esophagus has been diagnosed and who does not have adenocarcinoma when surveillance is established, it is apparent that there is a minimal impact of surveillance on the total number of deaths from esophageal adenocarcinoma. This reflects the fact that the vast majority of individuals who present with esophageal adenocarcinoma was not previously known to have Barrett's esophagus and was thus not in a surveillance program. Given the enormous expense and the potential usefulness of surveillance, a decrease in cost and the enhancement of practicality are critical societal and medical necessities if appropriate strategies for the management of adenocarcinoma risk are to be determined. Indeed, the cost of endoscopic surveillance could be dramatically curtailed if it were applied only to high-risk groups, such as men over the age of 50 years who have been suffering frequent heartburn for more than 10 years. Furthermore, the introduction of novel methods for the detection of dysplasia or early carcinoma might both greatly increase accuracy of diagnosis and reduce the cost of histopathology. The issue has been raised that chemoprevention, acid suppression, or even antireflux procedures might be effective management tools in facilitating even less frequent endoscopic surveillance, with an attendant enhancement of benefit versus cost.

The proposal that a normalization of esophageal acid exposure by PPI therapy might reduce the risk of conversion of Barrett's mucosa to adenocarcinoma is not supported by any direct data. Nevertheless, the control of acid reflux has been shown to greatly reduce the cox-II level in esophageal columnar metaplastic mucosa, thus suggesting that a putative effect may exist. Although the observation is tantalizing in its clinical extrapolation, it is premature to accept that the use of intensive high-dose PPI therapy to normalize or ablate esophageal acid exposure will benefit individuals with Barrett's.

In North America, there has been a surgical bias that antireflux surgery should be undertaken much more frequently to prevent the development of adenocarcinoma in patients with Barrett's esophagus. The rationale proposed claims that the prevention of the exposure of the metaplastic esophageal mucosa not only to acid but also to bile salts and other constituents of the gastric juice removes the inciting agents (sic) for this disease. Unfortunately, the primary hypothesis is flawed by the lack of evidence that the esophageal luminal environment is the principal component in facilitating the development of adenocarcinoma. A second issue that argues against this notion is the fact that many patients continue to have some degree of reflux of gastric juice into the esophagus after surgery, and the aggressiveness of action of this juice on the mucosa does not appear to be diminished by acid-suppressant therapy. Until recently, there existed only minimal anecdotal evidence demonstrating that adenocarcinoma developed after antireflux surgery. This information was quixotically interpreted by some as indicative of a protective effect of surgery. However, the publication by Lagergren in 2001 of a Swedish study of 65,000 patients has substantially refuted this whimsical notion of a protective effect of surgery by demonstrating no detectable impact of antireflux surgery on the risk of adenocarcinoma. Overall, at this time, it does not seem either prudent or reasonable to consider that the prevention of adenocarcinoma should be regarded as an established benefit of antireflux surgery.

Chemoprevention

A number of recent epidemiologic studies have demonstrated that aspirin or NSAID use is associated with a substantial reduction in the incidence of esophageal adenocarcinoma. The most recent study, by Farrow in 1998, is a U.S. population-based case-control study of 293 patients with esophageal adenocarcinoma. It reported that aspirin or nonaspirin NSAID use was associated with a substantially reduced odds ratio of 0.37 (confidence interval of 0.24 to 0.58) for the occurrence of esophageal adenocarcinoma when compared with individuals who were not using aspirin. A similar effect was noted with non-aspirin NSAIDs. These exciting epidemiologic data demonstrating a 60% reduction in the rate of conversion of Barrett's esophagus to adenocarcinoma by simple, inexpensive chemoprevention may, if proven correct, dramatically alter strategies for the surveillance of Barrett's esophagus. The biologic basis for such observations suggests that the protective effects of aspirin/NSAIDs may reflect the induction of apoptosis and the suppression of cox-II levels in esophageal columnar metaplastic epithelium. In support of this proposal are the data from a rat adenocarcinoma model that exhibit a 55% reduction of the conversion to cancer by cox-II inhibition.

To determine whether chemoprevention strategies of this type are valid and viable, it is necessary to establish large, direct intervention studies in which substantial cohorts of patients with Barrett's esophagus undergoing surveillance could be randomized to chemoprevention or placebo chemoprevention and then followed for several years. The risks of long-term aspirin administration in Barrett's esophagus patients need to be considered, although the fact that many will be using concurrent daily PPI therapy may, to a certain extent, obviate this issue.

Columnar mucosal ablation

The concept of removing the mucosa responsible for the development of the adenocarcinoma has been given serious consideration for more than a decade. In essence, it is proposed that such a measure would reduce the risk of development of adenocarcinoma. A variety of techniques have been considered as potentially effective, especially when combined with effective acid suppression or antireflux surgery. Unfortunately, little of this work has led to a rigorous or definitive assessment of whether ablation reduces the actual risk of adenocarcinoma, as most studies have not been adequately powered to determine this. Although there appears to be a degree of logic attached to the concept that ablation of Barrett's mucosa represents an acceptable surrogate for prophylaxis against conversion to adenocarcinoma, this statement is based more on belief than fact. A major flaw in the hypothesis is the fact that complete ablation of surface columnar metaplasia is difficult, if not impossible, to achieve in most cases and by the fact that there is clearly persistence of columnar metaplasia in all glandular structures buried under the squamous mucosa, irrespective of the type of ablative therapy used. The fact that adenocarcinoma may arise in buried glands that are not amenable to surveillance by endoscopic visualization and cytologic sampling presents a worrisome caveat to this mode of therapy.

Management guidelines

As might be predicted from the uncertainty pertaining to the biology of the disease, there is controversy regarding the optimal management strategy, and a variety of options have been hotly debated. As a result, a number of organizations have published guidelines regarding the management of Barrett's esophagus in an attempt to provide uniformity of care and define a standard. One of the most comprehensive summations provided by the American College of Gastroenterology is herewith provided in *précis* form. Treatment of esophageal reflux in patients with Barrett's esophagus should be the same as that in patients with GERD who do not have Barrett's esophagus. Patients with Barrett's esophagus should undergo surveillance endoscopy and biopsy at intervals that are based on the presence or absence and grade of dysplasia. Patients without dysplasia should undergo endoscopy every 2 to 3 years. When low-grade dysplasia is identified, endoscopy should be repeated after 6 and 12 months and then yearly thereafter if there is no histologic or endoscopic evidence of progression. When high-grade dysplasia is identified, the diagnosis should be confirmed by an independent experienced pathologist. If the diagnosis of high-grade dysplasia is confirmed, the American College of Gastroenterology endorses either intensive endoscopic surveillance (every 3 months) or esophagectomy.

A somewhat more aggressive approach, however, has been adopted by the International Society for Diseases of the Esophagus, the consensus panel of the Society for Surgery of the Alimentary Tract, the American Gastroenterological Association, and the American Society for Gastrointestinal Endoscopy. These groups have elected not to specifically endorse intensive endoscopic surveillance for high-grade dysplasia and instead recommend that fit patients with this lesion be considered for esophagectomy. It should be noted that the guidelines of the American College of Gastroenterology do not explicitly address the role of endoscopic ablative therapies for high-grade dysplasia, but the consensus panel concluded that these techniques require further study and should be limited to patients enrolled in clinical trials.

Summation

There is little doubt or debate that endoscopic screening for Barrett's esophagus should be considered for patients who have chronic symptoms (longer than 5 years) of GERD. In black or Asian women, the risk of cancer in association with Barrett's esophagus is so low as to probably not warrant even the minor risk associated with endoscopy, if the procedure is performed solely to screen for Barrett's esophagus. The group at highest risk for cancer consists of obese white men older than 50 years. Overall, current opinion would support the assessment that the evidence available to support the use of aggressive antireflux therapy to reduce the risk of cancer is insufficient to warrant the substantial expense and inconvenience of the therapy in routine clinical practice. Thus, antireflux therapy should be prescribed only as needed for the symptoms and signs of GERD.

Although there can as yet be no definitive management algorithm for Barrett's esophagus, it is worthwhile to provide a broad outline that encapsulates current practice. This cartoon is based on the working assumption (standard of care) that the idealized patient has undergone an initial endoscopic examination with biopsy specimens obtained in four quadrants at intervals of no more than 2 cm throughout the area of Barrett's esophagus. If for any reason the sampling of tissues during the initial endoscopy is inadequate, or if there is any question regarding the degree of dysplasia, the examination must be repeated. If it is the assessment of the histologist that inflammation is interfering with the assessment of the degree of dysplasia, intensive antireflux therapy (at the least, twice-daily treatment with a PPI) for 8 to 12 weeks should be given before repeat of the endoscopic biopsy to confirm the diagnosis. Although the American College of Gastroenterology has recommended that endoscopic surveillance be performed every 2 to 3 years in patients without dysplasia, this proposal may be overcautious based on currently available data. Thus, the initial recommendation was based on an estimated incidence of cancer in patients with Barrett's esophagus of 1% to 2% per year, whereas more recent studies suggest that the "true" incidence of cancer is approximately 0.5% per year. It therefore seems more reasonable to accept that less frequent surveillance—every 3 to 5 years—may be more appropriate in patients without dysplasia.

Because studies of intensive endoscopic surveillance for high-grade dysplasia are limited and have for the most part reviewed older patients, a degree of caution should be exhibited in applying the results of these studies to younger patients. Thus, more prolonged and intensive endoscopic surveillance may be

An algorithm for the management of Barrett's esophagus. (Adapted from Spechler SJ. Clinical practice. Barrett's Esophagus. *New Engl J Med* 2002;346:836–842.)

a valid alternative to immediate esophagectomy for older patients with high-grade dysplasia who can comply with this approach. Alternatively, in individuals who are old, infirm, or unwilling to undergo esophagectomy, endoscopic ablative therapy may be a potentially reasonable alternative if the procedure is performed by an expert involved in a formalized study protocol. A critical caveat, and of particular importance for both patient and physician, particularly as it applies to the issue of informed consent, is the fact that these recommendations have not been validated by studies demonstrating that this strategy prolongs survival or enhances the quality of life.

CHAPTER 6
CONSENSUS

Management consensus

GERD covers a spectrum of clinical disorders resulting from reflux of the gastric contents rostrally. The condition is increasingly common and making progressively increasing demands on the health service budget. The rise of GERD in the developed world over the last 50 years has paralleled the increase in obesity and sedentary behavior of our populations and shows no signs of abating. A rare complication of reflux disease, esophageal adenocarcinoma, is also being diagnosed more frequently and might be the price being paid for the indulgent and inactive lifestyle to which we have become accustomed. There are several contentious areas in the management of GERD, in particular the problems of accurately identifying the most specific symptoms of GERD and the management of patients whose symptoms are not abolished by potent acid-suppression medications. The problem of esophageal and extraesophageal nocturnal symptoms and their relationship to acid secretion, reflux, and impaired clearance of refluxate during the hours of recumbency and sleep are major areas of therapeutic interest.

As a consequence of the atypical manifestations of GERD and the association of Barrett's esophagus with esophageal adenocarcinoma, more attention has been drawn to GERD recently, which probably contributes in part to its increasing prevalence. Why else might GERD be becoming more prevalent? Is it only due to increased body mass in the developed world, or are our stomachs now producing more acid? Perhaps esophageal mucosal defenses are less adept than they once were?

There is no gold standard in diagnosing and staging GERD. Thus, the choice of a diagnostic strategy is based on symptoms, resources, and the clinical question posed. For example, in patients with alarm symptoms or who are older than 50 years of age, endoscopy is clearly important to identify complications or alternative diagnoses, whereas in patients with suspected extraesophageal manifestations, such as noncardiac chest pain, a 24-hour pH-recording study may be the most appropriate investigation. In many instances (e.g., in younger patients with a short history of typical symptoms), a therapeutic trial of a PPI at a high dose (often termed the *PPI test*) is sufficient to confirm a clinical diagnosis, especially in primary care. There is no consensus regarding how long this initial trial should be or the dosing strategy after a successful test. In

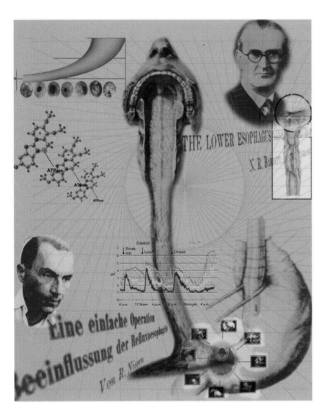

A collage of the evolution of the management of GERD. Therapy has evolved from the seminal notations of Barrett (top right), who first identified the pathologic problem at the lower end of the esophagus. Thereafter, a "surgical cure" using a wrap designed to obviate acidic reflux (bottom right) was envisioned and devised by Nissen (bottom left). The control of gastric acidity by PPIs such as pantoprazole (top left) has now largely superseded the surgical approach.

particular, it is not established that the PPI test has actual cost-saving advantages in practice over a strategy involving early endoscopy in practice, as theoretically predicted from a Markov model.

Definitions and symptoms

Gastroesophageal reflux may produce erosions (erosive GERD), no overt mucosal damage [nonerosive reflux disease (NERD)], or atypical manifestations of reflux, such as pulmonary diseases, noncardiac chest pain, reflux laryngitis, or dental erosions. However, the distinction between NERD and GERD becomes less important as microscopic esophageal damage is increasingly detected by chromoendoscopy and other methods.

The typical symptom of gastroesophageal reflux is usually described as a burning sensation radiating up from the sternum. This is commonly referred to as *heartburn* in English-speaking countries, but in other languages there is usually no cardiac reference. It is now becoming increasingly apparent that there is a large discrepancy between the intensity of the symptom of heartburn and the amount of acid regurgitation and objective evidence of pathologic gastroesophageal reflux. Indeed, the evidence that most patients treated "effectively" for ulcer healing still remain with a variety of persistent symptoms demonstrates our poor understanding of the cause of many heartburn-like symptoms. Whether these refractory symptoms represent "functional heartburn" or result from reflux of gastric contents is unclear. The recent decisions of British and Canadian gastrointestinal societies to include heartburn in the definition of dyspepsia, unlike that of the Rome II criteria, suggests that the symptom "heartburn" does not travel well across different cultures. This problem is also exemplified by the inability to understand a standard definition of GERD by a group of Scandinavian GERD patients.

Issues related to definitions of heartburn are likely to cloud clinical trials of therapy for GERD, particularly NERD, in which symptom relief is the main outcome measure. Development of an instrument that accurately evaluates specific esophageal and extraesophageal symptoms and that can be used to assess their prevalence and severity in studies of populations and in clinical trials is needed. GERD and NERD symptomatology might be best characterized by a multidimensional construct that would allow for a comprehensive assessment of the full gamut of symptoms, including the ability to document symptoms longitudinally, considering also external factors. Self-administered diaries that allow the patient to assess symptoms at multiple time points may provide the valid, reliable, responsive scale for the assessment of GERD symptom dimensions during therapy that is currently lacking.

Pathophysiology

There have been relatively few recent insights into the increasing prevalence or pathophysiology of GERD. An increased frequency of TLESRs is a well-recognized feature of GERD, and the recent demonstration that TLESRs may increase in the presence of a coexisting hiatal hernia may explain the association of hiatal hernia with GERD. More recently described phenomena include a more distensible gastroesophageal junction in GERD patients with hernias and the presence of a "pocket" of gastric juice in the gastric fundus that is much more highly acidic than the general gastric contents, which, therefore, may be particularly damaging to the mucosa at the gastroesophageal junction.

There are many known inhibitors of TLESR, including CCK antagonists, nitric oxide antagonists, atropine, morphine, cannabinoids, baclofen, and tegaserod; the newer members of this growing family of drugs are being actively investigated for their possible efficacy in primary or adjunctive therapy. However, the clinical usefulness of agents that promote LES contraction and the relative contribution of a low LES pressure to the pathogenesis of GERD remain uncertain in the absence of a clean pharmacologic agent whose actions are confined to this site. Similarly, although duodenal contents and pepsin are established injurious agents for the esophageal mucosa, the efficacy of potent acid suppression has drawn attention away from other toxic agents in gastric contents.

Barrett's esophagus

The metaplastic response of the esophageal mucosa to chronic damage, known commonly as *Barrett's esophagus*, is the subject of considerable current attention owing to its malignant potential. With the steady and inexorable rise in esophageal adenocarcinoma among white males in the developed world, it is important to understand the determinants responsible for the progression to and from Barrett's esophagus. Controversy surrounds almost every aspect of Barrett's esophagus—its true population prevalence, its relative contribution to the development of adenocarcinoma, and the rate of progression from Barrett's to dysplasia and cancer. Whether there are any strategies that may reduce this risk of progression and whether endoscopic surveillance is of any benefit in detecting lesions at an early enough stage to alter the natural history of adenocarcinoma are also unknown.

It is uniformly accepted that a critical issue in the management of GERD is the need to ensure appropriate effective therapy to minimize the risk of the development of Barrett's esophagus and to identify it accurately. Patients found to have Barrett's esophagus at biopsy but with no dysplasia should be placed in a surveillance program with approximately 5-year intervals between surveillance endoscopies. This opinion is to a large extent based on cost-effectiveness analysis data and may need to be modified with the significant alterations in endoscopic charges. If the pathologist diagnoses Barrett's esophagus and identifies the presence of dysplasia, then the material should be reviewed by two expert independent pathologists to confirm the diagnosis and to establish whether the changes conform to a pattern consistent with low- or high-grade dysplasia. The identification of low-grade dysplasia mandates repeat biopsy at 1 year to determine whether there is progression to high-grade dysplasia. If at the 1-year time point multiple biopsies fail to identify evidence of dysplasia, the patient should return to the normal surveillance program; if low-grade dysplasia persists, then endoscopy and biopsy should again be repeated in 1 year. If there is a diagnosis of high-grade dysplasia at the initial or any follow-up biopsy, then the patient should be treated with a high-dose

PPI for 3 months to rule out the possibility of inflammatory pseudodysplasia. If the repeat biopsy after 3 months confirms high-grade dysplasia, then the patient should be referred for consideration of surgery or ablative therapy. Some experts have expressed the opinion that very carefully repeated endoscopic surveillance of high-grade dysplasia can be performed to monitor for and biopsy any visible mucosal abnormality. Under such circumstances, surgery might be obviated until a carcinoma is discovered. However, the majority of authorities in this field are uncomfortable with this approach and express a preference for prophylactic surgery once the presence of a high-grade lesion had been reliably identified, provided the risk of surgery in a particular patient does not exceed that of the disease. Ablation therapy by laser, bicap, heater probe, or photodynamic therapy for Barrett's esophagus, dysplasia, or both, should be currently regarded as experimental.

In patients being endoscoped for any reason other than GERD, Barrett's esophagus may be much more prevalent than was previously thought (occurring in at least 10% of patients biopsied during diagnostic endoscopy). However, community-based studies are needed to define the age, sex, and race-related prevalences and other clinical features that may influence the risk of developing this lesion. Estimates of progression from Barrett's esophagus to adenocarcinoma of the esophagus in GERD patients have recently been downgraded to approximately 0.5% per year, but this figure may still be an overestimate, because most esophageal adenocarcinomas present *de novo* in patients without a prior diagnosis of Barrett's esophagus, and in some patients, Barrett's is not apparent at the time when the cancer presents.

Although there is little consensus regarding the merits of population screening to detect Barrett's, the practice in most developed countries is to survey GERD patients with Barrett's esophagus at intervals of 1 to 5 years, based on the hope that this will allow the detection of early cancers and thereby alter the natural history of the disease. How do we identify the small subset of Barrett's patients who may really benefit from surveillance? Studies currently in progress are likely in the near future to identify genetic markers in initial screening biopsies that will select from a large number of patients with Barrett's the small subset at increased risk of progressing to cancer, thus justifying costly continued surveillance in this small subset.

In the absence of such information, physicians may feel under some pressure to treat patients with Barrett's metaplasia empirically with acid-suppression medications. These forces derive from small studies demonstrating a potential normalization of surrogate endpoints, such as proliferation. Although the positive studies supporting such a policy are often emphasized, similarly designed studies that demonstrate no effect of these interventions on proliferation and other markers (including endoscopic and histologic factors) have frequently been ignored. Well-conducted, large prospective studies using as endpoints the progression of intestinal metaplasia to dysplasia or cancer are needed to definitively address whether acid inhibition, anti-cox drugs, or other potential chemopreventive interventions are of clinical value. Hopefully, in the future, there will be risk-stratified individualized approaches to screening, entry into surveillance programs, and possibly even treatment based on the demographic profile of the patient or on molecular markers in the at-risk mucosa as well as at the genomic level. These markers may also include real-time indicators of the state of the esophageal mucosa using, for example, optical coherence tomography, magnification, and chromoendoscopy.

Medical therapy

Most patients with GERD present to and are managed by general practitioners; some of the care for patients with GERD will require referral to a gastroenterologist and a surgeon. The management of GERD is a continuum, with management based on not only symptoms, but also on referral patterns and, more increasingly, financial constraints. The first step in the management of the patient with suspected GERD is a history and physical examination. A history of retrosternal burning-type chest pain radiating up from the epigastrium toward the throat is characteristic of GERD, and such symptoms have a high specificity for the diagnosis. If the patient has either atypical symptoms or any alarm symptoms such as dysphagia, anemia, weight loss, predominantly abdominal pain, or pain that does not respond to antacids or first develops symptoms after the age of 50 years, then prompt referral for endoscopy is necessary.

The majority of patients probably do not require endoscopy initially, and such patients should be counseled in regard to simpler antireflux measures, which may include elevation of the head of the bed, weight loss, and the avoidance of precipitating foods and drugs. It is of note, however, that there exist few rigorous data to support the concept that such measures are either of proven or long-term benefit in the management of GERD. The patient should also be advised to take antacids at the time of symptoms and to avoid heavy meals late at night or within 3 hours of retiring to bed. If symptoms persist after 2 to 4 weeks of these simple measures, or if antacids are needed often, if not daily, then formal therapy should be instituted. In the past, the first line of treatment was considered to be the use of an H_2 receptor antagonist, but the current, almost uniform, positive clinical experience with the use of PPIs at the standard (low) dose as initial therapy suggests that this strategy is more acceptable to both clinicians and patients. In circumstances in which the pain is a consistent component of the symptomatology, and particularly if there is a nocturnal component, the use of a PPI should be given unequivocal consideration.

If the symptoms are more suggestive of a motility problem, or it is felt that evidence of a motility component to the presentation is evident, a prokinetic drug, such as the $5-HT_4$ receptor agonist cisapride, may be considered. Such agents (motility) are, however, nonspecific in their site of gastrointestinal action and often display considerable adverse effects. These drugs should be given initially as a 1-month trial and then discontinued. If symptoms recur after this 4-week trial, or if they are not relieved during this treatment period, then the patient should be referred for endoscopy. Although the decision to undertake endoscopy at this time is somewhat arbitrary, it is consistent with the widely accepted position that a "once-in-a-lifetime endoscopy" in reflux disease is acceptable. Thus, an endoscopic evaluation can be included in the database of the patient before major and (possibly) long-term therapeutic decisions are made.

At the time of endoscopy, particular attention should be paid to the presence of erythema, erosions, and other signs of esophagitis, and the gastroesophageal

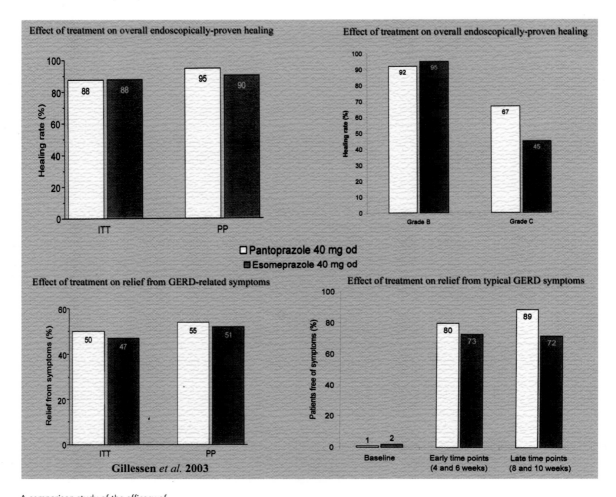

Effect of treatment on overall endoscopically-proven healing

Effect of treatment on overall endoscopically-proven healing

☐ Pantoprazole 40 mg od
▨ Esomeprazole 40 mg od

Effect of treatment on relief from GERD-related symptoms

Effect of treatment on relief from typical GERD symptoms

Gillessen *et al.* **2003**

A comparison study of the efficacy of pantoprazole and esomeprazole. Overall, endoscopically proven healing rates for patients receiving pantoprazole, 40 mg, and esomeprazole, 40 mg (top left), and endoscopically proven healing in patients according to their GERD grade (Los Angeles classification system) at baseline and treatment group (top right) show no significant differences between the two drugs. An examination of the overall relief of GERD-related symptoms for patients receiving pantoprazole and esomeprazole (bottom left) and those patients free of the GERD-related symptoms heartburn, acid regurgitation, and dysphagia according to treatment group at baseline, early and late time points (bottom right), demonstrate that pantoprazole and omeprazole have equal treatment efficacy.

junction should be examined carefully. If there is any suspicion of Barrett's esophagus, then four-quadrant biopsies should be taken at the gastroesophageal junction, but a gastroesophageal junction of normal appearance should not be biopsied routinely. Antrum and corpus biopsies should be taken for the diagnosis of *H. pylori* even in the absence of peptic ulceration, given the recent reports of accelerated gastric atrophy in patients with *H. pylori* taking long-term PPIs. Thus, prophylactic eradication of *H. pylori* in this group would be mandatory. There still exists a minority opinion that believes that because *H. pylori* infection is common, and in most circumstances does not lead to harm, establishing whether *H. pylori* was present may be irrelevant and potentially confusing.

In the absence of Barrett's esophagus or for Barrett's esophagus without high-grade dysplasia, the primary goal of treatment of GERD should be to relieve symptoms. Thus, with the identification of minimal or modest esophagitis at endoscopy and mild symptoms, a PPI should be the initial agent of choice. There is no longer much support for initial treatment with either an H₂ receptor antagonist or prokinetic agents, given their modest efficacy and the adverse effects noted, particularly at the high dosage levels needed to attain a consistently elevated pH. The cost to the patient in terms of lifestyle and work loss generated by initial failed therapy using such agents is no longer acceptable.

GERD Managment Algorithm

GERD presents as a complex set of clinical variables that require interpolation into a cohesive management strategy. PPIs are the most effective therapy, although surgery may have a role in a very small proportion of patients if rigorous and specific criteria are met. The usefulness of prokinetic agents remains ill defined.

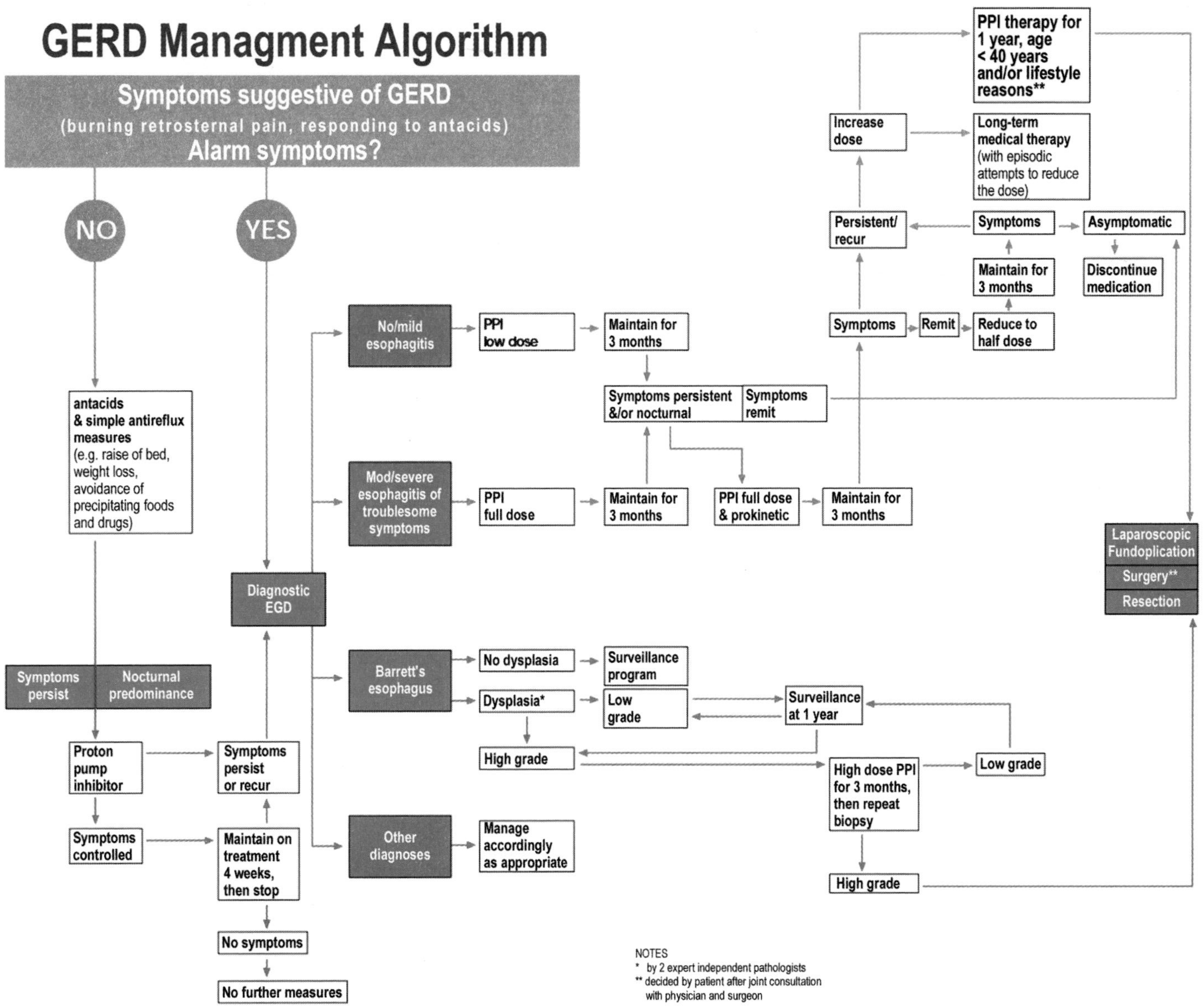

Symptoms suggestive of GERD
(burning retrosternal pain, responding to antacids)
Alarm symptoms?

NO

antacids & simple antireflux measures (e.g. raise of bed, weight loss, avoidance of precipitating foods and drugs)

Symptoms persist

Nocturnal predominance

Proton pump inhibitor

Symptoms controlled

Symptoms persist or recur

Maintain on treatment 4 weeks, then stop

No symptoms

No further measures

YES

Diagnostic EGD

No/mild esophagitis — PPI low dose — Maintain for 3 months — Symptoms persistent &/or nocturnal

Mod/severe esophagitis of troublesome symptoms — PPI full dose — Maintain for 3 months — Symptoms persistent | Symptoms remit — PPI full dose & prokinetic — Maintain for 3 months

Barrett's esophagus — No dysplasia | Dysplasia* — Surveillance program | Low grade | High grade — Surveillance at 1 year — Low grade | High grade — High dose PPI for 3 months, then repeat biopsy — Low grade | High grade

Other diagnoses — Manage accordingly as appropriate

Symptoms — Remit — Persistent/recur — Increase dose — PPI therapy for 1 year, age < 40 years and/or lifestyle reasons**

Long-term medical therapy (with episodic attempts to reduce the dose) — Symptoms | Asymptomatic — Discontinue medication — Maintain for 3 months — Reduce to half dose

Laparoscopic Fundoplication | Surgery** | Resection

NOTES
* by 2 expert independent pathologists
** decided by patient after joint consultation with physician and surgeon

431

There is uniform agreement that in the event of moderate or severe esophagitis or particularly troublesome symptoms, all patients should be treated with a PPI immediately. If a patient had been placed on H_2 receptor antagonist or prokinetic therapy and failed to resolve his or her symptomatology or relapsed, a PPI should be prescribed. Under such circumstances, it is well accepted that PPIs should initially be given at standard doses. In rare instances, when these fail to provide symptom relief for all patients, they may need to be increased to twice-daily dosing or even more to achieve full symptom relief. Based on currently available information, it is felt that the addition of a prokinetic agent to therapy in conjunction with a PPI is likely to be of only marginal benefit for GERD. Once a dose of an H_2 receptor antagonist, prokinetic agent, or PPI that relieves symptoms is identified, this dose should be maintained for a period of 3 months. After this time, an attempt should be made to reduce the dose, with the aim of maintaining a stable clinical status (asymptomatic) on half-dose PPIs or, alternatively, on alternative-day therapy. If symptoms recur, then the patient should resume the full dose of PPI and a plan should be formulated for long-term treatment.

The long-term treatment options are either medical therapy, with attempts to reduce the dose of medication occasionally, or consideration for surgery. With regard to patients who might enter long-term therapy, it should be noted that many, particularly those in the older age group, may already be taking several medications. Thus, careful attention should be directed to the drug-interaction profile of the various types of PPIs.

Antisecretory drugs

Together with implementing lifestyle modifications (whenever practicable), PPIs should be started as the drugs of choice for erosive esophagitis, achieving healing rates in clinical trials of over 80% at 4 weeks—significantly higher than for any other medication. Several recent publications have indicated that the optimal dose for healing moderate to severe erosive esophagitis is 40 mg of a PPI daily. Widespread use of PPIs testifies to the symptomatic benefits that they also offer in nonerosive disease. PPIs act by covalently binding to cysteine residues in H,K-ATPases (the proton pumps) in the membranes of the secretory canaliculi of parietal cells. Differences in the molecular structures of specific PPIs result in different cysteine residues being targeted. For example, all PPIs bind to *cys* 813; lansoprazole also binds to *cys* 321, and pantoprazole binds, in addition, to *cys* 822. Pharmacologic studies in a variety of test systems *in vitro* in animals and human experimental and pharmacodynamic data indicate that the ability of pantoprazole to target *cys* 822 may lead to a more prolonged effect. However, milligram for milligram, all drugs in this class appear comparable in their effects clinically, because human studies have not revealed significant or consistent differences between the drugs with regard to clinical or endoscopic end points or side-effect profiles. More detailed studies involving head-to-head comparisons between the various available drugs are needed to determine whether small pharmacokinetic differences between the PPIs translate into clinical practice. Improvement in PPI therapy is likely to result from a longer dwell time in blood or on the pump itself, since binding to *cys* 813 may be reversed in part by cellular gluthione. The improvement of esomeprazole, 40 mg, as compared to omeprazole, 20 mg, is attributed to a longer steady state of the S-enantiomer in the blood due to slower metabolism of this enantiomer as compared to the R-enantiomer. Other means of increasing the dwell time in the blood may be developed.

In comparing the results of clinical trials of PPIs, it may also be important to consider the metabolism of PPIs by cytochrome p450 CYP2C19. Clinically important polymorphisms of this enzyme have been described, occurring at varying frequencies in differing populations. Differences between clinical outcomes from studies performed in different parts of the world and an apparent failure of the drugs to control symptoms in some subjects may be explained and rationalized in some instances after a consideration of these polymorphisms. Ideally, agents lacking significant pharmacologic interaction with the cytochrome p450 enzymes are desirable, because many GERD patients are taking numerous other drugs for coexisting diseases and are at risk for drug interactions.

Because the proton pumps on the parietal cell are most accessible to PPIs when acid secretion is maximally stimulated after prolonged fasting, PPIs are most efficacious in inhibiting acid secretion when taken by patients shortly before a protein-rich breakfast. However, this may not be the case for many people who no longer eat such a meal on a daily basis or for those patients with dominant nocturnal symptoms. In these instances, might a better strategy be to take the drug before dinner instead of, or in addition to, the morning dose?

Future challenges to improving medical therapy include the problems of large-volume refluxers who experience symptoms despite reasonable neutralization of the intragastric pH and the optimal management of patients whose symptoms are predominantly nocturnal—any advantage in the addition of H_2 receptor antagonists to PPI dosing is rapidly lost due to the development of tolerance. In the future, the "on demand" use of PPIs for symptoms of heartburn in patients with nonerosive reflux disease may perhaps provide reasonable symptom relief with a considerable reduction in medication use compared with daily therapy. Additionally, such a strategy may provide a means to taper a patient from a daily dependence on PPIs without a severe acid/gastrin rebound effect.

The advent of intravenous PPIs has allowed for the achievement of more profound and more sustained predictable acid suppression in the absence of the development of any tolerance. This may provide clinical benefit for patients suffering from pathologic hypersecretory conditions, such as Zollinger-Ellison syndrome, or for those patients with severe erosive reflux disease who are unable to tolerate oral therapy, for example. However, with a paucity of rigorous data to support their usefulness, their role in the armamentarium of therapy is currently unclear.

Prokinetic agents

The impact of impaired esophageal or gastric motility on the development of reflux symptoms is conflicting and the prokinetic agents currently available disappointing in terms of efficacy and side effects. Thus, except for specific patients with documented motility abnormalities, there is little role for prokinetic agents in the treatment of GERD or NERD.

Nonmedical therapy

Surgical intervention for chronic reflux symptoms has been reported to give good results when performed by experienced surgeons in major centers. However, results from patients in community hospitals operated on by less-experienced surgeons indicate that the successful results of highly experienced surgeons are rarely achieved in ordinary practice. Surgery is a potentially attractive option for younger patients (younger than 40 years) and for patients who do not wish to take chronic medication for lifestyle reasons. Thus, individuals who require PPI therapy continually for a year are unlikely to be able to manage without these medications. Before surgery, patients should have the opportunity for a full and frank discussion with both their gastroenterologist and the surgeon, preferably together, regarding all the risks and benefits of long-term medical versus surgical therapy. Although the long-term data available are currently somewhat limited, laparoscopic fundoplication generally appears to be safe and preferable to open surgery if performed by an expert. Preoperative motility and pH studies are essential both to precisely delineate the state of the sphincter and to facilitate follow-up if there is any postsurgical relapse. The critical determinant of successful surgery is the choice of surgeon. The practice of surgery for the treatment of gastroesophageal reflux should be confined to those surgeons both experienced and expert in surgery for this condition. Current information supports the use of a wrap-type procedure, and no data exist to suggest that the addition of any form of vagotomy confers further benefit. (Indeed, given the cumulative experience of almost half a century of postvagotomy patients, it is probably malpractice to undertake such a procedure electively.) However, after the age of 60 years, the risks from surgery probably outweigh the benefits, and under such circumstances, the use of an appropriate PPI is probably safer than general anesthesia and violation of the peritoneal cavity. For patients with Barrett's esophagus as a component of intractable GERD symptomatology, it is essential to continue the surveillance program, even if the patient is asymptomatic after surgery, because progression of Barrett's esophagus after successful GERD surgery is well recognized.

A defective fundic wrap not only increases the costs of the surgical procedure but also significantly complicates further treatment and evidently increases risk if reoperation is undertaken. Published data indicate an incidence of defective fundic wrap of 7% after 7 months, of 23% after 77 months, and of 29% after 20 years. Thus, the reoperation rate may ultimately be as high as 5% to 10% for individuals who have previously undergone a Nissen procedure. Although questions have been raised about long-term medical therapy, the issue of the long-term viability of a fundic wrap may also require some consideration. A further problem with the surgical procedure is the postoperative dysphagia, which may require clinical treatment and occasionally even endoscopic management with dilation. The negative influences on the cost and outcome analysis of these events have yet to be precisely determined.

Currently under investigation are several endoscopic techniques designed to bolster antireflux barriers at the gastroesophageal junction. These methods include a variety of endoscopic suturing procedures, devices designed to cause scarring after thermal burns, and injections of inert substances into the mucosa superficial to the LES. The vast majority of publications report only short-term outcomes, often of few patients with mostly mild disease and usually with suboptimal study designs. Unfortunately, some of these devices already have been approved for patient use, although they are not yet established as being in patients' best interests. All these endoscopic methods should still be considered experimental, and we would strongly recommend that patients only receive such therapies in the context of well-controlled clinical trials conducted by well-trained endoscopists.

Helicobacter pylori

In the last 5 years, there has been considerable interest regarding the relationship of chronic *H. pylori* infection to the development and course of the symptoms and complications of GERD. Although in a large prospective trial, the response to therapy was significantly better in *H. pylori*–infected patients, post-hoc analysis of some large clinical studies, as well as observational data, led to the conclusions that there may be an inverse relationship between *H. pylori* infection and reflux esophagitis, that eradication of *H. pylori* may provoke or unmask reflux disease, and that carriage of *H. pylori* (particularly strains expressing the *cag* pathogenicity island) had a "protective" role against esophageal and cardia adenocarcinoma. However, with data accumulating from studies that were designed prospectively and specifically to evaluate the relationship between *H. pylori* and GERD, enthusiasm for such a beneficial effect of *H. pylori* in GERD is waning. Although means of results in large groups may not be predictive of effects in individual patients, depending on the extent of their gastritis and their ability to make acid, it is likely that for most patients, the presence or absence of *H. pylori* in the stomach has little or no influence on the development and natural history of GERD and its complications other than an effect on antisecretory medication requirements.

Nevertheless, there might be a need to consider the presence of *H. pylori* in patients taking long-term PPI therapy for GERD. Patients infected with *H. pylori* develop progression of gastritis, gastric metaplasia, and dysplasia over time, and a small percentage (less than 1%) get gastric cancer. Whether this progression is accelerated during long-term PPI therapy is not established and remains controversial. Lundell and colleagues clearly demonstrated that patients taking a PPI long term for reflux disease developed more gastric atrophy if *H. pylori* persisted, thus demonstrating that hypochlorhydria may accelerate the development of atrophy caused by *H. pylori*. Although the development of atrophy is a relatively early marker of the gastric preneoplastic process, the fact that it developed over only a few years is of concern. Larger and longer prospective studies to address this important issue are needed, as many gastroenterologists do not feel that the small theoretic risk of progression to cancer justifies eradication in all *H. pylori*–infected patients, regardless of whether they have GERD.

Conclusion

GERD is a highly and increasingly prevalent disorder. It impairs quality of life and sometimes leads to life-threatening complications. Physicians treating patients with GERD need to use the best currently available management options cost effectively. With regard to therapy, PPIs are excellent medications for patients who have erosive esophagitis, producing high healing rates of esophageal lesions rapidly and with very few side effects. For this condition, there appears to be no appreciable difference in clinical efficacy between different PPIs at equivalent doses. More challenging is the much larger group of patients who have NERD and symptoms of heartburn. In many of these patients, establishing a diagnosis and optimizing therapy continue to cause difficulty. In the future, heterogeneity in the patient population with regard to symptoms, risk of malignancy, and extraesophageal manifestations of GERD will dictate more individualized approaches. It is likely that better defining discriminating features in the patient's history and establishing alternative pharmacologic and molecular-based strategies will be needed to achieve optimal symptom relief and resource use. In the meantime, the development of agents with a more rapid onset of action than traditional PPIs and better methods to control nocturnal symptoms and problems related to the volume of refluxate are eagerly awaited.

Given the rate of scientific and medical advance at this time, it is not unreasonable to propose that more specific pharmacotherapeutic probes targeting the LES are likely to become available within the foreseeable future. In addition, the area of mucosal healing is a subject that is under extensive investigation, and the possibility of the development of agents capable of amplifying the healing process or altering the quality of the healed mucosa is significant (i.e., less likely to recur). Certainly, if one reviews medical advances made in the management of acid inhibition and the control of gastric mucosal inflammatory disease in the last 5 years, one might predict significant pharmacologic advances in the medical management of GERD in the upcoming time. In those patients who have indications that warrant surgery but are reluctant to undergo anesthesia and invasive procedures, physicians should adopt a cautiously optimistic but conservative posture.

The current vogue in the historical evolution of the management of the problem of reflux is represented by augmentation procedures for the LES. Rather than using a transperitoneal approach, these procedures are directed at the sphincter by the transesophageal route and include stitching, collagen injection, and radiofrequency-induced fibrosis. It is probable, however, that these techniques will suffer all the drawbacks of any mechanical intervention but somewhat decrease the morbidity of open, albeit minimally invasive, surgery. Similarly, a specific pharmacotherapeutic probe targeting the LES, although long fantasized, remains to be identified.

In all likelihood, it will transpire that reflux disease represents an electroconductive disorder of the gastric pacemaker that results in an ectopic gastric electric rhythm and intermittent valvular dysfunction (pylorus and LES) coupled with abnormal peristaltic activity. The effects of acid and pepsin or bile are simply adjunctive to an as-yet undefined gastric dysrhythmia and probably accentuated by as-yet undetermined food preservative agents that are now a common part of the twenty-first-century fascination with instant culinary products. Indeed, as the definition of abnormal cardiac electrophysiology led to the examination of a previously obscure clinical problem (cardiac arrhythmia—fainting, syncope, palpitations), it may be postulated that the delineation of the electrophysiology of the gastric cardia may similarly illuminate the definitive therapy of a disease that at present may be regarded as nothing less than God's Exquisite Revenge on Doctors!

SUGGESTED READING

Akerlund A. Hernia diaphragmatica: hiatus esophagei von Anatomishen und Roentgenologischen Gesichstpunkt. *Acta Radiologica* 1926;6:3–34.

Allgood PC, Bachmann M. Medical or surgical treatment for chronic gastroesophageal reflux? A systematic review of published evidence of effectiveness. *Eur J Surg* 2000;166:713–721.

Allison PR, Johnstone AS, Royce GB. Short esophagus with simple peptic ulceration. *J Thorac Surg* 1943;12:432–457.

Allison PR. Peptic ulcer of the esophagus. *Thorax* 1948;3:20.

Allison PR. Reflux esophagitis, sliding hiatal hernia, and the anatomy of repair. *Surg Gynecol Obstet* 1951;92:419–431

Allocca M, Mangano M, Colombo P, et al. Does loperamide decrease gastro-oesophageal reflux in patients with reflux disease [abstract]? *Gastroenterology* 1999;116:A1–11.

Anonymous. Guidelines for surgical treatment of gastroesophageal reflux disease (GERD). Society of American Gastrointestinal Endoscopic Surgeons (SAGES). *Surg Endosc* 1998;12:186–188.

Anvari M, Allen C. Laparoscopic Nissen fundoplication: two-year comprehensive follow-up of a technique of minimal paraesophageal dissection. *Ann Surg* 1998;227:25–32.

Armstrong D, Bennett JR, Blum AL, et al. The endoscopic assessment of esophagitis: a progress report on observer agreement. *Gastroenterology* 1996;11:85–92.

Ashcraft KW, Holder TM, Amoury RA. Treatment of gastro-esophageal reflux in children by Thal fundoplication. *J Thorac Cardiovasc Surg* 1981;82:706–712.

Bais JE, Bartelsman JF, Bonjer HJ, et al. Laparoscopic or conventional Nissen fundoplication for gastro-esophageal reflux disease: randomized clinical trial. *Lancet* 2000;355:170–174.

Bammer T, Hinder RA, Klaus A, et al. Five- to eight-year outcome of the first laparoscopic Nissen fundoplications. *J Gastrointest Surg* 2001;16:42–48.

Barrett NR. Chronic peptic ulcer of the œsophagus and "œsophagitis." *Br J Surg* 1950;38:175–182.

Bate CM, Richardson PDI. Cost-effectiveness of omeprazole in the management of gastroesophageal reflux disease in clinical practice. *Brit J Med Econ* 1994:7:81–97.

Baue AF, Belsey RHR. The treatment of sliding hiatus hernia and reflux esophagitis by the Mark IV technique. *Surgery* 1967;62:396–404.

Berenberg W, Neuhauser EBD. Cardio-esophageal relaxation (chalasia) as a cause of vomiting in infants. *Pediatrics* 1950;5:414–419.

Bernstein A. Hiatal hernia: a frequent and clinically important condition. *Univ W Ont JJ* 1947;17:159.

Bernstein LM, Baker LA. A clinical test for esophagitis. *Gastroenterology* 1961;34:1.

Bettex M, Kuffer F. Fundoplication in hiatal hernia—results after 10 years. *Progress in pediatric surgery.* Baltimore–Munich: Urban und Schwarzenberg, 1977:25–31.

Billard B. *Maladies des enfants nouveau-nés.* Paris, 1828.

Boeckxstaens GE, Hirsch DP, Fakhry N, et al. Involvement of cholecystokinin-A receptors in transient lower esophageal sphincter relaxations triggered by gastric distension. *Am J Gastroenterol* 1998;93:1823–1828.

Boulant J, Fioramonti J, Dapoigny M, et al. Cholecystokinin and nitric oxide in transient lower esophageal sphincter relaxation to gastric distention in dogs. *Gastroenterology* 1994;107:1059–1066.

Cameron AJ, Zinmeister AR, Ballard DJ, et al. Prevalence of columnar lined (Barrett's) esophagus. Comparison of population-based clinical and autopsy findings. *Gastroenterology* 1990;99:918–922.

Carlson MA, Frantzides CT. Complications and results of primary minimally invasive antireflux procedures: a review of 10,735 reported cases. *J Am Coll Surg* 2001;193:428–439.

Carlsson R, Dent J, Watts R, et al. Gastro-oesophageal reflux disease in primary care: an international study of different treatment strategies with omeprazole. International GORD Study Group. *Eur J Gastroenterol Hepatol* 1998;10:119–124.

Caro JJ, Salas M, Ward A. Healing and relapse rates in gastroesophageal reflux disease treated with the new proton-pump inhibitors lansoprazole, rabeprazole, and pantoprazole compared with omeprazole, ranitidine, and placebo: evidence from randomized clinical trials. *Clin Ther* 2001;23:998–1017.

Carré IJ. The natural history of partial thoracic stomach (hiatus hernia) in children. *Arch Dis Child* 1959; 34:344–353.

Castell DO, Katz PO. Acid control and regression of Barrett's esophagus: is the glass half full or half empty? *Am J Gastroenterol* 1997;92:2329–2330.

Castell DO. Aggressive acid control: minimizing progression of Barrett's esophagus. *Am J Manag Care* 2001;7:S15–S18.

Castell DO, Kahrilas PJ, Richter JE, et al. Esomeprazole (40 mg) compared with lansoprazole (30 mg) in the treatment of erosive esophagitis. *Am J Gastroenterol* 2002;97:575–583.

Cherry J, Margulies S. Contact ulcer of the larynx. *Laryngoscope* 1968;78:1937–1940.

Crawford JM. Membrane trafficking and the pathologist: esophageal dysplasia. *Lab Invest* 1997;77:407–408.

Crookes PF. Gastroesophageal reflux after partial gastrectomy. *Am J Gastroenterol* 1998;93:3–4.

Dallemagne B, Taziaux P, Weerts J, et al. Laparoscopic surgery of gastroesophageal reflux. *Ann Chir* 1995;49:30–36.

De Beaux AC, Watson DI, Boyle C, et al. Role of fundoplication in patient symptomatology after laparoscopic antireflux surgery. *Br J Surg* 1998;88:1117–1121.

De Caestecker JS. Measuring duodenogastro-oesophageal reflux (DGOR). *Eur J Gastroenterol Hepatol* 1997;9:1141–1143.

De Meester TR, Ireland AP. Gastric pathology as an initiator and potentiator of gastroesophageal reflux disease. *Dis Esophagus* 1997;10:1–8.

Dent J. Australian clinical trials of omeprazole in the management of reflux esophagitis. *Digestion* 1990;47:69.

Dent J. Roles of gastric acid and pH in the pathogenesis of gastro-esophageal reflux disease. *Scand J Gastroenterol* 1994;(Suppl 201):55–61.

Dent J. Patterns of lower esophageal sphincter function associated with gastroesophageal reflux. *Am J Med* 1997;103:29S–32S.

Dent J, Talley N. Heartburn and dyspepsia: diagnostic challenge, health care dilemma. *Aliment Pharmacol Ther* 1997;(Suppl 2):11.

Desta Z, Zhao X, Shin JG, et al. Clinical significance of the cytochrome P450 2C19 genetic polymorphism. *Clin Pharmacokinet* 2002;41:913–958.

De Trevisa J. *Bartholomeus d[e] proprietatib[us] re[rum].* (Westminster) V, xxiv, lf. 14/1. 1398.

Devesa SS, Bioty S, Fraumeni IF Jr. Changing patterns in the incidence of esophageal and gastric carcinoma in the United States. *Cancer* 1998;83:2049–2053.

Donahue PE, Larson GM, Stewardson RH, et al. "Floppy" Nissen fundoplication. *Rev Surg* 1977;34(4):223–224.

Donahue PE. Basic considerations in gastroesophageal reflux disease. *Surg Clin North Am* 1997;77:1017–1040.

Donahue D, Navab F. Significance of short-segment Barrett's esophagus. *J Clin Gastroenterol* 1997;25:480–484.

Donahue PE, Samelson S, Nyhus LM, et al. The floppy Nissen fundoplication: effective long-term control of pathologic reflux. *Arch Surg* 1985;120:663–668.

Duhamel B, Sauvegrain J, Masse NP. Les hernies par l'hiatus oesophagien et les malpositions cardiotubérositaires chez le nourrisson et chez l'enfant. *Le Pumon* 1953;1:33–45.

Economic evaluation of health care programs. Oxford: Oxford University Press, 1987.

Eggleston A, Wigerinck A, Huijghebaert S, et al. Cost effectiveness of treatment for gastro-oesophageal reflux disease in clinical practice: a clinical database analysis. *Gut* 1998;42:13–16.

Eissele R, et al. Pantoprazole 40 mg and esomeprazole 40 mg show equivalent healing rates in patients with GERD. *Gastroenterology* 2002;122(Suppl):W1181.

El-Serag HB, Sonnenberg A. Outcomes of erosive reflux esophagitis after Nissen fundoplication. *Am J Gastroenterol* 1999;94:1771–1776.

Eppinger H. *Pathologie des Zwerchfelles. Supplement zu Northmage Spezielle Pathologie und Therapie.* Wien und Leipzig: Holder, 1911.

Fackler WK, Ours TM, Vaezi MF, et al. Long-term effect of H2RA therapy on nocturnal gastric acid breakthrough. *Gastroenterology* 2002;122:625–632.

Fletcher J, Wirz A, Young J, et al. Unbuffered highly acidic gastric juice exists at the gastroesophageal junction after a meal. *Gastroenterology* 2001;121:775–783.

Galmiche JP, Janssens J. The pathophysiology of gastroesophageal reflux disease: an overview. *Scand J Gastroenterol* 1995;(Suppl 211):7–18.

Garrison FH. *An introduction to the history of medicine.* Philadelphia: Saunders, 1929.

Geagea T. Laparoscopic Nissen's fundal plication is feasible. *Can J Surg* 1991;34:313.

Giaretti W. Aneuploidy mechanisms in human colorectal preneoplastic lesions and Barrett's esophagus. Is there a role for K-ras and p53 mutations? *Anal Cell Pathol* 1997;15:99–117.

Gough AL, Long RG, Cooper BT, et al. Lansoprazole versus ranitidine in the maintenance treatment of reflux esophagitis. *Aliment Pharmacol Ther* 1996;10:529–539.

Harrington SW, Kirklin BR. Clinical and radiological manifestations and surgical treatment of diaphragmatic hernia with a review of 13 cases. *Radiology* 1938;30:147.

Harris RA, Kuppermann M, Richter JE. Proton pump inhibitors or histamine-2 receptor antagonists for the prevention of recurrences of erosive reflux esophagitis: cost-effectiveness analysis. *Am J Gastroenterol* 1997:92:2179–2187.

Hatlebakk JG, Johnsson F, Vilien M, et al. The effect of cisapride in maintaining symptomatic remission in patients with gastro-oesophageal reflux disease. *Scand J Gastroenterol* 1997;32:1100–1106.

Havelund T, Lind T, Wiklund I, et al. Quality of life in patient, with heartburn but without esophagitis: effects of treatment with omeprazole. *Am J Gastroenterol* 1999;94:178–179.

Hedbloom CA. Diaphragmatic hernia. *Ann Intern Med* 1934;8:256–276.

Heudebert GR, Marks R, Wilcox CM, et al. The choice of long-term strategy for the management of patients with severe esophagitis: a cost-utility analysis. *Gastroenterology* 1997:112:1078–1086.

Hillman AL. Economic analysis of alternative treatments for persistent gastro-oesophageal reflux disease. *Scand J Gastroenterol* 1994;29(Suppl 201):98–102.

Hirsch DP, Holloway RH, Tytgat GN, et al. Involvement of nitric oxide in human transient lower esophageal sphincter relaxations and esophageal primary peristalsis. *Gastroenterology* 1998;115:374–380.

Hirsch DP, Tiel-Van BUUI MM, Tytgat GNJ, et al. Effect of L-NMMA on post-prandial transient lower esophageal sphincter relaxations in healthy volunteers [abstract]. *Neurogastroenterol Motil* 1999;11:264.

Holtmann G, Cain C, Malfertheiner P. Gastric *Helicobacter pylori* infection accelerates healing of reflux esophagitis during treatment with the proton pump inhibitor pantoprazole. *Gastroenterology* 1999;117:11–16.

Hunt RH, Cederberg C, Dent J, et al. Optimizing acid suppression for treatment of acid-related diseases. *Dig Dis Sci* 1995;40:24S–49S.

Ingelfinger RJ. Esophageal motility. *Physiol Rev* 1958;38:533–584.

Jackson C. Peptic ulcer of the esophagus. *JAMA* 1929;32:369.

Jaup B. Gastroesophageal reflux after cure of *H. pylori* infection. *Gastroenterology* 1997;113:2019.

Johnsson F, Weywadt L, Solhaug JH, et al. One-week omeprazole treatment in the diagnosis of gastro-oesophageal reflux disease. *Scand J Gastroenterol* 1998;33:15–20.

Kahrilas PJ. Anatomy and physiology of the gastroesophageal junction. *Gastroenterol Clin North Am* 1997;26:467–486.

Kahrilas PJ. Laparoscopic antireflux surgery: silver bullet or the emperor's new clothes? *Am J Gastroenterol* 1999;94(7):1721–1723.

Kahrilas PJ, Shi G, Manka M, et al. Increased frequency of transient lower esophageal sphincter relaxation induced by gastric distention in reflux patients with hiatal hernia. *Gastroenterology* 2000;118:688–695.

Katashima M, Yamamoto K, Tokuma Y, et al. Comparative pharmacokinetic/pharmacodynamic analysis of proton pump inhibitors omeprazole, lansoprazole and pantoprazole, in humans. *Eur J Drug Metab Pharmacokinet* 1998;23:19–26.

Katz P. The ambulatory pH study is normal, but the patient is not—the importance of the symptoms index. *Am J Gastroenterol* 1998;93:129–131.

Kim SL, Wo JM, Hunter JG, et al. The prevalence of intestinal metaplasia in patients with and without peptic strictures. *Am J Gastroenterol* 1998;93:53–55.

Klinkenberg-Knol EC, Festen HP, Jansen JB, et al. Long-term treatment with omeprazole for refractory reflux esophagitis: efficacy and safety. *Ann Intern Med* 1994;121:161–167.

Klinkenberg-Knol EC, Nelis F, Dent J, et al. Long-term omeprazole treatment in resistant gastroesophageal reflux disease: efficacy, safety, and influence on gastric mucosa. *Gastroenterology* 2000;118:661–669.

Koerner T, Schuetze K, Van Leendert RJ, et al. Interim analysis of POE Trial, the Pantoprazole Omeprazole Equivalence Trial. Healing of lesions in patients with gastroesophageal reflux disease II/III after 4 weeks of treatment with pantoprazole 40 mg or omeprazole 40 mg once daily. *Gastroenterology* 2001;120(Suppl 1):2235.

Kromer W. Relative efficacies of gastric proton-pump inhibitors on a milligram basis: desired and undesired SH reactions. Impact of chirality. *Scand J Gastroenterol* 2001;234(Suppl):3.

Kronecker H, Meltzer S. Der schluckmechanismus, seine erregung und seine hemmung. *Arch Anat Physiol* 1883;(Suppl):328–362.

Kuipers EJ, Lundell L, Klinkenberg-Knol EC, et al. Atrophic gastritis and *Helicobacter pylori* infection in patients with reflux esophagitis treated with omeprazole for fundoplication. *N Engl J Med* 1996;334:1018–1022.

Labenz J, Blum AL, Bayerdorffer E, et al. Curing *Helicobacter pylori* infection in patients with duodenal ulcer may provoke reflux esophagitis. *Gastroenterology* 1997;112:1442–1447.

Labenz J, Tillenburg B, Peitz U, et al. *Helicobacter pylori* augments the pH increasing effect of omeprazole in patients with duodenal ulcer. *Gastroenterology* 1996;110:725–732.

Lagergren J, Bergstrom R, Lindgren A, et al. Symptomatic gastroesophageal reflux as a risk factor for esophageal adenocarcinoma. *N Engl J Med* 1999;340:825–831.

Laine L. *H. pylori* eradication in gastroesophageal reflux disease. *Gastroenterology* 1997;113:2019–2020.

Ledson MJ, Tran J, Walshaw MJ. Prevalence and mechanisms of gastro-oesophageal reflux in adult cystic fibrosis patients. *J Royal Soc Med* 1998;91:7–9.

Leggett PL, Churchman-Winn R, Ahn C. Resolving gastroesophageal reflux with laparoscopic fundoplication. Findings in 138 cases. *Surg Endoscopy* 1998;12:142–147.

Lidums I, Checklin H, Mittal RK, et al. Effect of atropine on gastro-oesophageal reflux and transient lower oesophageal sphincter relaxations in patients with gastro-oesophageal reflux disease. *Gut* 1998;43:12–16.

Lidums I, Lehmann A, Checklin H, et al. Control of transient lower esophageal sphincter relaxations and reflux by the GABA$_R$ agonist baclofen in normal subjects. *Gastroenterology* 2000;118:7–13.

Lundell L, Miettinen P, Myrvold HE, et al. Lack of effect of acid suppression therapy on gastric atrophy. Nordic GERD Study Group. *Gastroenterology* 1999;117:319–326.

Lundell L, Miettinen P, Myrvold HE, et al. Long-term management of gastro-oesophageal reflux disease with omeprazole or open antireflux surgery: results of a prospective, randomized clinical trial. *Eur J Gastroenterol Hepatol* 2000;12:879–887.

Lundell L, Miettinen P, Myrvold HE, et al. Continued (5-year) followup of a randomized clinical study comparing antireflux surgery and omeprazole in gastroesophageal reflux disease. *J Am Coll Surg* 2001;192:172–179.

Maziak DE, Todd TR, Pearson FG. Massive hiatus hernia: evaluation and surgical management. *J Thorac Cardiovasc Surg* 1998;115:53–60, discussion 61–62.

McDougall NI, Johnston BT, Collins JS, et al. Disease progression in gastro-oesophageal reflux disease as determined by repeat oesophageal pH monitoring and endoscopy 3 to 4.5 years after diagnosis. *Eur J Gastroenterol Hepatol* 1997;9:1161–1167.

Mittal RK, Balaban DH. The esophagogastric junction. *N Engl J Med* 1997;336:924–932.

Mittal RK, Holloway RH, Penagini R, et al. Transient lower esophageal sphincter relaxation. *Gastroenterology* 1995:109:601–610.

Modlin IM. *From Prout to the proton pump*. Konstanz: Schneztor, 1995.

Modlin IM. *A history of gastroenterology at the millennium*. Milano: NextHealth srl, 2001.

Modlin IM, Goldenring JR, Lawton GP, et al. Aspects of the theoretical basis and clinical relevance of low acid states. *Am J Gastroenterol* 1994;89:308–318.

Moss SF, Arnold R, Tytgat G, et al. Consensus statement for management of gastroesophageal reflux disease. *J Clin Gastroenterol* 1998;27:6–12.

Neuhauser EDB, Berenberg W. Cardio-esophageal relaxation as a cause of vomiting in infants. *Radiology* 1947;48:480–483.

Nissen R. Die gastropexie als alleiniger Eingriff bei hiatushernien. *Dtsch Med Wschr* 1956;81:185.

Nissen R. Operation zur Beeinflussung der Refluxoesophagitis. *Schweiz Med Wochenschr* 1956;86:590–592.

Nissen R. Gastropexy as the lone procedure in the surgical repair of hiatus hernia. *Am J Surg* 1956;92:389.

Nissen R. Reminiscences: reflux esophagitis and hiatal hernia. *Rev Surg* 1970;27:307–314.

O'Connor JFB, Provenzale D, Brazer S. Economic considerations in the treatment of gastroesophageal reflux disease: a review. *Am J Gastroenterol* 2000;95:3354–3364.

O'Connor JFB, Singer ME, Richter JE. The cost-effectiveness of strategies to assess gastroesophageal reflux as an exacerbating factor in asthma. *Am J Gastroenterol* 1999;94:1472–1480.

Orringer MB, Skinner DB, Belsey RHR. Long-term results of the Mark IV operation for hiatal hernia and analyses of recurrences and their treatment. *J Thorac Cardiovasc Surg* 1972;63:25–33.

Pandolfino JE, Shi G, Curry J, et al. Esophagogastric junction distensibility: a factor contributing to sphincter incompetence. *Am J Physiol Gastrointest Liver Physiol* 2002;282:G1052–G1058.

Paré A (1880), cited by Harrington SW. Diaphragmatic hernia, Part 2. *Arch Surg* 1928;16:386–415.

Parkman HP, Urbain JL, Knight LC, et al. Effect of gastric acid suppressants on human gastric motility. *Gut* 1998;42:243–250.

Patti MG, Gantert W, Way LW. Surgery of the esophagus. Anatomy and physiology. *Surg Clin North Am* 1997;77:959–970.

Pearson FG. Adventures in surgery. *J Thorac Cardiovasc Surg* 1990;100:639–651.

Penagini R, Bianchi PA. Effect of morphine on gastroesophageal reflux and transient lower esophageal sphincter relaxation. *Gastroenterology* 1997;113:409–414.

Penagini R, Hebbard G, Horowitz M, et al. Motor function of the proximal stomach and visceral perception in gastrooesophageal reflux disease. *Gut* 1998;42:251–257.

Peters JH, DeMeester TR, Crookes P, et al. The treatment of gastroesophageal reflux disease with laparoscopic Nissen

fundoplication: prospective evaluation of 100 patients. *Ann Surg* 1998;228:40–50.

Pettersson G. Hiatal hernia, brachy-esophagus and incompetence of the cardia in children. *Acta Chirurgica Scand* 1951;18:561–598.

Phillips C, Moore A. Trial and error-an expensive luxury: economic analysis of the effectiveness of proton pump inhibitors and histamine-antagonists in treating reflux disease. *Brit J Med Econ* 1997;11:55–63.

Potempski P. Nuovo processo operativo per la riduzione cruenta della ernie diaphragmatiche de trauma e per la sutura delle ferite del diaframma. *Bull Reale Accad Med Roma* 1889;15:191–192.

Provencale D, Kemp JA, Arora S, et al. A guide for surveillance of patients with Barrett's esophagus. *Am J Gastroenterol* 1994;89:670–680.

R. Copland Guydon's Quest Chirurg. Fijb, 1541.

Randolph J. Experience with the Nissen fundoplication for correction of gastro-esophageal reflux in infants. *Ann Surg* 1983;198:579–584.

Rantanen TK, Salo JA, Sipponen JT. Fatal and life-threatening complications in antireflux surgery: analysis of 5,502 operations. *Br J Surg* 1999;86:1573–1577.

Rantanen TK, Halme TV, Loustarinen ME, et al. The long term results of open antireflux surgery in a community based health care center. *Am J Gastroenterol* 1999;94:1777–1781.

Ravitch MM. Chalasia and achalasia of the esophagus. In: Benson CD (ed). *Pediatric surgery*. Chicago: Year Book Medical, 1962:299–300.

Richter JE. Extraesophageal presentations of gastroesophageal reflux disease. *Semin Gastrointest Dis* 1997;8:75–89 [published erratum appears in *Semin Gastrointest Dis* 1997;8:210].

Richter JE, Kahrilas PJ, Johanson J, et al. Efficacy and safety of esomeprazole compared with omeprazole in GERD patients with erosive esophagitis: a randomized controlled trial. *Am J Gastroenterol* 2001;96:656–665.

Ritvo M. Hernia of the stomach through the esophageal orifice of the diaphragm. *J Am Med Assoc* 1930;94:15–21.

Rokitansky K. *Handbuch der pathologishen anatomie*. Vienna: W. Braumuller, 1841.

Romagnuolo J, Meier MA, Sadowski DC. Medical or surgical therapy for erosive reflux esophagitis. Cost-utility analysis using a Markov model. *Ann Surg* 2002;236:191–202.

Rossetti ME, Liebermann-Meffert D. Nissen-Rossetti antireflux fundoplication (open procedure). In: Nyhus LM, Baker RJ, Fischer JE, eds. *Mastery of surgery*. Boston: Little, Brown and Company, 1997:743–762.

Sampliner RE. Practice Parameters Committee of the American College of Gastroenterology. Practice guidelines on the diagnosis, surveillance, and therapy of Barrett's esophagus. *Am J Gastroenterol* 1998;93:1028–1032.

Sandbu R, Hallgren T. The economics of laparoscopic antireflux operations compared with open surgery. *Eur J Surg* 2000;(Suppl 585):37–39.

Saslow SB, Thumshirn M, Camilleri M, et al. Influence of *H. pylori* infection on gastric motor and sensory function in asymptomatic volunteers. *Dig Dis Sci* 1998;43:258–364.

Shaheen N. Is there a "Barrett's iceberg?" *Gastroenterology* 2002;123:636–639.

Shaheen NJ, Crosby MA, Bozymski EM, et al. Is there publication bias in the reporting of cancer risk in Barrett's esophagus? *Gastroenterology* 2000;119:333–338.

Sharma P, Morales TG, Sampliner RE. Short segment Barrett's esophagus—the need for standardization of the definition and of endoscopic criteria. *Am J Gastroenterol* 1998;93:1033.

Shin JM, Sachs G. Restoration of acid secretion following treatment with proton pump inhibitors. *Gastroenterology* 2002;123:1588–1597.

Skinner DB, Belsey RHR. Surgical management of esophageal reflux and hiatal hernia: long-term results with 1030 patients. *J Thorac Cardiovasc Surg* 1967;v.53:33–54.

Skinner DB, Belsey RHR. Surgical management of esophageal reflux and hiatus hernia. *J Thorac Cardiovasc Surg* 1967;53:33.

Smit CF, Tan J, Devriese PP, et al. Ambulatory pH measurements at the upper esophageal sphincter. *Laryngoscope* 1998;108:299–302.

Smythe A, Bird NC, Troy GP, et al. Effect of cisapride on oesophageal motility and duodenogastro-oesophageal reflux in patients with Barrett's oesophagus. *Eur J Gastroenterol Hepatol* 1997;9:1149–1153.

Sonnenberg A. Motion—Laparoscopic Nissen fundoplication is more cost effective than oral PPI administration: arguments against the motion. *Can J Gastroenterol* 2002;16:627–631.

Sontag SJ, O'Connell S, Khandelwal S, et al. Most asthmatics have gastroesophageal reflux with or without bronchodilator therapy. *Gastroenterology* 1990;99:613–620.

Spechler SJ. Epidemiology and natural history of gastroesophageal reflux disease. *Digestion* 1992;51(Suppl 1):24–29.

Stein HJ, Balint A. Surgery for gastro-oesophageal reflux disease: laparoscopic versus traditional approach. *Ital J Gastroenterol Hepatol* 1997;29:391–394.

Stein HJ, Crookes PF, DeMeester TR. Three-dimensional manometric imaging of the lower esophageal sphincter. *Surg Ann* 1995;27:199–214.

Stewart MJ, Hurst AF. *Gastric and duodenal ulcer*. London: Oxford University Press, 1929:498.

Straathof JW, Lamers CB, Masclee AA. Effect of gastrin-17 on lower esophageal sphincter characteristics in man. *Dig Dis Sci* 1997;42:2547–2551.

Swanström LL. Motion—Laparascopic Nissen fundoplication

is more cost effective than oral PPI administration: arguments for the motion. *Can J Gastroenterol* 2002;16:621–623.

Talley NJ, Venables TL, Green JR, et al. Esomeprazole 40 mg and 20 mg is efficacious in the long-term management of patients with endoscopy-negative gastro-oesophageal reflux disease: a placebo-controlled trial of on-demand therapy for 6 months. *Eur J Gastroenterol Hepatol* 2002;14:857–863.

Thogersen C, Rasmussen C, Putz K, et al. Non-parametic classification of esophagus motility by means of neural networks. *Methods Inf Med* 1997;36:352–355.

Tileston W. Peptic ulcer of the esophagus. *J Am Med Sci* 1906;132:240–265.

Trus TL, Laycock WS, Wo JM, et al. Laparoscopic antireflux surgery in the elderly. *Am J Gastroenterol* 1998;93:351–353.

Vakil N, Trent S. The outcome of laparoscopic fundoplication for reflux disease in community practice in the USA [abstract]. *Gastroenterology* 2001;120:A16.

van Den Boom G, Go PM, Hameeteman W, et al. Cost effectiveness of medical versus surgical treatment in patients with severe or refractory gastroesophageal reflux disease in the Netherlands. *Scand J Gastroenterol* 1996;31:1–9.

Vandenplas Y. Commentary: oesophageal pH monitoring: how gold is the gold standard? *Ital J Gastroenterol Hepatol* 1997;29:302–304.

Vela ME, Tutuian R, Katz PO, et al. Baclofen reduces both acid and nonacid gastroesophageal reflux: a study using combined multichannel intraluminal impedance and pH [abstract]. *Am J Gastroenterol* 2001;96:542.

Vigneri S, Termini R, Leandro G, et al. A comparison of maintenance therapies for reflux esophagitis. *N Engl J Med* 1995;333:1106–1110.

Viljakka M, Nevalainen J, Isolauri J. Lifetime costs of surgical versus medical treatment of severe gastroesophageal reflux in Finland. *Scand J Gastroenterol* 1997;32:766–772.

Washington N, Steele RJ, Wright JW, et al. An investigation of lower oesophageal redox potentials in gastro-oesophageal reflux patients and healthy volunteers. *Physiol Meas* 1997;18:363–371.

Wilmer A, Van Cutsem E, Andrioli A, et al. Ambulatory gastrojejunal manometry in severe motility-like dyspepsia: lack of correlation between dysmotility, symptoms, and gastric emptying. *Gut* 1998;42:235–242.

Winkelstein A. Peptic esophagitis (a new clinical entity). *JAMA* 1935;104:906.

Yacyshyn BR, Thomson AB. The clinical importance of proton pump inhibitor pharmacokinetics. *Digestion* 2002;66:67–78.

Zhang Q, Lehmann A, Rigda R, et al. Control of transient lower oesophageal sphincter relaxation and reflux by the GABA$_R$ agonist baclofen in patients with gastro-oesophageal reflux disease. *Gut* 2002;50:19–24.

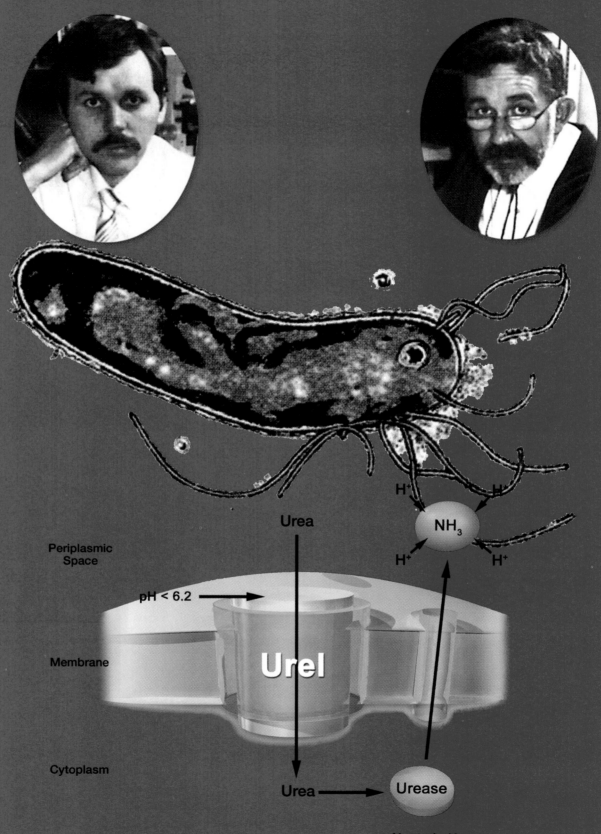

Periplasmic
Space

pH < 6.2 →

Membrane

UreI

Cytoplasm

Urea

Urea → Urease

NH₃

H⁺   H⁺

H⁺   H⁺

Neutral pH
Optimum Urease

SECTION 7

HELICOBACTER PYLORI

CHAPTER 1
HISTORY

Introduction

Although the association between *Campylobacter* (*Helicobacter*) *pylori* and ulcers was discovered by Robin Warren in 1979, and the organism was cultured by Barry Marshall in 1982, resulting in their seminal publications in *Lancet* in 1983, the historical origins of its discovery are rooted in the latter half of the nineteenth century. It was during this period that the eminent German bacteriologist Robert Koch proved scientifically that bacteria were the cause of certain diseases. Almost simultaneously, the Frenchman Louis Pasteur, having been galvanized by Koch's contributions, was in the process of developing vaccines against the microbes causing cholera and rabies. In Sicily, in a small homemade laboratory in Messina, an *émigré* Russian, Elie Metchnikoff, had discovered phagocytosis, thus initiating an entirely new vista of biologic investigation: host defense mechanisms.

Early bacteriology

Although Leeuwenhoek was probably the first to see both gastrointestinal and oral bacteria, it was O. F. Muller (1730–1784) of Copenhagen who provided the first definitive observations and descriptions of microorganisms; he also coined

Observations on Gastric Infection

Year	Individual	Observations
1875	G. Bottcher/M. Letulle	demonstrated bacteria in ulcer margins
1881	C. Klebs	bacterial colonization and 'interglandular small cell infiltration'
1888	M. Letulle	experimental induction of acute gastric lesions in guinea pigs (*S. aureus*)
1889	W. Jaworski	spiral organisms (*Vibrio rugula*) in gastric washings
1893	G. Bizzozero	identified spirochetes in gastric mucosa of dogs
1896	H. Salomon	spirochetes noted in gastric mucosa and experimentally transferred to mice
1906	W. Krienitz	spirochetes in gastric contents of patient with gastric carcinoma
1908	F.B. Turck	induced gastric ulcers in dogs by *Bacillus* (*Escherichia*) *coli*
1916	E.C. Rosenow	described streptococcus induced gastric ulcers
1917	L.R. Dragstedt	identified bacteria in experimental ulcers, no significant role identified
1921	J.S. Edkins	experimental physiology of *S. regaudi* (*H. felis*)
1924	J.M. Luck	discovered gastric mucosal urease
1925	B. Hoffman	described *B. hoffmani* - putative ulcerous agent
1930	B. Berg	partial vagotomy inhibits secondary infections in ulcers
1938	J.L. Doenges	spirochetes/inflammation in *Macacus* monkey and man
1940	A.S. Freedberg/L. Barron	identified spirochetes in man - no etiologic role
1940	F.D. Gorham	postulated gastric acidophilic bacteria as an etiologic agent in ulcer disease
1954	E.D. Palmer	no spirochetes detected using HE in 1,180 suction biopsies
1975	H.W. Steer	polymorphonuclear migration in ulcers - isolated *Pseudomonas aeruginosa*
1983	J.R. Warren	identified *Campylobacter* (*Helicobacter*) *pylori* in human gastritis
1983	B. Marshall	isolated and cultured *H. pylori*
1985-1987	B. Marshall/A. Morris	ingested and proved the infectivity of *H. pylori* (Koch's 3rd postulate)

A historical timeline of the individual contributions that led to the identification of *H. pylori*.

the terms *bacillus* and *spirillum*. Ferdinand Cohn (1828–1898) from Breslau, the botanist now regarded as one of the founders of bacteriology, classified microorganisms into several groups—*bacterial* (short, cylindric cells), *bacilli* (longer cells), *spirilla* (wavy or spiral forms), and *coccoid* (spheric)—and noted the fixity of bacterial species. Thus, even under varying conditions, he was never able to obtain cocci from bacilli and vice versa. In 1870, Cohn established his own journal, *Beitrage zur Biologie der Pflanzen*, and in this communication hosted most of the original, classic bacteriology papers, authored by both himself and his young *protégé*, Robert Koch. The classic postulates of the latter would subsequently form the logical basis for the investigation and identification of the disease-causing potential of bacteria. In 1872, Cohn published his mature exposition on bacteriology entitled *Untersuchungen über Bakteria*, wherein he further expanded the classification of bacteria into genera and species. He suggested an expanded classification into four groups: *sphaerobacteria* (cocci), *microbacteria*, *desmobacteria* (bacillus and vibrio), and *spirobacteria* (spirillum and spirochete). This work was well received and became so popular that it was reprinted in 1875 and again in 1876.

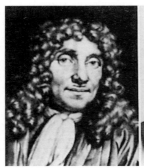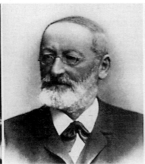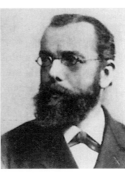

From left to right: Leeuwenhoek, Cohn, Koch. A. Leeuwenhoek (1632–1723), the enthusiastic pioneer of the biologic microcosmos, was the first to see gastrointestinal bacteria (mouth, colon) but due to his lack of medical training ascribed no pathologic importance to this new world. Once microscopes had sufficiently evolved, order was brought to the vague Linnaean genus of "Chaos" by F. Cohn's (1828–1898) morphologic classification of bacteria. Cohn's *protégé*, R. Koch (1843–1910), one of the founders of modern bacteriology, was also first to develop the correct theory of species-specific infectious diseases.

In 1878, the term *microbe* was introduced by C. E. Sedillot (1804–1883), a French surgeon who was responsible for undertaking the first gastrostomy and may have unwittingly happened on the organism. He proposed this term, derived from the Greek for "small life," with the caveat that such "small lives" must have the special ability to cause fermentation, putrefaction, or a disease process. This was a proposal much favored by T. Schwann (1810–1882), who had himself not only discovered pepsin in 1834 but also had written extensively on the role of fermentation, as well as the single-cell theory of disease.

Early data on gastric bacteriology

Careful analysis of gastric contents revealed that under fasting conditions, the normal stomach contained mucus, a few bacilli, and some yeast cells, whereas in stagnant gastric contents, obtained from patients with gastric disease, bacilli, micrococci, yeast, and fungus could readily be seen. Such early observations supported speculations regarding a putative causative role of these "foreign bodies" in gastric pathology. It was unclear, however, to these early, eager gastric bacteriologists whether a specific organism was the cause of a gastric disease entity or whether it was simply an abnormal accumulation of organisms in the stomach itself that culminated in gastric disturbances.

One of these first gastric bacteriologists was G. Bottcher, a German who, along with his French collaborator M. Letulle (1853–1929), could demonstrate bacterial colonies in the ulcer floor and in its mucosal margins. His convictions in regard to the disease-causing potential of ingested organisms were so ardent that by 1875, he had attributed the causation of ulcers to the bacteria that they could demonstrate. However, this was not a popular point of view, and in spite of an 1881 report by the pathologist C. Klebs of a bacillus-like organism evident both free in the lumen of gastric glands and between the cells of the glands and the tunica propria, with corresponding *"interglandular small round cell infiltration,"* the "bacterial hypothesis" fell into disuse. Bottcher was, however, probably the first to formally report the presence of spiral organisms in the gastrointestinal tract of animals, although spiral organisms were already well known and had been described as early as 1838 by Ehrenburg. The pathogenic properties of these particular organisms had similarly been recognized by Obermeier of Berlin, who, in 1872, could demonstrate their presence in the blood of patients with relapsing fever. An examination of the report of Klebs indicates that he had noted the presence of an inflammatory infiltration, although he made no specific comments with regard to its significance. However, could this have been the first notation, if not of *H. pylori* infectious gastritis, then at least of lymphoid tissue in the gastric mucosa?

In 1889, Walery Jaworski, professor of Medicine at the Jagiellonian University, Cracow, Poland, was the first to describe in detail spiral organisms in the sediment of washings obtained from humans. Among other things, he noted a bacterium with a characteristic spiral appearance, which he named *Vibrio rugula*. He suggested that it might play a possible pathogenic role in gastric disease. Jaworski supposed that these "snail" or "spiral" cells were only to be found in rare cases. However, Ismar Boas (Berlin), already a luminary for his gastrointestinal contributions and for the discovery of the "Oppler-Boas" lactobacillus, found these cells quite constantly in all "fasting" gastric contents containing hydrochloric acid. Further detailed analysis by Boas' assistant, P. Cohnheim, indicated that such "cells" could be induced by the reaction of bronchial or pharyngeal mucus and hydrochloric acid. This led to the suggestion that Jaworski had consistently observed acid-altered myelin and that similar secondary structures, threads, and small masses could also be induced by these simple chemical reactions. Cohnheim and Boas, therefore, inferred from their experiments that Jaworski's "cells" were most probably the product of gastric mucus and acid chyme.

The observations of Bottcher and Letulle had suggested a causative bacterial agent in ulcer disease, and by 1888, Letulle was actively searching for this postulated entity. A few years earlier, in 1881, the Scottish surgeon and bacteriologist, Alexander Ogston (1844–1929), had identified *Staphylococcus pyrogenes aureus* both in acute and chronic abscesses. Noting the similarity of this bacterium to their postulated entity, Letulle, in the time-honored tradition of his day, undertook a classic experiment. He used two modes of administration in guinea pigs: intramuscular injection of Ogston's pure, cultured *Staphylococcus* or oral intake of the agent. Not surprisingly, this resulted in the formation of acute gastric lesions per-

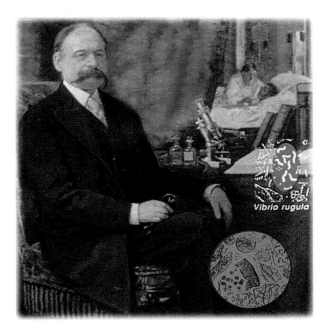

Vibrio rugula

In 1889, W. Jaworski discovered and postulated a pathogenic role for the spiral organisms (*Vibrio rugula*) that he found in gastric contents.

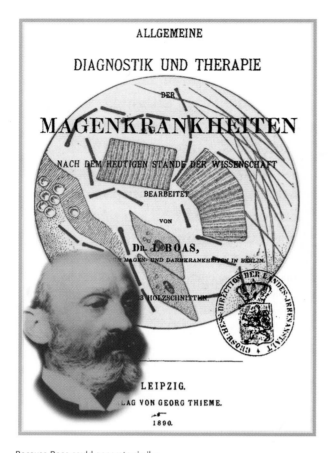

Because Boas could generate similar morphologic forms chemically, he suggested that Jaworski's cells were the result of the interreaction of gastric mucus and acid. Boas was responsible for the codiscovery of the Oppler-Boas bacterium, which he thought was implicated in the etiology of gastric carcinoma.

fectly consistent, at least to him, with the predictable mode of generation of gastric ulcers. Matters were, however, somewhat complicated by the fact that he obtained similar results with dysentery organisms and with pyrogenic *Streptococci*. Letulle was never able to experimentally discriminate between these different agents and was therefore not able to conclusively prove a role for bacteria in ulcer disease. Nevertheless, the experimental work of Letulle inspired a number of other scientists to follow his lead, and similar results were attained with *Lactobacillus*, diphtheria toxin, and *Pneumococcus*.

In a time frame contiguous to these sophisticated experiments, the Italian anatomist G. Bizzozero (1846–1901) was busily engaged in the extensive study of the comparative anatomy of vertebrate gastrointestinal glands with his adept and capable pupil, the future Nobel Prize winner Camillo Golgi. In specimens of the gastric mucosa of six dogs, Bizzozero noted the presence of a spirochete organism in the gastric glands and both in the cytoplasm and vacuoles of parietal cells. He commented that this organism affected both pyloric and fundic mucosa, and its distribution extended from the base of the gland to the surface mucosa. Although he neglected to ascribe any clinical relevance to these observations, he did, however, remark on their close association with the parietal cells.

Three years later, in 1896, in a paper entitled "Spirillum of the mammalian stomach and its behavior with respect to the parietal cells," H. Salomon reported spirochetes in the gastric mucosa of dogs, cats, and rats, although he was unable to identify them in other animals, including humans. In this early paper, Salomon undertook a series of somewhat bizarre experiments in which he tried to transmit the bacterium to a range of other animal species by using gastric scrapings from dogs. He failed to transmit it to owls, rabbits, pigeons, and frogs; however, the feeding of gastric mucus to white mice resulted in a spectacular colonization within a week, as evidenced by the series of drawings of infected gastric mucosa reproduced in the original paper. The lumen of the gastric pits of the mice were packed with the spiral-shaped bacteria, and invasion

G. Bizzozero, A. von Kolliker, and G. Golgi in Pavia, 1887. Bizzozero had a profound interest in the gut and inspired Golgi to study the canalicular apparatus of the resting and stimulated gastric gland. Although Bizzozero's main contribution was the identification of the platelets of the blood, it is clear that he noted the presence of spiral organisms in the gastric mucosa, although he unfortunately ascribed no particular significance to them. von Kolliker was later instrumental in securing the Nobel Prize for Golgi and Ramón y Cajal.

H. Salomon extensively studied *H. felis* in domestic animals. In this article, published in 1896, he described his unsuccessful attempts both at culturing the bacteria *in vitro* and at establishing the mode of transmission of the organism. Nonetheless, after failing in frogs, rabbits, and pigeons, he succeeded in infecting white mice with the bacterium. He also noted the invasion of the glands, as well as the close association with parietal cells. His studies refuted the then-current hypothesis that parietal cells were guards at the entrance of the stomach and acted to limit the entrance of microorganisms into the gastrointestinal tract.

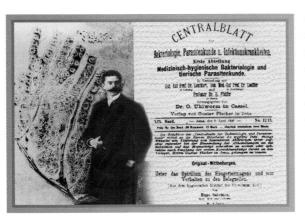

of the parietal cells was also noted. Almost 2 decades later, in 1920, Kasai and Kobayashi successfully repeated these experiments and, using spirochetes isolated from cats, demonstrated pathogenic results in rabbits. Histologic examination indicated both hemorrhagic erosion and ulceration of the mucosa in the presence of masses of the spirochetes.

Twentieth century

By the beginning of the twentieth century, physicians involved in the treatment of gastrointestinal disease were generally familiar with some infective processes of the digestive tract: the ulcerative processes of typhoid fever, a variety of dysenteric conditions, and tuberculosis. Kiyoshi Shiga had discovered a

J. Cohnheim (1839–1884) (top), born at Demmin in Pomerania and trained initially in Wurzburg and thereafter in Berlin as a pupil of Virchow before being, successively, Professor of Pathological Anatomy and Pathology at Kiel University (1869), a research collaborator at Carl Ludwig's "*Physiological Institute*" in Leipzig, and, in 1872, Professor of Pathological Anatomy at Breslau University. His major contributions were in experimental pathology; in particular, demonstrating that inflammation was an active, dynamic process. Cohnheim was among the first to describe the diapedesis of leukocytes and postulated that chemical factors played the critical role in the etiology of ulcers. Robert Koch (bottom) (1843–1910) was born at Clausthal in the Upper Harz Mountains, the son of a mining engineer. In 1862, he attended the University of Göttingen, where he studied medicine and was greatly influenced by the Professor of Anatomy, Jacob Henle, who had, as early as 1840, published that infectious diseases were caused by living, parasitic organisms. Having received an M.D. degree in 1866, Koch went to Berlin for 6 months of chemical study with Virchow. Koch demonstrated the results of his early bacterial work in 1876 to a research group including Ferdinand Cohn, Professor of Botany at the University of Breslau, and Julius Cohnheim. Both were deeply impressed by the work, and Cohn published Koch's material in the botanical journal of which he was the editor. Thereafter, Koch achieved fame as he successively pioneered the morphologic identification of bacterial-developed culture methods and the concept of the role of bacteria in the genesis of disease. Few remembered that it was Henle who, 30 years previously, had first proposed the criteria subsequently known as "Koch's postulates"!

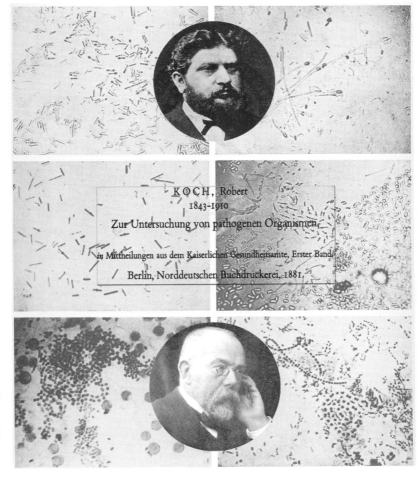

bacterium, erroneously recognized as *Shigella dysenteriae*, in 1898; an unspecified type of upper gastrointestinal (gastric) bacterial infection not accompanied by signs of active inflammation and designated as *bacterial necrosis* had also been annotated and was described in detail in Hemmeter's text of 1902. This pathology was characterized by the invasion of bacteria, usually into the lower depths of the mucous membrane, followed by bacterial growth and subsequent tissue necrosis.

J. Cohnheim (1839–1884), professor of pathology at Kiel, who as early as 1880 had prophesied that the young Koch would surpass all others in the field of medical bacteriology, had suggested that the formation of ulcers depended on chemical factors. Shortly thereafter, F. Reigel attributed hyperchlorhydria as the cause of chronic ulcers. The scientific foundations for the recognition of the role of gastric juice (acid) in the genesis of ulcer disease were laid first by A. Kussmaul (1822–1902), who had, in 1869, developed a method of intubation of the stomach, and second by the creation of the experimental gastric pouch preparation by I. P. Pavlov.

In 1906, Krienitz identified spirochetes in the gastric contents of a patient with a carcinoma of the lesser curvature of the stomach and commented that on microscopic examination, three types of spirochetes, including *Spirochete pallidum*, could be identified. He did not address the question of etiology. Spirochetal dysentery, as well as the presence of spirochetes in the stool of healthy

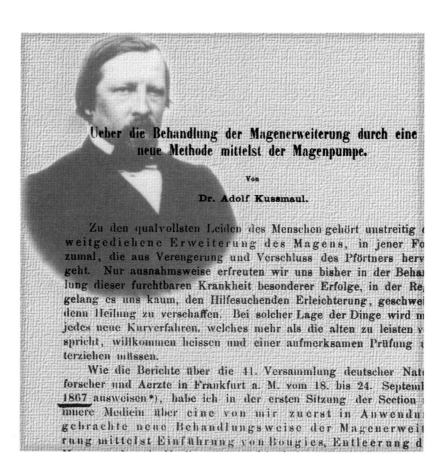

The foundations for the role of acid in the genesis of ulcers were laid by A. Kussmaul (1822–1902), who developed a method for intubating patients and who also advocated the use of bismuth subcitrate for the treatment of this disease.

individuals, were known, and Muhlens and, independently, Luger and Neuberger had all reported these organisms to be evident in the stomach contents of patients with ulcerating carcinomas of the stomach. The latter authors also noted the rarity of these organisms in the gastric mucosa and gastric juice of healthy individuals. Experimental biology, however, dominated gastric research, and in the same year, Turcke had undertaken an experiment in which he fed broth cultures of *Bacillus coli* to dogs for a number of months. This resulted in the development of chronic gastric ulceration. In an attempt to establish cause and effect, he thereafter cultured *B. coli* from the feces of ulcer patients, which was then injected intravenously into dogs without effect. However, when the animals ingested the microorganism, every single dog reacted with a spectrum of nonspecific gastric and duodenal alterations, which Turcke loosely called *ulcers*. When Gibelli attempted to repeat this work, he could not confirm the results obtained by Turcke.

In Cincinnati, Ohio, the American bacteriologist E. C. Rosenow, over a decade from 1913 to 1923, vehemently maintained that ulceration of the stomach could be reproduced in laboratory animals by *Streptococcus*. He isolated this bacterium from foci of infection in humans with ulcer disease and injected the culture into a wide range of animals, including rabbits, dogs, monkeys, guinea pigs, cats, and mice. A higher incidence of experimental lesions was identified using this particular inoculum than from cultures isolated from foci in other patients. Of additional interest was that *Streptococci* isolated from jejunal ulcers in Mann-Williamson–operated dogs also caused acute gastritis and duodenal ulcers that were limited to the upper gastrointestinal tract in experimental animals. Based on these observations, Rosenow postulated that "*gastric ulcer–producing* Streptococci" had a selective affinity for the gastric mucosa and produced a local destruction of the glandular tissue. He further proposed that, consequent on such damage, ulcers would thereafter form, given the autolytic capacity of gastric acid. Rosenow thought that the reservoirs for these bacteria were carious teeth and advanced the idea that a hematogenous bacterial invasion would result in the formation of an ulcer. These experiments were continued by Hardt in dogs and later by McGown in guinea pigs, with analogous results.

One of the early scientific interests of L. R. Dragstedt was the causation of gastroduodenal ulceration, although he would subsequently (1943) achieve renown as the surgeon who established the "physiologic" rationale for vagotomy as a treatment for duodenal ulcer disease.

As early as 1917, as a young physiologist, he had attempted to define the different mechanisms by which gastric juice could affect healing of acute gastric and duodenal ulcers. Aware of Rosenow's work and the question of the importance of the virulence of different bacterial strains in determining the chronicity of ulcers, he attempted to isolate and culture any bacteria he could find in the silver nitrate–induced ulcers of five experimental Pavlov-pouch dogs.

Bacteriologic examination revealed *Streptococcus*, *Staphylococcus*, and *Bacillus* species, which were similar to those types of bacteria isolated from clinical ulcers in humans.

Although trained as a physiologist in Chicago by A. Carlson, Lester Dragstedt (1893–1975) (left) realized that experimental surgical models provided a novel method to study gastrointestinal problems. Having been taught by Moorhead, a local surgeon, to create such models, he diligently explored the genesis of peptic ulcer disease and the regulation of acid secretion. The fact that he was never formally trained as a surgeon (despite being appointed Professor of Surgery) no doubt enabled him to maintain an open mind in respect to causality and therapy. Thus, early in his career, he believed that bacterial infection was the origin of gastroduodenal ulceration (top) but subsequently modified his views and concluded that neural regulation was critical and that the deleterious clinical consequences of excessive acid secretion could be surgically abrogated by vagotomy (bottom). In proposing both a bacterial and a neural etiology for peptic ulcer, Dragstedt twice crossed the intellectual Rubicon of his time.

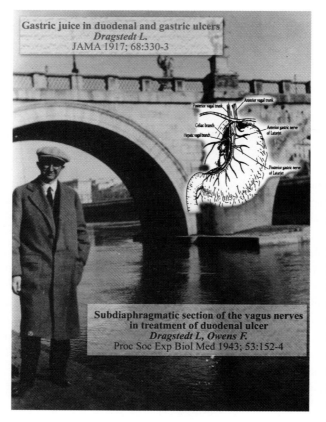

Gastric juice in duodenal and gastric ulcers
Dragstedt L.
JAMA 1917; 68:330-3

Subdiaphragmatic section of the vagus nerves in treatment of duodenal ulcer
Dragstedt L, Owens F.
Proc Soc Exp Biol Med 1943; 53:152-4

Dragstedt concluded that these bacteria colonized the damaged mucosa after ulcer formation and proposed that they had migrated up from the alimentary tract. He did not believe that they played a substantial role in the etiology of the disease and did not pursue these studies further, choosing rather to focus on the role of vagal innervation in acid-induced ulceration.

Fifteen years later, at the Mount Sinai Hospital, A. Berg used partial vagotomy to reduce "secondary" infections in ulcer margins. Soon thereafter, however, he turned his attention to the colon and, along with his collaborator, Crohn, became more famous for his role in the discovery of the etiology of this disease.

J. S. Edkins (1863–1940) of London made a significant contribution to the elucidation of gastric physiology by the discovery of gastrin. Motivated by his previous disappointment, incurred in the investigation of gastrin, Edkins still maintained his enthusiasm for the exploration of gastric pathophysiology. In contrast to the inoculation mode of experimental studies, he proceeded to investigate how the host itself might affect the prevalence and location of the spirochete organisms in different parts of the stomach. The organisms were named *Spirochete regaudi*, after Regaudi, who considered that the organisms of the gastric mucus layer of cats were morphologically analogous to the syphilis spirochete. Using the Giemsa stain to identify the organisms in stomach sections, Edkins identified them in both the fundus and the antrum and noted specific invasion of the epithelial cells of the fundic glands. It was also evident that the organism appeared to have a preference for the surface epithelium or for thick mucus of the feline experimental model. Of note was the demonstration of organisms not only in the subepithelial lymphoid tissue but also located within the phagocytic cells.

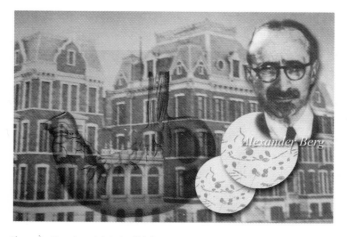

Alexander Berg

Alexander Berg (top right), the Chief of Surgery at Mount Sinai Hospital in New York, originally noted the presence of bacteria in stomachs he had resected for peptic ulcer disease (left) and proposed that a bacterial origin should be considered!

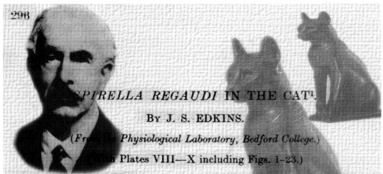

SPIRELLA REGAUDI IN THE CAT[1].

By J. S. EDKINS.

(*From the Physiological Laboratory, Bedford College.*)

(With Plates VIII—X including Figs. 1–23.)

THE spiral organism found in the stomach of various carnivora has been investigated by several observers (see the references at the end of this paper). Such studies have been mainly directed to the morphology of the organism, its infectivity and the part it plays in producing a pathological condition. In the present paper I have been concerned rather with the physiological condition of its host as influencing the prevalence and location of the organism in different regions of the stomach. I was anxious further to ascertain if the organism affected the normal processes of digestion in the stomach either to the advantage or the disadvantage of the animal entertaining it.

J. S. Edkins (1863–1940) is best known for his controversial (at the time) discovery of gastrin in 1905. What is less appreciated is his work on a spiral organism, most probably *H. felis*, in the stomach of cats. Apart from his critical contributions to the field of croquet, Edkins deserves credit for these two seminal observations in the field of gastroenterology.

He also described a "beaded form" of the organism in fasting cats, an observation consistent with the discovery of sporulation bodies. Gastric secretory activity did not appear to be compromised when the organisms were present and abundant, and indeed, there appeared to be a parallelism between the degree of acid and the abundance of the organisms.

In 1925, Hoffman investigated whether the causative agent of ulcer disease was a member of the bacillus family by the injection of 5 cc of gastric contents from a peptic ulcer patient into guinea pigs. He successfully produced gastric ulcers, from which he recovered gram-negative, fine, slender rods, which, when inoculated into another guinea pig, once again produced the same lesions. He modestly named his organism *Bacillus hoffmani*, but it was evident after further study that the lesion-producing capabilities of this bacterium were nonspecific. In 1930, Saunders demonstrated that the *Streptococcus* organism isolated from peptic ulcers in humans was of the alpha variety and identified specific antibodies against this agent in serum from patients. However, he was not able to produce ulcers in animals by injecting the inoculum and proposed that laboratory animals do not spontaneously form gastric ulcers, because they exhibited an innate resistance to this organism.

Based to a certain extent on the recognition of the widespread scourge of luetic disease, at approximately the beginning of the Second World War, spirochetes returned to gastric prominence.

J. L. Doenges observed the organisms to invade the gastric glands of every single one of the *Macacus* rhesus monkeys he studied and to be present in 43% of human gastric autopsy specimens. In contrast to the monkey, the organisms appeared to be difficult to identify in human gastric mucosa, and only 11 of the 103 specimens showed appreciable numbers.

Doenges' specimens, however, were autolytic, which precluded the attachment of any major significance to his observations. Of special note, however, was his observation that the organism was restricted to the gastric mucosa and not evident in the intestinal mucosa.

These reports prompted Freedberg and Barron, in 1941, to investigate the presence of spirochetes in the gastric tissue of patients who had undergone partial resection surgery. Both authors were familiar with the methods of identifying the organism and used the silver-staining method of DaFano, which they had previously successfully used (but not published) to identify spirochetes in dogs. In spite of such expertise, they were not able to identify

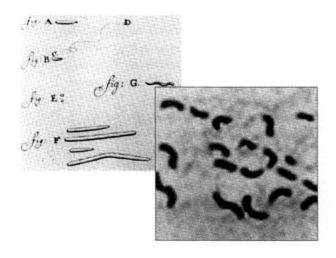

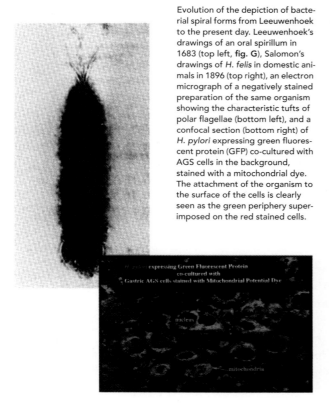

Evolution of the depiction of bacterial spiral forms from Leeuwenhoek to the present day. Leeuwenhoek's drawings of an oral spirillum in 1683 (top left, **fig. G**), Salomon's drawings of *H. felis* in domestic animals in 1896 (top right), an electron micrograph of a negatively stained preparation of the same organism showing the characteristic tufts of polar flagellae (bottom left), and a confocal section (bottom right) of *H. pylori* expressing green fluorescent protein (GFP) co-cultured with AGS cells in the background, stained with a mitochondrial dye. The attachment of the organism to the surface of the cells is clearly seen as the green periphery superimposed on the red stained cells.

the organisms, although they could demonstrate that spirochetes were more frequently present in ulcerated stomachs than in nonulcerated stomachs (53% versus 14%). Based on their own difficulties with adequate identification and the apparent histologic differences noted in Doenges' observations in the *Macacus* mucosa, they concluded that no absolute etiopathologic role for these organisms could be defined. It is with almost tragic irony that, in the report of the discussion of this paper, Frank D. Gorham, of St. Louis, Missouri, noted: *"I believe that a further search should be made for an organism thriving in hydrochloric acid medium (and variations of hydrochloric acid are normal in all stomachs) as a possible factor of chronicity, if not an etiologic factor, in peptic ulcer."*

Of interest is that Gorham also wrote that he had, over the previous 10 years, successfully treated patients who had refractory ulcer disease with intramuscular injections of bismuth! Although Gorham may have seemed to be ahead of his time, as early as 1868, A. Kussmaul had advocated the use of bismuth subnitrate for the treatment of gastric ulcer. In fact, the oral use of bismuth for gastrointestinal symptoms was well accepted, and as early as the late eighteenth century, reports of the therapy had begun to appear in the English literature. The antibacterial properties of bismuth, which may or may not have been known to Gorham, had already been successfully exploited by R. Sazerac and C. Levaditit in 1921, who used it to cure experimental syphilis in rabbits. Gastric syphilis had also been described, the ulcers associated with this disease were well known, and the infective agent, *Spirochete pallida*, had been successfully isolated and cultured from syphilitic abscesses.

The negative results of Freedberg and Barron and the ambivalent results of Doenges subsequently prompted E. D. Palmer, in the early 1950s, to investigate spirochetes in human gastric samples. He obtained gastric mucosal biopsies from 1,180 subjects using a vacuum-tube technique but, using standard histologic techniques, failed to demonstrate either spirochetes or any structures resembling them. Although Palmer did not attempt to identify the organisms with the more reliable silver stain, he concluded (confidently) that the results of all previous authors could be best explained as a postmortem colonization of the gastric mucosa with oral cavity organisms. He also postulated that spirochetes were normally occurring commensals of the mouth. Palmer's work may thus be credited with the enviable distinction of setting back gastric bacterial research by a further 30 years.

Ammonia and gastric urease

Although ammonia was noted in gastric juice as early as 1852, it was not until 1924 that Luck discovered gastric mucosal urease. His subsequent work and the work of others, especially the Dublin biochemist E. J. Conway, who specialized in investigations of the redox mechanism of acid secretion, confirmed the presence of gastric urease in a number of mammals. Histochemical studies demonstrated that enzyme activity appeared to be concentrated in the surface layers of the mucosa, in close conjunction with oxyntic cells. In addition, tissues surrounding gastric ulcers were found to be particularly rich in urease, whereas cancerous or achlorhydric stomachs were devoid of urease activity. These observations, as well as the long-standing observation of ammonia in gastric juice, prompted the proposal that urease activity was somehow coupled to hydrochloric acid secretion.

This hypothesis was, however, swiftly refuted on the demonstration that the mucosa could secrete acid in the complete absence of urea. Nevertheless, a clinical role for urea in gastric physiology was postulated by O. Fitzgerald (Conway's medical colleague), who thought that gastric urease functioned as a mucosal protective agent by providing ions to neutralize acid. This led to a number of studies (usually on medical students) in which the ingestion of urea-containing solutions was used to alter histamine-stimulated gastric acid secretion. Notwithstanding the unpleasant side effects of this administration (diarrhea, headache, polyuria, painful urethritis), Fitzgerald further applied his hypothe-

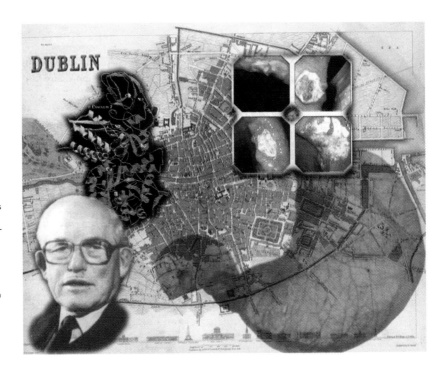

Fitzgerald of Dublin used urea solutions in the clinical setting in the 1940s to treat patients with ulcer disease (top right). This was based on the proposal that gastric urease (top left) functioned as a mucosal protective agent by providing ions to neutralize acid. Fitzgerald postulated that the ingestion of urea would alter histamine-stimulated gastric acid secretion by changing the gastric ionic milieu. While Fitzgerald considered this therapy satisfactory, the unpleasant side effects of administration prevented any further studies with this agent.

sis by treating ulcer patients with this regimen in 1949. Although he charitably summarized his results as *"in general, satisfactory,"* no further therapeutic studies were undertaken with this particular agent.

Within 5 years, investigators of gastric urease–containing tissue suspensions were also able to demonstrate the presence (contamination) of urea-splitting organisms. This led to the suggestion that gastric urease might actually be of bacterial origin. Preliminary feeding of antibiotics (penicillin and terramycin) to animals resulted both in reduced expiration of $^{14}CO_2$ from intraperitoneally injected ^{14}C-urea, as well as the abolition of urease activity in mucosal homogenates. Similar studies with analogous results were also performed in controls and subjects with uremia.

These observations, although establishing that gastric urease was of bacterial origin, failed to initiate an investigation of the relationship between urease-containing bacteria and ulcer disease. Indeed, the prevailing notion by the end of 1955 was that neither the bacterial gastric urease nor the bacteria played any essential role in gastric pathology. Interestingly, at the time, however, the clinical information derived suggested to some that antibacterial therapy could be used in patients with liver disease and elevated gastric ammonia levels. Antibiotic therapy was noted to reduce gastric urea and ameliorate the associated encephalopathy.

In 1975, Steer, while studying polymorphonuclear leukocyte migration in the gastric mucosa in a series of biopsy material obtained from patients with gastric ulceration, identified bacteria in close contact with the epithelium and suggested that white blood cells migrated in response to these bacteria.

In this seminal contribution, he not only clearly demonstrated bacterial phagocytosis but also provided electron microscopic images consistent with ingestion of a *Helicobacter*. Steer also attempted to isolate and culture the organism but, being unfamiliar with microaerophilic techniques, succeeded only in growing and identifying *Pseudomonas aeruginosa*.

Discovery of Helicobacter pylori and its etiologic role in peptic ulcer

By 1980, reports concerning an *"epidemic gastritis associated with hypochlorhydria"* had been published. These observations, coupled with Steer's findings of an apparent association between "active gastritis" and a gram-negative bacterium, suggested that the simultaneous occurrence of bacteria in the stomach and peptic ulceration might represent more than a correlatable epiphenomenon. Robin Warren, a pathologist at the Royal Perth Hospital, had for many years observed bacteria in the stomachs of people with gastritis. Although he was convinced that they somehow played a role in gastric disease, in the light of the prevailing dogma of acid-induced ulceration and the skepticism of his colleagues, he had been reluctant to discuss this controversial observation in the wider gastroenterologic community.

In 1982, a young gastroenterology fellow, Barry Marshall, was looking for a project to complete his fellowship. The iconoclastic hypothesis of Warren attracted Marshall, who persuaded Warren to allow him to investigate this further in the appropriate clinical setting. Later in the year, Marshall submitted an abstract detailing their initial investigations to the Australian Gastroen-

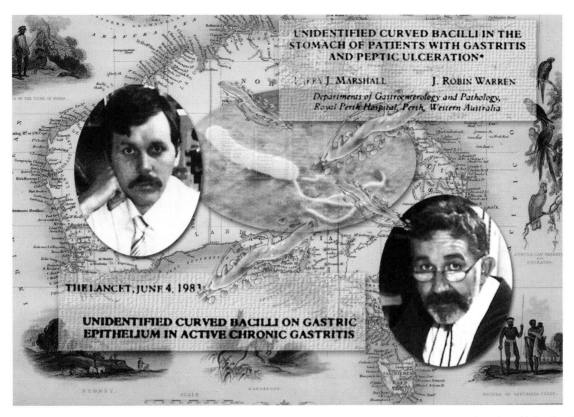

UNIDENTIFIED CURVED BACILLI IN THE
STOMACH OF PATIENTS WITH GASTRITIS
AND PEPTIC ULCERATION*

J. MARSHALL   J. ROBIN WARREN

*Departments of Gastroenterology and Pathology,
Royal Perth Hospital, Perth, Western Australia*

THE LANCET, JUNE 4, 1983

UNIDENTIFIED CURVED BACILLI ON GASTRIC
EPITHELIUM IN ACTIVE CHRONIC GASTRITIS

J. R. Warren (bottom right) observed the presence of a proliferating bacterium on the gastric mucosa from mucosal biopsies and established a close relationship to active chronic gastritis. B. J. Marshall (top left) successfully collaborated with Warren, resulting in the culture and classification of this new (old) gastric pathogen.

terology Association. It was flatly rejected, along with a handful of other abstracts. Young, unfazed, and seeking an alternative audience for the work, Marshall submitted the same abstract to the International Workshop of *Campylobacter* Infections, where it was accepted. Although the audience was skeptical of Marshall's and Warren's results, some members became interested enough to attempt to repeat some of their observations. Soon after the meeting, both Warren and Marshall published their initial results as two short letters in the *Lancet*. In the introduction to his seminal article on an S-shaped *Campylobacter*-like organism, Warren noted both the constancy of bacterial infection and the consistency of the associated histologic changes, which he had identified in 135 gastric-biopsy specimens studied over a 3-year period. He commented that these microorganisms were difficult to see with hematoxylin and eosin but stained well in the presence of silver. Furthermore, he observed the bacteria to be most numerous in an *"active chronic gastritis,"* in which they were closely associated with granulocyte infiltration. It is a mystery, he wrote, that bacteria in numbers sufficient to be seen by light microscopy were almost unknown to clinicians and pathologists alike! He presciently concluded, *"These organisms should be recognized and their significance investigated."*

Koch's second postulate states that *"the germ should be obtained from the diseased animal and grown outside the body."* In the same issue of the *Lancet*, Marshall described the conditions necessary to fulfill this requirement. Using the knowledge that these bacteria resemble the species of *Campylobacter* rather than spirochetes, he used *Campylobacter* isolation techniques

457

(microaerophilic conditions) to successfully grow isolates on moist chocolate agar. It is interesting to note that no organism growth was detected after 2 days' culture in the first 34 endoscopic biopsies Marshall tried to grow. The thirty-fifth plate, however, was left to culture over the long (6 days) Easter weekend, with positive results—serendipitously obtained!

To substantiate that the microorganism was actually a disease-causing agent, it was necessary to demonstrate that it could colonize normal mucosa and induce gastritis (Koch's third and fourth postulates). To prove pathogenicity, Marshall, looking back in time for guidance, decided to be his own guinea pig. Marshall, who had a histologically normal gastric mucosa and was a light smoker and social drinker, received, per mouth, a test isolate from a 66-year-old nonulcer dyspeptic man. Over the next 14 days, a mild illness developed, characteristic of an acute episode of gastritis, and was accompanied by headaches, vomiting, abdominal discomfort, irritability, and "putrid" breath. The infectivity of the agent was then successfully confirmed when, after 10 days, histologically proven gastritis was endoscopically documented. The disease process later resolved on its own accord by the fifteenth day. A fellow Australasian, Morris, later followed Marshall's lead, and in a similar experiment ingested the same inoculum of *H. pylori*. Although this initial ingestion did not establish a viable infection, a repeat challenge of the mucosa with a different, local (New Zealand) inoculum was more successful. In fact, it was so successful that a 2-month treatment of an antibacterial agent and bismuth was required to "eradicate" the organism. Morris and Nicholson established a direct effect of infection on acid secretion, but unfortunately for Morris, who had residual gastritis, a relapse was inevitable. Five years after the initial experiment, Morris was finally cured. There has been no recorded third experiment. Marshall went on to describe the urease of the organism and recognized its role in enabling survival of the organism in acidic media. Subsequent work showed that eradication of the organism reduced recurrence of duodenal ulcer to the level found with maintenance therapy with H_2 receptor antagonists, and acceptance of this organism as causative in association with acid is now universal.

The importance of these findings is enormous and must rank among the great iconoclasms in medicine. Some 15 years after the start of the modern *Helicobacter* era, many of the important issues remain unresolved. There is still a lack of knowledge about many aspects of the organism itself, its mode of transmission, how it causes disease, why only a select few develop ulcers, and what the correct clinical management of this infection should be, both in practice and as a public health issue. The following chapters highlight the areas of knowledge and uncertainty that represent the current information available on this ubiquitous and enigmatic organism and its effects on the human stomach.

CHAPTER 2
BIOLOGIC BASIS OF GASTRIC COLONIZATION BY *HELICOBACTER*

Introduction

The eradication of *H. pylori* for treatment of peptic ulcer disease not associated with NSAID use, steroids, or severe stress is now accepted as a necessary part of medical treatment of this set of illnesses. Perhaps less well accepted is the need for eradication of any infection by this gastric carcinogen. Since the early findings that infection was associated with fundic cell metaplasia and cancer, overwhelming data have been presented proving an association. For example, in Japan, where gastric carcinoma is the most common form of cancer, 3% of adult males older than 60 years who have infection have cancer, whereas none who are not infected has this lesion. A Swedish study showed a much higher probability of stomach cancer in patients undergoing hip transplant who were infected than in those who were uninfected. Even more germane, in a subgroup of patients who had been given high-dose antibiotics as coverage for this surgery, the incidence of cancer dropped precipitously, indicating that eradication is of benefit even after many years of infection.

Currently, therapy with PPIs and two antibiotics is the most frequently prescribed medication, with perhaps bismuth along with ranitidine and also two antibiotics as another possible therapy. The rationale for the need for the former combination is becoming clearer, but monotherapy would be more desirable, simplifying treatment and avoiding the use of antibiotics necessary for the treatment of other infections. To understand the biologic basis of this infection and pave the way for better treatment, the biology of *H. pylori* is being investigated on many fronts.

The nature of *Helicobacter pylori*

There has been much discussion about the pH of the environment inhabited by *H. pylori*. Although some would have the gastric surface neutral in spite of several hours with a luminal pH of approximately 1.0, most would agree that with a luminal pH of less than 2.0, surface pH is also 2.0 or less. Hence, *H. pylori* thrives in an acidic environment.

Bacteria can inhabit a variety of pH environments: acidic (acidophiles), alkaline (alkalophiles), and neutral (neutralophiles). In spite of the varying acidity of the environment, all bacteria harness the energy of the electrochemical proton gradient across their membranes to synthesize ATP. This gradient consists of a pH gradient and a gradient of electric potential difference. Hence, this gradient is modified by the different types of bacteria. Acidophiles already have an inward pH gradient under acidic conditions and modify their membrane potential so that it becomes internally positive to restrict inward proton movement. Alkalophiles increase their inside negative potential, so that the pH inward driving force is magnified. Neutralophiles grow best between pH 6.0 and 8.0 and do not grow outside this range.

The latter finding is also true of *H. pylori* in the absence of specific additions to the medium, such as urea. Neutralophiles are generally able to survive an acidic environment but do not grow in acid. Depending on whether they are in growth or log phase or in stationary phase, the response is considered acid tolerant or acid resistant. In either case, this allows the organisms to maintain viability. *H. pylori* and other gastric *Helicobacter* species are unique in that they not only survive but also grow in the gastric environment. These are, therefore, the only bacteria that have adapted to an acidic environment.

Aerobic bacteria (including microaerobes) synthesize ATP by coupling metabolic generation and oxidation of substrates to the formation of an electrochemical proton gradient across their cytoplasmic membrane (pH and membrane potential) and dissipation of this proton gradient through the cytoplasmic membrane's ATP synthase. The proton gradient is composed of two components: an actual pH gradient and a potential difference across the membrane. A balance of these two constituents of the proton energy charge of the membrane enables bacterial growth over a range of pH 2.0 to 11.0, depending on whether they are acidophiles, neutralophiles, or alkalophiles.

The outer membrane contains porins, which usually allow passage of protons. An acid-dwelling organism can either accept high acidity in the periplasmic space and regulate H^+ entry by changing the transmembrane potential or it can choose to regulate the pH of the periplasmic space, thus changing the pH component.

The circulation of protons across the cytoplasmic membrane is electrogenic, that is to say that export of protons by the redox pumps oxidizing substrate generates current and voltage cytoplasmic side negative. Uptake of protons through the F_1F_o ATPase driven by the pH and electrical gradient dissipates the potential and the pH and uses this to generate ATP from ADP and P_i.

Formally, the gradient of hydrogen ions is expressed as a function of the chemical and electrical potential, in which the electrochemical gradient of hydrogen ions is the driving force for ATP generation by the chemiosmotic mechanism first recognized by Peter Mitchell in 1961. The thermodynamic equation describing the electrochemical gradient (proton motive force) for H^+ is

$$\text{p.m.f (in mV)} = \Delta\bar{\mu}_H^+ = \Delta\psi + -RT/nF \ln[H^+_{out}]/[H^+_{in}] = -61\Delta pH + PD$$

where $\Delta\bar{\mu}_H^+$ is the electrochemical gradient for protons, R is the gas constant, T is the temperature in degrees Kelvin, F is the Faraday constant, n is the valence of the ion, and $\Delta\psi$ is the transmembrane potential, referred to in text as PD.

This relationship predicts that there is a reciprocal relationship between the pH gradient and the potential difference (i.e., as the inward pH gradient increases, the PD decreases, and vice versa, to maintain a relatively constant proton motive force). The chemiosmotic mechanism for ATP generation by a neutralophile is illustrated in the figure.

Because mean intragastric pH in people is 1.4, the issue arises as to the bioenergetic nature of *H. pylori*: is it an acidophile that has learned to colonize the human stomach? Or is it a neutralophile that has developed adaptive mechanisms to combat the variable acidity of its environment? Because it grows best between pH 6.0 and 8.0 and does not survive either pH less than 4.0 or pH greater than 8.2 in the absence of pH-regulatory enzymes such as urease, it is clearly a neutralophile but may have adopted some of the mechanisms of acidophiles to be able to inhabit the stomach.

ATP Synthesis by Electrochemical H⁺ Gradient in *Helicobacter*

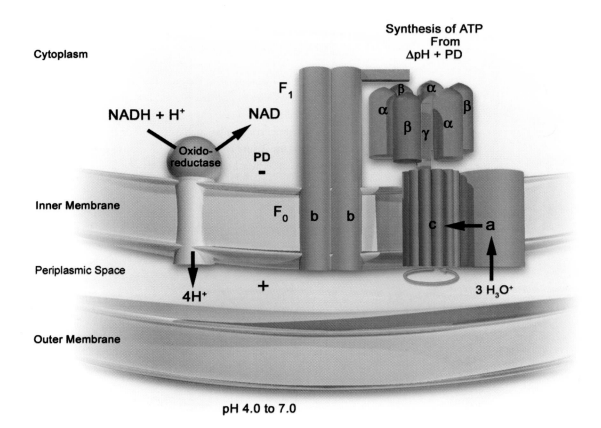

Synthesis of ATP From $\Delta pH + PD$

Cytoplasm

NADH + H⁺   NAD

Oxido-reductase

F_1

PD −

Inner Membrane F_0 b   b

c ← a

Periplasmic Space

4H⁺   +   3 H₃O⁺

Outer Membrane

pH 4.0 to 7.0

A schematic representation of the generation and use of electrochemical gradients of protons by gram-negative aerophilic bacteria. Redox pumps generate a chemical and electrical gradient across the inner membrane (negative inside), thus generating an inward driving force for H⁺. This drives the proton through the ATP synthase; the mechanism of ATP synthesis is gradient-dependent rotation of the c subunit of the membrane-embedded F_0 complex that allows transmission of three protons per ATP synthesized to the rotary $\alpha\beta$ trimer of the F_1. As illustrated, this mechanism defines the limits of acid adaptation of the organism in the absence of urea in the environment. In this illustration, a, b, and c are components of the F_0 complex: c is a rotary proton conductor, and a and b are membrane-stabilizing subunits.

H. pylori is a motile, gram-negative organism that can be cultured in microaerobic (low O_2) conditions, although it adapts to high O_2 at higher culture densities. As such, it has an outer membrane, the outer leaflet of which is lipopolysaccharide, a cell wall and periplasm, an inner membrane, and cytoplasm. The bioenergetic survival of the organism depends on the maintenance of an adequate proton motive force between the periplasmic space and the cytoplasm across its inner or cytoplasmic membrane.

The organism is helical or spiral in shape and possesses six to eight flagella at one end. Flagellar function depends on the activity of a flagellar motor also driven by the proton motive force generated across the cytoplasmic membrane of the organism. Given the two-membrane structure of the organism, control of periplasmic and cytoplasmic pH is vital for survival and growth of the organism.

Modern molecular biologic methods for defining the genome have been applied to the genetic structure of *H. pylori*. The genome contains approximately 1,500 genes, 300 of which encode membrane proteins, many of as-yet unknown function. The genome contains sequences encoding for membrane proteins, such as the F_1F_0 ATP synthase complex, and various oxidoreductases,

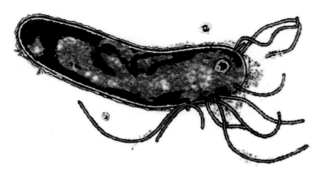

Electron micrograph of *H. pylori*, showing outer and inner membranes separated by the periplasm and the polar location of the flagellae.

such as cytochrome o, several transporters, and a variety of two component signaling systems (the equivalent of eukaryotic receptors). Some of the recognized transporters are illustrated in the figure on the previous page.

The organism contains enzymes for glucose metabolism but lacks β-galactosidase (and hence is unable to metabolize lactose) and some of the enzymes of the Krebs cycle (no isocitrate dehydrogenase). The genome also encodes for several outer membrane proteins (OMPs), some of which are porins, able to allow movement of a variety of molecules into or out of the periplasmic space. Some of these have a higher isoelectric point than those of neutralophiles such as *E. coli* or *B. subtilis*, which may enable resistance to acute acidic changes of pH, because proton permeability is expected to be less because they are more positively charged.

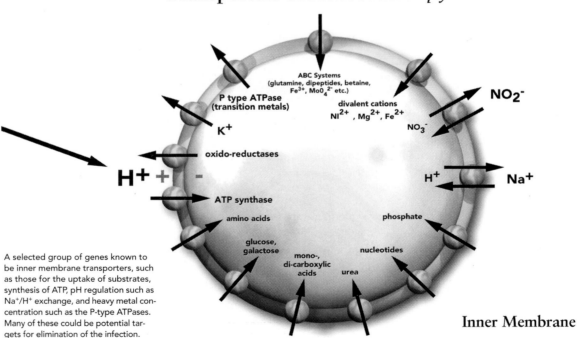

Transporters of *Helicobacter pylori*

A selected group of genes known to be inner membrane transporters, such as those for the uptake of substrates, synthesis of ATP, pH regulation such as Na^+/H^+ exchange, and heavy metal concentration such as the P-type ATPases. Many of these could be potential targets for elimination of the infection.

Inner Membrane

Acid and *Helicobacter pylori*

The survival and growth of organisms as a function of medium pH is diagnostic of their bioenergetic profile. For example, neutralophiles such as *E. coli* characteristically are able to survive between pH 4.0 and 8.0 and grow well between pH 6.0 and 8.0. When these properties of *H. pylori* are measured as shown in the figure, it seems that this organism shares survival and growth characteristics with *E. coli*, a neutralophile with acid tolerance and resistance mechanisms but not acid-adaptive mechanisms.

A plot of survival or growth of *H. pylori* at different medium pH in the absence of urea. In blue is shown the finding that the organism can survive between pH 4.0 and 8.0 but grow only between pH 6.0 and 8.0. These data are obtained in the absence of urea. Also illustrated is the concept that sensitivity to antibiotics such as amoxicillin and clarithromycin is found only during growth; hence, where survival is present without growth, these antibiotics will not affect the organism.

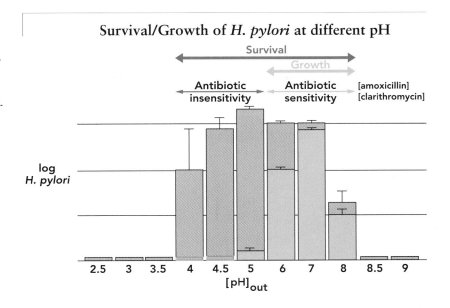

From the measurement of survival, which is found at a medium pH only when greater than 4.0, it is obvious that without specialized acid-adaptive mechanisms, *H. pylori* would not be found in the stomach. It is also clear that any colonization without adaptive mechanisms would be impossible given the pH characteristics of growth. A similar conclusion can be derived from measurements of protein synthesis *in vitro*, where a correlation is found between protein synthesis and growth, as illustrated.

The organism must have mechanisms preventing a fatal decrease of the proton motive force in acid to survive and even mechanisms for enabling elevation of periplasmic pH in acid to grow in the stomach. Some of these have been identified by both *in vitro* and *in vivo* experiments.

Illustration of protein synthesis as a function of fixed medium pH in the absence and then the presence of urea. Optimal protein synthesis is found at pH 7.0 and declines at pH 6.0 and is absent at pH 5.0 and 3.0 in the absence of urea. In the presence of urea, there is no effect at pH 7.0 but enhancement at pH 6.0 and a marked increase at pH 5.0 and 3.0. The role of urea and urease will be discussed in detail. UreA and UreB are the structural subunits of the bacterial urease. (SOD, superoxide dismutase.)

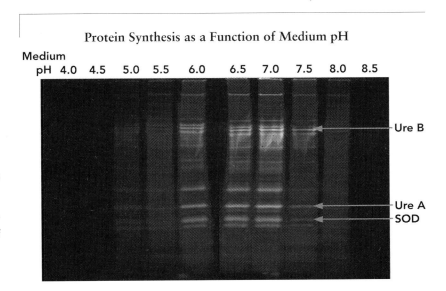

Knowledge of the potential difference and pH gradient across the cytoplasmic membrane of *H. pylori* as a function of medium pH would also enable conclusions as to the nature of the membrane homeostatic machinery necessary for gastric habitation by this organism. The organism is too small for microelectrode measurements of pH or potential difference, but less direct methods using dye probes of these parameters have proved successful.

For example, a dye, bis-carboxyethylcarboxyfluorescein acetomethoxy ester, is loaded into the microorganisms and becomes fluorescent. When this dye is used to measure internal pH at a medium pH of 7.0 using what is called a *null point method* (i.e., comparing change of fluorescence with all other gradients equal when intracellular pH is made equal to medium pH with the addition of an equilibrating ionophore), internal pH is found to be 8.4 at a medium pH of 7.0. This is equal to a potential difference of approximately −90 mV. A similar measurement of internal pH in *E. coli* gives an internal pH of approximately 7.8, somewhat lower than that found in *H. pylori*.

Fluorescent dyes have also been used to measure transmembrane potential. A lipophilic fluorescent dye, the cation di-S-C_3-(5), is taken up, and its fluorescence quenches as a function of an internal negative potential. The membrane potential is also calibrated by a null point method, in which the K^+-selective ionophore, valinomycin, is added to set the membrane potential to that generated by the transmembrane K^+ gradient. Then K^+ is added until there is no fluorescence quench (i.e., PD = 0), and then the internal K^+ is known, because when there is no membrane potential, $[K^+]_{in} = [K^+]_{out}$. From this known value of $[K^+]_{in}$, the membrane potential with the addition of valinomycin and then before addition of valinomycin can be calculated.

At pH 7.0, it is −131 mV (a value also found by studies of distribution of a lipophilic cation). The proton motive force across the inner membrane of this gastric denizen is therefore −221 mV, the sum of the pH gradient and the membrane-potential difference.

The inner membrane potential as a function of medium pH, showing that as the pH gradient increases (more acidic outside), membrane potential becomes less negative inside, and that outside the range of survival in the absence of urea, there is no membrane potential. An absence of such a potential is therefore lethal to the organism. Thus, the organism is unable to survive a pH <3.5 in the absence of urea and >8.5, and if urease activity generates such an external pH, it is also lethal to the organism.

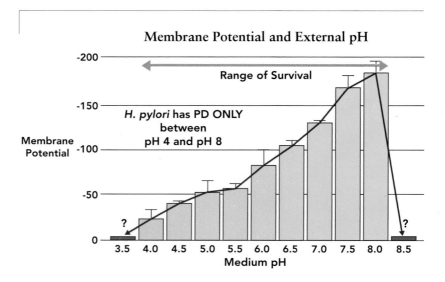

When membrane potential was measured as a function of medium pH, a potential difference was found between a fixed medium of pH 4.0 and pH 8.0, exactly the pH range over which the organism survives, as shown in the earlier illustration. Again, for gastric survival and growth, the pH range over which a membrane potential can be generated must be extended. The reciprocal relationship between medium pH and membrane potential is that predicted by the proton motive force equation. The mechanism whereby external pH controls membrane potential remains undefined.

Effects of acute changes of medium pH

From the illustration, there is an absence of membrane potential and, thus, no survival at pH less than 4.0 and greater than 8.0. Gastric acidity undergoes rapid changes as a function of the rate of acid secretion and buffering of gastric contents. The duration of survival of the organism at the extremes of pH is therefore highly relevant in terms of the rate at which it has to adapt to acid. An experiment in which this was tested is shown in the illustration below.

Here the bacteria were added to an acidic medium at pH 3.5 and their membrane potential measured by the dye-uptake method outlined earlier. No membrane potential was found at that pH. After 5 minutes, buffer was added to elevate medium pH to 6.2, and no restoration of the potential was found, indicating death of the organism. On the other hand, when buffer was added almost immediately to bring the pH back to 6.2, there was a slow recovery of membrane potential to the control value expected for a medium pH of 6.2. Hence, *H. pylori* is able to survive only short exposure to acid, and its acid-adaptive response must happen relatively quickly. Again, this shows that acid-adaptive mechanisms are essential even for survival of the organism with exposure to mild acidity.

Survival of *H. pylori* to acid exposure can be correlated with the ability of the organism to generate an inner membrane negative inward potential. This experiment shows that when the bacteria are added to a buffered solution of pH 3.5, there is no transmembrane potential as shown by the red line. If, however, there is a rapid increase of external pH to 6.2 by the addition of buffer of pH 8.5 as shown by the blue arrow, membrane potential is restored over a period of approximately 10 minutes. However, if addition of the buffer to elevate pH to 6.2 is delayed by 5 minutes (*red arrow*), there is no recovery of membrane potential, and the organism is dead. At the end of the experiment, the protonophore, tetrachlorosalicylanilide (TCS), is added to show that the blue curve is measuring bacterial inner membrane potential difference. Thus, only short exposure to pH 3.5 in the stomach is sufficient to eradicate the organism in the absence of acid-adaptive mechanisms such as urease and UreI.

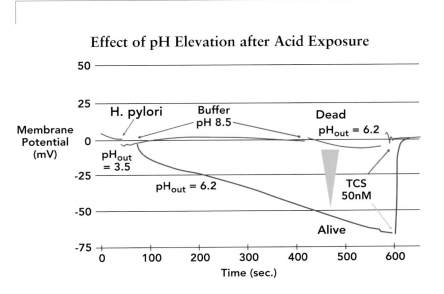

Effect of pH Elevation after Acid Exposure

Metabolism as a function of medium pH

Bacterial metabolism should also correlate with survival and, therefore, the pH range of the proton motive force. There are various ways of measuring metabolism, such as oxygen consumption, CO_2 production from labeled glucose, or incorporation of radioactivity into protein. A particularly convenient means that is also adaptable to monitoring of survival is the measurement of pH changes induced by a bacterial suspension. The metabolism of microorganisms generates metabolic acid; hence, acidification indicates metabolism.

A microphysiometer is an instrument capable of very sensitive measurement of pH changes in a flow-through system, which avoids the use of strong buffers to maintain a constant pH environment. This reflects the conditions in the stomach in the postdigestive phase, in which there is little buffering of secreted acid, and gastric luminal pH falls to as low as 1.0.

A light addressable pH sensor is computer controlled to measure the pH within eight chambers simultaneously that contain approximately 10^5 immobilized bacteria in soft agar through which solution is pumped. The pH change is read out in mV per second as the pump is stopped for 16 seconds in a 40-second pump cycle. This pH change indicates the ability of the bacteria to metabolize the glucose or glucosamine in the superfusion solution during the time that the pump is stopped.

The bacteria are able to acidify the medium at neutral pH between pH 6.0 and 8.5 due to the production of metabolic acid and alkalinize the medium below pH 6.0 down to pH 4.0 due to reabsorption of H^+ for ATP synthesis, as shown. Below pH 5.5, metabolism results in mild alkalinization of the medium, probably due to uptake of protons through the F_1F_o ATPase. The range of metabolism displayed here again corresponds to what is found using either standard survival measurements or measurement of the range over which the organism maintains a PD across its inner membrane. There is no recovery of acidification potential when the organisms are superfused with solutions at a pH lower than 4.0 that do not contain urea, whereas exposure to a medium pH greater than 8.2 is also lethal to the bacteria.

From these different approaches, *H. pylori* is a neutralophile and displays no evidence for general acidophilic mechanisms that would enable survival at the highly

Metabolism of *H. pylori* at different medium pH in the absence of urea. The bacteria are superfused with a weakly buffered solution containing either glucose or glutamine at the pH indicated on the X-axis and the pH change monitored during brief periods when superfusion is stopped. Below a pH of approximately 4.0, there is no change of medium pH, indicating that the organisms are no longer viable. At a pH above this, at first, there is alkalinization until pH 5.5 due to absorption of protons. After that, the organisms acidify the medium, indicating metabolic activity. Therefore, *H. pylori* are unable to survive weak acidity, as monitored by metabolic capability. Glucose alone is not as effective as with glutamine, perhaps because glutamine can be hydrolyzed to glutamic acid and NH_3. TGE

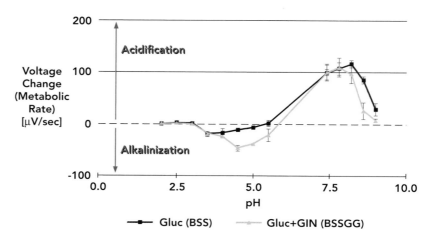

Metabolism of *H. pylori* at Different Medium pH

acidic pH that gastric contents must reach severally during the day. Regulation of the pH of the periplasm and cytoplasm environment is important for the organism.

Acid-adaptive mechanisms in *Helicobacter pylori*

Urease

H. pylori expresses the highest level of urease seen in bacteria. The urease activity was recognized as an important parameter enabling acid survival early on in research on the gastric mechanisms of *H. pylori*. Urease-negative mutants cannot colonize animal stomachs nor survive acidity below pH 4.0. It is therefore essential for acid adaptation by this gastric pathogen.

Urease activity

The action of urease is shown below.

$$\text{CO (NH)}_2 + H_2O \xrightarrow{\text{urease}} NH_3 + NH_2COOH$$
$$NH_2COOH \rightarrow NH_3 + CO_2$$

The first step is the urease-dependent catalysis of the generation of ammonia and carbamic acid. In the absence of buffer, the pH of the medium will rapidly reach the pK_a of the NH_4^+/NH_3 couple, namely 9.25. The second step, the spontaneous breakdown of carbamate, produces ammonia and carbon dioxide. Both gases can diffuse across the inner membrane of the organism and then, in the periplasm, generation of bicarbonate by the periplasmic carbonic anhydrase and protonation of the ammonia results in the formation of ammonium bicarbonate, buffering the periplasm.

Location of urease

The enzyme is found both in the cytoplasm and loosely associated with the cell surface, presumably binding to the lipopolysaccharide of the outer leaflet of the outer membrane. It had been thought that this external urease was responsible for elevating the microenvironment outside the organism to a level compatible not only with life (pH greater than 4.0) but also with growth (pH greater than 6.0). This was attributed to a cloud of ammonia generated by urease activity. This concept, although attractive, is now known to be incorrect for many reasons that have been established experimentally in several laboratories.

pH profile

The pH optimum of *H. pylori* urease lies between pH 7.5 and 8.0, far higher than the environment often encountered by the bacteria. Therefore, surface-bound urease has a mildly alkaline pH optimum, but its activity also declines until the pH reaches 4.5, and below that, there is no detectable urease activity, and in fact, there is irreversible inactivation. Hence, unless the pH of the bacterial environment is greater than 4.0, surface urease activity will have no effect on acid survival of the organism.

The pH-activity curve of surface urease and urease activity of intact bacteria in buffer. Surface urease activity has a pH optimum of approximately 7.5, and activity declines to zero as medium pH falls to pH 4.0. However, in intact bacteria, there is low activity at neutral pH, but there is an approximately 20-fold increase of activity between pH 6.5 and 5.5 and maintained activity down to at least pH 2.5, showing that there is an acidic medium activation of intrabacterial urease due to acid enhancement of urea entry to this urease compartment.

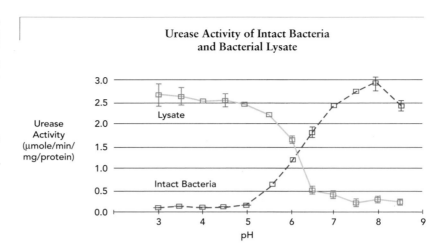

Urease Activity of Intact Bacteria and Bacterial Lysate

The situation is quite different when urease activity is measured in the intact organism. There is little measured activity until pH 6.5 is reached, and then there is a greater than 20-fold increase in urease activity, with a steady state of urease activity being held down to a pH of 2.5. There is, therefore, medium acidity activation of urease activity in the intact bacteria. The maintained intrabacterial urease activity in acid is a major factor in the acid adaptation of *H. pylori*. It is predicted, then, that intrabacterial urease activity will be able to buffer both periplasm and cytoplasm in gastric acid. These measurements are made by determining the amount of $^{14}CO_2$ released from ^{14}C urea in buffer.

The rate of alkalinization is measured in a chamber containing *H. pylori* after superfusion at the different pH values indicated at the top of the figure and stopping the superfusion using a pH sensor. There is no alkalinization in a weakly buffered solution containing glucose, but when 2.5 mM urea is present in the medium, there is an increase of pH at all the pH values. The increase is limited until pH 3.0, at which there is a 40-fold increase in alkalinization due to intrabacterial urease activity; an increase is still seen at pH 2.5. The large increase in urease activity seen at pH 3.0 is due to the inability of the urease activity to restore periplasmic pH so as to shut down the acid-activated urea channel, UreI.

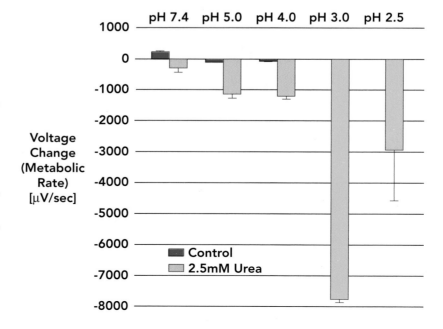

Urease Activity Measured by Alkalinization of Perfusing Medium

Most previous measurements of *H. pylori* urease activity have been done using the rate of change of pH of an unbuffered medium; as pH increases, urease activity is lost, hence, blinding the investigator to the acid activation of intra-bacterial urease.

A similar activation of urea hydrolysis is seen when pH measurements are made in the cytosensor and the rate of alkalinization correlated with urease activity, as shown in the figure on the opposite page. This also differs from previous investigations, because acid is constantly added to the organisms, and inactivation of the mechanism for enhancement of urease activity does not occur. There is approximately a 40-fold activation of urease activity as the pH falls to below 4.0. At higher pH, in the small volume of the chamber, urease activity is able to elevate chamber pH very rapidly; hence, urease activity is only transient. At a pH of 3.0, the level of acid is sufficient to require significant levels of urease activity to attempt to elevate pH. These

Above is shown the arrangement of the urease gene cluster of *H. pylori*, consisting of seven genes. The first two are the structural subunits of the enzyme; the last four are required for the insertion of Ni^{2+} into the UreA-B apoenzyme, and the third gene of the cluster, UreI, is a urea transporter. Below is shown the effect of deletion of UreI from the organism where, although there is full urease activity in bacterial lysate of the deletion mutant, all acid activation of urease is lost. This shows that UreI is responsible for the increase of urease activity in the intact organism.

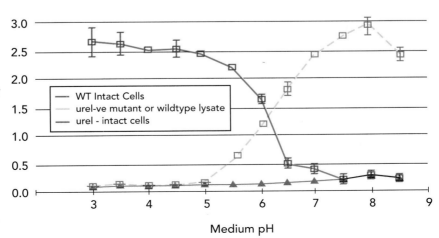

The Urease Gene Cluster in *H. pylori*

ureA   *ureB*   *ureI*   *ureE*   *ureF*   *ureG*   *ureH*

Structural Genes

Putative Membrane Protein

Accessory Genes for Urease Assembly

Intact Bacteria

Urease Activity (μmole/urea/min/mg/protein)

— WT Intact Cells
— urel-ve mutant or wildtype lysate
— urel - intact cells

Medium pH

data also show that intrabacterial urease is activated by acidification of the medium but stays relatively inactive at neutral pH.

Reality of surface urease

The finding that there is bound urease on the surface of the organism rests largely on data after centrifugation of intact bacteria. *H. pylori* is a fragile organism, and when care is taken to separate the medium and the intact organism, surface urease is not detected.

Role of UreI in activity of intrabacterial urease

The most likely explanation for the increase in urease activity seen with acidification is that there is a urea transporter in the bacteria. The urease gene cluster contains seven genes. There is a promoter followed by genes encoding the structural subunits, UreA and UreB. There is then a second promoter and then genes encoding UreI, -E, -F, -G, and -H. The last four are genes required for the assembly of active urease from the UreA-B apoenzyme by insertion of nickel, an essential cofactor in urease activity. UreE and -G and UreF and -H form heterodimers, and then a complex with UreA-B and nickel insertion occurs.

UreI, however, encodes an inner membrane protein with six transmembrane segments and is likely to be the transporter that is acid activated, enabling urea access to intrabacterial urease. Hence, in the absence of activation of this urea transporter, urea has slow, bilayer permeability–determined access to the urease, and there is low activity of the urease above pH 6.5. With activation, there is a large increase in urea entry and, thus, increase in intrabacterial urease.

The nature of UreI

When UreI is expressed in *Xenopus* oocytes, there is a large increase in urea uptake that is pH dependent. There is no increase at neutral pH but a large increase with acidification down to pH 4.0, the limit of survival of oocytes. The pH-transport curve can be overlaid on the pH-urease activity curve of intact bacteria. Half-maximal transport occurs at a medium pH of 5.9. The increased uptake is energy independent, temperature independent, and nonsaturable, properties indicating that UreI is a urea channel. This allows extremely fast transport of urea across the inner membrane of the bacteria. Complementation of UreI deletion mutants with wild-type UreI in *H. pylori* also restore urease activation at acidic pH, showing that UreI is a urea transporter in both the heterologous oocyte expression system and in the native organism.

Analysis of the structure of UreI shows that it is an integral inner membrane protein containing six transmembrane segments, with both ends in the periplasm. Examination of the amino acid residues shows that there are several histidines and carboxylic acids in the periplasm. There are two other known variants of the UreI of *H. pylori*, the UreI of *H. hepaticus* and the UreI of *S. salivarius*. The former is also pH sensitive, the latter pH insensitive. Site-directed mutagenesis and chimer constructs involving swapping of

Uptake of labeled urea into *Xenopus* oocytes expressing UreI. There is no enhancement of urea uptake at neutral pH but an approximately 20-fold increase at pH 5.0 that is not changed in the presence of 100 mM urea, showing that transport by UreI is nonsaturable, indicating a channel-like property.

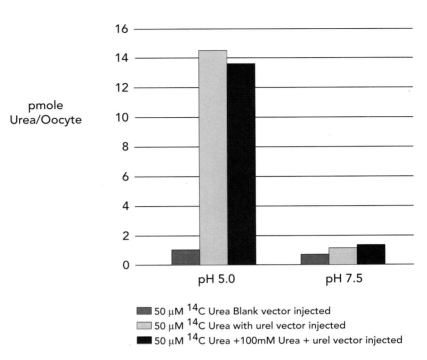

The Effect of UreI on Urea Transport in *Xenopus* Oocytes

pmole Urea/Oocyte

■ 50 µM ^{14}C Urea Blank vector injected
☐ 50 µM ^{14}C Urea with urel vector injected
■ 50 µM ^{14}C Urea +100mM Urea + urel vector injected

various periplasmic loops have allowed the conclusion that protonation of the periplasmic domain in acid alters the conformation of this region, which is transmitted to the membrane domain, allowing opening or closing of the channel as a function of periplasmic pH, in the case of gastric *Helicobacter* species such as *H. pylori* or with *H. hepaticus*. There are no functional protonatable groups in *S. salivarius*, nor are there conformational changes in its membrane domain.

Recent data on the mutation of UreI of *H. hepaticus* show that two periplasmic histidines and two periplasmic carboxylic acids are involved in the proton-dependent increase of open probability of the channel. This is illustrated in the accompanying figure on the next page. Presumably, a similar mechanism involving histidines and carboxylates is present in the UreI of *H. pylori*.

Role of UreI in gastric survival and colonization

UreI is probably the most important adaptation used by *H. pylori* for gastric colonization. This acid-activated urea transporter appears essential not only for survival in acidic media but also for survival in the stomach at its site of colonization.

The Secondary Structure of 3 Bacterial Urea Channels

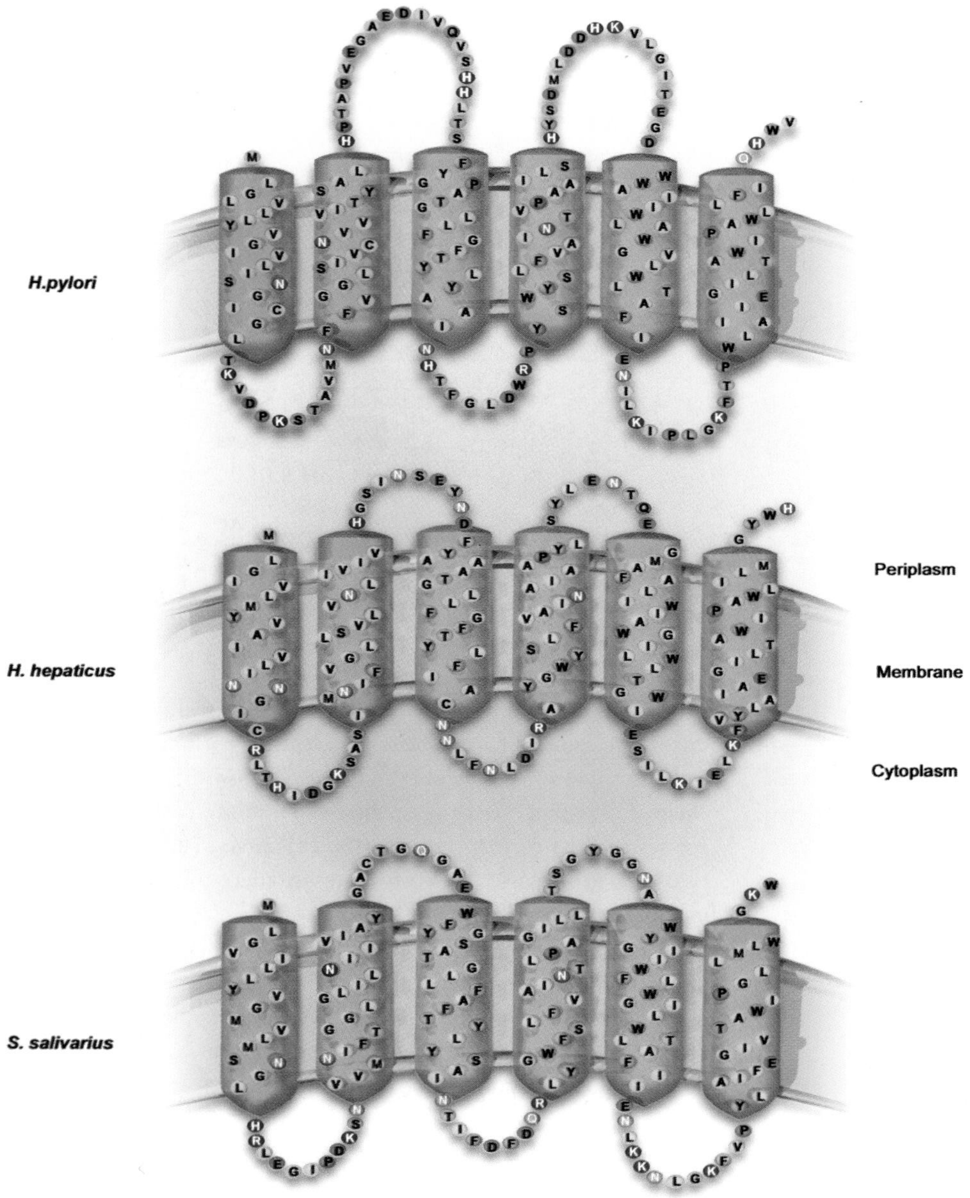

H.pylori

H. hepaticus

S. salivarius

Periplasm

Membrane

Cytoplasm

The secondary structure of three bacterial urea channels. On the bottom is that of *Streptococcus salivarius*. This channel has strong homology in the membrane and cytoplasmic domains with the other two urea channels, but only a single protonatable amino acid (glutamic acid, E) in the periplasmic domain. It is not acid activatable. *Helicobacter hepaticus* probably evolved its UreI from this with the addition of five protonatable amino acids in the periplasmic domain and became acid activated. This periplasmic domain was further refined by *Helicobacter pylori* with now 14 protonatable amino acids in the periplasmic domain. The urease activity of the latter is much higher, and the channel is essentially entirely closed at neutral pH to prevent overalkalinization in the absence of acid secretion. This property optimized its ability to colonize the stomach under all physiologic conditions. The amino acids are in single-letter codes and are colored dark blue for basic amino acids and red for acidic amino acids to show these residues in the periplasmic domain.

When the properties of bacteria containing UreI and those with UreI deleted are compared in a medium of pH 2.5 at different urea concentrations, it is found that with UreI present, the organisms are able to survive pH 2.5, with half-maximal survival seen at a urea concentration of 1 mM within the physiologic range of gastric juice urea. With the deletion mutants, there is no survival in acid until a concentration of 100 mM urea is reached, and half-maximal survival is seen at a urea concentration of 250 mM. Hence, there is an approximately 300-fold increase of urea permeability in *H. pylori* due to expression of UreI at an external pH of 2.5. Because UreI is in the inner membrane and plays no role in the function of the putative surface urease, the latter compartment does not play a role in acid survival *in vitro*.

The survival of *H. pylori* at pH 2.5 at varying concentrations of medium urea. On the left are the data for wild-type bacteria; on the right the data for *UreI*-deletion mutants, showing the loss of acid survival at physiologic urea concentrations when UreI is not expressed.

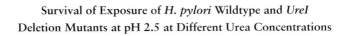

Survival of Exposure of *H. pylori* Wildtype and *UreI* Deletion Mutants at pH 2.5 at Different Urea Concentrations

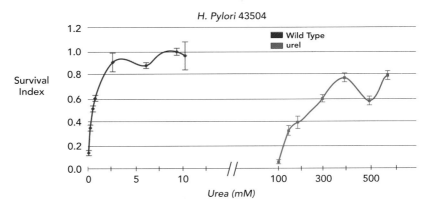

These *in vitro* data can be extended to the *in vivo* situation. UreI-deletion mutants of *H. pylori* were not able to infect the mouse stomach, and further, were not able to infect or colonize gerbil stomachs, whose intragastric pH is similar to the human stomach. Mutants in which UreI deletion was complemented with wild-type UreI had the properties of the normal wild type.

In the gerbil, however, when acid secretion was inhibited by a PPI or an APA, infection by both wild-type and UreI-deletion mutants occurred. When acid secretion was allowed to return, wild-type organisms continued to colonize the stomach, but UreI-deletion mutants were eradicated. These data show that UreI is an essential gene for gastric colonization but not for growth at neutral pH *in vivo*. Moreover, these data demonstrate that the normal gastric environment of *H. pylori* is less than pH 4.0, the limit of survival of UreI deletion mutants. Hence, the idea that the environment of *H. pylori* is neutral is not correct, and "surface" urease has no role in gastric infection or colonization. The data for the experiments in the gerbils are shown in the following table.

Intragastric pH of the gerbil stomach is 1.6. *H. pylori* wild-type strain infects the gerbil stomach, but *H. pylori* UreI knockouts do not. Inhibition of the gastric acid pump raises the intragastric pH to 6.0, allowing infection by the UreI knockout strain. Because *H. pylori* UreI deletion mutants cannot survive at pH of less than 4.0; these results show that the site of infection is at pH 4.0 or lower. Condition I, no acid inhibition (red); condition II, acid inhibition only during inoculation (black); condition III, acid inhibition during all phases of the experiment (blue); ++, more than seven animals positive; +, four to seven animals positive, (+), one to three animals positive; -, no animals positive. Two tests for the presence of *H. pylori* were used: measurement of urease activity and the more sensitive PCR reaction for the presence of the constitutive gene, *flaA*.

UreI is Essential for Gastric Survival and Infection

Urease Test	Wild-type antrum	Wild-type Corpus	*urel* Knockout antrum	*urel* Knockout Corpus	*urel* Knockout [pAAB37] antrum	*urel* Knockout [pAAB37] Corpus
I	++	(+)	-	-	++	(+)
II	++	(+)	-	-	not deter	not deter
III	+	++	+	++	not deter	not deter

PCR *flaA*	antrum	Corpus	antrum	Corpus	antrum	Corpus
I	++	(+)	-	-	++*	(+)*
II	++	(+)	-	-	not deter	not deter
III	+	++	+	++	not deter	not deter

Activation of Helicobacter pylori *urease in the human stomach*

From the above, it would be expected that acidification of a test meal would increase intrabacterial urease activity and, hence, improve the results of the urea breath test. This is a measurement of the CO_2 released either from ^{14}C- or ^{13}C-labeled urea. It is known that acidification does in fact do this. At one time, this was thought to be due to the slowing of gastric emptying due to the acidification and, thus, longer exposure of the bacteria to urea. However, when the rate of emptying was measured, no change was found, and the effect of acidification of the test meal is more likely due to the activation of UreI and a resulting increase in urease activity in the stomach. Therefore, the data in which the activation of intrabacterial urease has been analyzed *in vitro* and in animal models applies also to the infected human stomach.

The effect of acidification on the rate of gastric emptying on the right and the urea breath test (UBT) on the left. It can be seen that there is an improvement in the UBT either with apple juice (pH 3.0) or acidification of a test meal (Ensure) but that apple juice is emptied more quickly and that there is no difference in the emptying of either neutral or acidified Ensure.

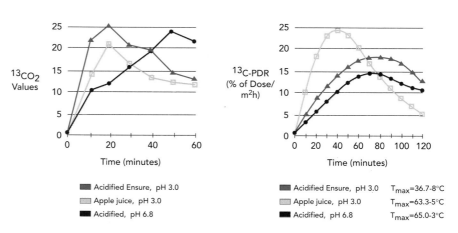

Gastric Acidity and Urea Breath Test

$^{13}CO_2$ Values — Time (minutes)

^{13}C-PDR (% of Dose/m^2h) — Time (minutes)

■ Acidified Ensure, pH 3.0
▢ Apple juice, pH 3.0
■ Acidified, pH 6.8

■ Acidified Ensure, pH 3.0 T_{max}=36.7-8°C
▢ Apple juice, pH 3.0 T_{max}=63.3-5°C
■ Acidified, pH 6.8 T_{max}=65.0-3°C

Regulation of urease assembly

The above methods of urease regulation relate to rapid changes in urease activity. Other means of regulation of urease have also been developed by the organism. Exposure to mild acidity increases urease assembly without changes in protein levels, and the promoter in front of UreI also allows regulation of the level of expression of the four genes implicated in urease assembly.

A simplified model illustrating the means of regulation of intrabacterial urease activity is shown below, emphasizing the central role of UreI in this process.

Acid activation of urea transport through the pH-gated urea channel UreI increases intrabacterial urease activity, and the ammonia produced buffers cytoplasm and periplasm.

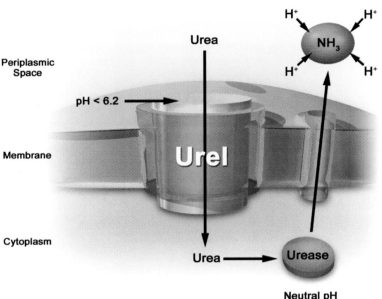

Adaptation of *Helicobacter* Urease

Urease association with the inner membrane

Immunoprecipitation of urease or blue native gel electrophoresis established that urease apoenzyme is associated with the membrane protein, UreI, raising the possibility that the NH_3 released during urease activity is able to diffuse rapidly through the inner membrane into the periplasm, decreasing the possibility of excessive alkalinization of the cytoplasm.

Further, electron microscopic examination of immunostained sections of *H. pylori* with antibodies against UreI and UreB shows that at acidic medium pH, there is increased association of urease with UreI. This is shown in the figure.

Hence, the means whereby the organism has used a neutral pH optimum intrabacterial urease to survive gastric acidity is not only by expressing a pH-gated urea channel but also by ensuring the most rapid access of urea entering the channel during acidification to urease, increasing the rapidity of the response and confining the response to the membrane region.

UreI as a target for monotherapy

Because expression of this protein is essential for survival of the bacteria in acid or in the stomach, a compound that would inhibit channel opening would proba-

Localization of UreB and UreI
at Neutral and Acidic pH

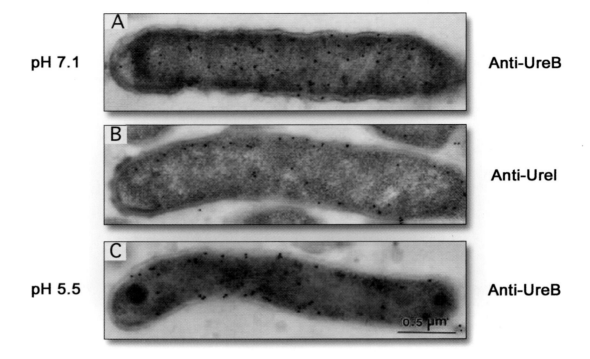

pH 7.1   Anti-UreB

Anti-UreI

pH 5.5   Anti-UreB

0.5 µm

Wong & Sano

Electron micrographs of postsectioning staining using immunogold particles with antibody against UreB (large particles), showing, in the first image, general cytoplasmic distribution. The second image shows, using smaller gold particles, staining for UreI localized to the inner membrane. Strikingly, at a medium pH of 5.5, UreB is now associated with the inner membrane.

bly be useful as monotherapy for eradication. This histidine-aspartate-glutamate-histidine interaction mechanism and the three-dimensional structure of this region of the protein presumably would form the target domain of any such drug.

Other acid-adaptive mechanisms

The exact concentration of urea at the site of bacterial infection is not known, but dependent on the level of colonization, variation in blood concentration, and location of the organism with respect to the surface of the stomach, there may well be times when urea concentration is insufficient to cope with the acidity of the environment. Hence, the bacteria use a variety of ancillary systems to improve their chances of acid survival.

Various other genes that increase acid resistance have been identified either by intuition or screening methods. These include the heat shock protein, Hsp70, *Cag*A, as well as a gene involved in outer wall composition. Ten genes were found by random mutagenesis that were required for growth at pH 4.8: four had unknown function; others were *lep*A, which is a membrane-bound GTPase; three were involved in H^+ transport; and two were similar to those found in other organisms (*ucr*A and *atp*F'). Gamma glutamyl transpeptidase was shown to be essential for colonization. *fur*, a ferric iron uptake regulator,

Gene Expression as a Function of Medium pH

CLUSTER ANALYSIS

Columns (left to right): pH7.4, pH7.4, pH6.2, pH6.2, pH6.2, pH6.2, pH5.5, pH5.5, pH5.5, pH4.5, pH4.5, pH4.5, pH4.5

HP0537-cag pathogenicity island protein (*cag16*)
HP0528-cag pathogenicity island protein (*cag8*)
HP0019-chemotaxis protein (*cheV*)
HP0048-transcriptional regulator (*hypF*)
HP0115-flagellin B (*flaB*)
HP0541-cag pathogenicity island protein (*cag20*)
HP0325-flagellar basal-body L-ring protein (*flgH*)
HP0540-cag pathogenicity island protein (*cag19*)
HP1399-arginase (*rocF*)
HP0727-"transcriptional regulator, putative"
HP1186-carbonic anhydrase (periplasmic)
HP0542-cag pathogenicity island protein (*cag21*)
HP1067-chemotaxis protein (*cheY*)
HP0792-sigma-54 interacting protein
HP1559-flagellar basal-body rod protein (*flgB*))
HP0393-chemotaxis protein (*cheV*)
HP0520-cag pathogenicity island protein (*cag1*)
HP0166-response regulator (*ompR*)
HP0278-guanosine pentaphosphate phosphohydrolase
HP0082-methyl-accepting chemotaxis transducer (*tlpC*
HP1557-flagellar basal-body protein (*fliE*)
HP0070-urease accessory protein (*ureE*)
HP0071-urease accessory protein (*ureI*)
HP0752-flagellar hook-associated protein 2 (*fliD*)
HP0532-cag pathogenicity island protein (*cag12*)
HP1287-transcriptional regulator (*tenA*)
HP0601-flagellin A (*flaA*)
HP0543-cag pathogenicity island protein (*cag22*)
HP0004-carbonic anhydrase (*icfA* cytoplasmic)
HP1192-secreted protein involved in flagellar motility
HP0315-virulence associated protein D (*vapD*)
HP1572-regulatory protein DniR
HP0294-aliphatic amidase (*amiE*)
HP0751-polar flagellin (*flaG*)
HP0165-signal-transducing protein, histidine kinase
HP0723-L-asparaginase II (*y*)

A cluster analysis of genes showing a more than twofold upregulation after exposure to pH 4.5 for 30 minutes, as a function of gradual change in medium pH from 7.4 to 4.5. Each column represents a separate experiment, and the data show that some genes are already upregulated at a medium pH of 6.2, some begin to show upregulation at pH 5.5, and some only at pH 4.5. Increasing intensity of red implies upregulation; black, no change. Cy3 was used for control and cy5 for acidic pH. Colors in text to the right indicate different functional categories of genes.

impaired growth in acid. pH-regulatory enzymes, such as arginase and amidase, increase acid survival *in vitro*.

Differential display of *H. pylori* grown for eight passages at pH 5.5 and 7.4 showed elevation of eight genes, including *ureB*, *atoE*, and *flaA*. These data might explain the increase of infectivity of the organism as a function of passage. A microarray analysis at pH 7.0 and 4.0 identified eight genes upregulated and three as downregulated under these conditions using PCR amplification of the hybridization spots. Among these, there was *cagA*, as well as a lipid-biosynthesis enzyme involved in LPS biosynthesis (HP1052) and a component of the membrane-secretory apparatus (*secF*). Analysis of gene expression after incubation for 48 hours at pH 7.2 and 5.5 showed 80 genes as more than fivefold upregulated. These included subunits of the F_1F_0 ATPase, an Na^+-dependent transporter, amidase, flagellin B homolog, flagellar biosynthesis protein, thioredoxin reductase, and methyl-accepting chemotaxis protein, *Omp11*, and arginase.

A general method is to identify genes that change expression progressively as medium acidity increases using technology such as microarrays. Several genes were found that are upregulated at a medium pH of 6.2, and these genes were still upregulated in the presence of 5 mM of urea, indicating that their regulation depends on periplasmic rather than cytoplasmic pH. Microarray methods are based on labeling of the cDNA generated by reverse transcription of the RNA isolated under neutral pH conditions with one fluorophore and labeling the cDNA generated by reverse transcription of the RNA isolated from acidic conditions with another fluorophore. The two cDNAs are hybridized to a slide containing the microarray representing all the genes of the organism.

In this way, more than 100 genes were found to be upregulated by exposing the bacteria to a medium of pH 4.5 in the presence of 5 mM of urea. Some of these were pH-regulatory genes such as amidase, arginase, and periplasmic carbonic anhydrase. These results show the breadth of adaptation of *H. pylori* to gastric acidity. A means of displaying these data is to use cluster analysis and determine the degree of upregulation of genes at acidic pH that show increased labeling with the red fluorophore—cy5—as compared to the genes at neutral pH labeled with the green fluorophore, cy3. This powerful method allows identification of all the genes that respond to acid, and systematic knockout of these genes will allow definition of genes essential for acid survival and gastric colonization.

As shown in the cluster array image, there are categories of genes that are upregulated. In green text are genes from the pathogenicity island, in black text are genes regulating bacterial pH, and in blue text are genes regulating transcription. It is already known that motility and regulation of urease activity is essential for infection and, hence, some of these genes might become targets for monotherapy.

CHAPTER 3
PATHOGENESIS

With the recognition that gastric infection was associated with ulcer disease also came the realization that infection was five times more frequent than ulcers. Much effort has been expended in attempts to identify the culprit genes responsible for the pathogenic consequences of infection. This is probably going to be extended to identifying genes also responsible for carcinogenesis.

Pathogenicity is either due to the organism itself being able to enter cells in the stomach or is the result of proteins released by lysis or secretion from the organism and then taken up by the cells or being injected into the cells of the gastric epithelium. There is no evidence that the first process takes place; hence, the lytic, secretory, or injected products of *H. pylori* must play the central role in the response of the surface epithelium of the upper gastrointestinal tract to infection.

However, although symptomatic disease is an infrequent outcome of infection, gastritis is a universal response. The inevitable gastritis that results from infection may well relate to the generation of NH_3 by bacterial urease. The finding that the vast majority of urease activity results from acid activation of internal urease promotes the idea of synergism between the organism and acid in causing initial damage. An increase of NH_3 on the surface of gastric cells results in an increase of intracellular pH. In turn, this results in an increase of intracellular calcium and initiation of calcium signal–dependent phenomena. These could be the harbingers of arrival of inflammatory cells that, in turn, produce the cytotoxic effects observed.

For *H. pylori* to establish and cause gastritis, it is likely that specific adhesion must occur to the surface membrane of gastric cells. The organisms tend to bind at regions of contact between cells *in vivo* and *in vitro*. These regions may contain specific receptor proteins for the organism, such as cadherins, integrins, or Lewis-type antigens. Such points of contact can result in pedicle formation and changes in intracellular distribution of cytoskeletal elements, perhaps aiding initiation of cell pathology.

The first unique protein identified as increasing host response was *CagA*, a protein of approximately 120 to 140 kDa. Its function is unknown, but it is part of what has been called a *pathogenicity island*. As for other bacteria, this region, which contains approximately 40 genes, appears to affect virulence. This island in *H. pylori* and other organisms contains DNA with a different base composition compared to the rest of the genome and is thought to have been acquired by horizontal transfer from another organism. Another product that is coexpressed with *CagA* is *VacA*. There are several variants in this region, showing that this gene is a mosaic. Another gene more recently identified with virulence is *iceA*. There appears to be a relatively clear relationship between expression of those genes and clinical outcome.

Within the pathogenicity island, there are a number of membrane-inserted proteins, many thought to be involved in export of proteins. The most frequently used protein-secretory pathway is that involving the secretory mechanisms, which relates to cotranslational insertion of a cleavable signal sequence into the translocon. After insertion of this sequence, the rest of the protein is externalized, and the signal sequence is cleaved outside the inner membrane, resulting in export of the protein.

For externalization of the flagella, a different system is used—the type III secretory system. The flagellar motor proteins are part of this, and a specialized protein is also present in the outer membrane that allows extrusion of the flagellar protein in proper orientation through both membranes. That type IV secretion exists in the organism, with direct injection of bacterial protein into host cells, has also been suggested.

Protein secretion by *H. pylori* may be a minor player in pathogenicity, however. A comparison of the protein composition of the organism with the medium in which it was grown showed a remarkable similarity, indicating that most of the medium proteins had arisen by lysis of the organism. This was confirmed further by showing that the pattern of *de novo* synthesized proteins in the presence of ^{35}S-methionine was very similar in the organism and in the medium. This experiment shows that few of the major proteins appear to be secreted. Rather, whole-cell lysis is the major mechanism for release of intracellular proteins. There is, however, a class of secreted proteins that may play an important role in pathogenesis.

	Identities of Putative Secreted Proteins Using Mass Spectrometry			
No. in the 2D gel	Name	pI*	Mwt. (kDa)	Single Peptide
1	Vacuolating toxin (VacA)	9.37	87.0	Yes
2	Hypothetical protein (JHPO839)	7.50	11.0	No
3	Hypothetical protein (JHPO766)	9.71	9.4	No
4	Probable thioredoxin (JHP1351)	8.17	11.7	No
5	Hypothetical protein (HPO305)	9.73	20.0	Yes
6	Hypothetical protein (HPO721)	8.42	17.6	Yes
7	Outer membrane protein (HP1564)	9.29	30.2	Yes
8	Hypothetical protein (HPO231)	9.35	29.5	Yes
9	Hypothetical protein (HPO973)	9.69	39.8	Yes
10	Conserved hypothetical secreted protein (HP1286)	9.37	20.6	Yes
11	Hypothetical protein (HPO129)	9.51	16.2	Yes

*: Isoelectric point of each protein

This table shows the proteins identified to be secreted by *H. pylori* by comparing radioactivity in the supernatant and intact bacteria after pulse change labeling with ^{35}S-methionine, 2D gel electrophoresis (IEF and SDA), and mass spectrometry.

Using protein labeling and two-dimensional gel electrophoresis of the medium and the organism, it was possible to identify proteins enriched in the medium—hence, candidates as secreted proteins. Shedding of plasma membrane vesicles was avoided by inhibiting cell division without inhibition of protein synthesis, and approximately 11 proteins were identified as being explicitly secreted rather than released. Their role in pathogenesis as compared to proteins released during lysis has yet to be established.

The figure shows the relative enrichment of each of the proteins in the above table in the medium, as compared to the intact organism, relative to a protein known to be released only by lysis (UreB).

The result of inflammation caused by *H. pylori* infection has become increasingly difficult to predict based on its genomic composition as more data are obtained from different geographic regions. In Asia, in contrast to Western countries, expression of *CagA* is not a marker for pathogenesis. On the other hand, to consider the possibility that the organism is a commensal ignores the universal gastritis that is found with infection. Probably, there is a complex relationship between microbe and host that determines the outcome of inflammation.

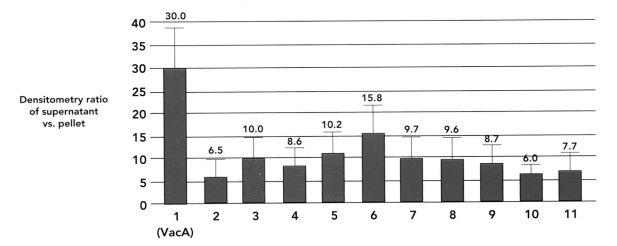

Secreted Proteins of *H. pylori*

Densitometry ratio of supernatant vs. pellet

$$\text{Relative Secretion Index} = \frac{\text{Candidate}_{SN}}{\text{Candidate}_{Pellet}} \times \text{UreB lysis correction factor}$$

Relative enrichment of 11 proteins in the medium, identified as being secreted by *H. pylori*. VacA is the major protein secreted, but the others are also clearly secreted. The numbers correspond to those shown in the table above.

CHAPTER 4
INFECTION AND
ITS CONSEQUENCES

Gastric acid secretion after infection

Acute phase

In early infection, acid secretion decreases, and at least two acid-inhibitory substances have been purified from *H. pylori*, with one partially sequenced. It appears to represent a metabolic gene. There is inevitably an acute gastritis observed in animal models, with ingress of a variety of inflammatory cells into the submucosa. The reason for the gastritis is obscure, but it is found after infection by any strain of *H. pylori*. It seems possible that NH_3 production is the explanation, because all strains that are infective produce large quantities of NH_3 that would tend to alkalinize the interior of gastric epithelial cells.

The addition and removal of NH_4Cl has large effects on cell pH. With addition, NH_3 is rapidly permeable across cell membranes relative to NH_4^+ and, on entering a cell, is protonated to NH_4^+, hence alkalinizing the cell. When the salt is removed, NH_3 leaves the cell, and acidification results. Alkalinization of the cells increases intracellular Ca^{2+}, which in turn could result in the production and secretion of cytokines such as IL-8 and others, resulting in the inflammation. From the urease properties defined above, NH_3 production would be much larger and constant between pH 6.2 and 2.5. However, at acidic pH, the NH_3/NH_4^+ ratio would decline, resulting in lower concentrations of the permeable NH_3. But if there were periods of elevated pH or regions where gastric acid containing NH_3 were rapidly neutralized, then the concentration of NH_3 would rise, permeate cells, and elevate internal pH and, thus, intracellular calcium. This hypothesis suggests that NH_3 production in parallel with varying acidity could account for many of the sequelae of infection.

Chronic phase

It has been known for many years that duodenal ulcer patients have, on the average, higher acid output than do patients without duodenal ulcer. Gastric ulcer patients tend to have lower than normal acidity. Counting the number of parietal cells has shown that duodenal ulcer patients have more parietal cells, thus explaining the acid-output data.

The gastric effects of *H. pylori* depend in part on the site of infection, be it antral or fundic. Infection, therefore, results in either antral or fundic gastritis. In the case of antral infection, there is a decrease of somatostatin or the D-cell population, accompanied by hypergastrinemia. The latter is thought to be trophic for parietal cells, thus accounting for the higher acid output in duodenal ulcer patients. In the case of infection of the gastric corpus, there is often gastric atrophy with loss of acid-secreting cells. This would result in a reduced level of acid secretion in those patients with gastric atrophy.

H. pylori Disease Profile

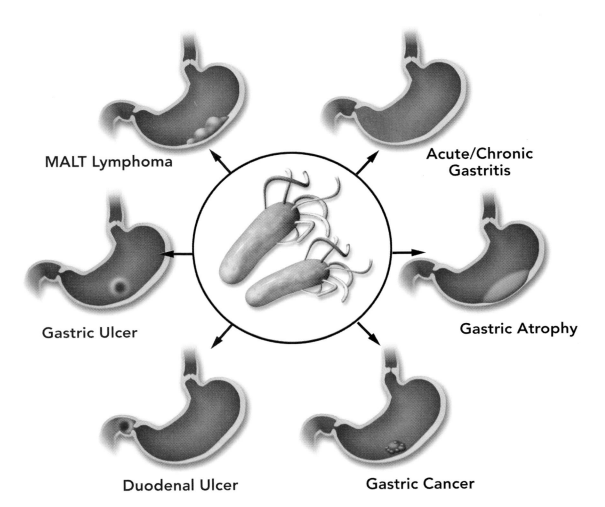

MALT Lymphoma

Acute/Chronic Gastritis

Gastric Ulcer

Gastric Atrophy

Duodenal Ulcer

Gastric Cancer

The different potential clinical and pathologic manifestations of infection with *H. pylori* in the gastroduodenal area. Mucosal infection with the organism results in a number of different events, including active chronic inflammation, lymphoid follicle reaction, development of atrophy, and intestinal metaplasia. In addition, it appears that the organism is also the common denominator in the development of duodenal ulcer, gastric ulcer, MALT gastric lymphoma, and, in some circumstances, gastric adenocarcinoma. The latter diverse pathologic events are multifactorial disease processes, and their evolution to some extent is dependent upon the host-response to infection. Thus, host versus *H. pylori* interactions and the effects on gastric physiologic functions (acid secretion, mucosal integrity, inflammatory response) and exogenous diverse environmental factors together determine the final expression of the disease in a particular individual.

Pathogenic strains

As discussed above, all strains result in gastritis at the site of colonization, but only approximately 20% of infected individuals acquire peptic ulcer disease. This may be due to variation in the organism or in the host or due to other factors.

The finding that eradication appears to increase acid reflux that, in turn, may associate with Barrett's esophagus suggests to some that there may be a benefit to gastric infection. It is true that some frequent human genetic abnormalities may confer protection, such as sickle cell hemoglobin-A mutation providing antimalarial properties or cystic fibrosis transport regulator against typhoid. It does appear unlikely that gastric inflammation is of real benefit to the host.

***Helicobacter pylori* and ulcer site**

The duodenal ulceration site is in the first part of the duodenum, usually at a site where it might be supposed that the highest acidity is found. Even now, it has not been established that *H. pylori* is actually present at the site of ulceration or whether gastric metaplasia and ectopic parietal cells are associated with the presence of *H. pylori* at that locale.

The site of gastric ulceration is usually in the transition zone between fundus and antrum. In this region, there are still parietal cells and chief cells that may mainly secrete type II pepsinogen. The organism is clearly found in association with gastric ulcers, and it may be that this region of the stomach is more susceptible to the consequences of infection than the more hardy fundus and the non–acid-secreting antrum.

The presence of acid is as important as that of the organism in the generation of peptic ulcers, and given that the apical membranes of gastric cells are relatively acid impermeable, it is likely that the first site of damage is the tight junction between the epithelial cells. This effect may well be due to inflammation. Once the tight junction is damaged, allowing acid back diffusion, further damage can result in the back diffusion of pepsin.

The combination of infection, inflammation, and acid and pepsin back diffusion results in ulcer development.

Helicobacter pylori and its gastric environment

The organism is found at the gastric surface and within the gastric mucus. There is a degree of controversy about the most frequent site of habitation and as to what the conditions are at the site of habitation. Many believe that the gastric surface is close to neutrality, thus allowing colonization. However, direct measurement has shown that at a luminal pH of 2.0 or less, no pH gradient can be detected at the gastric surface. Because mean diurnal pH is 1.4 in normal people, it is likely that at times during the day, the environment of the organism is genuinely acidic, and its acid-adaptive mechanisms must come into play. Further, because UreI-deletion mutants can inhabit the stomach when acid secretion is inhibited but disappear when acid secretion is allowed to return, clearly the pH of the environment must be less than 4.0 for some considerable time.

It is not known where the first site of colonization is found after infection. It seems that infection often occurs in childhood, perhaps before acid secretion reaches adult levels, and, therefore, either antral or fundic infection could occur. It also seems that infection per se transiently reduces acid secretion by the human stomach, thereby enabling better colonization.

The organisms are found with mainly antral colonization when antral gastritis arises (the more frequent manifestation) or with fundic colonization (when fundic gastritis arises, perhaps a later stage of the disease). They are also often associated with the tight junction regions, perhaps because of the higher urea concentration. Organisms are attached to cells by a pedicle with morphologic alterations at the cellular side of the pedicle. Whether there are specialized outer-membrane proteins then associated with the pedicle, enabling more direct entry of NH_3, or perhaps even proteins by type III secretion, is not known.

Several papers have claimed that treatment with PPIs reduces the number of organisms in the antrum and increases their level in the fundus. Inhibition

The nature of alterations in acid secretion and different stages of mucosal inflammation that may occur consequent upon *H. pylori* infection. In patients with a high gastric acid output, colonization may be limited to the antrum, whereas patients with a low gastric acid output are characterized by a body (corpus)-predominant gastritis. The former is associated with a downregulation of somatostatin (SST) secretion, a concomitant increase in gastrin, and a continued high acid secretory response, which may ultimately evolve into a duodenal ulcer phenotype in some patients. Infection of the corpus and a low acid secretory response is associated with mucosal alterations such as atrophy and an increased risk of neoplasia.

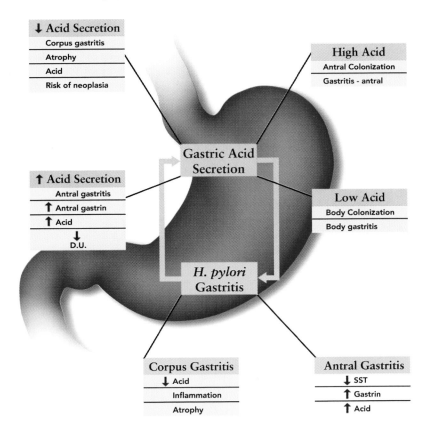

H. pylori, Acid and Gastritis

of acid secretion to the level expected from PPI treatment in principle could reduce acidity on the antral surface to a level at which urease activity could be toxic to the organism. An increase of pH on the fundic surface, improving the habitat there for the bacteria, could increase bacterial frequency in this region of the stomach. Because there is variation in the response to PPIs, there may also be variation in the effect of PPIs on localization of *H. pylori* in the stomach.

Most agree that fundic infection is able to lead to atrophy, metaplasia, and perhaps cancer. If, indeed, PPI treatment results in relocation of infection to the fundus, there is a strong case to be made for eradication in those patients undergoing chronic therapy with PPIs for GERD.

Serial biopsies taken over many years from patients infected with *H. pylori* indicate that the long-term consequences of infection may include gastric atrophy and intestinal metaplasia, and, by implication from earlier studies, these may lead to dysplasia and gastric cancer. Although controversial, the concept that decreased acid secretion and gastric atrophy are intimately related is an old one. Although it was previously held that acid inhibition was the result and not the cause of atrophic gastritis, recent data have suggested that if infec-

The organism affects a number of cell types in both the antrum and the fundus. These include at least the neuroendocrine G, D, and ECL cells and the immune system. Stimulation of G-cell function (increase in gastrin release) activates the ECL cell to produce histamine that drives parietal cell acid secretion. This effect may be further modulated by the cascade of cytokines that are released by epithelial cells damaged by the organism or its products. Of the neuroendocrine cell acid regulators, ECL cell function is impaired by interleukins. In addition, the gastric T-cell immune response is directed towards the Th1 pathway, which is associated with an enhanced cell-mediated immunity that results in damage (atrophy) to the gastric epithelium.

Gastric Cellular Effect of *H. Pylori* Infection

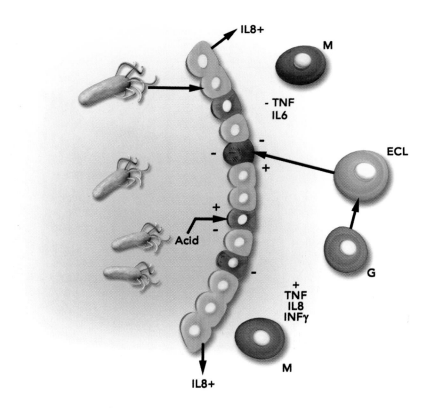

tion with *H. pylori* is present, acid inhibition may result in accelerated atrophy. The mechanism of this effect remains obscure, but pharmacologic and surgical reductions of gastric acid secretion are both associated with a more severe inflammatory response to *H. pylori*, which may lead to more severe epithelial cell damage. Interpretation of the data remains difficult, in part because of the problems in defining gastric atrophy and in part because of age mismatch in the cohorts studied.

The recent publication of the updated Sydney system for the classification and grading of gastritis may be helpful in future studies of atrophy. However, whether this scheme will be more clinically useful than its predecessors remains to be evaluated. Nevertheless, the attempt to objectively define gastritis using visual analog scales is a significant advance and may add considerably to the objectivity of the assessment. However, there is still considerable debate concerning the reversibility of atrophy, whether functional or morphologic; most would argue that atrophy is not reversible. Unfortunately, due to potential sampling errors in follow-up biopsy studies, convincing data are still lacking, and, therefore, debate on this issue will still continue.

Many studies have established that infection with *H. pylori* and the secondary mucosal inflammatory response increase gastric epithelial cell prolif-

Gastritis

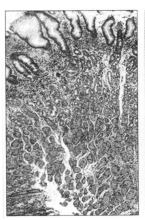 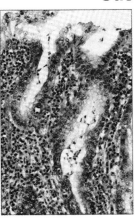 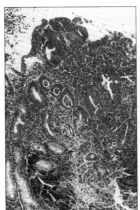 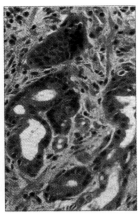

Superficial   *Active*   *Active chronic*   *Atrophic*

The different histologic types of gastritis identifiable during various stages of *H. pylori* infection of the gastric mucosa. Superficial gastritis is followed in the majority of patients with active and chronic active gastritis. This is followed, over time and only in a subset of patients, with the development of intestinal metaplasia and atrophy. It has been established that both environmental and host-related factors play significant roles in the evolution of the patient's gastritis "profile."

eration. This may be a necessary step in the process of gastric carcinogenesis, as for many other malignancies. *H. pylori* probably does not increase proliferation directly; increased cell proliferation is more likely a response to apoptosis (programmed cell death) induced by the organism or the inflammatory response. After a compensatory hyperproliferative response, the balance between apoptosis and proliferation may determine whether ulcers and atrophy develop or, conversely, whether mucosal mass grows in an unrestrained fashion. Some information is available from animal models. For example, *H. felis* infection in mice increases cell proliferation, particularly of mucous neck cells, but decreases the number of parietal cells. The hyperproliferative response is more extreme in animals that are homozygous for p53, suggesting that *H. pylori* may act in concert with other oncogenes and tumor-suppressor genes to produce neoplasia. Although little is known about the effect of *H. pylori* on the normal gastric cell cycle, it has been demonstrated that the lipopolysaccharide of *Helicobacter* displays synergism in gastrin-mediated increased DNA synthesis in ECL cells.

Because the ECL cell is a crucial link between gastrin and acid in the normal stomach, the interaction of *H. pylori* with this cell may throw light on some of the discrepant information regarding the effects of *H. pylori* on gastrin and acid secretion. Whether the ECL cells are exposed to *H. pylori* lipopolysaccharide directly is unclear, because the ECL cells are not thought to be in communication with the gastric lumen. Nevertheless, lipopolysaccharide is present in measurable quantities in the blood stream and may impinge on the ECL cell in the same fashion that gastrin does. It is possible that mucosal damage induced by *H. pylori* and disruption of tight junctions may also facilitate access. Either way, it may be that the population of ECL cells does increase in *H. pylori* infection, and, in combination with PPIs especially, micronodular carcinoids may develop.

H. Pylori Lipopolysaccharide-Mediated ECL Cell Proliferation

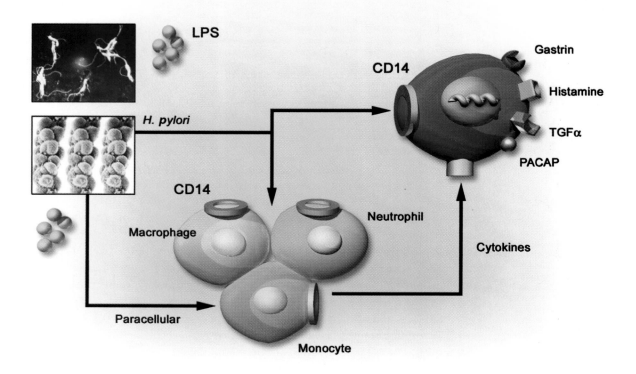

A cartoon of the possible mechanisms by which *H. pylori* lipopolysaccharide may result in stimulation of ECL cell proliferation and secretion.

Acid activation of urease in the stomach will result in the production of NH_3, which will rapidly convert to NH_4^+. At pH 4.0, for example, with a pK_a of 9.0, there will be a 10^5-fold excess of NH_4^+. However, if acid secretion slows or a 10-mM NH_4Cl solution is emptied into the duodenum at pH 7.0, there will be a 1,000-fold increase in NH_3 concentration. This would be sufficient to alkalinize the cell and elevate intracellular calcium, perhaps to levels at which cytotoxic effects could be observed, as shown in the following figure.

A conceptual model of the means whereby ammonia production from urease activated by gastric acidity may damage the mucosa. In acid, the impermeant ammonium ion is generated, but then with neutralization, the concentration of the diffusible ammonia increases. Entry of this into cells will result in alkalinization and perhaps cytokine release.

H. pylori Urease and Toxicity

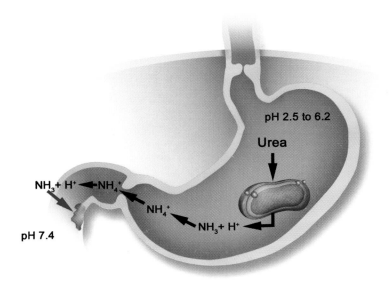

pH 2.5 to 6.2

Urea

$NH_3 + H^+ \leftarrow NH_4^+$

NH_4^+

NH_4^+

$NH_3 + H^+$

pH 7.4

Mucosal-associated lymphoid tissue (MALT) lymphoma

H. pylori vaulted into a position of considerable clinical relevance with the recognition of its critical association with gastroduodenal ulceration. The further observation that the resolution of the genesis of mucosal ulceration might lie with its eradication almost paled in significance when it became evident that the organism was the probable cause of a form of gastric neoplasm. Indeed, the link between *H. pylori* infection and gastric MALT lymphoma is similar to that between the putative small intestinal infection and IPSID (*immuno proliferative small intestinal disease*). Because the normal stomach possesses no mucosa-associated lymphoid tissue, the origin of gastric lymphoma is enigmatic. Nevertheless, it is apparent that as a sequel of *H. pylori* infection, MALT, comprised of lymphoid follicles and a lymphoepithelium, accumulates in the gastric mucosa. The organism has been identified in gastric lymphoma, and the presence of *H. pylori* in the stomach is directly associated with MALT lymphoma. Furthermore, in areas where there is a high prevalence of *H. pylori* infection, the likelihood that individuals will develop gastric lymphoma is significantly increased. Because the stomach normally possesses no lymphoid tissue in the gastric mucosa, the accumulation of MALT is almost pathognomonic of *H. pylori* infection. The proposed role of *H. pylori* presented antigens in driving the lymphoid tissue hyperplasia, and its transformation into a neoplasm is consistent with current clinical observations. Thus, early antibiotic therapy has been associated with eradication not only of the *H. pylori* but also of the lymphomatous disease. Alternatively, if the lymphoma has reached an *H. pylori*–independent phase or has transformed from

Pathogenesis of MALT Lymphoma

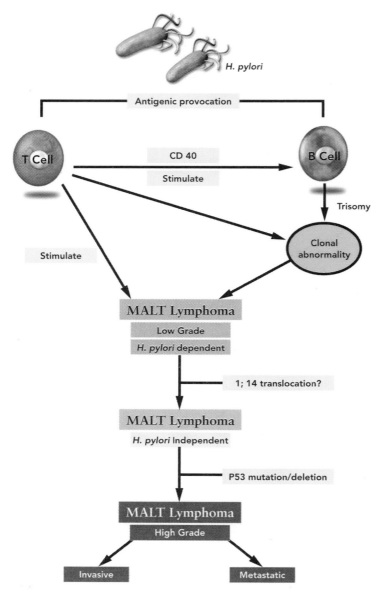

A schematic outline of the pathogenesis of MALT lymphoma due to stimulation of B- or T-cell proliferation by *H. pylori* antigens, followed by neoplastic transformation.

its low-grade status to a high-grade MALT lymphoma, eradication therapy is not effective.

The gastrointestinal tract is the most common site of primary extranodal lymphoma, and gastric lymphoma accounts for the majority of cases. It is of importance to differentiate primary gastric lymphoma from secondary involvement of the stomach by nodal lymphoma, which occurs relatively commonly. The precise incidence of primary gastric lymphoma is difficult to ascertain, given the widely different diagnostic criteria that have been used as well as the considerable geographic variation in incidences. Overall, there is evidence to support the fact that gastric lymphoma may be increasing in incidence, although the incidence of *H. pylori* is decreasing. It is necessary, however, to define *primary gastric lymphoma* as lymphoma occurring in the stomach with or without the presence of regional lymph nodes, with the stomach being the site of the majority of the disease, if not the only site.

Hodgkin's disease rarely occurs in the stomach, and the great majority of primary gastric lymphomas are B-cell tumors. Nevertheless, T-cell lymphomas do occur, although they are extremely rare. For the most part, the histopathologic features of low-grade primary gastric lymphoma—MALT—recapitulate the structure of Peyer's patches rather than lymph nodes. In certain instances, low-grade MALT lymphomas may transform to high-grade disease, and it is likely that most instances of this entity represent evolution, because the tumors are derived from the same B-cell lineage. What is apparent, however, is that gastric MALT lymphomas do not share any of the features common to nodal lymphomas but instead exhibit a marked increase in the frequency of trisomy 3. Similarly, the gastric MALT lymphomas differ from their nodal counterparts in that their behavior is usually quite favorable.

The low-grade gastric lymphomas, which have been characterized as MALT, usually occur in individuals older than 50 years, with a peak in the seventh decade. Nevertheless, instances of such disease have been described at almost all ages. There appears to be a slight male predominance (1.5:1.0). More often than not, the symptoms are of a nonspecific nature, with a central dyspeptic component rather than any specific signs, as might occur with a gastric adenocarcinoma. At endoscopy, the findings are usually those of a nonspecific gastritis with erosions or ulceration, although a mass lesion is occasionally identifiable. It is unusual to be able to detect extraabdominal dissemination, although such events have been recorded. In contrast to the low-grade MALT lymphomas, patients presenting with the high-grade B-cell gastric lymphomas usually do so at a slightly older age (64 years versus 55 years). In these patients, the clinical presentation more commonly represents that of a gastric adenocarcinoma with pain, weight loss, and anemia being the most common presentations, although perforation rarely may occur as the initial clinical event. At endoscopy, an obvious tumor mass is usually evident, with ulceration in many instances. For the most part, gastric lymphomas involve the antrum, but they may occur at any site in the stomach. The low-grade MALT lymphomas usually are flat infiltrative lesions, which are often difficult to diagnose and often require multiple or double-level biopsies. The high-grade gastric lymphomas are more commonly large and bulky tumors with considerable infiltration.

The low-grade MALT lymphomas produce a histologic appearance closely simulating that of a Peyer's patch. Thus, the lymphoma infiltrates around and between reactive follicles in the region corresponding to the marginal zone of a Peyer's patch and spreads diffusely into the surrounding mucosa. Tumor cells are usually small to medium in size, with moderately abundant cytoplasm with nuclei that have an irregular outline closely resembling the nuclei of centrocytes. An important histologic feature of low-grade MALT lymphomas is the presence of lymphoepithelial lesions formed by the invasion of individual gastric glands by aggregates of tumor cells. At a later stage, this is associated with disintegration of the glandular epithelium and eosinophilic degeneration. Occasionally areas of a low-grade lymphoma may be replaced by a high-grade lymphoma, suggesting transformation from one form to the other. The presence of confluent clusters or sheets of transformed cells is strongly indicative of transformation to a high-grade lymphoma lesion.

Low-grade MALT lymphomas are seldom disseminated at the time of diagnosis and rarely involve lymph nodes or bone marrow. As a result, prolonged survival is common, with figures reaching as high 91% at 5 years and 75% at 10 years if surgical resection is used. Nodal low-grade B-cell lymphomas are usually widely disseminated at diagnosis, with the majority of patients having

H. pylori
Gastric Carcinogenesis

Sequence · Histology

H. pylori Infection

Chronic Gastritis

Gastric Atrophy

Intestinal Metaplasia

Dysplasia

Adenocarcinoma

Possible histology of the sequence of events due to infection by H. pylori leading to gastric adenocarcinoma.

bone marrow involvement. Treatment is usually ineffective, and most patients die within 7 to 10 years, often as a result of high-grade transformation. There is controversy as to whether high-grade MALT lymphomas have as favorable a prognosis. On balance, it appears that the higher the grade of lymphoma, the less favorable the outcome is likely to be.

Low-grade MALT lymphomas commonly involve the local draining lymph nodes; if peripheral spreading occurs, it is a late event. This results in a favorable prognosis quite unlike that of the indolent yet progressive disease pattern associated with disease-disseminated low-grade B-cell lymphomas of lymph nodes. In fact, low-grade MALT lymphomas tend to remain localized to their site of origin for prolonged periods, although the reason for this is not clearly defined. It has been proposed that this type of lesion may not even be a malignant lymphoma but represents either a hyperplasia or a "pseudolymphoma." One suggestion is that the proliferation of the MALT represents the presence of a local antigen presented by *H. pylori*, and the process may be a lymphocyte-homing phenomenon. Nevertheless, MALT possesses many of the criteria that are used to define a malignant tumor. It is monoclonal, demonstrates the presence of a clonal genetic abnormality, and displays various degrees of invasiveness and dissemination. The low grade of the MALT lymphomas, and especially the gastric lymphoma, suggests some form of immunologic control that may be influenced by a local antigen—in this case, *H. pylori*. This might well explain the tendencies of such lymphomas to remain localized, because lymphoma cells disseminating to peripheral locations would then fail to proliferate in the absence of a specific antigen. Indeed, low-grade gastric lymphomas exhibit variable numbers of transformed tumor cells and show plasma cell differentiation, which tends to be maximal beneath surface epithelium. This characteristic would be consistent with a luminal or epithelial antigen causing such effects. Similarly, the phenomenon of "follicular colonization," in which lymphoma cells migrate to centers of reactive B-cell follicles, is also evident and consistent with a manifestation of an antigen effect.

Antibiotics would presumably sterilize the gastric lumen, removing the bacterial antigen, which is responsible for driving the proliferation of lymphoma cells. In this context, the success noted in treating gastric MALT lymphomas with antibiotics would be consistent with removing the *H. pylori* antigen or product responsible for driving the proliferation of lymphoma cells. Support for this hypothesis reflects not only clinical material but also experimental studies in which cells from individual cases of low-grade gastric lymphoma were stimulated to divide and secrete tumor-specific immunoglobulin by specific strains of *H. pylori*. The response of the lymphomatous B-cells is mediated via contact with *H. pylori*–specific T-cells, and considerable practical support has been provided for the organism-driven proliferative theory in studies in which patients with MALT gastric lymphoma treated with antibiotics exhibit regression of the lesion as well as eradication of the organism. Nevertheless, it is apparent that in more aggressive forms of gastric MALT lymphoma, particularly in those that exhibit more deeply invasive lesions, the lymphoma does not completely regress on eradication therapy. Whether this

Diagnosis of *Helicobacter pylori*

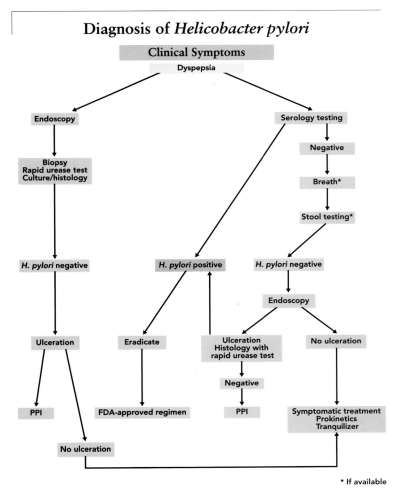

A flow diagram outlining the steps to diagnose infection.

represents transformation of the neoplastic phenotype into a different mode or failure to completely eradicate the organism is not certain. It has been suggested that the phenotype of gastric lymphomas that have disseminated beyond the stomach and local lymph nodes may have altered, such that their growth would be independent of *H. pylori*–stimulated T-cells.

There are still a considerable number of unanswered questions relating to the issue of MALT lymphoma. A number of studies have concluded that in up to 80% of patients with low-grade gastric MALT lymphoma, remission may be predicted after cure of *H. pylori* infection using a treatment regime consisting of a PPI, a nitroimidazole, and an antibiotic. It is not yet certain whether such high remission numbers are reproducible or whether the histologic and endoscopic remission will remain stable in the long term. In the majority of patients in whom antibiotic and PPI therapy fails, a high-grade lymphoma (autonomous) is often detectable at surgery. In this respect, it may be important to use endoscopic ultrasonography to determine the extent of lymphoma. In those lesions that have invaded the deeper parts of the gastric wall, the likelihood of high-grade lymphoma is higher, and the possibility of therapeutic failure should be considered early in the disease course to obviate delay. Overall, patients with MALT lymphomas in stage E1 appear curable, whereas those in stage EII do not benefit and may require alternative treatment strategies, including surgery.

Difficulties exist with the distinction between induction of remission and cure in patients with low-grade MALT lymphomas. The use of polymerase chain reaction assay to determine the presence of rearranged immunoglobulin heavy chaining indicative of B-cell lymphoma often remains positive, even when clinical appearance of complete remission has been attained. Adequate predictive data from long-term follow-up studies to determine whether the ongoing presence of monoclonal bands in the polymerase chain reaction assay are indicative of a high risk of developing a relapse of the disease are not available.

Diagnosis

Endoscopy cannot be justified merely to diagnose *H. pylori* infection. As a noninvasive test, the urea breath test is extremely useful, particularly in establishing whether active infection exists or if eradication therapy has been successful.

The breath test is the only currently available accurate nonendoscopic way to check for successful eradication. Although current practice guidelines may recommend the use of confirmatory breath testing for individuals with complicated ulcer disease, the issue of whether confirmatory testing should be performed in uncomplicated cases with continued symptoms is controversial.

Testing to confirm eradication in these patient groups as well as individuals who are asymptomatic after eradication therapy will be driven by cost, accessibility, accuracy, and patient demand for diagnostic certainty. However, given the risk of gastric cancer, it should always be performed. The major drawbacks of the ^{13}C urea breath test are its cost and limited availability worldwide. It is currently being purposively marketed at a price only slightly below endoscopy and is significantly more expensive in the United States than elsewhere in the world. However, the newly FDA-approved ^{14}C urea breath test is under $100, thus indicating that market forces may play a critical role in further decreasing the costs of breath tests. Nevertheless, if either breath test is to be used as the initial noninvasive diagnostic test, it must surpass the convenience and accuracy of office-based serologic or stool antigen tests, which, even if not quite as sensitive or specific as laboratory-based serology, are inexpensive, quick, and easy to use, but only for diagnosis, not for eradication.

Antibody-based tests should be specific and respond rapidly to eradication. Perhaps novel antigens could be used to improve both specificity and analysis of loss of organism. It should be remembered that only a few organisms in a special niche in the stomach could result in false analysis of eradication, because these could regrow after some considerable period. Hence, at least 1 month should be left in between therapy and eradication testing.

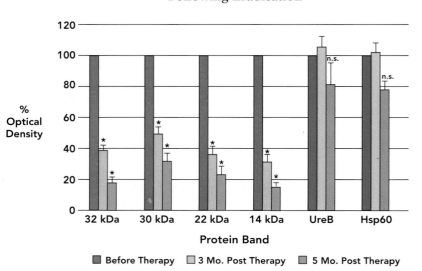

Diagnostic Decrease in Antibody Response Following Eradication

Diagnostic analysis of nine patients' sera before and after eradication, comparing the response to eradication of the antibody response to four low-molecular-weight antigens and to the large UreB and Hsp60, which persist much longer. These bands have been identified by mass spectrometry and Western analysis of recombinant proteins. Hence, immunoreactivity of patient sera to these proteins indicates infection and also allows analysis of success of eradication therapy in a noninvasive office procedure.

Recently, three low-molecular-weight antigens have been found in *H. pylori* that are accurate for diagnosis of infection, and also, the antibody response disappears rapidly after eradication. If developed for widespread use, this test would provide a cost-effective means of identifying the organism and its disappearance after therapy.

Three of these, expressed as recombinant proteins (32 kDa-HpaA, 30 kDa-Omp18, and 22 kDa-HP0596), reacted specifically with sera from infected patients, whereas the 14 kDa-RPL7/L12 cross-reacted with one out of five sera from *H. pylori*–negative patients. Because these are readily available as recombinant proteins, strip tests could be constructed and used for office testing of infection and eradication.

However, because there is no current gold standard for the diagnosis of *H. pylori*, the choice of diagnostic test depends more on local resources, experience, and cost-effectiveness than small differences in sensitivity and specificity. Probably, serology will be used to establish infection and breath test for efficacy of eradication. However, the accuracy of many of the current serology tests could be improved. False positives lead to needless expense, false negatives to inappropriate peace of mind on the part of either patient or physician.

Given that urease activity is largely dependent on acid, breath tests should not be administered immediately after a PPI. But in any case, it is probably best to administer the urea in conjunction with citric acid to activate intracellular urease so as to obtain maximal sensitivity of the breath test, as discussed above.

Relevance as a disease entity

In 1994, the National Institutes of Health consensus statement declared that all patients with peptic ulcers associated with *H. pylori* should have the organism eradicated. In addition, it was stated that more work was needed to evaluate the link between *H. pylori* and nonulcer dyspepsia before treatment is recommended for these patients. In 1997, the scientific message is basically unchanged, but clinical practice has altered appreciably. Thus, in the mid-1990s, only die-hard *H. pylori* aficionados would commonly use eradication therapy, even for patients with documented ulcer disease. Currently, primary care physicians are comfortable with using eradication therapy for a wide variety of indications, whereas some practitioners choose not to even test for the organism that is to be killed.

It is of interest to reflect on how such a confusing situation has evolved. Of particular concern is whether it will ever be possible to perform the studies necessary to establish cause and effect for nonulcer dyspepsia. Practicing evidence-based medicine while adopting cost-effective approaches to this potential public health problem may even be mutually exclusive. For example, some models suggest that the simplest way to manage a patient with ulcer-like dyspepsia, and perhaps even the asymptomatic patient with *H. pylori*, is by *H. pylori*–eradication treatment. Thus, although there is still no hard evidence that *H. pylori* is associated with nonulcer dyspepsia, it is unlikely that current practice modes will ever allow us to revert to a time in which a symptom could be evaluated carefully in the context of the patient's general health. Indeed, it is apparent that a new world of marketing and public domain information has led to the situation that *H. pylori* eradication has so permeated the minds of both physicians and the public that neither group is probably prepared to contemplate living with this potential carcinogen in their stomachs.

In retrospect, it seems probable that the 1994 announcement by the International Agency for Research on Cancer of the World Health Organization that *H. pylori* is a definite carcinogen may have been somewhat premature. Although accepting the epidemiologic association between *H. pylori* and gastric cancer, a recent reappraisal of a much wider data base has emphasized the need to keep an open mind on this critical question. Indeed, skeptics have raised the philosophic question as to whether it may be possible that not all *H. pylori* are bad. It has been noted that the recent increase in the diagnosis of reflux esophagitis and adenocarcinoma of the lower esophagus and gastric cardia has accompanied the natural decline in *H. pylori* infection in the West over the last 50 years. Thoughtful individuals have questioned whether such observations and phenomena may be related. In general, esophagitis and fundic gastric cancer are not associated with *H. pylori* infection, and in fact, a negative association may exist. Labenz and coworkers have reported that eradicating *H. pylori* from duodenal ulcer patients may even precipitate reflux disease.

H. pylori and NSAIDs are independent risk factors in the etiology of ulcers. This may, however, be an oversimplistic interpretation of studies that have excluded some patients most at risk for NSAID ulcers. In addition, some of these reports have relied on relatively insensitive serologic assays whose performance may be altered by NSAID use to identify the presence of *H. pylori*. A consequence would be an underestimate of the contribution of *H. pylori* in patients taking NSAIDs who develop ulcers in many studies in which serology is the sole criterion for the diagnosis of *H. pylori* infection. It has been reported that in patients anticipating treatment with naproxen, prophylactic *H. pylori* eradication decreased the risk of ulcers, suggesting that the bacterium and NSAIDs may be synergistic.

Epidemiology

The epidemiology of *H. pylori* has been extensively studied and the risk factors for the acquisition of infection determined. It is clear that most infection occurs in childhood and that infection or reinfection is not a clinical problem for most adults, in developed countries at least. How *H. pylori* is transmitted, however, remains unclear, and it remains possible that more than one route exists. The evidence for fecal-oral transmission is based mainly on a small group of children in Africa, on contaminated water supplies, and by analogy with hepatitis A. Although the organism has been cultured from feces in the developed world, most researchers have only found *H. pylori* in the stool by polymerase chain reaction. Alternative methods of transmission include the oral-oral route, perhaps lurking in dental plaque or by regurgitation of gastric contents, or waterborne. *H. pylori* has been identified by polymerase chain reaction in the water supply occasionally, not only in Peru, but also in Scandinavia. Apart from some early attempts by enthusiastic investigators to fulfill Koch's postulates by drinking *H. pylori* or occasional episodes of epidemic achlorhydria related to sharing common inadequately sterilized endoscopes or gastric tubes, documented transmission from person to person has been largely elusive. It appears that the routine use of high-level disinfection for endoscopes and reusable biopsy forceps should eliminate iatrogenic transmission of *H. pylori* by physicians.

Perhaps the use of animal models, of which there are many, may clarify the issue of transmission. The earliest animal models required the use of gnotobiotic pigs, but more recently, many other animals (cats, ferrets, gerbils, hamsters, rats, and mice) have been infected with a variety of *Helicobacter* species, both nonhuman *Helicobacter* and *H. pylori*. Some of these animals have developed pathology similar to that found in human disease. For example, *H. mustelae* in ferrets produces a multifocal atrophic gastritis. Gastric ulcers can be produced by infection with *H. heilmanii* (formerly *Gastrospirillum hominis*) in mice or by *H. pylori* in gnotobiotic pigs. It is of considerable interest that some animals even develop MALT lymphoma and cancer. The outcome of infection in certain animal models has been shown to be dependent not only on the bacterium inoculated but also on the animal's genotype. Ultimately, animal models may be useful not only for the development of vaccines but also for determining the natural history of *Helicobacter* infection. They may be of use in the evaluation of the bacterial and host factors that determine clinical outcome and in the elucidation of the mechanism of the association between *H. pylori* and gastric malignancy.

Treatment

Whom to treat

The identification of the individual who should be treated is probably the most controversial aspect of *H. pylori* at this time. Because most agree that a diagnosis of *H. pylori* infection should not be sought unless treatment is to be undertaken, a more pertinent question may be the decision of who should be tested. To date, the only proven benefit in eradicating *H. pylori* is for patients with ulcers. Nevertheless, there are a number of arguments, economic and emotional, not purely scientific, that in practice dictate that many more patients than only those with ulcers should receive treatment. In view of the fact that health policy and management recommendations continue to evolve at a rapid rate, it may never be possible to complete the necessary studies to determine whether *H. pylori* eradication would benefit certain categories of nonulcer patients. For example, the European Consensus Meeting held in the fall of 1996 at Maastricht suggested considerably extending the 1994 National Institutes of Health and Wellness consensus indications for treatment. In addition to all ulcer patients, *H. pylori* eradication was recommended, not surprisingly, for early MALT lymphomas (preferably in expert centers, in the context of clinical trials) and also for all patients who had undergone gastrectomy, whether for cancer or ulcers. The argument for treating cancer patients was the persuasive study of a relatively limited number of Japanese patients who had an early gastric cancer resected. In those who thereafter had *H. pylori* eradicated, a reduced chance of a second cancer was noted.

The question of whether treatment can be recommended based on a single report or, alternatively, whether it is acceptable to delay responding to such information pursuant on the availability of more extensive information that might take years to assemble raises both moral and ethical issues. In addition to these indefinite indications for treatment, the European experts also considered other types of patients in whom *H. pylori* eradication therapy might be deemed to be desirable. These included patients with nonulcer dyspepsia, severe (defined macro- or microscopically) gastritis, intestinal metaplasia types II and III, dysplasia, and even atrophy (although there exists no definitive evidence that any of these early precancerous lesions will regress). Furthermore, the European consensus concluded that there was probably a need to treat patients who were receiving maintenance PPIs (at variance with the recent conclusions by the FDA), patients with a family history of gastric cancer, patients taking or about to take NSAIDs, and finally, all patients who desire treatment. It was not discussed which patient, if any, would not choose to eradicate the organism that has been so vilified in the popular press. Indeed, the media, educated carefully by corporate marketers, has virtually empowered patients to determine their therapeutic preferences. Thus, complex deliberations in regard to which particular groups of patients ought to have their *Helicobacter* eradicated may be a purely academic exercise, because the desires of patients may be the prime consideration as to whether they are treated. This scenario, however, may not be the final one, because in the age of managed care, the ultimate and perhaps definitive arguments about who receives therapy may not come from clinicians or patients but from those who hold the purse strings. Treatment of gastric cancer is vastly more expensive than eradication of the organism.

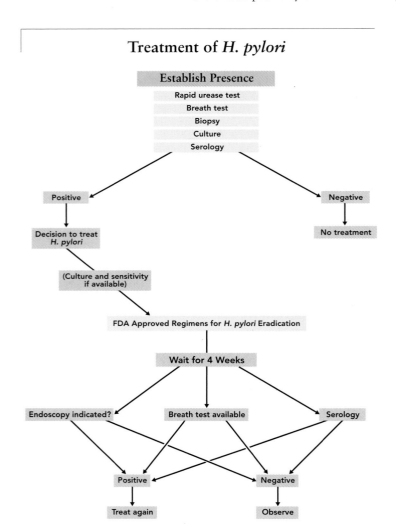

Treatment of *H. pylori*

Establish Presence
Rapid urease test
Breath test
Biopsy
Culture
Serology

Positive → Negative

Decision to treat *H. pylori* → No treatment

(Culture and sensitivity if available)

FDA Approved Regimens for *H. pylori* Eradication

Wait for 4 Weeks

Endoscopy indicated? — Breath test available — Serology

Positive — Negative

Treat again — Observe

A flow diagram outlining possible therapeutic approaches to *H. pylori* infection.

The recent overwhelming data establishing the much-increased risk of gastric cancer is moving opinion to eradication of any serologically positive individual. For worldwide implementation, a simple method for testing of efficacy of eradication is also desirable. If simple monotherapy were to become available, then testing of all individuals for the presence of infection would become economically feasible.

Economics

In recent times, an increasing number of analyses have been performed aimed at determining the cost and benefit of a variety of different management strategies for the *H. pylori*–infected patient. Almost all have used modeled best-available estimates to a theoretic population; few have closed the loop by reapplying the recommended approach to a real population. All agree that for peptic ulcers associated with *H. pylori*, eradication therapy is not only the most clinically efficacious but also the most cost-effective long-term treatment. It is, however, still unclear what to do with patients with dyspepsia in whom a definitive diagnosis is not available. Should they be screened for *H. pylori* and treated according to the *H. pylori* result (either with or without an endoscopy), or should they be treated blindly with anti–*H. pylori* medications or antisecretory therapy, or both? Alternatively, would it be cost effective to test and simply eradicate *H. pylori* from all, including the asymptomatic? Even as algorithms are being developed and used (e.g., suggesting referring to gastro-enterologists for endoscopy only those patients who may have a malignancy or who fail conventional treatment), the pressure is on primary care physicians to test and treat all. For example, one recent analysis concluded that the "treat and see" approach will always be less expensive than doing endoscopy in *H. pylori*–positive patients, unless endoscopy costs can be reduced by 90% or more. However, these models are only as good as the data on which they are based. It is uncertain that someone who has had *H. pylori* eradicated for ulcer disease will never have ulcers or ulcer-like symptoms again. *H. pylori*–negative duodenal ulcers do exist, and rather than being a great rarity, they may comprise as much as one-fourth of all duodenal ulcers in the United States. Further unknowns complicate the model systems. For example, is it really of no consequence to miss the occasional gastric cancer? How predictable and how expensive to society will be the emergence of non-*Helicobacter* bacterial resistance secondary to the indiscriminate use of antibiotics?

There are persuasive arguments that the eradication of *H. pylori* should be viewed as a public health measure to prevent future gastric cancer. Again, computer-derived evidence suggests that screening for *H. pylori* in the middle-aged population and eradicating *H. pylori* from those who test positive could be relatively cost effective, certainly no more expensive than other cancer-prevention strategies, if eradication reduces the gastric cancer risk by more than 20%. However, it may be unrealistic to expect that eradicating *H. pylori* from middle-aged people will reduce the gastric cancer risk at all—there is no good evidence that gastric preneoplasia is reversible. Thus, prospective randomized trials of large numbers of patients followed for many years will be necessary to answer this important question. It may be that intervening in children is the only way to prevent the long-term impact of infection.

Finally, it should be noted that we should beware of falling into the trap whereby we blame *H. pylori* for all of our ills. The idea of an alien invading and living in our stomachs and causing disease may be popular for those who would like to blame unhappiness and pain on an external agent. In scapegoating this bacterium and closing our minds to other possibilities, we may be deluding both ourselves and our patients. It should be remembered that our previous long-term obsession with acid soured our judgment in the past, and we should be cognizant of the potential relevance of pepsin and the possibility of both inherent mucosal defects and other putative infective agents in the genesis of esophagogastroduodenal mucosal disease.

Methods of treatment

With the gradual establishment of the role of *H. pylori* in peptic ulcer disease, there were initially trials on a small number of infected individuals with a variety of protocols claiming various degrees of success. At the time of writing this chapter, it has become accepted that the best controlled clinical trials, in which intention-to-treat was the analytic criterion, involving an adequate number of patients, showed that a 7-day treatment with a combination of a PPI, such as omeprazole, and two antibiotics, such as amoxicillin and metronidazole and clarithromycin, reached between 85% and 90% eradication efficacy. This triple therapy is given twice per day. Trials using other PPIs, such as lansoprazole or pantoprazole, produced essentially the same results. Another protocol that has received approval is a combination of ranitidine and bismuth subcitrate with two of the above antibiotics. Ulcer disease is then treated with continuation of the secretory inhibitor for the approved length of time, although some studies suggest that eradication on its own is all that is required.

Although earlier approval was granted to a combination of a PPI and a single antibiotic, current thinking is that this regimen is relatively ineffective.

The results of some large studies analyzing a variety of combinations are summarized in the bar graph.

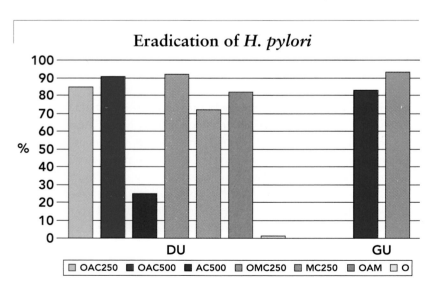

A summary of the results of a series of double-blind multicenter studies on eradication of *H. pylori* comparing a number of twice-a-day regimens, showing the need for two antibiotics and a PPI.

In trials so far performed with pantoprazole or lansoprazole, equivalent efficacy has been shown. It can be seen that any two of the three antibiotics in combination with omeprazole reach the eightieth percentile eradication. However, only those containing clarithromycin reach the ninetieth percentile. It is also clear that two antibiotics are ineffective, as is omeprazole alone. There is now more evidence that resistance to clarithromycin is increasing, and some instances of resistance to amoxicillin have been found. Metronidazole resistance is found rather frequently in those populations in which treatment with the nitroimidazoles for other diseases was prevalent. It must be admitted, however, that outside the clinical trial setting, eradication rates fall to approximately the seventieth percentile. Also, resistance to clarithromycin is also increasing.

Role of PPIs in Eradication of *H. pylori*

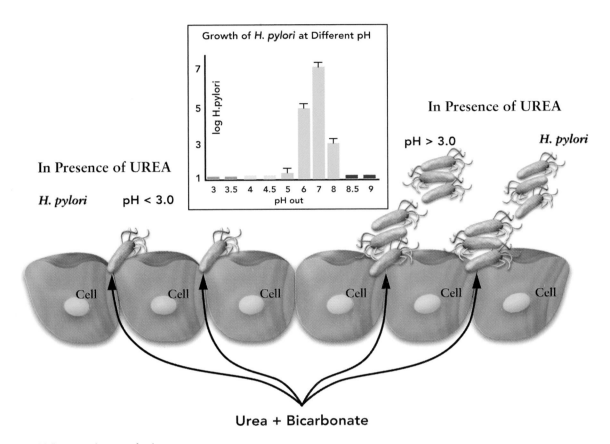

Growth of *H. pylori* at Different pH

In Presence of UREA

H. pylori   pH < 3.0

In Presence of UREA

pH > 3.0   *H. pylori*

Cell   Cell   Cell   Cell   Cell   Cell

Urea + Bicarbonate

A model illustrating the reason for the use of a PPI in combination with growth-dependent antibiotics such as amoxicillin and clarithromycin. With normal secretion, many of the organisms will be in stationary phase, as shown on the left. With inhibition of acid secretion, more organisms move into log-phase growth and become susceptible to these antibiotics. Hence, PPIs are necessary for eradication with these antibiotics but do not improve eradication due to metronidazole and other DNA-targeted antibiotics.

Rationale for proton pump inhibitors in combination therapy

The two antibiotics with which PPIs synergize are amoxicillin and clarithromycin. The former antibiotic inhibits cell wall biosynthesis by inhibiting peptidyl transferase and by binding to other proteins in the cell wall biosynthesis pathways. Cell division is therefore required for the bactericidal action of this class of antibiotic. Clarithromycin binds to the 23S RNA and thereby inhibits protein synthesis. Hence, protein synthesis is required for the action of this antibiotic. Metronidazole is reduced to the hydroxylamine derivative, which then binds to DNA, hence not requiring cell division or protein synthesis for its efficacy. PPIs do not synergize with this antibiotic. Resistance to metronidazole develops by decrease of the level of reducing enzyme and, therefore, may be relative or absolute. Resistance to clarithromycin occurs by a base mutation at the binding site on the RNA and is usually absolute.

Any maneuver that increases the population of *H. pylori* undergoing division will make the bacteria relatively more susceptible to either amoxicillin or clarithromycin or both (because they have biochemically distinct targets). Remembering the survival and growth data previously shown, the organism survives over a much wider pH range than that found for growth. So, if antibiotic is given where many of the organisms are nondividing, poor eradication will be found. If, however, PPIs are coadministered to decrease the fraction of the population in the nondividing state, synergism will be observed. Some consider that PPIs increase the gastric bioavailability of these antibiotics, but evidence for this is scanty. These considerations are modeled in the illustration.

In the future, alternative therapies will become available, such as monotherapy targeted at a unique gene or unique feature or vaccination may be successful. Both approaches are the focus of active research.

SUGGESTED READING

Andrutis KA, Fox JG, Schauer DB, et al. Inability of an isogenic urease-negative mutant strain of *Helicobacter mustelae* to colonize the ferret stomach. *Infect Immun* 1994;63:3722–3725.

Atherton JC. The clinical relevance of strain types of *Helicobacter pylori*. *Gut* 1997;40:701–703.

Axon ATR. Eradication of *Helicobacter pylori*. *Scand J Gastroenterol* 1996;31:47–53.

Blaser MJ. *Helicobacter pylori* and gastric diseases. *Br Med J* 1998;316:1507–1510.

Blaser MJ. Hypothesis on the pathogenesis and natural history of *Helicobacter pylori* induced inflammation. *Gastroenterology* 1992;102:720.

Bode G, Malfertheiner P, Lenhardt G, et al. Ultrastructural localization of urease of *Helicobacter pylori*. *Med Microbiol Immun* 1993;182:223–242.

Chalk PA, Roberts AD, Blows WM. Metabolism of pyruvate and glucose by intact cells of *Helicobacter pylori* studied by C-13 NMR spectroscopy. *Microbiology* 1994;140:2085–2092.

Chan FKL, Sung JY, Chung SCS, et al. Randomised trial of eradication of *Helicobacter pylori* before non-steroidal anti-inflammatory drug therapy to prevent peptic ulcers. *Lancet* 1997;350:975–979.

Chey WD, Fey D, Scheirman JM, et al. Role of acid suppression in the effects of lansoprazole and ranitidine on the 14C urea breath test. In: Graham DY, Blazer MJ, eds. *Developments in* Helicobacter *research*. 1997:17–18 (abstract).

Clyne M, Labigne A, Drumm B. *Helicobacter pylori* requires an acidic environment to survive in the presence of urea. *Infect Immun* 1995;63:1669–1673.

Current European concepts in the management of *Helicobacter pylori* infection. The Maastricht Consensus Report. *Gut* 1997;41:8–13.

Dixon MF, Genta R, Yardley JH, et al. Classification and grading of gastritis: the upgraded Sydney system. *Am J Surg Pathol* 1996;20:1161–1181.

Domiguez-Munoz JE, Leodolter A, Sauerbruch T, et al. A citric acid solution is an optimal test drink in the 13C urea breath test for diagnosis of *Helicobacter pylori* infection. *Gut* 1997;40:459–462.

Dunn BE, Cohen H, Blaser MJ. *Helicobacter pylori*. *Clin Microbiol Rev* 1997;10:720–741.

Eaton KA, Krakowka S. Effect of gastric pH on urease-dependent colonization of gnotobiotic piglets by *Helicobacter pylori*. *Infect Immun* 1994;62:3604–3607.

Eissele R, Brunner G, Simon B, et al. Gastric mucosa during treatment with lansoprazole: *Helicobacter pylori* is a risk factor for argyrophil cell hyperplasia. *Gastroenterology* 1997;112:707–717.

European *Helicobacter* Study Group Current European concepts in the management of *Helicobacter pylori* infection. The Maastricht Consensus Report. *Gut* 1997;41:8–13.

Faraci WS, Yang BV, O'Rourke D, et al. Inhibition of *Helicobacter pylori* urease by phenyl phosphoramidates: mechanism of action. *Bioorg Med Chem* 1995;3:605–610.

Feljou JF, Bahame P, Smith AC, et al. Pernicious anemia and *Campylobacter*-like organisms: is the antrum resistant to colonisation? *Gut* 1989;30:60–64.

Fendrick AM, Chernew ME, Hirth RA, et al. Alternative management strategies for patients with suspected peptic ulcer disease. *Ann Intern Med* 1995;123:260–268.

Ferrero RL, Labigne A. Organization and expression of the *Helicobacter pylori* urease gene cluster in *Helicobacter pylori*: biology and clinical practice. In: Goodwin CS, Worley BW, eds. Florida: CRC Press, 1993:171–195.

Ferrero RL, Lee A. The importance of urease in acid protection for the gastric colonizing bacteria, *Helicobacter pylori* and *Helicobacter felis*. *Microbial Ecol Health Dis* 1996;4:121–134.

Goodwin CS, Carrick J. Peptic ulcer disease and *Helicobacter pylori* infection. *Curr Opin Gastroenterol* 1991;7:108–1115.

Graham DY. *Campylobacter pylori* and peptic ulcer disease. *Gastroenterology* 1989;96:615–625.

Graham DY. *Helicobacter*: its epidemiology and its role in duodenal ulcer disease. *J Gastroenterol Hepatol* 1991;6:105–113.

Hawtin PR, Stacey AR, Newell DG. Investigation of the structure and localization of the urease of *Helicobacter pylori* using monoclonal antibodies. *J Gen Microbiol* 1990;136:1995–2000.

Hong W, Sano K, Morimatsu S, et al. Medium pH-dependent redistribution of the urease of *Helicobacter pylori*. *J Med Microbiol* 2003;52:211–216.

Kidd M, Miu K, Tang LH, et al. *H. pylori* lipo-polysaccharide stimulates histamine release and DNA synthesis in rat ECL cells. *Gastroenterology* 1997;113:1110–1117.

Kim N, Weeks DL, Shin JM, Scott DR, et al. Proteins released by *Helicobacter pylori* in vitro. *J Bacteriol* 2002;184:6155–6162.

Koop H, Stumpf M, Eissele R, et al. Antral *Helicobacter pylori*-like organisms in different states of gastric acid secretion. *Digestion* 1991;48:230–236.

Kuhler TC, Fryklund J, Bergman NA, et al. Structure-activity relationship of omeprazole and analogues as *Helicobacter pylori* urease inhibitors. *J Med Chem* 1995;38:4906–4916.

Kuipers EJ, Klinkenberg-Knol EC, Vandenbroucke-Grauls CM, et al. Role of *Helicobacter pylori* in the pathogenesis of atrophic gastritis. *Scand J Gastroenterol* 1997;(Suppl 223);28–34.

Kuipers EJ, Lundell L, Klinkenberg-Knol EC, et al. Atrophic gastritis and *Helicobacter pylori* infection in patients with reflux esophagitis treated with omeprazole or fundoplication. *N Engl J Med* 1996;334:1018–1022.

Labenz J, Blum A, Bayerdorffer E, et al. Curing *Helicobacter pylori* infection in patients with duodenal ulcer may provoke reflux esophagitis. *Gastroenterology* 1997;112: 1442–1447.

Labenz J, Tillenburg B, Peitz U, et al. *Helicobacter pylori* augments the pH-increasing effect of omeprazole in patients with duodenal ulcer. *Gastroenterology* 1996;110:725–732.

Labigne A, Cussac V, Courcoux P. Shuttle cloning and nucleotide sequences of *Helicobacter pylori* genes responsible for urease activity. *J Bacteriol* 1991;173:1920–1931.

Lee A, Dixon MF, Danon SJ, et al. Local acid production and *Helicobacter pylori*: a unifying hypothesis of gastroduodenal disease. *Eur J Gastroenterol Hepatol* 1995;7:461–465.

Li H, Andersson EM, Helander HF. *Helicobacter pylori* infected rats; a study on infection, inflammation, immunology, apoptosis, cell proliferation and gastric ulcer healing. *Gastroenterology* 1997;112:A198.

Lind T, Bardhan KD, Bayerdorffer E, et al. Mach 2 Study: optimal *Helicobacter pylori* therapy needs omeprazole and can be assessed by UBT. *Gastroenterology* 1997;112:A200.

Lind T, Veldhuyzen van Zanten SJO, Unge P, et al. The MACH 1 study: optimal 1 week treatment for *H. pylori* defined? *Gut* 1995;(Suppl 1):A4.

Lind T, Veldhuyzen van Zanten S, Unge P, et al. Eradication of *Helicobacter pylori* using one-week triple therapies combining omeprazole with two antimicrobials: the MACH I Study. *Helicobacter* 1996;1:138–144.

Malfertheiner P, Ditschuneit H. Helicobacter pylori, *gastritis, and peptic ulcer.* Berlin: Springer Verlag, 1990.

Marshall BJ, Barett LJ, Prakash C, et al. Protection of *Campylobacter pyloridis* but not *Campylobacter jejuni* against acid susceptibility by urea. In: Kaijser B, Falson E, eds. Campylobacter *IV.* Göteborg, Sweden: University of Göteborg Press, 1988:402–403.

Marshall BJ, Barrett LJ, Prakash C, et al. Urea protects *Helicobacter (Campylobacter) pylori* from the bactericidal effect of acid. *Gastroenterology* 1990;99:697–702.

Masubuchi N, Takahashi S, Utsunomiya K, et al. Effects of ecabete sodium and benzohydroxamic acid on *Helicobacter pylori* infection in the cynomolgous monkey. *Gastroenterology* 1994;106:A2513.

McGowan CC, Cover TL, Blaser MJ. *Helicobacter pylori* and gastric acid: biological and therapeutic implications. *Gastroenterology* 1996;110:926–938.

Megraud F. Transmission of *Helicobacter pylori*: faecal-oral versus oral-oral route. *Aliment Pharmacol Ther* 1995;9(Suppl 2):85–89.

Mendz GL, Hazell SL, Burns BP. Glucose utilization and lactate production by *Helicobacter pylori*. *J Gen Microbiol* 1993;139:3023–3028.

Mendz GL, Hazell SL, Vangorkom L. Pyruvate metabolism in *Helicobacter pylori*. *Arch Microbiol* 1994;162:187–192.

Meyer-Rosberg K, Scott DR, Rex D, et al. The effect of the environmental pH on the proton motive force of *Helicobacter pylori*. *Gastroenterology* 1996;111:886–900.

Miederer SE, Grubel PG. Profound increase of *Helicobacter pylori* urease activity in gastric antral mucosa at low pH. *Dig Dis Sci* 1996;41:944–949.

Misiewicz JJ, Harris AW, Bardhan KD, et al. One week triple therapy for *Helicobacter pylori*: a multicentre comparative study. Lansoprazole *Helicobacter* Study Group. *Gut* 1997;41:735–739.

Mitchell P. Chemiosmotic coupling in oxidative and photosynthetic phosphorylation. *Biol Rev* 1966;41:445–502.

Mobley HLT, Island MD, Hausinger RP. Molecular biology of microbial ureases. *Microbiol Rev* 1995;59:451–480.

Mollenhauer-Rektorschek M, Hanauer G, Sachs G, et al. Expression of UreI is required for intragastric transit and colonization of gerbil gastric mucosa by *Helicobacter pylori*. *Res Microbiol* 2002;153:659–666.

Moss SF, Calam J, Agarwal B, et al. Induction of gastric epithelial apoptosis by *Helicobacter pylori*. *Gut* 1996;38:498–501.

Neithercut WD, Greig MA, Hossack M, et al. Suicidal destruction of *Helicobacter pylori*: metabolic consequence of intracellular accumulation of ammonia. *J Clin Pathol* 1991;44:380–384.

Olso ER. Influence of pH on bacterial gene expression. *Mol Microbiol* 1993;8:5–14.

Parsonnet J, Friedman GD, Vandersteed DP, et al. *H. pylori* infection and the risk of gastric cancer. *N Engl J Med* 1991;325:1131.

Parsonnet J, Harris RA, Hack HM, et al. Modelling cost-effectiveness of *Helicobacter pylori* screening to prevent gastric cancer: a mandate for clinical trials. *Lancet* 1996;348:150–154.

Pei ZH, Ellison RT 3rd, Blaser MJ. Identification, purification, and characterization of major antigenic proteins of *Campylobacter jejuni*. *J Biol Chem* 1991;266:16363–16369.

Peterson WL. *Helicobacter pylori* and peptic ulcer disease. *N Engl J Med* 1990;324:1043.

Phadnis SH, Parlow MH, Levy M, et al. Surface localization of *Helicobacter pylori* urease and a heat shock protein homolog requires bacterial autolysis. *Infect Immun* 1996;64:905–912.

Rauws EA, Tytgat GN. Cure of duodenal ulcer associated with eradication of *Helicobacter pylori*. *Eur J Gastroenterol Hepatol* 1990;6:773–777.

Report of the Digestive Health Initiative International Update Conference on *Helicobacter pylori*, February 1997. Presented at: Digestive Disease Week, Washington, DC, May 1997.

Sachs G. Gastritis, *Helicobacter pylori* and proton pump inhibitors. *Gastroenterology* 1997;112:1033–1036.

Sachs G, Weeks DL, Melchers K, et al. The gastric biology of *Helicobacter pylori. Annu Rev Physiol* 2003;65:349–369.

Scott DR, Weeks D, Hong C, et al. The role of internal urease in acid resistance of *Helicobacter pylori. Gastroenterology* 1998;114:58–70.

Talley NJ. A critique of therapeutic trials in *Helicobacter pylori*-positive functional dyspepsia. *Gastroenterology* 1994;106:1174–1183.

Tomb J-F, White O, Kerlavage AR, et al. The complete genome sequence of the gastric pathogen *Helicobacter pylori. Nature* 1997;388:539–547.

Tsuda M, Karita M, Morshed MG, et al. A urease-negative mutant of *Helicobacter pylori* constructed by allelic exchange mutagenesis lacks the ability to colonize the nude mouse stomach. *Infect Immun* 1994;62:3586–3589.

Tytgat GNJ. Endoscopic transmission of *Helicobacter pylori. Aliment Pharmacol Ther* 1995;9(Suppl 2):105–110.

Tytgat GNJ, Lee A, Graham DY, et al. The role of infectious agents in peptic ulcer disease. *Gastroenterol Intern* 1993;6:76.

Uemura N, Mukai T, Okamoto S, et al. Effect of *Helicobacter pylori* eradication on subsequent development of cancer after endoscopic resection of early gastric cancer. *Cancer Epidemiol Biomarkers Prev* 1997;6:639–642.

Verdu EF, Armstrong D, Idstrom JP, et al. Effect of curing *Helicobacter pylori* infection on intragastric pH during treatment with omeprazole. *Gut* 1995;37:743–748.

Voland P, Weeks DL, Vaira D, et al. Specific identification of three low molecular weight membrane-associated antigens of *Helicobacter pylori. Aliment Pharmacol Ther* 2002;16:533–534.

Walsh JH, Peterson WL. The treatment of *Helicobacter pylori* infection in the management of peptic ulcer disease. *N Engl J Med* 1995;333:984–991.

Warren JR, Marshall B. Unidentified curved bacilli on gastric epithelium in active chronic gastritis. *Lancet* 1983;1:1273–1275.

Weeks DL, Eskandari S, Scott DR, et al. A H+ gated urea channel: the link between *Helicobacter pylori* urease and gastric colonization. *Science* 2000;287:482–485.

Yeomans ND, Brimblecombe RW, Elder J, et al. Effects of acid suppression on microbial flora of upper gut. *Dig Dis Sci* 1995;40:81S–95S.

Yousfi MM, El-Zimaity HMT, Cole RA, et al. Metronidazole, omeprazole and clarithromycin: an effective combination therapy for *Helicobacter pylori* infection. *Aliment Pharmacol Ther* 1995;9:209–212.

THE TWENTY-FIRST CENTURY

It is foolish to imagine that we, as mere mortals viewing the new millennium, may be able to predict either the logical or the serendipitous progress of science. Imagine the turn of the nineteenth century. Certainly, Darwin and Mendel had made their epochal discoveries, but physics was Newtonian, subatomic structure undreamed of, the periodic table of the elements unspecified, biochemistry almost nonexistent, and the radio not even imagined. Although the introduction of the telephone, electricity, and the automobile had revolutionized humanity's concepts of communication and transport, civilization was still a brittle affair governed by power as much as, if not more than, understanding. Who might have even dreamed of the contributions of the first 20 years of the last century, let alone have predicted the advances of the last 20 years? Although contemporary evaluation of progress always suggests that a lesser challenge has been surmounted, the recent advances in the pharmacotherapeutic targeting of disease processes may be measured among the most salutary accomplishments of humankind.

In this context, there was a major revolution in the understanding and treatment of gastrointestinal ulcer disease in the last quarter of the twentieth century. The progenitors of this late-breaking revolution reflected both individual perspicuity and the evolution and application of sophisticated technology. This reflected advances in the understanding of the physiologic regulation of acid secretion and its cellular mechanisms, improved visualization of the lesions using flexible endoscopes, more precise surgical approaches, and the burgeoning arena of sophisticated pharmaceutical research. The discovery of *H. pylori* and its implication in ulcer disease provided a further insight into an expanding biologic world of contemporary clinical relevance, whereby bacteria and acid were recognized to have synergistic roles in the pathogenesis of mucosal disease. And this bears witness to only a fraction of the progress that has been made. . . .

We are still arguing about the personality of *H. pylori*. Is it always a pathogen? Is it merely a commensal on occasion, hindering rather than helping to initiate disease? The early part of the twenty-first century should provide an answer to this conundrum. Whether it will resolve some of our other dilemmas is not as certain. Thus, although treatment of acid related disease has been particularly successful, the treatment of gastric or esophageal malignancies has failed to progress with similar accomplishment. A causative factor in this tardiness has been the relative lack of success in the elucidation of the basic biologic processes governing cell transformation. Robotic surgery coupled with imaging technology may amplify the level of precision associated with excision and facilitate levels of curative extirpation impossible at this time. Nevertheless, the cell as a target for antineoplastic therapy is likely to be more viable from the therapeutic point of view than is organ ablation, irrespective of the technology used to accomplish this process.

We now have the complete human genome with its 30,000 or so genes. The surprise in this was the finding that there are many more proteins than genes due to either alternative splicings of the gene or posttranslational modification. This makes the task of identifying all organ- or cell-specific proteins more daunting than was thought. Nevertheless, methods will be worked out to achieve this end. Such information may enable us to diagnose the presence of, or to predict one or more of, life's many ills. Such information will almost certainly provide a crowd, if not a host, of novel therapeutic targets. At this time, however, the number and variety of oncogenes that have been described and the various cell growth and multiplication cascades still confuse and obfuscate as much as they illuminate. But it is predictable and assured that with genomics, proteomics, and their offshoots, better and more detailed descriptions of tumor generation will emerge. From such knowledge, one can be assured that more rational and targeted therapy of malignancies will evolve.

The era of small-molecule agonists and antagonists dawned in the last quarter of the last century, and perhaps little is to be discovered there. However, peptidomimetics have yet to make their entrance onto the stage of novel therapeutics. Control of transcription by way of gene insertion, RNA, or antisense nucleotide oligomers awaits efficacious, reliable, and safe methods. Undoubtedly these will come. The challenges of the future extend into novel cancer therapeutics and the control of aging of organs or the individual.

Eternal youth, dying old while young, eternal life? Dare we anticipate these? Whose names, whose pictures will illustrate the historical part of this book 100 years from now? In the immortal words of Pontius Pilate, *Quod scripsi, scripsi*!

INDEX

The second edition of *Acid Related Diseases: Biology and Treatment* was written by Irvin M. Modlin, M.D., Ph.D., F.R.C.S.(Ed), F.R.C.S.(Eng), F.C.S.(SA), F.A.C.S., and George Sachs, M.B., Ch.B., D.Sc., and composed by Lisa Cunningham, Silverchair Science + Communications, Inc. in Sabon and Avenir. The cover conception was the product of Irvin M. Modlin and George Sachs and was designed by Lou Moriconi, Lippincott Williams & Wilkins. The interior design of the book is by Sudler & Hennessey. Illustrations were provided by Steve Lustig, BioDesign Communications; George Sachs; Irvin M. Modlin; and Mark Kidd. Printed by Walsworth Publishing Company.